# CRANIAL MRI AND CT

# CRANIAL MRI AND CT

## FOURTH EDITION

## Editors

**S. Howard Lee, M.D.**

*Clinical Professor of Radiology*
Robert Wood Johnson
Medical School
*Director of Neurosciences Center*
Muhlenberg Regional Medical Center
Plainfield, New Jersey, and
Somerset Medical Center
Somerset, New Jersey

**Krishna C. V. G. Rao, M.D.**

*Professor of Radiology*
Uniformed Services University
of the Health Sciences
Bethesda, Maryland
*Neuroradiologist*
Walter Reed Army Medical Center
Washington, D.C.

**Robert A. Zimmerman, M.D.**

*Professor of Radiology*
University of Pennsylvania
School of Medicine
*Chief of Neuroradiology and
Magnetic Resonance Imaging*
Children's Hospital of Philadelphia
Philadelphia, Pennsylvania

**McGRAW-HILL**
Health Professions Division
New York   St. Louis   San Francisco   Auckland
Bogotá   Caracas   Lisbon   London   Madrid   Mexico
Milan   Montreal   New Delhi   Paris   San Juan
Singapore   Sydney   Tokyo   Toronto

## McGraw-Hill

A Division of The **McGraw·Hill** Companies

**CRANIAL MRI AND CT, 4/e**

Copyright © 1999, 1992, 1987, 1983 by The McGraw-Hill Companies, Inc. All rights reserved. Printed in the United States of America. Except as permitted under the United States Copyright Act of 1976, no part of this publication may be reproduced or distributed in any form or by any means, or stored in a database or retrieval system, without the prior written permission of the publisher.

1234567890     QPKQPK     99

ISBN 0-07-037689-1

This book was set in Garamond by Progressive Information Technologies, Inc.
The editors were James T. Morgan III, Martin J. Wonsiewicz, and Peter J. Boyle;
the production supervisor was Richard C. Ruzycka;
the book designer was Judy Allan / The Designing Woman Concepts;
the page layout and cover design were done by José Fonfrias;
the indexer was Barbara Littlewood.
Quebecor Printing/Kingsport was printer and binder.

**Library of Congress Cataloging-in-Publication Data**

Cranial MRI and CT / editors, S. Howard Lee, Krishna C. V. G. Rao,
   Robert A. Zimmerman. —4th ed.
     p.    cm.
    Includes bibliographical references and index.
    ISBN 0-07-037689-1
    1. Skull—Magnetic resonance imaging.    2. Skull—Tomography.
I. Lee, Seungho Howard.    II. Rao, Krishna C. V. G.    III. Zimmerman,
Robert A.
    [DNLM:  1. Skull—radiography.    2. Brain Diseases—diagnosis.
3. Magnetic Resonance Imaging.    4. Tomography, X-Ray Computed.    WE
705 C8893   1998]
RC936.C73   1999
6187.5′107548—dc21
DNLM/DLC
for Library of Congress                        97-28648
                                        CIP

TO OUR PARENTS
WITH LOVE AND GRATITUDE

# CONTENTS

# CONTRIBUTORS

**Larissa T. Bilaniuk, M.D.**
Professor of Radiology
University of Pennsylvania School of Medicine
Children's Hospital of Pennsylvania
Philadelphia, Pennsylvania
*Chapter 16*

**Andrew R. Bogdan, Ph.D.**
Senior Physicist
Analogic Corporation
Peabody, Massachusetts
*Chapter 3*

**D. W. Fellows, M.D.**
Assistant Professor of Radiology
Uniformed Services University of the Health Sciences
Bethesda, Maryland
Neuroradiologist
Walter Reed Army Medical Center
Washington, D.C.
*Chapter 17*

**Debra A. Gusnard, M.D.**
Washington University School of Medicine
Barnes Hospital
St. Louis, Missouri
*Chapter 5*

**Carl E. Johnson, M.D.**
Assistant Professor of Clinical Radiology
Department of Radiology
St. Luke's–Roosevelt Hospital Center
Columbia University College of Physicians and Surgeons
New York, New York
*Chapter 9*

**Michele H. Johnson, M.D.**
Associate Professor of Radiology
Section of Neuroradiology
Medical College of Virginia Hospital
Virginia Commonwealth University
Richmond, Virginia
*Chapter 13*

**Wayne S. Kubal, M.D.**
Assistant Professor of Radiology
Section of Neuroradiology
Medical College of Virginia Hospital
Virginia Commonwealth University
Richmond, Virginia
*Chapter 13*

**S. Howard Lee, M.D.**
Clinical Professor of Radiology
Robert Wood Johnson Medical School
University of Medicine and Dentistry of New Jersey
Director of Neurosciences Center
Muhlenberg Regional Medical Center
Plainfield, New Jersey, and
Somerset Medical Center
Somerset, New Jersey
*Chapters 3, 7, and 11*

**Krishna C. V. G. Rao, M.D.**
Professor of Radiology
Uniformed Services University of the Health Sciences
Bethesda, Maryland
Neuroradiologist
Walter Reed Army Medical Center
Washington, D.C.
*Chapters 4, 6, 12, and 15*

**John Rees, M.D.**
Neuroradiologist
Department of Radiology
Orlando Regional Medical Center
Orlando, Florida
*Chapter 7*

**Hector A. Robles, M.D.**
Clinical Assistant Professor of Radiology
Radiology Department
University of Miami
Neuroradiologist
VA Medical Center
West Palm Beach, Florida
*Chapter 15*

**James G. Smirniotopoulos, M.D.**
Chairman, Radiology Department
Professor of Radiology and Neurology
Department of Radiology and Nuclear Medicine
Uniformed Services University of the Health Sciences
Bethesda, Maryland
*Chapter 7*

**Gordon Sze, M.D.**
Professor of Radiology
Yale University School of Medicine
Chief of Neuroradiology
Yale-New Haven Hospital
New Haven, Connecticut
*Chapters 9 and 11*

**Karel G. TerBrugge, M.D.**
Professor of Radiology
Head, Division of Neuroradiology
The Toronto Hospital
University of Toronto
Toronto, Ontario, Canada
*Chapter 12*

**Theodore Villafana, M.D.**
Professor and Head, Radiation Physics
and Safety Division
MCP Hahnemann University School of Medicine
Philadelphia, Pennsylvania
*Chapters 1 and 2*

**John B. Weigele, M.D.**
Division of Neuroradiology
Department of Radiology
Johns Hopkins Hospital
Baltimore, Maryland
*Chapter 14*

**Robert A. Zimmerman, M.D.**
Professor of Radiology
University of Pennsylvania School of Medicine
Chief of Neuroradiology and Magnetic Resonance Imaging
Children's Hospital of Pennsylvania
Philadelphia, Pennsylvania
*Chapters 5, 8, 10, 14, and 16*

**S. J. Zinreich, M.D.**
Associate Professor of Radiology
Department of Neuroradiology
Johns Hopkins University Medical Center
Baltimore, Maryland
*Chapter 17*

# PREFACE

Since the third edition of this book was published in 1992 rapid advancement of MR technology and its clinical applications has taken place. The field of neuroradiology has become a fast-moving, demanding, and exciting multidisciplinary activity. As with all previous editions, the fourth edition is intended to be a useful source of practical information on utilizing cranial CT and MR technology and is designed to be a reference guide for students, residents, fellows, and clinicians in the field of neuroscience.

We are deeply indebted to all the authors, our colleagues and friends. Their contribution and sacrifice made this a worthwhile and proud endeavor.

We would like to thank Lucinda Bauer, James Morgan III, Anna Ferrera, Martin J. Wonsiewicz, Richard Ruzycka, and José Fonfrias in the Health Professions Division of McGraw-Hill. Special thanks to Peter Boyle at McGraw-Hill, Dr. Charles E. Swallow in Bethesda, Maryland, and our colleagues and technologists in the neuroradiology departments. Rachel Zimmerman, Valerie Vigna, Michele Lee, and Jennifer Lee deserve separate mention for their tireless and unwavering support of this project.

Without the understanding and encouragement of our families, the book would not have been born. We again thank them immensely.

# CRANIAL MRI AND CT

# 1 PHYSICS AND INSTRUMENTATION: COMPUTED TOMOGRAPHY

*Theodore Villafana*

## CONTENTS

A wealth of radiological information was overlooked in classic radiology and tomography. In fact, CT and MRI as now known are probably just the beginning of what will come. Radiologists, of course, are caught in this imaging revolution. They must become increasingly familiar with the physical principles, instrumentation, and technical limitations of these modalities to make accurate and precise diagnostic interpretations. The purpose of Chaps. 1 and 2 is to provide a fuller understanding of the basic CT and MRI scanning principles of direct importance to the clinician. The presentation consists first of a brief overview of the basis and the limitations of classic radiographic imaging. Second, the use of classic tomography as an attempt to overcome some of the problems of classic radiography is also briefly discussed. Finally, computed tomography and its limitations are discussed fully. Chapter 2 addresses MRI.

## BASIC X-RAY IMAGE FORMATION

The basic aim of diagnostic radiology is to record on a film (or display on a monitor) a pattern of densities (or illumination levels on a monitor) which corresponds to and conveys diagnostic information about the size, shape, and distribution of the anatomic tissues within a patient. For instance, Fig. 1-1 shows a beam of x-rays penetrating a "simplified patient" consisting simply of a square block of tissue surrounded by a different but uniform tissue background. As the x-rays pass through the patient, they are attenuated; that is, they are both absorbed and scattered within the patient. Attenuation

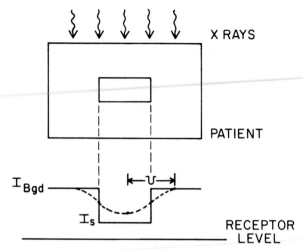

**Figure 1-1**  An intensity profile of the x-ray beam as it emerges from the patient. Here a hypothetical square-edged anatomic structure ideally casts a shadow ($I_s$) relative to the adjoining background tissue ($I_{Bgd}$). The relative depth of the shadow or subject contrast, $C_s$, depends on the difference in attenuation between the two areas. Factors such as scatter, motion, and focal spot size tend to degrade both subject contrast and the edge character of the pattern (dashed curve). $U$ is the resulting unsharpness or distance over which edge is blurred.

depends on the type of tissues present, the patient thickness, and the x-ray beam energy. Finally, the x-rays emerge from the patient and arrive at the image receptor level, where they are detected or recorded.

Figure 1-1 depicts one particular x-ray intensity profile across the simplified patient. It is important to realize that this profile is the sum total of the transmitted primary beam and the scattered radiation reaching the receptor level. Each point along the final profile thus depends on the x-ray attenuation that occurred along each ray path within the patient as well as the scatter generated. Note also that the final two-dimensional image is composed of the collection of all such intensity profiles within the patient for the entire exposed field.

The further study of the representation of radiographic images by intensity profiles is the key to understanding CT technology. Figure 1-1 shows that this profile exhibits a certain depth (subject shadow) as well as a certain edge character. It should be clear that if the anatomic square structure under study had been more similar in atomic number and density to the background medium, the pattern depth or shadow would have been diminished and visualization would have been poorer. The relative x-ray intensity difference between the background and the anatomic structure of interest is referred to as the *subject contrast*.

$$C_s = \frac{I_{Bgd} - I_s}{I_{Bgd}} \qquad (1)$$

where $C_s$ = subject contrast, $I_{Bgd}$ = background intensity, and $I_s$ = subject intensity.

Subject contrast (also referred to as tissue contrast) depends on a number of factors, of which the beam energy is one of the most important. Beam energy in turn is governed by the operating kilovoltage and the beam filtration present in the beam. The second factor is the atomic number difference between the background and the anatomic structure in question. Figure 1-2 plots subject contrast as a function of beam energy for various combinations of anatomic tissues. Note that subject contrast diminishes as beam energy increases and as tissues become more similar. The practical importance of the $C_s$ measure and how it limits routine radiography can be illustrated by the case of blood vessels within soft tissue surrounds. Visualization of brain vasculature in radiography, for instance, is essentially impossible. However, introduction of contrast media into the blood vessel drastically increases its attenuation properties compared with the surrounding tissues, and the blood vessels "light up." Visualization is markedly improved.

In addition to subject contrast, a second important aspect of the x-ray image is its edge character. Figure 1-1 shows the ideal case, in which the x-ray image has exactly the same well-defined edges as the structure itself. In practice, this is not the case in that unsharp edges usually appear. Deviation from a well-defined edge is quantitated with the concept of *unsharpness* (or *blur*), which is a measure of resolution.

Unsharpness represents the spread around the edge and is simply expressed as the linear distance from the

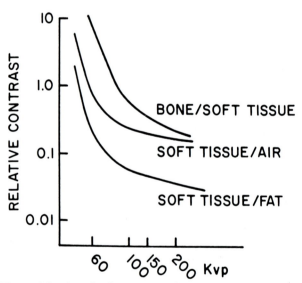

**Figure 1-2**  Plot of subject contrast between typical tissues as a function of energy. Note how subject contrast diminishes with increasing energy and increasing similarity in tissue densities. (*Adapted from Meredith and Massey 1972.*)

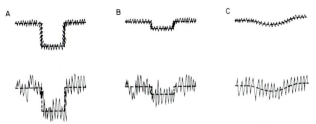

**Figure 1-3**  The effects of x-ray noise (quantum mottle) on x-ray intensity profiles. **A.** Ideal intensity profile with relatively high subject contrast (deep shadow). Increasing amounts of noise mask the x-ray image, but it may still be detected. **B.** Ideal profile with relatively low subject contrast. Increasing amounts of noise readily obscure pattern. **C.** Unsharp and low subject contrast pattern is also readily obscured by noise.

point of maximum intensity to the point of minimum intensity. A number of factors affect unsharpness in the x-ray image. The most important are anatomic and patient motion, focal-spot size, and the relative geometry of the patient and the x-ray source. The concept of unsharpness can be applied not only to the x-ray image but also to the final recorded and visible image by incorporating the recording-system image-degrading effects.

In addition to subject contrast and unsharpness, a third aspect of the x-ray image is *quantum mottle* (or *x-ray image noise*). Quantum mottle can be simply defined as the relative fluctuation in photon number arriving at the image plane. Figure 1-3 illustrates how quantum mottle can seriously obscure both the edge character and the depth character of a given image, especially for low subject contrast and small object sizes. Quantum mottle arises from the fact that there are random fluctuations in the x-ray emission spectrum of the x-ray source as well as in the interactions the x-rays undergo within the patient.

To minimize the effect of quantum mottle in the x-ray image, the overall number of photons utilized at the image plane must be increased. This can be accomplished by increases in x-ray tube current, or kilovoltage, or by a decrease in distance from the x-ray source to the image receptor. Attempts to decrease quantum mottle in such a manner, however, may result in an increased radiation dose to the patient.

## CLASSIC RADIOGRAPHY

In classic radiography, the clinician attempts to record directly the x-ray intensity profiles in the form of a density distribution on a film. This process, though simple and direct, forms the major limitation for classic radiography. The reason for this limitation is clear when considering that the patient is made up of a complex distribution of different tissues and structures. Any particular

x-ray intensity profile emerging from the patient is thus the compounded sum of the attenuation which occurred in the patient along a particular ray path (the superimposition effect). Under these conditions contour can interfere with contour and shadow with shadow. What is finally most prominent in the recorded image is the anatomic structure with the greatest absorption. Thus lesions can be "lost" behind the ribs or the heart shadow or, in the skull, behind the fossa as well as along the base of the calvarium. In practice, this information loss is compensated for in part by obtaining two views perpendicular to each other, such as anterior-posterior and lateral views, or by obtaining oblique views.

Other limitations in classic radiography include the presence of scatter and the use of nonlinear receptors. Scatter is a major source of image degradation; hence, scatter-eliminating grids are generally used. It is true that the use of high-ratio grids reduces scatter as much as 95 to 98 percent, depending on patient thickness and grid ratio. However, it is also true that the difference in subject contrast between such structures as gray matter and white matter is of the order of 0.5 percent. As a result, even a small percentage of scatter can obscure visualization of subtle tissue differences.

In the case of nonlinear receptors, the basic problem is the fact that low subject contrast structures may have densities falling in the nonlinear response region of the receptor. These nonlinear regions yield less film contrast and, consequently, low image contrast. This can be seen in the H&D response curve and the corresponding film contrast curve illustrated in Fig. 1-4. Here, film contrast is merely the slope of the H&D response curve and determines the actual density differences seen on the film. Note that the point of maximum film contrast occurs at about the middle of the linear region. This means that slight exposure or x-ray intensity differences at this level of the H&D curve result in the greatest displayed density differences. Film contrast progressively falls toward both the high-density and low-density sides of the linear region. Final displayed density difference ($\Delta B$) is referred to as *image, radiographic,* or *broad-area* contrast.

Figure 1-4 illustrates these ideas graphically. Here a given slight exposure difference along $B$ is finally displayed with a density difference $\Delta B$. If exposures had been such that tissue structures of interest were in the low-density region, that is, along $A$, then final displayed contrast would be $\Delta A$ and the observed density difference would be less than that obtained along the center of the H&D curve. Basically, visualization is poor in both the underexposed and the overexposed regions of the film. Radiographically, this can be seen in Fig. 1-5A, where a bullet is not visible in an approximately correctly exposed chest film, which usually

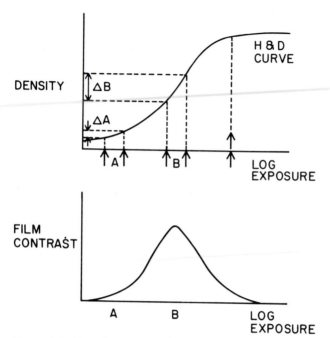

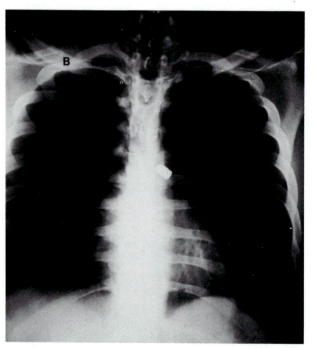

*Figure 1-4*  Typical H&D curve plotting log exposure versus resulting optical density. Nonlinearity of this curve results in a variable film contrast as seen in the lower figure, where the film contrast at any point of the curve is plotted as merely the slope of the H&D curve at each point. Slight differences in exposure along *B* lying on the linear portion of the H&D curve are displayed with the greatest difference in densities or image contrast (Δ*B*) and thus are better visualized. Exposures at the lower densities (*A*) are visualized at lower image contrast (Δ*A*). This is also true for exposures at higher densities.

leaves the mediastinum area at relatively low densities and thus low display contrast. Figure 1-5*B* shows the same patient but with exposures sufficiently high so that structures of interest are displayed at higher densities and thus higher display contrast; the presence of the bullet then becomes obvious.

One last observation should be made here: Even if the exposure factors (kilovoltage and milliamperage) are selected optimally for a given tissue or subject contrast, one may still be limited by a relatively small final display contrast (difference in illumination on the display monitor). In CT scanning using linear detectors under computer control, one can increase and optimize the display contrast, utilizing the full black-and-white capability of modern cathode ray tube (CRT) monitors. This is referred to as *windowing*. For instance, exposures along *B* in Fig. 1-4, rather than being displayed with display contrast Δ*B,* can be windowed in such a way to arbitrarily assign them any desired gray-scale values, including the full range of white to black. This important feature is discussed further in a subsequent section.

The following limiting factors of classic radiography as seen in this section can be summarized as follows:

1. Superimposition of three-dimensional information onto two dimensions causes the loss of low-tissue-contrast anatomic structures.

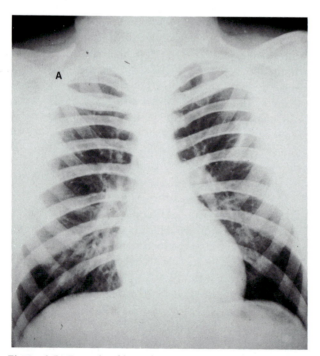

*Figure 1-5*  Example of loss of important image details in classical radiography as a function of density on the film. **A.** Correctly exposed chest film leaving heart shadow and mediastinum at low density and thus low image contrast. **B.** Bullet obviously present when film is exposed to higher density levels where image contrast is higher. However, note the loss of details in lung areas.

2. Presence of scatter obscures low-tissue-contrast anatomic structures.
3. Presence of nonlinear film receptors limits display contrast at high and low densities; furthermore, display contrast is not adjustable on film by the observer.

## CLASSIC TOMOGRAPHY

Classic tomography was formulated in an attempt to minimize the problem of the superimposition of three-dimensional information onto two dimensions. It is based on moving the x-ray source and film cassette relative to each other in such a way that the recorded images of anatomic structures within the patient are blurred. However, one anatomic layer (referred to as the *focal, fulcrum,* or *pivot plane*) within the patient remains stationary relative to the film and is recorded unblurred. Thus the third dimension (patient thickness, or depth) is removed via blurring, and presumably only the specified or pivot layer is recorded at full contrast and sharpness. It is clear, however, that the scatter problem is still present, as are the limitations of nonlinear film and screen systems. Finally, even the blurring within the nonfocal plane layers is never total. It depends on a number of geometric factors as well as the contrast of the objects being blurred.

Classic tomography has been reviewed in depth (Littleton 1976), and the reader is referred to the literature already available. What must be emphasized here is that tomography has certain inherent limitations that result in less than optimal information acquisition. These limitations can be summarized as follows:

1. There is incomplete tomographic blurring of the nonfocused planes. This means that obscuring anatomy is never completely and totally removed. The degree of blurring depends on the subject contrast of the object being blurred as well as distance from the focal plane. Therefore, structures near the focal plane affect the image to a greater extent than do structures far from the focal plane. Likewise, structures nearer to the film side produce less of a tomographic effect than do structures on the far side of the pivot level.
2. Some blur occurs within the focal plane itself, obscuring the anatomy sought to be visualized, since theoretically only an infinitesimally thin plane is truly in focus. This may be overcome in part by scanning over wide-arc angles (thin-section tomography). Finally, some blur also may occur within the focal plane because of mechanical vibration of the moving apparatus.
3. Tomographic blur is dependent on the direction of motion relative to the shape of the anatomy to be blurred. For example, linear tomography does not blur structures whose boundaries are parallel to the direction of arc motion; rather, only structures whose margins are at an angle to the arc motion are blurred.
4. Even though unwanted structures are blurred, they contribute fog background density to the film, which lowers the relative contrast of the structures within the pivot plane.
5. Since the whole body section is irradiated, large amounts of image-degrading scatter are generated.

## COMPUTED TOMOGRAPHY

CT has in great measure overcome the various limitations of both classic radiography and classic tomography. This has been accomplished by

1. Scanning only a thin, well-defined volume of interest, which serves to minimize the superimposition effect
2. Minimizing scatter by collimating down to relatively thin volumes
3. Using linear detectors with computerized windowing functions

The final success of the diagnostic task hinges on how well the image displays or conveys diagnostic information on the distribution of anatomic structures within the patient. In classic radiography the emerging x-ray beam is recorded directly, with an intensifying screen-film combination. The emerging beam, however, represents the total attenuation which occurred within the patient cross section, and as discussed previously, the superimposition effect is present. Ideally, a point-by-point characterization of the anatomic cross section under study (transaxial image) would be displayed. The characterization used in CT scanning is that of x-ray attenuation in tissue. Historically, a host of other characterizations and different radiation types have been proposed and studied. These include the atomic number and electron density (Phelps 1975a; Rutherford 1976; Latchaw 1978), ultrasound acoustic impedance (Carson 1977; Kak 1979), microwaves (Kak 1979; Maini 1980), neutrons (Koeppe 1981), *and* protons (Cormack 1976). CT reconstructions based on fluoroscopic techniques have also been developed (Baily 1976; Kak 1977). Proton magnetic resonance, has been extremely successful and is discussed in Chap. 2. Finally, single photon emission computed tomography (English 1995, Madsen 1995) and positron emission tomography (PET) have also been highly successful.

The computed tomography approach consists in isolating a specific planar volume within the patient. This plane, or slice, has a thickness $z$, as seen in Fig. 1-6.

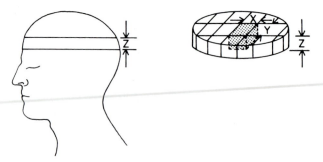

**Figure 1-6** Cross-sectional slice across patient. The expanded view shows arrangement of pixels (or picture elements) of dimensions *x* by *y* in a grid array. Volume element (or voxel) is formed in a third dimension (*z*) due to the finite slice thickness.

## Table 1-1    Attenuation Coefficients and CT Numbers for Biological Tissues at 60 keV

| TISSUE | ATTENUATION COEFFICIENT $\mu$ (CM$^{-1}$) | CT NUMBER |
|---|---|---|
| Bone | 0.400 | +1000 |
| Blood | 0.215 | +100 (approx.) |
| Brain matter | 0.210 | +30 (approx.) |
| CSF | 0.207 | +5 (approx.) |
| Water | 0.203 | 0 |
| Fat | 0.185 | −100 (approx.) |
| Air | 0.0002 | −1000 |

*Adapted from Phelps 1975b.*

The x-ray beam to be utilized passes through only this volume; thus superimposition and scatter effects are greatly minimized but not totally eliminated. Final characterization of tissues within the scanned volume are expressed and displayed for each element area given by *x* and *y*, as seen in Fig. 1-6. This element area is referred to as a *pixel* (*pic*ture *el*ement). The volume formed by virtue of the slice having some thickness *z* is referred to as a *voxel* (*vo*lume *el*ement). In practice, the whole patient part is arbitrarily broken down into a matrix array of such pixels. The pioneer EMI Mark I unit consisted of an 80 × 80 array in which each pixel corresponded to a 3 mm × 3 mm area within the patient and had a slice thickness of 13 mm. Matrix sizes of modern units are 256 × 256 or 512 × 512. Pixel sizes can now correspond to less than 1 mm by 1 mm within the patient. Different CT units have different pixel configurations. In most cases, however, the critical parameter is not the number of pixels but the area and volume they correspond to within the patient. This in turn depends on the field of view employed for a particular scan protocol.

## Attenuation Coefficients and Algorithms

The tissue type within each pixel is characterized by the tissue's ability to attenuate x-rays. Attenuation is defined simply as the removal of x-ray photons from the beam. This removal can be accomplished either by absorption (energy deposited at or near the site of photon interaction) or scatter events (energy removed from the site of photon interaction). Tissues in general have different attenuation properties, depending on their atomic number and physical density and the incident photon energy. The attenuation of a material can be described in terms of the *attenuation coefficient,* usually symbolized by the Greek letter $\mu$ and having units of cm$^{-1}$. The attenuation coefficient is quite familiar to radiological scientists and, with the advent of CT scanning, has taken on special importance to the

clinical radiologist. Table 1-1 lists typical biological tissues of interest and their corresponding attenuation coefficients. Also shown is their representation on an arbitrary scale on which bone is specified as +1000, air as −1000, and water as zero. This scale is referred to as the *Hounsfield scale* in honor of the inventor of computed tomography, Godfrey N. Hounsfield (1972). More commonly, the numbers are simply referred to as *CT numbers.* (For extensive tabulation of attenuation coefficients and CT numbers see Phelps 1975b). The CT number of any tissue is given by Equation (4).

The decision to characterize tissue types by CT numbers still leaves the problem of actually determining the value of the CT number for each pixel within that patient. Figure 1-7 shows a simplified 3 × 3 matrix array containing nine pixels, each having specific but unknown values of attenuation. The task is to determine the attenuation for each pixel. If x-rays are passed through ray path *A,* a total attenuation corresponding to, for instance, 12 units is determined. This value is referred to as a *ray sum* and represents the total attenuation occurring from the sum of the attenuation in all the pixels along that ray. Likewise, ray paths *B* and *C* yield totals of 7 and 4, respectively. The process is repeated from another angle perpendicular to the first (ray paths *D, E,* and *F*), and ray sums of 9, 8, and 6 are found. Now the task is to assign or reconstruct values for each pixel which conform with ray sums experimentally found from the two angles used. It is possible in fact to "play" with the numbers and finally arrive at the correct distribution, such as that indicated in parentheses in Fig. 1-6. In practice, ray sums also have to be taken at various angles to assure unique and accurate reconstructions.

In the case of matrix arrays which are, for instance, 512 × 512 in extent, ray scans must be determined over a complete contour of the patient and the amount

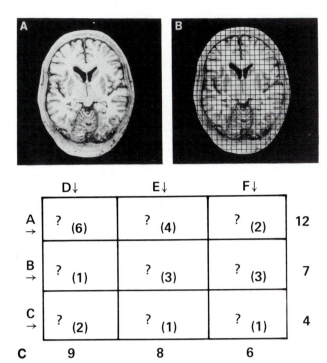

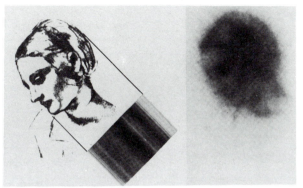

**Figure 1-8** Example of back-projection technique using a pictorial view of a face. The value of the density along each line is given by the average along each line. In this case the average is obtained via a smearing motion (equivalent to back projection). When all such projections are summed, the original face is, surprisingly enough, reconstructed. (*After Gordon 1975.*)

**Figure 1-7** **A.** Cross-sectional slice of brain showing structures to be imaged. **B.** Grid array of pixels superimposed over brain slice. The task in CT scanning is to determine tissue type within each pixel. **C.** As an example of how pixel values are determined, here is an unknown $3 \times 3$ array of pixels. Each pixel has some number value. Even though the interior values are unknown, the total exterior sums along the horizontal paths A, B, and C and vertical paths D, E, and F as well as along various angles can be determined (transmission values when using x-rays). Mathematical techniques (algorithms) are available to reconstruct the true interior values from this type of exterior data even for a very large number of pixels. (Solutions to pixel values are shown in parentheses.)

of data to be collected is formidable—so much that a computer is necessary to keep track of the data and perform the actual calculations necessary for a successful reconstruction. The model, or calculation scheme used for reconstruction, is referred to as an *algorithm*. The most popular algorithm for commercial scanners is the filtered back-projection algorithm. In this algorithm the ray sum for each row of pixels for a first approximation is assigned to each pixel along that row (this is called *back projection*). As each new set of data corresponding to a new angle of scan is determined, it is also back-projected and averaged into each pixel. Such a procedure, though not directly intuitive, does in fact, as seen in Fig. 1-8, result in a successful image reconstruction. Note in Fig. 1-8 that back projection is accomplished by linearly smearing (back-projecting) the image for a number of different angles, and the sum, or superimposition, of all the views represents a reconstruction of the original image.

In practice, before back projection is implemented, each intensity profile is modified or filtered to minimize starlike artifacts caused by the use of a finite set of angular images made to correspond to a square

pixel. A number of *filter functions* are incorporated in the algorithms that have been used or proposed, and the reader is referred to various reviews in the classic literature (Gordon 1974; Brooks 1975). These filter functions, which are sometimes called *kernels,* can also incorporate varying degrees of *smoothing* and edge enhancement. Smoothing may sometimes be of value when noise limits the detail visible in the image. Many CT units have a number of filter functions available, and the user should be aware of possible improvements in the images and the possibility of decreasing patient dose with their use. It should, however, also be realized that the smoothing operation degrades image resolution and thus limits the smallest sizes that can be displayed. It should be considered only as a noise suppressant in imaging relatively large structures.

## Data-Collection Geometry

The reconstruction process involves the collection of x-ray transmission values outside the patient. These transmission values are an index of how much the radiation was attenuated in passage through the patient. The collection of such data from a number of different angles around the patient is used to calculate the attenuation occurring at each picture element within the patient. Various data-collection schemes have been employed for the acquisition of x-ray transmission data. All schemes involve some geometrical pattern of scanning around the patient coupled with use of a suitable radiation detector. The signal from the radiation detector is digitized by the use of an analog-to-digital (A/D) converter and passed on to the computer for processing. After the reconstruction is completed, the results are displayed on a video monitor. Interim storage of the images is via hard disk. Long-term storage is accomplished either on magnetic tape or on optical disks. The overall layout is illustrated in Fig. 1-9.

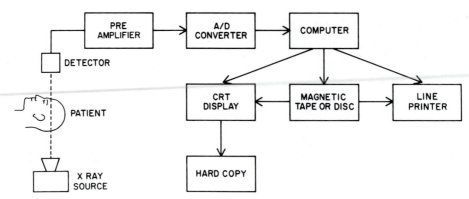

**Figure 1-9** Block diagram of a typical CT system. After x-rays emerge from the patient, they are detected, amplified, and digitized with an analog-to-digital (A/D) converter. After computer processing, the reconstruction results are assigned a gray scale and displayed on a CRT video monitor from which hard-copy views may be obtained. Since CRTs are analog devices, the image data must be converted from digital form back to analog form. CT number data can also be outputed to a line printer for quantitative analysis. Normally a tape or disk system is also used for storage of data for later redisplay and/or image manipulation.

## TRANSLATE/ROTATE GEOMETRY

The first successful clinical CT scanner was based on a translate-rotate gantry geometry. Although this technology is now obsolete, it is discussed since because of its simplicity it illustrates the basic principles of CT scanning.

In this type of system the x-ray beam is collimated down to the desired slice thickness and to a narrow slit. The resulting x-ray pattern is referred to as a *pencil beam*. The pencil beam is then passed through the patient and is incident on a radiation detector, as seen in Fig. 1-10. The quantity of radiation arriving at the detector for each ray path depends on the total attenuation that occurs along the ray path for each volume element (voxel) traversed.

To determine the ray-attenuation sums for each row of voxels, the pencil beam is made to linearly scan, or translate, across the patient. During the translate motion the detector, being rigidly connected to the x-ray tube, moves in such a manner that it always intercepts the x-ray pencil beam. The signals detected during the translation motion form a profile representing the ray sums along all voxel rows.

To determine the ray-sum profiles at different angles, the unit must sequentially rotate and perform a translation movement across the patient for each angle of rotation. The original EMI Mark I system rotated a total of 180°, one degree at a time (the configuration usually referred to as *first-generation geometry*). These movements required a total of 5½ to 6 minutes to complete a scan. Unfortunately, patient motion and resulting mismatch between patient position and pixel position resulted in severe image streaks. To reduce overall patient examination time, two detectors were placed side by side in the $z$ (or slice thickness) direction and the x-ray beam was made wide enough to include both detectors. This had the effect of providing two image slices simultaneously and shortening the overall time needed to obtain all the slices desired as well as minimizing patient motion between slices.

Individual slice scan times can be reduced significantly by providing for multiple pencil beams, with each beam directed at its own detector. This has the effect of obtaining ray sums from different angles on one translation (the configuration referred to as *second-generation geometry*). This is illustrated in Fig. 1-11 for a three-pencil-beam system. Here the pencil beams are configured to be at a 1° angle to one another. Consequently, during one translation, data are collected for three different angles, and the unit can be rotated 3° instead of 1° as needed for a single-pencil-beam configuration. Scan times can thus be reduced approximately by three since the unit has to complete only one-third the number of rotations and translations. (Sixty rotations at 3° increments will still provide for 180° around the patient and 180 ray-sum profiles.) Additionally, the clinician may again provide for a sec-

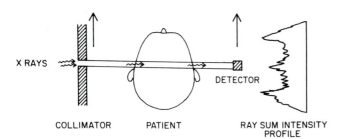

**Figure 1-10** First-generation CT configuration. A pencil beam is formed with a collimator and passed through the patient at a particular angle onto a detector traversing the patient along with the x-ray pencil beam. A ray sum intensity profile is thus detected and channeled to the computer for processing. The process is repeated at 1° intervals for 180°.

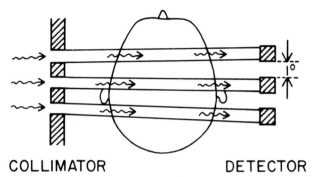

**COLLIMATOR**       **DETECTOR**

***Figure 1-11*** Configuration for second-generation gantry systems. A series of pencil beams pass through the patient at an angle, for instance, of 1° to one another. To obtain 180° of information, the number of translations across the patient is then reduced to 180/N, where N is the number of detectors. When possible, another row of detectors is added to obtain a second slice simultaneously with the first.

ond bank of detectors identical with the first to detect and process two slices simultaneously. To further reduce scan times even more pencil beams may be incorporated, each with its own detector. Thus 10 beams will require 10 detectors and only 18 rotations, 20 beams will require 9 rotations, etc. In fact, given sufficient beams and detectors, scan times can be effectively reduced to a few seconds. In this latter case, since scan times are relatively short, the second bank of detectors may be eliminated for a considerable cost saving.

## ROTATE-ONLY GEOMETRY

The logical extension of using more and more pencil beams is to open up the x-ray beam in the transverse plane to produce a fan beam large enough to encompass the entire patient. This is the so-called third-generation geometry. This fan beam is incident on a whole array of detectors which move along with the fan, as in Fig. 1-12. In this process the time-consuming translation motion is entirely eliminated. Note that not only must detectors number at least 180 (one for each of the 180° of view), but actually even more detectors are needed, since the array must be large enough to include a wide range of patient diameters. It is also necessary to include additional detectors to monitor and to correct for any variations in x-ray output. Modern

third-generation units use up to 800 or more detectors, with subsecond scan times possible. At these scanning times it is not necessary to have a second array of detectors for simultaneous two-plane scanning, as was common with single-pencil and some multiple-pencil systems. This reduces the cost and complexity of the equipment considerably.

One problem, however, with third-generation configuration is related to the detector calibration problem. The reconstruction process requires extremely high precision, and slight variations (as low as 0.1%) in x-ray output or in detector electronics must be corrected for. Each individual detector must then be calibrated to assure constancy and uniformity of response as compared with adjacent detectors. In first- and second-generation systems, because of the translation motion, the detectors were out from behind the patient and were directly exposed through air to the x-ray beam at the extreme ends of their travel during each scan motion. They could thus be easily calibrated in air before traversing the patient again. Third-generation systems preclude the possibility of frequent calibrations in that detectors are always behind the patient and cannot be calibrated between individual scans. The result is the formation of artifactual ring structures, with each ring corresponding to a drift in one or more detectors, as seen in Fig. 1-13. Ring artifacts can be minimized with certain algorithm corrections; however, sta-

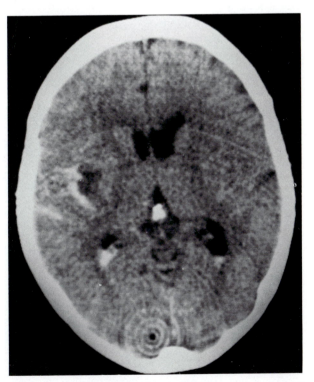

***Figure 1-13*** Demonstration of typical third-generation ring artifacts. These ring structures are caused by slight detector calibration drifts (typically less than 1 percent).

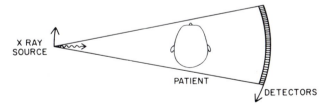

***Figure 1-12*** Configuration for a third-generation gantry system. Here an entire fan of x-rays is passed through the patient onto the array of detectors. Since all portions of the patient are viewed, translation motion across the patient is eliminated entirely.

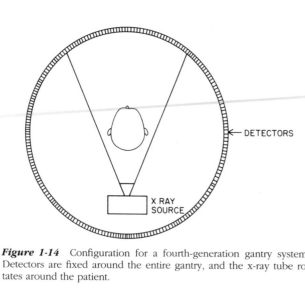

***Figure 1-14*** Configuration for a fourth-generation gantry system. Detectors are fixed around the entire gantry, and the x-ray tube rotates around the patient.

bility in the detector system and uniformity of detector response are crucial. In fact, detector drifts of much less than 1 percent can cause visible artifacts.

One possible method of avoiding detector-calibration problems, as found in third-generation configurations, is to use a ring of detectors fixed around the entire periphery of the gantry (*fourth-generation geometry*). This configuration is seen in Figs. 1-14 and 1-15. In such an arrangement the x-ray beam rotates around the patient and always radiates a freshly calibrated detector. The added complexity and cost of fixing many detectors around the entire gantry periphery and the associated electronics are obvious. Variations on the fourth-generation configuration include putting the x-ray tube outside the detector array. This allows the use of a

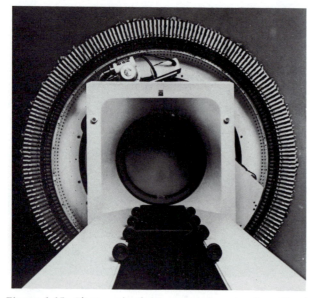

***Figure 1-15*** Photograph of detector configuration for a fourth-generation gantry system.

smaller detector ring as well as more closely packed smaller detectors, which result in enhanced resolution and possibly lower costs. In this configuration, provision is made for continuously moving the detector ring out of the direct x-ray beam path.

## ELECTRON BEAM GEOMETRY

One gantry configuration that is being called by some a fifth-generation system consists of a stationary gantry-detector system with a moving electron beam sweeping across an extended anode target arranged semicircularly around the patient (Boyd 1982; Lipton 1985, 1986). In this approach there are actually multiple target layers so that electrons sequentially sweeping across each result in the formation of multiple successive fan beams of x-rays. The result of all this is that one can acquire multiple image slices within a very short period of time. Additionally, dual detector banks are present which allows for dual slice acquisition. Present configuration of this system provides for four target arcs with dual detector sampling yielding eight image slices in rapid succession. This high-speed image acquisition (about 50 milliseconds per image) allows for cine-type scan sequences. Additionally, flow phenomena can also be studied. Application of this scanning concept was originally limited to cardiac imaging. It is now, however, available for general scanning (Brundage 1985; Lipton 1986; Villafana 1991). For general CT use it has been commercially available under the name Imatron, Fastrack (Picker Corporation), or more recently, Evolution (Siemens Corporation).

## Detectors

Various types of radiation detectors are commonly used in CT scanning. Two general types have emerged, the scintillation crystal-photodiode detector and the pressurized ionization chamber detector. Each of these is briefly discussed.

### SCINTILLATION DETECTOR-PHOTODIODE

This consists of a solid scintillation crystal which has the property of emitting light when x-ray or gamma photons are incident upon it. This emitted light falls on a photodiode surface that converts the light to an electronic signal, which in turn is amplified. In CT scanning the signal is then digitized and transmitted to the computer for processing. Solid state detectors are very efficient in absorbing x-ray photons (up to 98%) but do have afterglow properties which may limit their performance. The original detector configuration in early CT units consisted of coupling the solid state scintillation detector to a photomultiplier instead of a photodiode. Photomultipliers, however, are large, expensive, and easily subject to drift and are no longer used. Examples of typical scintillation crystals used in such configurations are seen in Table 1-2.

## Table 1-2   CT Detectors

| DETECTOR TYPES | CHEMICAL FORM |
| --- | --- |
| Scintillation crystals plus photomultiplier* | Sodium iodide NaI (TI)* |
| | Calcium fluoride $C_aF_2$* |
| | Bismith germanate* |
| | $Bi_4Ge_3O_{12}$ (BGO)* |
| Scintillation crystals plus photodiode | Cadmium tungstate $CdWO_4$ |
| | Cesium iodide CsI ($N_a$) |
| | Hi-Light Detector† |
| Ionization chamber | Xenon (under pressure) |

*Now obsolete technology.
†General Electric Corporation proprietary technology.

## PRESSURIZED IONIZATION CHAMBERS

One of the requirements for CT detectors is that they be small and capable of being configured very close to one another to provide for full capture of the incident radiation. The ionization chamber approach comes very close to providing these features. Such a chamber consists of one large assembly having very thin walls defining each small collection region, as in Fig. 1-16. This configuration yields a very high packing density of these small detectors. Additionally, xenon gas is perfused evenly throughout the assembly to ensure uniformity of response. Some disadvantages include the fact that xenon, being a gas, does not provide for as much absorption efficiency as do solid-state detectors. To compensate for these losses, ionization chambers are pressurized at 10 to 30 atmospheres (providing more gas molecules for absorbing the x-ray beam) and are constructed with relatively deep depths (providing greater path length for x-ray photons to be absorbed). Unfortunately, some attenuation loss is experienced within the relatively thick face plate needed to withstand the high xenon gas pressure, and this reduces detection efficiency.

## DETECTOR REQUIREMENTS

To be effective in CT scanning applications, detectors should have the characteristics listed in Table 1-3. The need for *high absorption efficiency* is self-evident. This provides for maximum utilization of the photons incident on the face of the detector. Here the important factors are the physical density, atomic number, size, and thickness of the detector. *Conversion efficiency* relates to the ability of the detector to convert the absorbed x-ray energy to a usable electronic signal. *Capture efficiency* means that the size of the detector and the distance to adjacent detectors should be such that as many as possible of the photons passing through the patient are incident on (or captured by) the detector face. The total detector efficiency is merely the running product of these three individual efficiencies. Total detector efficiency is also referred to as *dose efficiency*. Typical dose efficiencies fall between 50 and 70 percent for gaseous detectors and better than 95 percent for solid state detectors. It is unfortunate that the conversion efficiency from light to an electrical signal at the photodiode is not nearly as high and overall efficiency of solid state detector is reduced though still higher than that of gaseous detectors. The *temporal response* of a detector should be as fast as possible in that in a scanning configuration each detector sees the radiation for a relatively short time measured in milliseconds. Within this time, the signal must be processed and the detector must be ready for the next measurement. It is clear that the performance of a unit would be severely degraded if the detector had a significantly delayed response, sometimes referred to as *phosphorescence* or *afterglow*. With significant afterglow, correlation between the specific voxel the x-ray beam is traversing and the signal received by the computer would be lost. Afterglow would be especially limiting for fast, dynamic scanning. Because of the relatively poor temporal response of the earlier detectors such as NaI (TI) and $CaF_2$, these are no longer used in modern scanners. *Wide dynamic range* refers to the ability of the detector to respond linearly to a wide range of x-ray intensities. When scanning patients, the x-ray beam sometimes passes through air having negli-

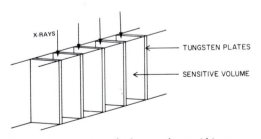

*Figure 1-16*  Close-up view of adjacent plates within a pressurized xenon gas detector. The small size of these detectors allows for very small data-sampling distances; also, there is minimal information loss between detector cells (high capture ratio).

## Table 1-3   Favorable Detector Characteristics

High absorption efficiency
High conversion efficiency
High capture efficiency
Good temporal response (little afterglow)
Wide dynamic range
High reproducibility and stability

gible attenuation and consequently forming a very intense signal at the detector. On the other hand, the beam may then traverse a thick patient or body part having a high beam attenuation. The x-ray signal formed at the detector would then be very low. Ideally a detector should respond linearly between these two extremes; a dynamic range of more than 100,000 to 1 should be minimal. Finally, *high reproducibility and stability* are required to avoid drift and resultant detector fluctuation or noise.

## CT Image Display and Recording

What the computer understands to be an image consists merely of an array of CT numbers, one number corresponding to each pixel. For the viewer to see a "real" image, this array of numbers must be displayed on a suitable medium such as a video monitor or hardcopy film. Three considerations must be taken into account for the proper display and storage of CT images:

1. Adjustment of the video monitor display characteristics of brightness and display contrast, that is, the video gray scale
2. Selection of settings (center and window) to optimize the display of anatomic tissues of interest within the given video gray scale
3. Recording of the image for long-term storage

### VIDEO GRAY SCALE

Every video device has its own gray scale. The gray scale refers to the manner in which the device goes from its darkest to its brightest illumination. The gray scale usually is displayed as a graded series of steps, at one end representing the darkest and at the other end the brightest illumination. Steps in between, therefore, have intermediate values of gray, and the rapidity with which they go from light to dark is the video monitor contrast. Rather than steps, some units have a continuous illumination strip. In any case, the result is the same, namely, the actual display brightness and contrast of the monitor can be observed. Adjustments can be made exactly as the monitor display characteristics are controlled during image-intensified fluoroscopy, ultrasound video, or home video viewing. These settings are usually chosen initially and remain fixed thereafter. The basis for actual settings varies with the individual viewer. Usually, however, the final gray scale should display both the very darkest and the very brightest that the monitor can display as well as a relatively uniform gradation of gray between these two extremes. All installations have a monitor for direct viewing and a means to obtain hard-copy films. In the latter case, the gray scale should be adjusted to optimize the image, taking into account the characteristics of the film which will be used to record the image. Selection of film and the monitor brightness and contrast used to record the film are not trivial matters, and care must be taken to assure the best possible film images.

Variations in optimal window and center settings reported between CT sites are usually due in part to differences in initial gray-scale settings and differences in video monitor display characteristics.

### CENTER AND WINDOW SETTINGS

One of the biggest differences between radiographic film viewing and CT viewing is the ability in the latter to *window* the anatomic tissues of interest. By this is meant that the viewing of particular tissues of interest can be optimized by assigning to them the full range of blacks and whites available on the CRT monitor. For example, the center setting assigns the video midgray value to the CT number (or tissue) desired; the window setting defines the CT number range which will occupy the scale from black to white. To illustrate, consider a head CT scan viewed at a center of +50 and a window of 200 CT units. The +50 corresponds to the approximate CT number of gray and white matter, and it is these tissues that are displayed with the midgray illumination. A window of 200 CT units implies that the range will be from +150 (100 above 50) to −50 (100 below 50). Consequently all tissues having CT numbers of 150 or above will be displayed as white, whereas all tissues at −50 and below will be displayed as black. On these settings, bone calcifications and blood pools will appear light, and ventricular volumes will appear darker. The above settings may be ideal for a head scan, but different settings are needed for body scanning, since body scanning involves a greater range of tissue types, so that a greater window range must be selected. Likewise, a bone window is defined with center above +500 and lung windows with centers below −500.

The power of the windowing function is appreciated when it is recalled that in film radiography the user must accept whatever exposure was made and is limited to what is seen on the film. Film, however, is nonlinear and thus results in different image contrast at each image point, depending on its density level. Additionally, films may be underexposed or overexposed. In either case, as discussed previously, information is lost at both the low- and high-density regions of the film. There is no such limitation for digital imaging. Figure 1-17 illustrates the role of windowing using linear detectors. If the full tissue range of −1000 to +1000 is displayed, note that the particular tissues of interest in the previous example (−50 to +150) would be limited to a relatively small range of grays, and visualization would be poor. However, with windowing as in Fig. 1-17B, the full black-and-white range is assigned

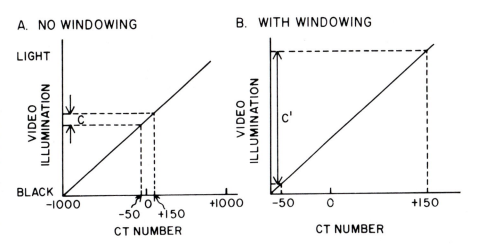

**Figure 1-17** On a scale of −1000 to +1000, if no windowing is available, a given CT number difference such as −50 to +150 is displayed with only a limited range of gray values (low image contrast C). With windowing invoked, the same CT number range can be displayed with up to the maximum video range from white to black (high image contrast C'): that is, −50 can be assigned full dark and +150 is assigned to full light.

between the −50 and +150 CT values, and visualization of these particular tissues is optimal in that the greatest illumination difference results.

## LONG-TERM STORAGE MEDIA

It has always been necessary to record the final image for patient records and subsequent comparisons and for referring physicians. Such recording can be done on film as for classic radiography. However, it is advantageous to record the actual computer image consisting of all the pixel values since pixel values, if available, can allow for subsequent windowing and redisplay and for computer manipulations such as magnification, CT number, or tissue identification and various image-enhancement routines. Thus magnetic tape and magnetic disk systems are usually incorporated into the basic CT instrumentation. In fact, the basic image-recording configuration of a clinical scanner may consist of some or all of the items listed in Table 1-4.

### Film

Film continues to be the most popular and economic long-term storage medium. It should be realized that the films used in CT imaging are quite different from the films used in radiography inasmuch as an image is being recorded either off a video monitor (multiformat camera) or via a laser beam scanner (laser printer). The film usually consists of a single emulsion sensitive to either the light-emission spectrum of the video-screen phosphor for the multiformat camera or to the laser beam light. Additionally, these nonscreen films tend to be linear. Multiimage-format cameras consist of a self-enclosed video monitor with independent access to the computer pixel image information. The arrangement is such that the camera exposes the film to the particular size format desired. For instance, four views (or image slices) on an 8 × 10 film and nine views on a 14 × 17 film are quite popular. The laser printer has

now become the recording system of choice. Here, the data are recorded via laser on film directly from the computer, bypassing the video system entirely. Since the video system is a relatively poor imaging component, its elimination results in significant image quality improvement.

Polaroid film originally had three drawbacks: limited film contrast range, expense, and the need for mounting for permanent records. To a lesser extent there was also the nuisance of paper wrappers, the wait for development, and the need for coating. Newer Polaroid film emulsions have extended film contrast range and do not need coating. This form of image recording, however, will probably still remain limited to relatively low patient-volume sites where the capital cost of multiimage cameras, laser printers, or tape recorders is a

## Table 1-4  Storage Media

| MEDIUM | PIXELS RECOVERABLE? | COMMENTS |
|---|---|---|
| Film | No | Convenient, various sizes available |
| Polaroid film | No | Relatively expensive; relatively poor contrast scale |
| Magnetic tape | Yes | Access time long, good for long-term storage |
| Floppy disk | Yes | Convenient size and format; relatively expensive; limited capacity |
| Magnetic disks | Yes | Expensive but fast |
| Optical disks | Yes | Greatly expanded storage capacity |

factor and sites where rapid film processing equipment is not available.

### Magnetic Tape

Magnetic tape recording of computer outputs is a well-established technology. Pixel values as well as patient identification data can be readily recorded in relatively short times. This means that images can be redisplayed at any subsequent time, and different computer manipulations of the images, including windowing, are possible. Additionally, the fidelity of the images is excellent. A number of drawbacks, however, exist. For example, storage space is limited to around 300 images per tape, depending on the number of pixels in the image. A $256 \times 256$ pixel array demands four times less tape space than a $512 \times 512$ pixel array. A capacity of a few hundred images, in the case of a busy site, means that only 1 or 2 days' worth of patient images may be stored on one tape. In practice, this is a severe limitation because accessing patient images on different tapes requires an inordinate amount of time, because of the need for loading and reloading tapes, and because of the relatively slow search times characteristic of magnetic tape systems. Finally, the number of tapes accumulated and the required floor storage space have dictated the recycling of tapes. Thus it is not uncommon to find tapes covering only 6 to 12 months or even less at a particular site.

### Disk-Based Systems

Three basic approaches to disk imaging have evolved. One approach uses so-called floppy disks. These disks are relatively small and flexible. In some cases a full patient examination or more can be recorded on one disk and can be conveniently transported to another room or site for image review at an independent viewing station. Disk search time is essentially negligible. However, the cost of each disk is such that many sites rely on magnetic tape recording for long-term storage and use floppy disks only for recent patients or for particularly interesting cases. Floppy disks have very limited capacity. For instance, they can only hold a few $512 \times 512$ images.

Another disk-based system consists of a bank of large disks (referred to as hard disks or Winchester disks) capable of storing thousands of images. These are random-access devices, so that stepping through every image in the file to find the required one is not necessary and search and access times are minimal. Viewing at remote consoles is possible only via direct data-link connection to the computer. The overall costs of such a system are relatively high. Every CT scanner, however, is outfitted with such disks for short-term storage of image data.

The third disk system is the optical disk. The optical disk expands storage capability to many thousands of images. It is now emerging as a cost-effective long-term archival modality. Image information is stored on these disks by producing a computer-coded pattern of micron-sized holes with a laser beam. Typical capacity is in the gigabyte range per optical disk and these are capable of storing thousands of images. Multioptical disk systems are available (jukeboxes) which greatly expand image storage capacity.

## Artifacts in CT Scanning

CT scanning, like any imaging modality, has artifacts unique to it. Many artifacts have multiple causes, and their complete description requires rigorous mathematical techniques. Here are presented a number of the more significant artifacts that the clinician should be aware of. Artifacts can manifest themselves either visibly in the form of streaks or quantitatively in the form of inaccurate CT numbers.

Streaks arise in general because there is an inconsistency in a particular ray path through the patient. This inconsistency can be due either to an error along the ray or to inconsistencies between rays. Table 1-5 summarizes the various sources of artifacts. Classification of artifacts has been troublesome (Joseph 1981). For purposes here, artifacts are classified according to what is happening to the data. Each of the artifacts listed in Table 1-5 is discussed in turn.

### DATA FORMATION

This section is concerned with how data are formed as x-rays pass through the patient. As previously discussed, the transmitted x-ray beam detected in CT scanning is an index of the degree of attenuation that

## Table 1-5 Sources of CT Artifacts

| SOURCE AREA | CAUSE |
|---|---|
| Data formation | Patient motion |
| | Polychromatic effects |
| | Equipment misalignment |
| | Faulty x-ray source |
| Data acquisition | Slice geometry |
| | Profile sampling |
| | Angular sampling |
| Data measurement | Detector imbalance |
| | Detector nonlinearity |
| | Scatter collimation |
| Data processing | Algorithm effects |

has occurred as the beam passed through the patient. Reference to Fig. 1-6 shows that the patient contour is arbitrarily divided into pixels. To accomplish the CT scan process, ray paths along different angles around the patient are obtained. Thus data are collected for the attenuation at each point in the field from different angles. If such ray-path data are inconsistent—that is, if the pixel does not contribute the same attenuation regardless of the particular angle of view—then streaks result. The most familiar example of data inconsistency is that caused by patient motion.

## Patient Motion

Motion has plagued CT scanning from the beginning. The original CT scan units took up to 6 minutes of scan time. The inordinate amount of time allowed for considerable patient motion during the course of the examination. When such motion occurs during the scanning process, the computer has no means of keeping track of where the pixels are in space and which ray-path sums belong to which row and column. This inconsistency results in severe streaking and is especially aggravated by the presence of high-density structures. In early CT units, the long scanning time necessary was so limiting that it provided the impetus to develop faster and faster scanners. Modern scanners can routinely perform scans in a few seconds and are capable of even subsecond scans.

It should be clear that motion not only introduces artifactual streaks but, as in classic radiography, may cause both a loss of *spatial resolution* (the ability to visualize fine spatial detail) and a loss of *tissue resolution,* or low contrast resolution (the ability to visualize small differences in tissue densities). These losses are usually minimal compared with the presence of streaks. To minimize motion artifacts the clinician may, in addition to scanning faster, provide for immobilization of the patient. Another approach used in earlier scanners involves overscanning. Here the patient was typically scanned 40° to 60° beyond the normal 180° or 360°, the rationale being that one is then collecting repeat, or redundant, views. For instance, if the patient has moved between the beginning of the scan and the end, there will be a discrepancy between the data collected on the 0° pass and the 180° pass. If the patient has not moved during the scan, these two views should be identical; any difference detected is entirely due to patient motion. Under computer control these differences can be averaged (or feathered) out. One obvious drawback to overscanning is the fact that scan times are longer, introducing the possibility of further motion artifacts. In spite of this, however, overscanning may be useful under certain circumstances.

## Polychromatic Effects

Probably the best-known polychromatic artifact referred to in clinical practice is the beam-hardening artifact. The basis for this artifact is the fact that in the reconstruction process the clinician attempts to assign an attenuation coefficient value to each voxel within the patient. However, attenuation coefficients are highly dependent on x-ray beam energy. Photons in x-ray beams do not have a unique energy but rather are polychromatic; that is, they are made up of photons having a wide distribution of energy. As the beam passes through the patient, the lower-energy photons are preferentially absorbed, and it is said that the beam becomes harder. (This is similar to the rationale for the use of filters in diagnostic radiology to reduce the patient dose.) Any given voxel within the patient is, however, viewed along different ray paths for each different angular projection. Consequently, the x-ray beam, having experienced different degrees of beam hardening, will have a different energy as it passes any particular voxel along these different ray-paths (Fig. 1-18). The overall result will be a general decrease in the CT numbers, since higher energies imply lower attenuation coefficients. This effect is most notable along ray paths containing thicker and denser bony structures, as along the orbit-base views. The visual result is dark streaks, since higher energies result in the display of CT numbers denoting less dense tissues. The best example of this effect is the interpetrous bone hypodensity streaks seen in Fig. 1-19. This particular artifact is also caused in part by the nonlinear partial volume effect (Glover 1980).

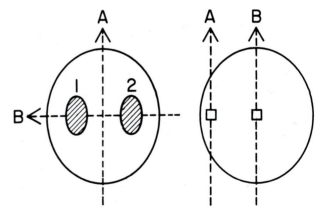

**Figure 1-18** Demonstration of beam hardening in CT scanning. *Left:* Interpetrous bone hypodensity artifact. Ray A suffers a different degree of beam hardening from ray B, which travels through bony structures 1 and 2. The result is an inconsistency in the CT numbers calculated, and streaks result between the bony structures. *Right:* Cupping artifact. Rays such as A, passing through the periphery of a uniform structure, suffer less attenuation than do rays such as B, passing through the center of that structure. The result is an apparent cupping, or increase in tissue density toward the periphery.

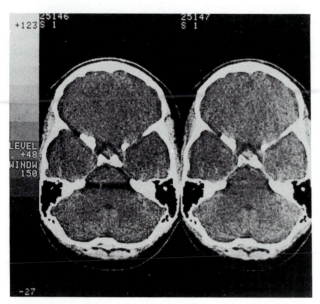

**Figure 1-19**  *Left:* Interpetrous bone artifact. *Right:* Same view after bone corrections are performed.

Beam hardening also leads to a spillover effect near the interface of bony structures with adjoining softer tissues. This is evident at the edge of the skull and was originally interpreted as the cerebral cortex (Ambrose 1973). Its artifactual nature was demonstrated by Gado and Phelps (1975), and it is now referred to as the *pseudocortex.* The basis for this effect, which is also referred to as *cupping,* is illustrated in Fig. 1-18: rays passing through the periphery of the patient cross section suffer less hardening. Since they are less hardened, they have lower energy and are more easily attenuated. Rays passing through the thicker center of the patient have been hardened and are less easily attenuated. The reconstruction process interprets this as a tissue through which radiation easily penetrates. The central regions thus are displayed as having lower CT numbers and appear darker. A similar effect is seen in the apical artifact discussed in the CT number accuracy section and illustrated in Fig. 1-26. The original EMI Mark I water bag system circumvented many of the problems of beam hardening as well as dynamic range of the detectors by providing for an essentially equal path length for all rays in all projections. Another approach to minimize beam-hardening effects is to add filtration to the beam or to add specially shaped compensating attenuators such as bow-tie filters to the beam. These approaches are discussed further in the section on CT number variations.

Beam hardening has been discussed at length, and a number of algorithms are available to correct for it (Brooks 1976a; Joseph 1978b). Typical CT scanners include within their reconstruction algorithm a so-called water correction based on the linearization of the data

collected. Bone or calcium correction algorithms represent a more complete correction but usually involve a longer reconstruction time.

### Equipment Misalignment

Mechanical misalignment of the x-ray source and radiation detectors may lead to artifactual streak formation. The basic problem is that of isocenter location. If an aluminum pin is placed at the isocenter and scanned, its position will be isocentric for all views and projections. If a misalignment of the isocenter is present, an inconsistency results between angular views, and streaks sometimes referred to as "tuning fork" streaks result. These streaks are more pronounced at dissimilar tissue boundaries such as between air and soft tissues or soft tissues and bone.

### Faulty X-Ray Source

If the x-ray output varies during the scan process, an obvious inconsistency in data immediately arises, since detectors cannot distinguish between increases or decreases in radiation level due to increases or decreases in x-ray output and those due to increased or decreased absorption along the ray path. All CT units include reference detectors to detect output variations for the purpose of correcting for such changes. These corrections, however, are for data from a single angular view. If variations are present between angular views, streaks criss-crossing the image field and forming moiré patterns result (Joseph 1981; Stockham 1979). These are assumed to be most likely related to the speed of anode rotation, which is also called *anode wobble.* Other possible x-ray source problems include momentary high-voltage arcing and fluctuations, which may reduce or increase instantaneous x-ray output. Again, such changes, though detected by reference chambers, still may result in inconsistencies between angular views, and streaks result.

## DATA ACQUISITION

In this section, artifactual effects resulting from the manner in which the data are collected are studied.

### Slice Geometry

The thickness of the slice scanned determines a very significant, though nonvisible, artifact: the partial volume effect. To understand this effect and its significance in practice, remember that the pixel displayed represents a volume in the patient given by both the area size and the slice thickness (the voxel). The voxel representing some finite patient volume may contain more than one tissue type. What happens is that if tissues are relatively similar (small CT number differences), the total contents of the voxel are for small CT number differences, in effect linearly averaged rather

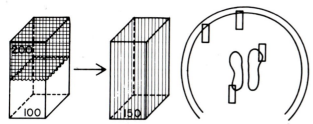

**Figure 1-20** *Left:* Example of the partial volume artifact. Here, if a particular voxel contains different tissues, the final computed value will be characterized by the average CT number. If the CT numbers are very different from each other, the summing average process is exponential and therefore nonlinear, and streaks may result. *Right:* Cross-sectional view of voxel positions at various levels within the skull, showing a varying degree of partial volume averaging for different tissue-structure boundaries.

than exponentially averaged. It is this average CT number value that is assigned to the voxel. Figure 1-20 illustrates this effect. For instance, if half the pixel is filled with a tissue having a CT number of 100 and the other half with a tissue having a CT number of 200, the average of the two is 150, and this voxel will be displayed as if it were filled with a tissue type of CT number 150, which in fact is not present within the voxel.

This effect is significant for relatively small anatomic structure sizes or for tissue volumes which are rapidly changing in size. Examples are the orbital base level and regions near the calvarium. Additionally, vascular structures, blood clots (Lim 1977), thin flat structures, as well as optic nerve visualization (Salvolini 1978), are subject to the partial volume effect. The result of the partial volume effect is the loss of tissue and spatial resolution and not necessarily streaks. In many instances, however, volume averaging is nonlinear in that tissue types within the voxel may have widely different CT numbers. This in turn results in large exponential, nonlinear absorption differences. An example of this would be the bony structures of the petrous ridges and the adjacent brain matter. The result is the interpetrous ridge lucency artifact, which has been discussed previously. At first this artifact was thought to be entirely due to beam-hardening effects. However, these artifacts were subsequently shown to be partly due to the nonlinear partial volume effect, which in turn is related to the sampling slice thickness (Glover 1980). Thus this artifact can be minimized by diminishing the slice thickness, although it cannot be eliminated entirely unless beam hardness is also corrected.

The basis for the nonlinear partial volume effect is that the detector response varies nonlinearly with the degree of bony intrusion into any given volume element; that is, the net signal at the detectors depends on the relative amount of soft tissue and bony tissue within the voxel. However, this dependence theoretically, does not vary linearly, since attenuation in each material is an exponential function. These nonlinearities result in an inconsistency in the data collected as the volume element is viewed from various angles around the patient, and it is this inconsistency that creates the streaks observed. These streaks appear not only across the petrous bones but also from the occipital protuberance and wherever there are relatively large, abrupt variations in tissue or structure densities such as air-liquid interfaces and metallic objects. To minimize this artifact, merely reduce the slice thickness, in which case the clinician must contend with more image noise because of fewer photons being detected. Alternatively, x-ray tube factors may be adjusted upward, resulting in a greater patient dose for the thinner slices.

Another slice-geometry artifact is that associated with the fact that the x-ray beam is diverging as it passes through the patient. This causes some interesting effects. For instance, where is the slice thickness indicated? Figure 1-21 shows that there is no unique slice thickness; thickness varies throughout the scanned volume. By convention, we specify the thickness at the center of rotation (isocenter) of the CT unit. If the scan is completely around the patient (360°), the volume actually being imaged may be symmetrically depressed in the center depending on the geometry of the scanner. The consequences of this effect are as follows:

1. Partial volume effects are then a function of position in the field as well as whether 360° or less than 360° scans are obtained. Also, greater spatial and tissue resolution are found in the center than at the periphery since these parameters depend on slice thickness.

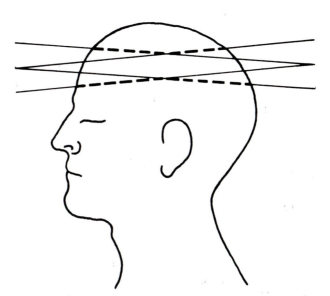

**Figure 1-21** Beam diverges as it passes through patient. As beam rotates around patient, it forms not a parallel-sided slice but a concave slice (given by dashed lines) with the center thinner than the periphery.

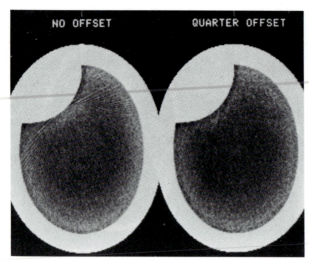

**Figure 1-25**    Verification of the removal of aliasing streaks, seen on the left, by quarter offset or shift of the central detector in a third-generation geometry array. (*After Brooks 1979.*)

need, according to Equation (3), to obtain two samples per detector width $d$ (a frequency of $2/d$); the quarter offset provides exactly this sampling interval, and aliasing streaks are markedly reduced, as seen in Fig. 1-25. Finally, undersampling in the $z$ direction can be reduced by using thinner slices.

### Angular Sampling

Just as a particular profile can be undersampled as discussed above, the number of profiles or angular view samples around the patient can be deficient. Such angular undersampling also leads to the formation of streak artifacts. However, these streaks, although radiating from small, dense objects or sharp edge objects, always occur at some distance from the object. Edges of patient stretcher are specifically shaped so that such artifacts are not cast directly over and onto patient image. It has been shown that undersampling along the profile (governed by the number of detectors) is more important and leads to more severe aliasing streaks compared with undersampling the number of angular views around the patient (Brooks 1979). Streaks due to view undersampling usually lead to artifacts in the image emanating from the undersampled structure but first appear at some distances from that structure.

To summarize this section, data acquisition or sampling schemes play a key role in the quality and accuracy of the final image. Sampling includes the thickness of the slice, the sampling along each profile (detector size), the number of angular views around the patient, and the matrix size. Effects can range from simple inaccuracies in the CT number to severe streaks obliterating the desired diagnostic information. Some of the ways to minimize aliasing streaks include thinner slices, closely packed small detectors, and quarter-

shifted detector geometry, larger matrix size (smaller pixels), and greater number of angular views.

## DATA MEASUREMENT
### Detector Imbalance

It has already been emphasized that detectors should have high efficiency and high reproducibility. Of importance also is that each detector in an array of detectors be matched in response compared with the other detectors in the array. When an imbalance occurs, for instance, in a third-generation system, ring artifacts such as those in Fig. 1-13 result. Imbalance may result from individual detector gain shifts. Shifts as low as 0.1 percent can result in visible streaks. Furthermore, the appearance of streaks is more severe if detector error affects only one ray path or a small group of ray paths, such as in third-generation systems. Fourth-generation system detector errors affect the whole view (each detector sees every point of the whole patient), and as a result, inconsistency is smoothed and averaged over the whole image, detector matching is not as critical, and ring artifacts are absent.

When shifts occur, they can be calibrated out. This calibration is performed whenever the detector is out from behind the patient. Calibration is automatic for fourth-generation systems. This is because detectors at the leading edge of the fan beam can be recalibrated before they move in behind the patient. Third-generation systems, however, present a problem in that the detectors are behind the patient throughout the examination. The resulting ring artifacts (Fig. 1-13) are particularly troublesome. To minimize these ring artifacts, these units must be calibrated between patients—typically every few hours, especially for solid-state detector systems.

### Detector Nonlinearities

Ideally, the response of a detector should be directly proportional to the quantity of radiation incident on it. In CT scanning, the range of x-ray intensities may be as high as 100,000 to 1 or even higher. The detector should have a dynamic range at least this high. Some factors contributing to detector nonlinearity (Joseph 1981) are dark current or leakage (current flow in the absence of radiation), saturation (detector output is at its maximum, and higher intensities do not evoke higher output), and hysteresis (detector continues to respond after irradiation ends). One form of hysteresis is the afterglow of scintillation detectors. All these may lead to inconsistency in data and can result in streaks. The severity of these streaks is related to the contrast of the structure as well as the presence of abrupt discontinuities in its shape. One way to minimize the detector nonlinearity problem is to reduce the range of intensities arriving at the detector. This was accomplished by placing the patient within a water box to provide equal ray paths in the original EMI Mark I system. More commonly, a compensating wedge-shaped filter (bow tie filter) can be used (Fig. 1-27).

### Scatter Collimation

Scatter present at the detector plane is similar to that from leakage in the detector. This can be appreciated by considering a very dense object. The primary x-ray intensity behind this object is expected to be low; however, small amounts of scatter at the detector indicate a higher than actual transmission. The resulting data are inconsistent with data from ray paths not traversing the high-contrast object, and streaks can result. Scatter is less of a problem in third-generation systems, where scatter-rejecting collimation can be incorporated into detectors. In fourth-generation systems, however, stationary detectors must accept radiation from a wide range of angles, and collimation cannot be used. Consequently, this latter system is more susceptible to scatter image degrading effects.

### DATA PROCESSING

The final step to be considered here is how the data are processed within the computer. The specific algorithm used may introduce artifacts into the final image that are not due to sampling or measurement factors. Examples of this are the use of an edge-enhancement algorithm, which can result in a false subarachnoid space. Another example is that originally described by Hounsfield (1977), as well as Stockham (1979), and Joseph (1981), involving scanning long, straight-edged, bony, or high-contrast structures. Approximations normally used in algorithms lead to the formation of streaks along the edge of such structures. These streaks can be minimized by using narrower collimators and smaller detectors as well as the use of hardened (filtered) x-ray beams. Needless to say, algorithm-induced artifacts are mathematically complex, and further discussion is beyond the scope of this chapter.

## CT Number Accuracy

In the previous section the factors resulting in mainly visible streak artifacts were studied. In this section the factors affecting actual accuracy of the CT numbers are considered.

A number of factors limiting the absolute accuracy of CT numbers are listed in Table 1-6. As discussed in an earlier section, the CT reconstruction process computes a value for the linear attenuation coefficient of each volume element within the patient scanned. In all CT designs, the computer then assigns to the attenuation coefficient a value based on the arbitrary $-1000$ for air to $+1000$ for bone scale. (Modern units are capable of accurately computing and displaying values up to

### Table 1-6  Factors Affecting CT Number Accuracy

X-ray beam kilovoltage and filtration
Patient thickness and shape
Tissue type and location
Partial volume effect
Algorithm and calibration shifts
Field calibration accuracy

$+3000$ and above.) These CT number values represent quantitative data from which tissue identification can be made. In general, they are related to the attenuation coefficient of water ($\mu_w$) as follows:

$$CT\ no. = \frac{\mu - \mu_w}{\mu_w} \times 1000 \qquad (4)$$

where $\mu$ is the attenuation coefficient of the material the CT number is specified for. Table 1-1 gives a short list of CT numbers for typical tissues. All CT scanners have provisions for determining the CT number for any specified point or region of points in the image field either by direct interaction with the video display or using a region-of-interest (ROI) indicator.

Since CT numbers characterize the tissue or its chemical composition, it is not surprising that considerable effort has been expended to use these quantitative data. This involves not only identifying gross tissue type but, among other more sophisticated applications, the determination of bone mineral content (Exner 1979; Revak 1980; Genant 1985A and B) and the identification of calcified versus noncalcified pulmonary nodules (Siegelman 1980; Checkley 1984; Zerhouni 1982). In fact, CT scanning can be configured to determine directly the effective atomic numbers or electron densities (tomochemistry) instead of the attenuation coefficients (McDavid 1977b; Latchaw 1978).

The question of validity must be posed before undue reliance is placed on CT numbers. A number of factors affect the validity of correlating directly the CT number obtained from a particular CT machine and the tissue it is supposed to characterize. Specific factors to be considered are given in Table 1-6, from which it is easy to see that the CT numbers from one machine cannot be expected to match those from another exactly. One reason is that CT numbers are dependent on x-ray beam energy. Thus correlation cannot be rigorously expected between units operated at different kilovoltage even between similar units operated by the same nominal kilovoltage because of kilovoltage calibration inaccuracies. CT number anomalies can also occur for the same unit whenever the kilovoltage shifts. In general, the CT number of any material will shift as a function of the difference between the atomic number of that material and the atomic number of water: it will increase for materials with an atomic number less than water and decrease for materials with an atomic number greater than water. A tight quality-assurance program monitoring daily the constancy of CT numbers for a given unit is necessary as well as frequent system calibration by service engineers.

Beam filtration also affects the energy distribution of the x-ray beam. In general, the greater the filtration. the harder the beam (or the greater the effective beam energy); also, the beam becomes more monochromatic and therefore less subject to further hardening. This means that CT numbers are subject to variation between units depending on the degree of beam filtration incorporated in each unit as well as the calibration and shift effects discussed above. It is also interesting to note that some CT units provide for two filtration modes—one for head scans and a relatively thicker filtration for body scans—the rationale being that the greater tissue-path lengths in bodies would produce greater beam hardening. Greater initial filtration would then reduce this effect in that the beam is prehardened via the additional filter and is closer to a monochromatic beam before it enters the patient. Patient thickness is crucial in determining the CT numbers finally computed. Again, beam hardening is involved in that different patient thicknesses yield different beam paths and different degrees of beam hardening. This is illustrated in Fig. 1-26. It can also be seen that results will depend on the shape of the body parts. Figure 1-26 also illustrates the so-called apical artifact (DiChiro 1978), in which CT number variations occur between the slice levels scanned owing to varying head thickness and thus different degrees of beam hardening.

It has already been noted that the original EMI Mark I unit provided a water box surrounding the patient's head. This meant that all ray paths were more nearly equal, as seen in Fig. 1-27, for any orientation around the head. With such a configuration, beam hardening is minimal. Figure 1-27 also shows one attempt to provide for a fixed path length by providing for a "bow tie" compensating filter. Here added filter thickness toward the periphery of the bow tie presumably compensates for decreased peripheral patient thickness. Patient centering here will obviously be important, and the configuration will not be as effective as a water box, though it is certainly simpler. Some advanced designs provide for varying the shape of this bow tie as a function of reconstruction field size to more accurately accomplish equalization of the ray paths. Figure 1-27 also shows how the presence of dense structures adds to the beam-hardening problem. Discrepancies for ray

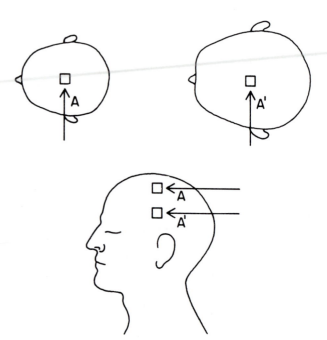

**Figure 1-26**  Different degrees of beam hardening yielded by different patient thicknesses and the effect on CT number accuracy. Ray path A to any particular pixel is shorter in the smaller patient on the left than ray path A′ in the larger patient on the right. As shown in the lower figure, even in the same patient path length to any given pixel can differ depending on slice level (apical artifact). All these effects are further compounded when the beam rotates around the patient and path length is a function of ray angle.

paths close to the tangent of the edges of the structure in fact result in severe image streaking.

The partial volume effect also strongly influences CT number accuracy. This was discussed in a previous section.

Finally, the question of algorithms must be addressed. Each CT manufacturer attempts to minimize the beam-hardening problem and to calibrate its CT number scale to maximize accuracy. Such algorithms vary between manufacturers, and the actual field calibrations on any given unit at any given time vary.

An additional application of the quantitative use of CT number data is in dynamic scanning. In this approach the absolute value of the CT number is unimportant; rather, it is the relative change in the CT numbers at a point which is observed. Here a given tissue slice is repeatedly scanned while contrast or some treatment regime is being administered. A region of interest is defined, and a plot of the average CT number within that ROI versus time is obtained. Note that beam hardening is not a problem since measurements are made within the same region. Presumably, the CT number variation here, for instance, is proportional to the time concentration of contrast within the ROI, which in turn is a function of the blood flow and vascularization properties of the tissue within that ROI (Michael 1985; Som 1985).

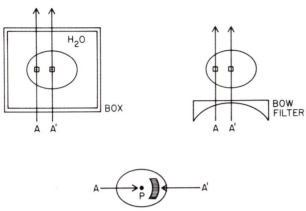

**Figure 1-27** *Left:* In original CT units a water bath providing a fixed path length for any and all ray paths, such as A and A', resulted in minimal beam-hardening effects on CT numbers. *Right:* In an attempt to equalize ray paths A and A' without a water bath one can provide for a "bow tie" filter arrangement. Here varying filter thickness results in attenuation matching the curvature of the patient. *Bottom:* Presence of dense structures (shaded region) aggravates the beam-hardening problem between ray paths A and A', since the beam through a point such as P suffers different beam hardening along the two paths indicated. This is particularly severe for ray paths falling along the edges of the structures, and image streaks are usually formed.

To accomplish dynamic scanning the CT x-ray tube must be capable of withstanding high heat loads because of the need for rapid successive scan acquisition. One software approach which extends capability for obtaining data at short time intervals is that of segmental scanning. That is, the data from a 360° scan, which normally produces only one image, are divided and reallocated into a multiple number of overlapping shorter angular segment scans. Thus, for instance, one 360° scan can be reconstructed as three images (or more) at shorter intervals of time, with data from one angular interval overlapping the other. Finally, the accuracy and frequency of system calibration plays an important role in CT number accuracy.

This section can be summarized simply by stating that great caution must be exercised in using CT numbers, not only between and within different manufacturers' models but also for the facility's own unit, as a function of the factors listed in Table 1-6. When quantitative CT number data are desired, it is best to scan a phantom with calibrated CT number materials.

## CT Reconstruction Performance

As already seen, CT performance is a complex area of study. A number of different aspects of it requires further discussion (Table 1-7). Attention is drawn to a very comprehensive but somewhat mathematical and technical text (Newton 1981).

## Table 1-7  Aspects of CT Reconstruction Performance

*CT number performance*
  CT number accuracy
  CT number linearity
  Spatial independence of CT numbers
  Sensitivity to artifactual effects
  Contrast scale
*Geometric and mechanical factors*
  Divergence of beam
  Focal-spot penumbra
  Source and detector collimation and alignment
  Dual-slice effects
  Slice location and table incrementation
  Mechanical vibration
*Imaging performance*
  Spatial resolution
  Tissue resolution
  Noise characteristics
  Pixel sizes and zoom
  Data sampling
*Patient dose*
  Single-slice dose
  Multiple-slice dose
  Dose profile

## CT NUMBER PERFORMANCE
### CT Number Accuracy

CT numbers have been discussed at length in previous sections, especially as they relate to factors causing artifactual variations in their reproducibility and accuracy. To quantitate the accuracy of CT numbers, merely scan a collection of plastics having known attenuation coefficients (or CT numbers) in a water bath. The CT numbers computed are then compared with the known values. In addition, these data when plotted should form a straight line (CT number linearity). The National Council on Radiation Protection and Measurements (NCRP 1988) recommends $0 \pm 1.5$ CT numbers for the CT number value of water and $-1000 \pm 3$ for air as a performance standard covering day-to-day variations in CT numbers. Each site should actually set its own limits, taking into account the manufacturer's recommendations. It should again be noted that CT numbers vary with beam energy. Thus kilovoltage and beam filtration as well as size of the phantom used affect the CT number. Proper field service calibration of the unit, however, will assure that water gives a CT number of zero for a given reconstruction scan circle or field size and that the known plastics scanned also display their correct CT numbers.

area must be used. However, this then affects image quality since ideally walls should be as thin as possible and placed as close to each other as possible. Because of the relatively inefficient quantum absorption of the gas, long chamber walls are required to maintain low patient dosage. This in turn may make the chamber susceptible to further vibration.

## CT Imaging Performance

In addition to the problem of artifact sensitivity, as discussed previously, there are three basic descriptors of CT imaging performance: spatial (or high-contrast) resolution, image noise, and tissue (or low-contrast) resolution.

### SPATIAL RESOLUTION

Spatial resolution is the ability of a CT scanner to record fine, high-contrast detail. Various measures of spatial resolution are available (Table 1-8). What they all have in common is essentially 100 percent contrast and noise-free conditions. These measures, however, do not necessarily predict the actual performance of a CT unit when imaging tissues having similar attenuation coefficients (low contrast condition). The resolution-bar pattern is probably the most familiar test objects used in general radiology. It can be configured for CT scanning (Goodenough 1977), for instance, with a series of Plexiglas strips (or similar material) in a water bath in such a manner that equal widths of Plexiglas alternate with equal spaces of water. These Plexiglas widths form a *line pair* with the adjoining water space, and each line pair is made progressively narrower; that is, a greater number of line pairs per millimeter (higher line-pair frequency) is formed. The resolving power of the system is that line-pair frequency which is just barely visible on the image.

A variation of the basic resolution bar pattern is the sunburst phantom (Goodenough 1977), in which alternate radial strips and spaces are arranged in a tapered manner around a circle like wheel spokes to provide

## Table 1-8   Spatial Resolution Measures (100 Percent Contrast and Noise-Free Conditions)

| MEASURE | MATHEMATICAL EQUIVALENT |
| --- | --- |
| Resolution bar and pin pattern | Zero cutoff of MTF |
| Sunburst pattern | Zero cutoff of MTF |
| Point-spread function (PSF) | Basic response function |
| Line-spread function (LSF) | Integral of PSF along line |
| Edge-response function (ERF) | Integral of LSF along line (slope of ERF = LSF) |
| Modulation transfer function (MTF) | Fourier transform of LSF |

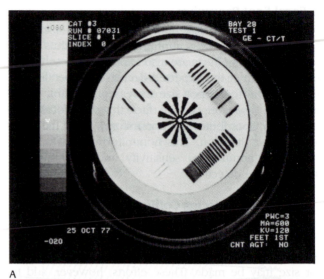

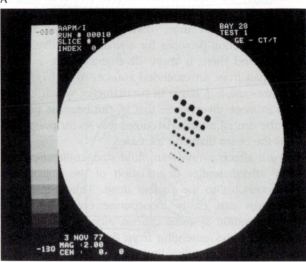

*Figure 1-29*  Examples of spatial resolution test-scan results for two popular phantom configurations. **A.** Starburst and bar pattern scans. Four different bar patterns of differing subject contrast can be displayed on the Catphan phantom (Goodenough 1977). **B.** Phantom made up of Plexiglas with different-diameter holes in each row (AAPM phantom; AAPM 1978). Both of these phantoms have a variety of test objects in addition to those shown here for evaluating the full range of CT system performance as well as for ongoing quality control tests.

for continuously varying frequencies (Fig. 1-29A). Resolution is given by the distinctly visible tapered pattern closest to the center. This approach was actually used to also approximate the modulation-transfer function of early CT systems (MacIntyre 1976). Instead of repetitive bar patterns, a series of varying-diameter Plexiglas high-contrast pins in a water bath can be used to assess spatial resolution. Alternatively, one can have holes of varying diameters in Plexiglas. Figure 1-29 shows the results for two popular phantoms incorporating various spatial-resolution patterns.

A number of other spatial-resolution descriptors are shown in Table 1-8. Though each is distinct, they are all interrelated. The *point-spread function* (PSF) is the most fundamental measure and is defined as the response of a system to a point object. The PSF can be measured by scanning a high-contrast wire pin which is perpendicular to the long axis of the slice. The *line-spread function* (LSF) is the response of the system to a line object lying within or along the long axis of the slice plane. Mathematically, the LSF can be obtained from the PSF by integrating the PSF along a line. The *edge-response function* (ERF), in turn, is merely the mathematical integration of the LSF along a plane. Experimentally, the ERF may be obtained directly by scanning a sharp edge object.

In addition to the resolution-bar and pin patterns, the *modulation-transfer function* (MTF) (Villafana 1978*a*) approach is probably the most commonly cited descriptor of spatial resolution. The MTF is defined as the response of the system to a sinusoidally varying object. Because of the difficulty of constructing objects with sinusoidally varying CT numbers, usually the PSF (Goodenough 1977), the LSF (Bishop 1977), or the ERF (Judy 1976) is measured and then mathematically converted to the MTF. For instance, the LSF may be subjected to a Fourier transform operation and converted to an MTF. For the interested reader, Jones (1954) has reviewed in depth the various mathematical relationships between these measures.

The point at which the MTF goes to zero can be used as a single number description of overall resolution. However, owing to the presence of noise and the difficulty of locating the zero cutoff, the resolution measure is many times specified at the 10 or 20 percent MTF response.

To illustrate the use of MTFs, Fig. 1-30 shows for comparison purposes of the MTF for the early GE CT/T 7800 and 8800 systems as well as the more recent 9800 system. The 8800 system has a detector aperture nearly one-half the size of the 7800. As a result, the MTF of the 8800 system is correspondingly better (about twice as good). This can be seen from the fact that the MTF response of the 8800 system drops at higher frequencies than the drop for the 7800 system.

The ideal MTF would correspond to a unit (MTF = 1) response regardless of frequency. Such comparisons can be of great value in assessing performance. Comparisons can also be made between different manufacturers' models and even between subcomponents of a given model CT. This latter application has been admirably demonstrated by Barnes (1979), as shown in Fig. 1-31, where it is seen that for the particular CT unit under study, the algorithm (or filter function) represents the limiting system component, since its MTF drops to zero the most quickly, and the focal spot is the component least limiting CT performance. The overall total or composite curve is obtained from the

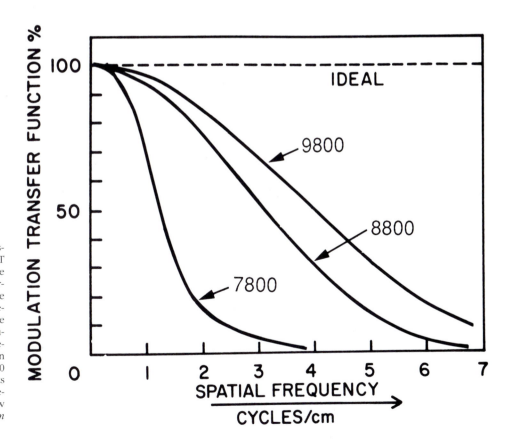

**Figure 1-30** The modulation-transfer functions (MTF) for the GE CT/T 7800, 8800, and 9800 systems. The GE 8800 system has a detector aperture size nearly half as large as the 7800, and the detectors are correspondingly more closely spaced. The improvement in the MTF is significant (nearly two times). Further reduction in detector size yields even greater improvement for the 9800 system. The ideal curve represents the situation in which the system response is unity regardless of how high the frequency is. (*Adapted from GE brochures.*)

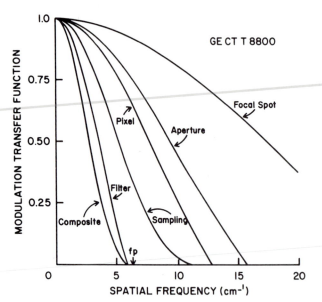

**Figure 1-31** Comparison of individual-component MTFs for a given CT system. System shown is the GE CT/T8800 for a 24-cm-diameter patient circle, 0.78-mm pixel size. (*Adapted from Barnes 1979.*) Here the sampling and the algorithm filter function would be the limiting component, while the focal spot would be the least limiting. Also shown is the composite or total MTF curve, which is the product of all the component curves. Note that the composite is poorer than any individual component.

product of the MTFs of all the system components at each frequency; that is, in the general case,

$$\text{MTF}_{\text{TOT}} = \text{MTF}_1 \times \text{MTF}_2 \times \text{MTF}_3 \times \ldots \qquad (6)$$

Note that the composite MTF is in general lower than, and at most equal to, the lowest MTF response component in the system. Attempts to improve the spatial resolution of a system should be directed toward improving the lowest-response link in the system. In the specific case shown in Fig. 1-31, the sampling MTF would be the next most advantageous component to improve after the filter function.

As previously seen, insufficient sampling results in aliasing and artifactual streak formation. Even if algorithms are available to remove such artifacts, a generalized loss of spatial resolution will still be present as predicted by the sampling MTF in Fig. 1-31. The pixel MTF refers to the fact that choice of pixel size or pixel matrix will affect the resolution of the final image. For instance, a smaller patient or reconstruction circle results in a smaller effective pixel size and higher resolution. This relation is given by

$$\text{Pixel size} = \frac{\text{reconstruction diameter}}{\text{matrix size}} \qquad (7)$$

For example, a 256 × 256 matrix applied over a 400-mm reconstruction diameter results in a pixel size of

400 mm/256 = 1.56 mm. Likewise, a 512 × 512 matrix for the same diameter results in a pixel state of 400 mm/512 = 0.78 mm, or half the pixel size of a 256 matrix. Finally, the aperture (or collimator) MTF in Fig. 1-31 refers to the physical opening at the detector.

It should be noted that some systems with relatively large detectors provide for an absorbing pin which can be placed in front of the detector to reduce its effective size and thus improve its MTF or resolution response. Here again, component MTF curves can predict the possible success of such a maneuver. For instance, such an absorbing pin would be essentially futile for all third-generation xenon ionization chamber systems, since such systems can be configured with small detector face area and the aperture MTF is not particularly limiting.

Finally, we again caution that MTF data do not of themselves predict actual clinical performance, since they are defined for 100 percent contrast and for essentially noise-free conditions. Consequently, they should be used for comparative purposes only and for the imaging of high-contrast structures.

**NOISE**

In detecting low-contrast tissue structures (tissues of similar CT numbers), noise plays a dominant role; it is in general the limiting factor in CT scanning, since in many applications diagnosis hinges on the visualization of tissue structures with very similar CT numbers. For instance, gray- and white-matter tissues are separated by only 5 to 10 CT numbers. Noise can be defined as the standard deviation in CT numbers in a scanned uniform water bath. All CT scanners provide for an ROI selector where the standard deviation of the CT numbers falling within the selected area (usually about 25 pixels in size) can be read out automatically. To make the noise measure independent of the particular CT unit and contrast scale [Equation (5)], the following expression is used:

$$\text{Noise} = \frac{\text{CS} \times \sigma_w}{\mu_w} \times 100 \qquad (8)$$

where $\mu_w$ = the linear attenuation coefficient of water (0.195 cm$^{-1}$ for 70 keV) and $\sigma_w$ = the observed standard deviation for a uniform water-bath region.

It is crucial to note that image noise is directly related to the number of photons received and processed at the detectors. Consequently, to decrease CT noise, the number of photons passing through the patient and available at the detectors must be increased. This, of course, increases the patient dose. The statistical variation in the photon number in a uniform beam that is finally detected is given by the standard deviation of that photon number as follows:

$$\sigma_N = \sqrt{N} \qquad (9)$$

where $\sigma_N$ is the fluctuation in the photon number $N$ (which is related to patient dose) and must be distinguished from $\sigma_w$ as specified for the standard deviation in CT numbers of the final reconstructed uniform water field, the difference between these two being the contribution of algorithm noise.

From Equation (9) emerges an underlying and crucial conclusion: *CT imaging performance depends on patient radiation dose.* This is true because the number of photons at the detector is directly related to the number of photons passing through the patient, which in turn determines patient dose. Because of the dependence of image quality on patient dose, the patient dose associated with any image performance specification must be specified. Stated another way, an image may be of very high quality but may have been obtained at the cost of an unacceptably high radiation dose to the patient. Haaga and coworkers (1981) have illustrated how photo levels of different milliamperage affect actual visualization.

The statistical noise $\sigma_N$, pixel size $w$ (representing the limiting resolution measure), slice thickness $t$, dose $D$, and the fractional attenuation of the patient $B$ are related as follows:

$$\sigma_N = \left( \frac{KB}{w^3 tD} \right)^{1/2} \qquad (10)$$

where $K$ is a proportionally constant for any given CT unit. Equation (10) reveals that in general, as the slice thickness decreases, the noise value increases. This is evident, since less thickness $b$ implies a narrower beam and consequently the delivery of fewer photons to the detector. A similar statement is true for the patient-dose factor $D$ in that a lower dose to the patient (for instance, less tube milliamperage or scan time) results in fewer photons at the detector. Both these factors vary as the square root, which means that halving either one results in a $\sqrt{2}$ times greater noise level. The noise dependence on pixel size, on the other hand, is as the third power. Thus halving the pixel size (which may result in doubling the resolution) results in an eightfold increase in dose to maintain the same level of noise! Not only does CT image performance depend on noise, but attempts at increasing performance by reducing noise may result in a very considerable dose increase to the patient.

If noise is in fact limiting CT performance and not spatial resolution, the operator may opt, for instance, to increase pixel size. Such a move would reduce noise and might improve visualization of large but low-contrast structures, but care must be taken since a net reduction of spatial resolution would also result. As discussed above in Equation (10), noise dependence varies with slice thickness to the $\frac{1}{2}$ power. Thus increases in slice thickness also reduce noise, but not nearly to the same degree as increases in pixel width, which vary to the $\frac{3}{2}$ power. The rationale for the noise dependence on pixel width and slice thickness is simply that reduction in these sizes causes a reduction in the number of photons available to make up the image for each pixel. A reduced number of photons in turn creates greater statistical variation, and image noise is increased.

An interesting approach to reducing final noise without increase in dose to the patient is by mathematical smoothing. Algorithms can be configured to include various smoothing routines (referred to as *kernels* or algorithm filters). Such smoothing, however, usually results in blurring and thus a loss of spatial resolution. However, if accomplishment of a particular task is limited by the presence of noise, smoothing may in some circumstances yield significant results.

Finally, it should be stated that other descriptors of noise even more complete and general are available. For instance, noise power spectra can be constructed. These describe noise as a function of spatial frequency; hence, they are similar to and can be combined with the MTF descriptor. For further details, the reader is referred to the literature (Barnes 1979; Hanson 1981; Riederer 1978).

## TISSUE RESOLUTION

Tissue, or low-contrast, resolution may be defined as the smallest object or pin size detectable under low-contrast conditions. Low contrast is considered to exist when scanning CT number differences of less than 0.5 percent or 5 CT numbers. (For a $-1000$ to $+1000$ CT system, each CT number represents 0.1 percent difference.) Phantoms used are similar to the bar and pin object types already discussed. Recent CT units have a tissue resolution of 4 to 5 mm, compared with a spatial high-contrast resolution of 0.5 mm or less. Tissue resolution is also called *low-contrast detectivity* or *low-contrast sensitivity.*

The tissue-resolution measure is more accurate in predicting clinically expected performance, since low-contrast conditions are more clinically relevant. Also, since low-contrast conditions are specified, the influence of noise is incorporated. Because of crucial interplay among noise, performance, and patient dose, tissue-resolution specifications must be accompanied by statements of pixel size, patient dose, phantom diameter, kilovoltage or filter, and other reconstruction details.

Another approach describing system resolution has been introduced which uses so-called contrast-detail curves (Cohen 1979*a,b*). In this approach both the low-contrast and high-contrast resolution responses of a system are specified. Figure 1-32 shows a contrast-

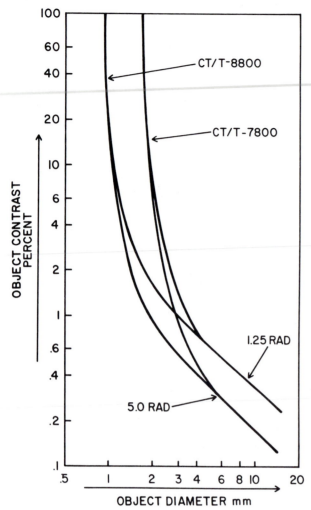

**Figure 1-32** Detail-contrast curves. Plot of object diameter visible on both the GE 7800 and the GE 8800 versus object contrast for two different dose levels. At high contrast the smallest possible object diameter is visible (the resolution limit) independent of dose or noise. At low contrast, noise becomes a significant factor and results are highly dependent on dose. (*Adapted from Cohen 1979a,b.*)

detail curve for two levels of radiation dose and two different earlier CT systems. In this figure, at high contrast, spatial resolution is better for system A compared with system B and is independent of dose or noise. Note that in both cases spatial resolution still does not get better than a certain minimum detectable size (called the *resolution limit* and occurring at 100 percent contrast). As contrast decreases, resolution becomes poorer. That is, objects have to be larger to be seen. At low-contrast levels, curves tend to flatten out (this is referred to as the *noise limit*). Note from Fig. 1-32 that if noise levels are reduced (dose increased), detectable size decreases at low-contrast levels but not at high-contrast levels.

Finally, mention should be made of still another approach to quantitating the performance of CT equipment. This consists in using receiver- (or reader)

operator-characteristic (ROC) curves. Here, an attempt is made to compare the numbers of false-positive and false-negative detection rates as a function of reader bias and decision criteria. The interested reader is referred elsewhere for further details (Goodenough 1974; Goodenough 1981).

## PIXEL SIZES, ZOOM, AND CT PERFORMANCE

Various aspects of pixels have been previously discussed. Since much discussion concerning CT units centers on statement of pixel sizes, some pertinent facts are summarized as follows: (1) Pixels are the basic building blocks of the CT image. They represent an element or area of the view over which the reconstruction process has calculated a CT number. (2) Pixels represent a weighted nonlinear average CT number of the various tissues which fall within a given volume element (voxel) within the patient (volume-averaging or partial volume effect) and as a result may be artifactual, especially in regions of the patient where tissue type and structure are rapidly changing. The original EMI Mark I pixel sizes were relatively large in that they represented a $3 \times 3 \times 13$ mm$^3$ volume ($80 \times 80$ matrix array). (3) Currently, pixel sizes can be configured to less than 1 mm on a side and are given by Equation (7), for example, by the ratio of the reconstruction circle size to the matrix size. (4) Changing pixel sizes can indeed improve CT images in that the partial volume effect is reduced and, consequently, both spatial and low-contrast tissue resolution can improve. Improvement in the latter, however, is dependent on whether there is a corresponding increase in photon levels to overcome the greater noise levels inherent with smaller pixels (that is, smaller pixel sizes imply a greater number of pixels and thus fewer photons per pixel) and whether the imaging limitation was in fact the pixel size. It is clear that other components, such as motion, focal-spot size, and detector-aperture size, may be limitations, in which case pixel-size reduction may result only in either image degradation due to noise and corresponding low-contrast resolution loss or an increase in patient dose if photon levels are increased to overcome the higher noise levels associated with smaller pixel sizes.

Other features that affect pixel size and imaging performance are magnification and zoom. There are a variety of ways in which magnification and zoom can be accomplished. These are referred to as geometric zoom, interpolated zoom, and reconstructed zoom.

### Geometric Zoom

Geometric zoom refers to image enlargement accomplished by varying geometric factors such as sampling distances, number of detectors used for the reconstruction process, and mechanical configuration of the gantry. For instance, if a smaller reconstruction area is chosen and if the number of pixels is the same, the patient volume size corresponding to each pixel decreases, and the size of the image increases. This may result in an increase in system performance. For instance, if a particular system is configured for displaying $256 \times 256$ pixels for a reconstruction circle of 400 mm, each pixel represents $400/256 = 1.56$ mm. If the reconstruction circle is reduced to 200 mm, each pixel represents $200/256 = 0.78$ mm. To exploit this, CT units have selectable reconstruction circles or field of view over which data can be collected, selection being based on the size of the patient. One must be careful to distinguish between the gantry opening (or patient window), which is the physical opening within which the patient is placed, and the reconstruction circle, which is that region within the gantry opening over which the data are actually collected and processed. For the best images, the CT operator should select the smallest possible reconstruction circle. In general, modern scanners provide for various scan protocols (such as for head or body scans). Selection of a particular protocol automatically chooses an appropriate reconstruction circle. Actually, in some applications where resolution is critical, a reconstruction circle even smaller than the patient size is selected and is centered on a particular region of interest, as in scanning the cervical spine.

Sometimes this latter approach is also referred to as *region-of-interest* scanning and is still a form of geometric zoom. In ROI scanning, caution must be observed in interpreting the resulting CT numbers, since inaccuracies may be introduced by the contribution of patient volumes outside the ROI. As already stated, the pixel size for small reconstruction circles represents a smaller volume in the patient. As a consequence, the actual size of the patient image on the display screen is enlarged. Furthermore, this represents a true zoom in that enlargement of the image is accomplished with each pixel still representing actual patient data.

In third- and fourth-generation systems, the detectors see the full patient contour, and the millimeters of patient per pixel and thus data sampling distances are fixed; thus the use of small detectors is especially necessary. These units, however, still have a selectable reconstruction circle and different possible degrees of final display magnification in that the smaller regions scanned can still be imaged over the full display with the total pixels available. Image quality is again usually improved, but such improvement will depend on the relative role of the sampling and pixel size MTFs.

One interesting variation of geometric zoom which vendors have provided for in the past is a configuration providing for variable magnification within the gantry. For example, the detector array, along with the x-ray source, can be moved closer to or farther away from the patient in such a manner that the full array of detectors is always used. When the x-ray source is closer to the patient (and detectors far), the smaller patient diameters can be viewed with the greater number of detectors (smaller beam diameter and finer ray sampling). For larger patient diameters, the source is placed farther away to assure the full field of view. In either case, all the detectors are utilized. With this arrangement, the sampling distances and therefore the image quality can always be optimized in addition to having images with variable magnification.

### Interpolated Zoom

This is quite different from geometric zoom. Interpolated zoom enlarges the image of a relatively small region of interest within an already processed image and, under computer control, expands it to fill the entire display by averaging the CT numbers in each particular pixel over the neighboring pixels. Therefore, although the final pixels represent a smaller patient volume, they do not represent unique and true patient data but arithmetic averages (or interpolations) over adjacent pixels. It is always performed on a finished image after the reconstruction routine. As the ROI decreases, the image appears larger, but spatial resolution is progressively degraded.

### Reconstructed Zoom

This type of zoom depends on original data being available to allow reconstruction over a smaller area. Typically, reconstructed zoom can be performed with optimal results when scan sampling distances are smaller than the pixel display sizes. For example, if a scanner is used with a $512 \times 512$ calculation matrix but final reconstruction results are condensed and displayed on a $256 \times 256$ pixel array, then if original data are still available, a reconstructed zoom of at least two times can be invoked on the original image. This is a true zoom in that original patient data are reconstructed and displayed.

In summary, it can be stated that pixel size is indeed an important parameter determining CT imaging performance. A statement of array size by itself it not, however, sufficient. Rather, it is important to state what size (or volume) the pixel actually represents in the patient. There are various ways to enlarge or magnify the image which correspond to decreasing the volume each pixel represents. Such zooming may or may not lead to an increase in perceived image quality.

### Data Sampling

We have seen that detector size and sampling frequency are important parameters. Some recent CT designs incorporate various features to enhance the imaging performance of CT scanners by affecting these two

bles and connections were not fixed on the x-ray tube. Rather, such connections were made via rings rotating with the tube but sliding in contact with rings supplying the electrical energy. This is not an easy task since high voltage between 110 and 140 kV had to be transferred across the rings. Some CT models currently incorporate the high-voltage transformer within the gantry to rotate with the x-ray tube which helps alleviate, somewhat, the problem since only low voltage would then have to be transferred across the rings. This latter approach would require the high-voltage transformer to be of the high-frequency type to allow small enough size and low enough weight. Even with slip rings, the scan protocols called for acquiring a 360° scan for one single slice then stopping the x-rays (while tube was still rotating) incrementing the patient into the gantry, then reinitiating x-rays to acquire the next slice. In essence, this maintains the problem of slice-to-slice acquisition but with a shorter interscan delay time. Another major advantage gained was that the very heavy x-ray tube/detector bank did not have to be accelerated to constant velocity around the patient, come to an abrupt stop at end of scan, and accelerate back in opposite direction for the rewind trip. The concept of continuously incrementing the patient through the gantry with the x-rays continuously on and acquiring data as the tube spiraled around the patient was finally introduced in 1990 in a commercial scanner (Kalender 1990; Kalender 1992).

In spiral scanning (sometimes referred to as helical scanning), the patient uniformly moves through the gantry opening while the x-ray beam is continuously on. As a result, of these two motions, data acquired does not correlate with any particular plane but represents data over a three-dimensional volume. The actual spiral path of the beam over the patient is seen in Fig. 1-35. In spiral scanning, during the passage of the beam around the patient every point in the patient has had radiation pass through it and this represents true three-dimensional acquisition. However, there is no specific image plane defined in this continuous acqui-

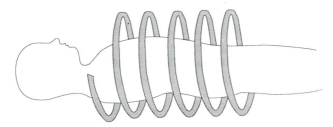

**Figure 1-35** Spiral motion of x-ray tube around patient as the patient continuously moves through gantry. As a result of these two motions, all points in the patient are interrogated by the x-rays.

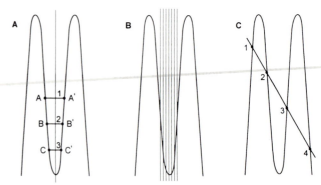

**Figure 1-36** Interpolation of spiral data to obtain desired slice plane. **A.** Data are interpolated between data points A and A′ to obtain point 1 in the desired plane. Likewise, interpolation is performed between B and B′ for point 2 and C and C′ for point 3. Simple averages are not taken; rather weighted average is taken, depending on which data point is closest to the desired plane. For example, point 3 falls closer to data point C: therefore, the average will be more weighted to this value. **B.** Multiple planes can be interpolated between data points down to submillimeter spacing if desired. **C.** Interpolation can be performed for any orbitrary angle plane (or curved surface).

sition. To line up points along a particular plane, the clinician must interpolate between the data acquired. Various interpolation schemes have evolved. Figure 1-36 illustrates the simplest approach. Here we see that to obtain points along plane P, it is necessary to identify the corresponding points on the measured data. For example, in Fig. 1-36A the available data for point 1 is A and A′. Note that point 1 is exactly halfway between data points A and A′. Thus a simple average would suffice. Likewise, the same process is followed for determining point 2 by averaging between data points B and B′. This time, however, the average must be weighted toward data point B since it is closer to point 2. The interpolation scheme used in spiral scanning in fact consists of determining each point in the desired plane by performing linear weighted averaging between available data points. Just as one plane can be interpolated between spiral arms, likewise, an arbitrary number of planes can be interpolated for multiplanar and three-dimensional reconstructions down to submillimeter spacings as would be required, for instance, in inner ear studies (Fig. 1-36B). Extending this concept further, any plane at any angle (or even a curved surface) can be interpolated and corresponding images reconstructed (Fig. 1-36C). A certain unsharpness is introduced into the image since each point represents an average over a finite distance. Different interpolations schemes introduce varying degrees of unsharpness as seen by broadened sensitivity profiles and resulting loss of resolution in the image. Slice sensitivity profiles are a measure of how thick a slice section is actually scanned. The broader the sensitivity profile, the poorer the resolution and structure detectivity. Originally 360° interpolations were performed, which yielded poorer resolution images. Currently, 180° interpolation is used, which results in much improved image quality. The 180° interpolation is obtained since each anatomic point in the scanned volume is actually viewed from two opposing sides of the patient. This allows for a calculation of a second spiral midway between the first. Interpolation is thus accomplished over 180° rather than 360° The result is an improvement in the sensitivity profile and final image quality. Figure 1-37A illustrates this. Figure 1-37B shows the effects for different table incrementation values on the sensitivity profiles for 180° interpolation: the larger the incrementation velocity the greater the broadening of the sensitivity profile.

After obtaining the interpolated image points, the reconstruction process proceeds as for conventional CT using the filtered back-projection algorithm. It should be noted that there is no loss of resolution (no broadening of sensitivity profile) within the scan plane (Kalender 1994). One drawback (though not unsurmountable) to 180° interpolation as compared with 360° interpolation is that more quantum mottle is expected by a factor of $\sqrt{2}$ since only half the available data range is being utilized. This yields a total noise increase of $\sqrt{4/3}$ or 1.15 as compared with a conventional single slice CT image. Since x-ray tubes are on continuously, the problem of tube heat load arises. Tubes must have sufficient heat capacity to stay on at high peak kilovoltage [kV(p)] and high milliamperage (mA) for at least a breath hold. Some x-ray tubes are now available for spiral scanning that have a capacity of more than 5 million heat units. Heat unit capacity is a measure of how much heat energy a tube can withstand and is proportional to the product of the operating kV(p), mA, and time of exposure. [Heat units = $1.44 \times$ kV(p) $\times$ mA $\times$ second.]

## Image Quality in Spiral Scanning

Figure 1-34 shows the problem of missed structures and partial contrast structures as a function position relative to slice level for conventional single-slice scanning. To overcome this problem or to enhance resolution along the slice direction for three-dimensional imaging, overlapping slice-by-slice scans would have to be taken. This results in significantly greater patient dose as well as significantly greater scan times and x-ray tube load. These problems are avoided in spiral CT scanning, the reason being that three-dimensional information, in fact, is being acquired in a continuous manner and can be reconstructed at any level desired retrospectively. Also, scans can be overlapped to any arbitrary degree down to 1 mm or less scan increments with no additional dose to patient. This also avoids misregistering artifacts along contours which are rapidly changing in slice direction due to respiration. In addition, the sensitivity profile is broadened in spiral scanning with consequent image quality degradation compared with slice by slice acquisition. This broadening is minimized using the 180° interpolation algorithm. Image quality degradation can be calculated in terms of MTFs given the sensitivity profile (Kalender 1994). Another factor contributing to broadening is table feed velocity, that is, how fast the patient is moving through gantry. This was illustrated in Fig. 1-37B.

Until now, no mention has been made of the effects of slice thickness on spiral scanning. Obviously, this is as important image quality factor for spiral scanning as it is for conventional CT scanning. Slice thickness ($t$) and table feed per 360° rotation affects on image quality are correlated. These two can be combined using table feed expressed in distance ($d$) traversed in one 360° rotation into one parameter referred to as the Pitch $P$;

$$P = \frac{d}{t}$$

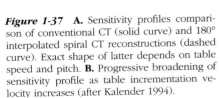

*Figure 1-37* **A.** Sensitivity profiles comparison of conventional CT (solid curve) and 180° interpolated spiral CT reconstructions (dashed curve). Exact shape of latter depends on table speed and pitch. **B.** Progressive broadening of sensitivity profile as table incrementation velocity increases (after Kalender 1994).

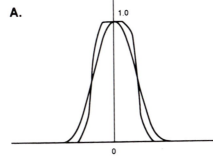

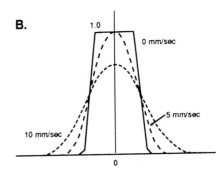

run 10 to 40 mGy (Conway 1992). Furthermore, dose at the surface compared with dose at the center of the patient is nearly equal for head scans, whereas for body scans the difference is typically 50 percent lower for the center. These results are based on the fact that as patient thickness increases, there is an expected increase in dose, due to the inverse square law, to the skin since it is nearer the x-ray source. However, the beam penetration through the patient and the addition of dose to the other side are exponentially reduced by the added tissue thickness. Thus, there is a somewhat complex interplay between the inverse square law and exponential attenuation, as well as scatter characteristics and beam penetrating ability as governed by the peak kilovoltage and filtration characteristics of the x-ray beam.

## KILOVOLTAGE

The x-ray tube kilovoltage determines the energy of the x-rays produced. It affects the dose in two possible ways. If kilovoltage is increased, more x-ray photons are produced at the x-ray tube and the patient dose is also increased. The second effect is that increased peak kilovoltage also yields more energetic, more penetrating x-ray photons. A dose decrease is possible only if increasing kilovoltage allows a greater proportional decrease in the milliamperage. This relative decrease possibility comes about because the number of photons arriving at the detector is greater owing to the higher penetrating ability of the higher kilovoltage beam.

In practice, the kilovoltage is usually fixed for a given unit at between 120 and 140 kV(p). For pediatric patients a lower voltage may be considered.

## FILTRATION

Added beam filtration always leads to lower patient doses. The reason for this is the same as in clinical radiography: Filtration removes the softer, low-energy photons that are readily absorbed in the patient and have little probability of penetrating through to the detectors. Selection of filters on CT scanners, however, is not only to provide for dose saving but also to harden the beam to avoid beam-hardening effects within the patient. Filters used are usually 5 mm or more of aluminum and are placed directly within the x-ray beam near the x-ray tube. Bow tie filters are in addition to filtration discussed here; such added filtration is selected for scanning large body parts, compared with scanning heads. (The filtration referred to here should not be confused with software filters incorporated in the computer algorithm, and which are part of the mathematical reconstruction process.)

## TUBE CURRENT AND SCAN ON TIME

Tube current represents the flow of electrons across the x-ray tube, and along with the scan time and peak kilovoltage controls the final quantity of x-rays emitted. By convention it is measured in milliamperes. Scan "on time" refers to the period of time the tube current is actually flowing and x-rays are actually on. Some CT units are used to provide for continuous x-ray production throughout the scan. Pulsing units are more the norm now and are configured to fire or turn on x-ray pulses for various intervals of time (pulse length). These pulses are repeated at various angles as the x-ray tube rotates around the patient. Each pulse constitutes a projection through the patient. The product of the tube current and the on time (the milliamperage second product) is the important dose-determining factor. Many CT units offer a fast scan at low image quality and a slower scan at higher image quality (if patient motion is not limiting). Typically, the faster scans are accomplished by pulsing at fewer intervals around the patient or by an overall reduction in scan times. Likewise, a partial scan (less than 360° rotation) may be provided. Since the milliamperage product will be lower for such fast scans, the dose also will be lower. The actual "beam on" scan time is usually smaller than the nominal overall scan time. This is true since radiation is delivered in pulses as the x-ray tube circles the patient. The actual beam on time is then the product of the number of x-ray pulses multiplied by the pulse length time.

## FOCAL SPOT SPREAD

Figure 1-28 illustrates the fact that there is a spread of radiation across the slice and beyond the slice borders. This spread affects the dose overlapping from one slice into another, which then affects the overall dose to the patient. The smaller the focal spot, the less the penumbral spread beyond slice borders and the better the dose characteristics of the scanner. Remember, however, that smaller focal spots unfortunately also result in diminished x-ray tube capacity.

## BEAM COLLIMATION

Typically, CT scanning involves the use of highly collimated beams. Fan beams, as used in third- and fourth-generation systems, are opened along the horizontal direction. Actually two collimating systems are used, one near the source and one near the detectors. As far as dose is concerned, the important idea is that the x-ray beam should be collimated down to yield a field incident on the patient which corresponds to the desired slice thickness and to the field actually arriving at the detector. Figure 1-39 shows examples of a poorly collimated beam and a well-collimated beam. Note that

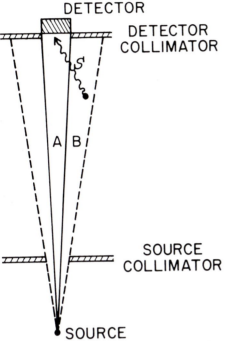

*Figure 1-39*  Well-collimated beam (A) along slice direction confined to the dimensions of the detector. Poorly collimated beam (B). Radiation passing through the patient is not utilized at the detector. Additionally, scatter (*S*) from the patient may degrade image quality.

for poor collimation the region which extends beyond the active area dimensions of the detector unnecessarily adds to the patient dose and forms a region of overlapping dose when the adjacent slice is scanned. To study this in more detail, dose profiles are usually obtained across the patient in a direction perpendicular to the slice plane (along the *z* axis). These can be obtained by the use of thermoluminescent dosimeters (TLD),* for instance, placed on tissue-equivalent phantoms or on patients directly. Alternatively, ionization chambers on phantoms or film dosimetry can also be used.

One of the prime means of evaluating the dose characteristics of a CT scanner is to compare the dose profiles with the sensitivity profiles. The sensitivity profile is the response of the CT system along the perpendicular (*z* direction) to the scan plane. The dose profile is

*TLD detectors usually consist of a small lithium fluoride chip (typically about 1.0 mm × 3 mm × 3 mm), which has the advantage of being small and tissue-equivalent; however, it has a low-energy dependency and must be calibrated very carefully. The TLD detector is based on the principle that electrons liberated by the incident radiation are trapped at certain impurity centers, or electron traps, within the crystal. When the crystal is heated, the electron traps are emptied and light is emitted as the electrons fall back to the ground state. This emitted light is proportional to the original incident radiation.

the radiation distribution along the same direction but measured at the patient. Ideally, the dose profile should be identical with the sensitivity profile for a particular set of scan parameters when both are compared at the patient level. Thus the ratio of the two should be 1.0, or 100 percent. This ratio is referred to as *dose utilization*. The practitioner is cautioned that a particular CT unit may have a high dose utilization yet also result in a relatively high dose to the patient, since dose utilization indicates how efficiently the radiation was detected but does not yield the magnitude of the actual dose received.

## SLICE WIDTH AND OVERLAP

As slice width decreases, the penumbral region of the field becomes relatively more important, because the tails of the dose profiles then represent a proportionately larger fraction of the dose distribution, and overlapping on multiple scans becomes correspondingly more serious. Additionally, some degree of slice overlap may be incorporated into the scan sequence. Thus a 1.5-mm slice width being scanned may be incremented, for instance, by a 1.4-mm distance. This results in a 1-mm scan overlap, which drives the patient dose even higher. Figure 1-40 shows how total dose distribution for a series of consecutive scans can be obtained by summation of a single-scan dose profile incremented by a known amount; it also shows the case in which peaks may appear in dose distribution, depending on the extent of the tails in the dose profile and the degree of overlap incorporated in the scan sequence. Evaluation of CT dose performance must be specific as to whether the minimum, the average, or the peak doses are being specified.

If a space is left between slices (incrementation is greater than slice thickness), the radiation dose will be reduced, since part of the patient may receive little, if any, radiation and possibility of dose profile tails overlapping is reduced.

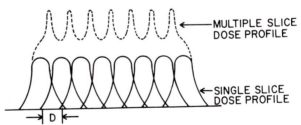

*Figure 1-40*  Determination of dose distribution over an extended body part when multiple scans are obtained. Appropriate summation of the dose profiles is accomplished by superimposing the dose profiles with incrementation distance D. Because of the tailing off of the dose profiles and the degree of overlap in incrementation, dose peaks may appear in the distribution.

## Table 2-1    MR Properties of Certain Nuclei

| NUCLEUS | SPIN QUANTUM NUMBER | NATURAL ABUNDANCE, % | GYROMAGNETIC RATIO (MHZ/TESLA) | RELATIVE SENSITIVITY FOR EQUAL NUMBER OF NUCLEI AT CONSTANT FIELD (RELATIVE TO $^1$H), % |
|---|---|---|---|---|
| $^1$H | ½ | 100 | 42.56 | 100 |
| $^{13}$C | ½ | 1.1 | 10.7 | 0.25 |
| $^{14}$N | 1 | 99.6 | 3.1 | 0.20 |
| $^{15}$N | ½ | 0.36 | 4.3 | 0.10 |
| $^{19}$F | ½ | 100 | 40.1 | 0.94 |
| $^{31}$P | ½ | 100 | 17.2 | 0.41 |

*Adapted from House 1983.*

tude of the magnetic field associated with any particular nucleus depends on the degree to which the magnetic fields of the individual nucleons add to or cancel each other. In general, nuclei with an even number of protons and an even number of neutrons ("even-even" nuclei) have zero spin magnetic moment. Examples of these are $^{12}$C, $^{16}$O, $^{32}$S, and $^{40}$Ca. Odd-atomic-numbered nuclei with an odd number of protons have much stronger magnetic fields associated with them. These "odd-odd" nuclei are most amenable for imaging. Examples include $^1$H, $^{13}$C, $^{19}$F, and $^{31}$P. Odd-even and even-odd nuclei tend to have intermediate-strength magnetic fields.

The magnetic resonance process depends critically on the net magnetic moment of the nucleus. Of the biologically important nuclei, the hydrogen nucleus provides the greatest overall sensitivity to the MR process (Table 2-1). This is because of both its large magnetic moment and its great abundance in the body in the form of water and other biologically important molecules. Though much research is certainly going on in sodium imaging as well as imaging of other biologically important nuclei, all practical clinical MR imaging is currently done with hydrogen nuclei. It can be understood why MRI is so much more sensitive than CT scanning when it is realized that the differences in water content (and thus hydrogen content) of biological tissues are much greater than the corresponding differences in x-ray attenuation upon which CT depends.

We have established that a magnetic field may exist around any given nucleus. The particular configuration of this magnetic field is always of the dipole type; that is, there are distinct north and south poles. The alignment of the north and south poles defines what is referred to as a *magnetic vector*. Thus, a nucleus has a magnetic vector which will always have some magnitude and will be aligned in some particular direction in space. In the case of a spinning nucleus, the vector is aligned perpendicular to the plane of spin, as seen in

Fig. 2-1*A*. In an extended medium all the various nuclei, because of random interactions with neighboring nuclei and with thermal environments, have their magnetic vectors aligned at random in all directions throughout the medium. These vectors add to or cancel each other (Fig. 2-1*B*). Being random means that all directions are equally present and at any instant of

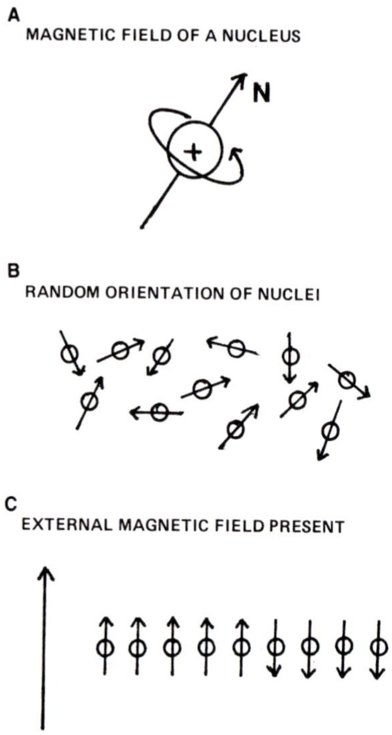

*Figure 2-1*   **A.** Individual nucleus possessing spin manifests a magnetic field directed perpendicular to the plane of spin. This defines a magnetic dipole with north and south poles, and it is said the nucleus has a magnetic moment or vector. **B.** In a medium, individual nuclei with their individual magnetic vectors align randomly. There is no net external magnetic field since they will all cancel each other. **C.** When an external magnetic field ($B_0$) is present, the nuclei of hydrogen, for instance, line up either in the same direction as $B_0$ (parallel) or in the opposite direction of $B_0$ (antiparallel). There is only a slight excess aligned in the parallel direction.

time any one vector in one particular direction cancels with another one oriented in the exact opposite direction. As a result, the overall medium does not have an external magnetic field because all the nuclei cancel each other within that medium. Such is the case for biological tissues, which do not normally have externally detectable magnetic fields. Yet the potential for magnetic effects is there since tissues in fact contain nuclei that have magnetic vectors which, if properly manipulated, can be made to be externally detected.

If the medium is placed in a strong external magnetic field (usually referred to as the $B_0$ field), the magnetic vectors of the individual nuclei will tend to align with this external magnetic field. Hydrogen, for instance, has two possible alignments: one for the magnetic vector lining up in the same direction as the external magnetic field (referred to as a parallel alignment) and the other for the magnetic vector aligning in the direction opposite to the magnetic field (antiparallel alignment), as seen in Fig. 2-1C. The parallel direction is a lower-energy state, and as a result a slight excess number of protons are aligned in this direction compared with the antiparallel direction. Since these two vectors are in opposite directions, they tend to cancel out. Because of the slight excess in the parallel directions, however, some net magnetization will remain in the parallel direction. The magnitude of this net magnetization increases with the strength of the $B_0$ field since it would then take even more energy to align antiparallel. In general these result in only about one to three excess parallel aligned protons for every million protons in the medium. Only this relatively small fraction of residual protons enters into the MR process.

One additional very important phenomenon occurs when the nuclear magnetic vectors are under the influence of an external magnetic field: The magnetic vectors will not only line up parallel or antiparallel but will also precess around that magnetic field. That is, the vector will circle around the $B_0$ direction, as seen in Fig. 2-2A. This precession occurs with a particular frequency. Equation (1) shows the relationship between the frequency of precession and the applied external magnetic field.

$$F = KB_0 \qquad (1)$$

In this equation, $B_0$ is the magnitude of the external magnetic field and $K$ is a constant for each different nucleus called the gyromagnetic ratio constant. For hydrogen the gyromagnetic constant equals 42.56 megahertz per tesla (MHz/T). Equation (1), also referred to as the Larmor equation, is a fundamental relationship governing the MR process. The tesla is a unit of magnetic field strength and is numerically equal to 10,000 gauss (G). The gauss is also a measure of magnetic

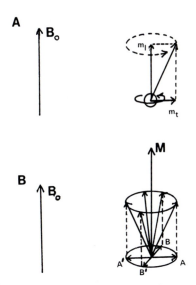

**Figure 2-2 A.** Individual nuclear magnetic vector precessing around the $B_0$ field. There will be only a couple of protons out of every million whose magnetic field will remain uncanceled and precession parallel to the external field. Each of these nuclei will have a transverse ($m_t$) and a longitudinal ($m_l$) component to the precessing magnetic vector at any instant. **B.** When the ensemble of all nuclei in a particular region of space is considered, each is in a random position in its precessional cycle. As a result, all the transverse components will cancel ($A$ cancels with $A'$, $B$ with $B'$, etc.) There will, however, be a net longitudinal component since vectors all add up in this direction. This resulting longitudinal component is called the bulk magnetization vector ($M$).

field strength. To give a sense of magnitude for this unit, the natural magnetic field around the earth is approximately 0.5 G.

Table 2-1 shows the constant $K$ as well as other physical data for various isotopes of interest in medical practice. Note the relatively large sensitivity for hydrogen nuclei. This high sensitivity coupled with hydrogen's very high abundance in the body in the form of water and other biologically important molecules makes it ideal for imaging. In general, isotopes, having an odd number of protons and neutrons, have the greatest MR sensitivity.

Figure 2-2B shows that the magnetic vectors for the ensemble of all participating nuclei at any one region in space precessing around the static external magnetic field essentially form a cone of vectors. These randomly rotate around the external field. Looking at the projections of each of these vectors onto the transverse plane (the horizontal plane), it can be seen that each vector precesses in a random orientation relative to every other vector. Again, since there are no preferred directions in space, there are just as many vectors in one direction as there are in any other direction. In this case, then, all these vectors cancel in the transverse plane. (In Fig. 2-2B, $A$ cancels with $A'$, $B$ with $B'$, etc.) As a result, for any point in the medium, an equilibrium is established where no net magnetic vector

## Table 2-2  Summary of the MR Preparatory Phase

1. Each hydrogen nucleus in the medium possesses a magnetic moment caused by the inherent spin of its nucleus.

2. The medium possesses no overall externally detectable magnetization since all the individual nuclei are aligned randomly and cancel each other's magnetic fields.

3. When placed in a strong external magnetic field, the nuclear magnetic moments align themselves in either the parallel or the antiparallel direction and in addition precess around the external field direction with frequency given by the Larmor equation ($F = KB_0$).

4. A slight excess population of nuclear magnetic vectors aligned in parallel direction do not cancel out with antiparallel vectors. This yields a net magnetization in the parallel direction (direction of the magnetic field).

5. The magnetic vectors will have their transverse plane projections all cancel out at each point in space because of their random motions. The vectors, however, add up in the longitudinal direction, giving the medium a bulk magnetization along the applied external magnetic field direction. This is the equilibrium or relaxed state.

6. No signal will be detected when the system is in the equilibrium state since no transverse magnetic component exists. However, a signal will be produced when the system is disturbed away from the equilibrium state.

---

exists in the transverse plane. However, when looking at the projections of the vectors on the longitudinal (up and down or vertical) axis, it can be seen that each vector in fact adds to every other vector along this longitudinal axis and that a large net longitudinal vector results, composed of the sum of all the various precessing vectors. This net magnetization, also called the bulk magnetization vector ($M$), is seen to lie entirely in the longitudinal direction. At this point the system is in dynamic equilibrium and is relaxed. At equilibrium each point in the image field will contain a net magnetization along the longitudinal direction but no magnetization in the transverse plane, for example

$$\left.\begin{array}{l} M_l = \text{maximum} \\ M_t = \text{zero} \end{array}\right\} \text{at equilibrium}$$

The detection of signals is discussed at length in another section, but suffice it to say here that a signal will be generated whenever there is a net transverse magnetization component. In the equilibrium condition just described, there is no net transverse component to the bulk magnetization and no net signal is detected. However, any displacement from equilibrium will shift some magnetization from the longitudinal direction onto the transverse plane and then a signal will be generated. The preparatory process steps are summarized in Table 2-2.

The next step in the MR process is to excite the nuclei, purposely causing a displacement away from the longitudinal alignment, and thus increase transverse magnetization.

## THE EXCITATION PROCESS

It has already been shown that under equilibrium conditions no net signal is detected since the net bulk magnetization vector is entirely along the longitudinal direction. A signal will be detected only if there is some net magnetization along the transverse axis. In the MR process, the intent is to purposely excite nuclei away from the longitudinal alignment into the transverse plane and thus create a signal. As the nuclei relax (return to equilibrium), this signal decays at a time rate characteristic of the particular chemical and tissue milieu of the hydrogen nuclei and will convey information about the tissue properties at each point in the medium.

What form of energy can be utilized to excite these hydrogen nuclei and their magnetic vectors as they precess around the direction of the external field? Radiofrequency electromagnetic waves are capable of doing just that. The reason for this can be understood by going back to Equation (1), the Larmor relationship. The precessional frequency in megahertz specified there is the key to exciting the nucleus. That is, if magnetic energy is varied at exactly the Larmor frequency, a resonance absorption effect occurs in which energy is transferred to the nucleus and the nucleus becomes excited. The frequency expressed in the Larmor relationship in fact lies in the electromagnetic radio-frequency (RF) range for nuclei of clinical interest. To further understand this resonance effect, remember that electromagnetic radiation does in fact have electric and magnetic properties. The magnetic component of these waves having magnitude called $B_1$ is of interest here. Additionally, it is known that this magnetic component varies sinusoidally. If the frequency of the RF sinusoidally varying $B_1$ field exactly matches the Larmor frequency, resonance absorption of RF energy occurs. The net effect is that the bulk magnetization vector is tipped in space away from the longitudinal alignment and into the transverse plane. Additionally, where before all the individual vectors were randomly precessing around the $B_0$ direction, they now become bundled together so that not only are they tipped toward the transverse plane but they are all spinning in phase relative to each other (phase coherence). Therefore, instead of many vectors randomly precessing, the vectors are spinning together as one. This means that the individual vectors no longer cancel in the transverse plane. Rather, there is now a very large net transverse plane magnetization. Depending on the amplitude and duration of the exciting RF energy, the tip angle will increase. Thus, the vector can be tipped to any angle such as 90°, 180°, or 270°, as seen in Fig. 2-3A. The actual manner in which the magnetization vector is displaced is also seen in this figure. Essentially what occurs is that the RF wave provides a torque on the bulk vector such that a spiraling precessional motion of the vector away from the original longitudinal alignment results. This motion traces the surface of a sphere as the vector is rotated from equilibrium (0°) to the desired tip angle. As the magnetization vector spirals down, the longitudinal magnetiza-

### A.  RF EXCITATION: STATIONARY FRAME

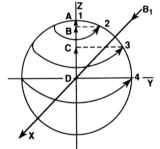

### B.  RF EXCITATION: MOVING FRAME

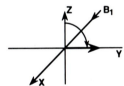

### C.  LONGITUDINAL AND TRANSVERSE MAGNETIZATION

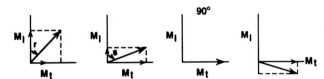

*Figure 2-3*  **A.** When a radio-frequency wave of appropriate frequency is incident on the nuclei at equilibrium, the magnetic field component $B_1$ of that RF wave provides a torque such that the magnetization vector precesses in spiral fashion away from the original longitudinal alignment. Longitudinal magnetization goes from maximum (position 1, tip angle 0°) to zero (position 4, tip angle 90°). At intermediate positions (2 and 3) longitudinal magnetization is of intermediate value. Corresponding to each position, the transverse magnetization builds up from zero at position 1 to maximum at position 4. **B.** It is common to use the moving frame representation of excitation by which the original magnetization vector is tipped directly from the original longitudinal alignment to any tip angle. Here we have a tip angle of 90°. **C.** During excitation over any angle (*r* or *s*, for instance) $m_l$ steadily decreases while $m_t$ steadily increases. At 90°, $m_l$ is zero and $m_t$ is maximum. Beyond 90°, $m_l$ assumes negative values while $m_t$ begins to decrease.

tion is reduced. For instance, as seen in Fig. 2-3A, at equilibrium (position 1) full magnetization (vector height A) exists. At positions 2 and 3 there is only a partial longitudinal magnetization projection (vector heights B and C). Notice that we now also have some signal-producing transverse magnetization present (vector lengths B-2 and C-3). At position 4 (90° tip angle) there is zero longitudinal and maximum transverse magnetization (vector length D-4). For simplicity's sake, it is common to depict this spiraling precessional motion as viewed from a moving frame of reference, that is, as if one were riding on the vector. In such a frame of reference the magnetic vector is represented as directly rotating from the longitudinal z axis to the transverse axis y, as seen in Fig. 2-3B.

What is important to realize in this section is that RF energy can in fact excite the nuclei of interest and that such excitation results in the perturbation of the equilibrium longitudinal alignment to create a transverse component where there was none before. This transverse component can generate a detectable electrical signal. The RF excited state for a 90° flip angle can then be described as

$$M_l = 0$$
$$M_t = \text{maximum}$$

Note that the excited state here is just the opposite of the equilibrium relaxed state. It should also be noted that the RF energy incident on the tissues is of such low energy and frequency that it does not disturb the electrostatic bonds of the constituent atoms and molecules within the tissues, so that these will not perturb the MR process.

When the RF field is turned off, the hydrogen protons will be at some given state of excitation manifested by the magnetic vector at some angle relative to the longitudinal axis and generating some signal from the transverse magnetization induced. Individual nuclei will gradually revert to the longitudinal alignment by losing excitational energy to the overall thermal environment. Such interactions are called spin-lattice interactions. Nuclei can also exchange energy between themselves and the immediately neighboring nuclei. These interactions cause a dephasing of the individual spinning vectors; that is, nuclear spins which were originally in phase (e.g., moving together as one) immediately after excitation interact with each other and rapidly lose their phase coherence and revert back to the random orientation in the transverse plane. As phase coherence is lost, so is the signal. Phase coherence is lost via spin-spin interactions, and they involve interaction of the protons with their immediate neighbor proton within the atom or molecule. The time constant associated with recovery of the longitudinal mag-

## Table 2-3    Summary of the MR Excitation Phase

1. Magnetic component ($B_1$) of an RF wave with frequency exactly matching the Larmor precessional frequency.
2. Magnetization vector begins to precess in a spiraling motion away from the longitudinal alignment. As a result, the longitudinal magnetization is reduced and the transverse magnetization increases.
3. Nuclei will return to the relaxed original state (longitudinal alignment) with relaxation times ($T_1$ and $T_2$) characteristic of the particular tissue milieu nuclei sit in.
4. Transverse magnetization component provides a detectable signal allowing the determination of spin relaxation rates as the system returns to the equilibrium state.

netization (spin-lattice interactions) is given by $T_1$, and the time constant associated with loss of phase coherence (spin-spin interactions) is given by $T_2$. Both of these processes lead to the loss of transverse magnetization and a consequent loss in the detected signal. Table 2-3 summarizes the MR excitation phase.

# SIGNAL DETECTION AND SIGNAL DECAY PROCESSES

It has already been seen that RF energy can excite the nuclear spin system, causing the magnetization vector to reorient in space, and thus create some transverse magnetization and consequently a detectable signal. But just how is this signal detected? Figure 2-3C shows the magnetization vector $M$ at some intermediate tip angle ($r$). Note that the vector has projections in both the longitudinal axis ($m_l$) and transverse axis ($m_t$). At a greater tip angle ($s$), $m_t$ is larger and $m_l$ smaller. At the 90° angle $m_t$ is at a maximum whereas $m_l$ is zero. If $M$ is tipped beyond 90° then $m_t$ decreases while $m_l$ starts assuming negative values. The relative amount of transverse magnetization (the signal) can be determined by providing a coil of wire nearby. As the magnetization vector precesses, it induces an electrical signal in the wire coil. This is merely the phenomenon of electromagnetic induction that governs, for instance, the operation of electrical transformers and other devices familiar in x-ray instrumentation. The magnitude of the induced signal is dependent on the angle that exists at a particular moment between the vector and the wires in the coil. A maximum signal is induced when the vector is cutting across the coil at 90°, which corresponds with the situation when transverse magnetization is maximum. As the magnetization angle de-

creases, the transverse component ($m_t$) decreases and consequently the signal decreases. It is crucial to emphasize that the signal detected in MR always depends entirely on the amount of transverse magnetization present. This therefore forms the basis for signal detection and provides the means of determining $m_t$ and $m_l$, as will be seen shortly. As the nuclei return to the ground state by losing energy to the thermal lattice environment (via spin-lattice interactions), the magnetic vector gradually returns to the original longitudinal alignment. But as this occurs, the projection on the transverse axis would be expected to gradually diminish and the possible signal detected would also gradually diminish. The actual manner in which the signal is expected to diminish is exponential.

$T_1$ relaxation is defined in terms of the longitudinal magnetization recovery; specifically, $T_1$ is defined for

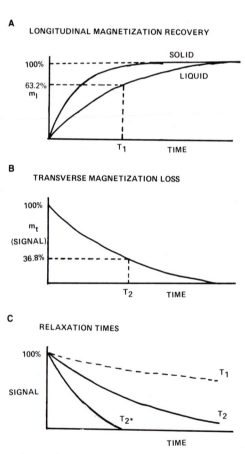

***Figure 2-4*** **A.** After a 90° RF excitation pulse the longitudinal magnetization begins to recover. $T_1$ represents the time constant of this recovery and is defined for 63.2 percent recovery. Also shown is the expected elongation in $T_1$ for a liquid compared with a solid. **B.** Loss of transverse magnetization (the signal) is principally due to dephasing and is usually very rapid compared with recovery of the longitudinal magnetization. $T_2$ is the time necessary for signal to decay to 36.8 percent of its original value. **C.** $T_2^*$ decay rate is due mainly to local nonhomogeneities of the magnet. It is the dominant dephasing mechanism and drives the detected signal to zero very quickly. True $T_2$ signal is shown for the case where $T_2^*$ is absent. $T_1$ (dashed curve), is relatively long, and its signal would normally not be seen.

63.2 percent recovery, as seen in Fig. 2-4$A$. This figure also shows the different $T_1$ recovery times expected for a semisolid compared with a liquid. In a semisolid, molecules are closer and are more directly coupled to each other. More importantly, however, is the condition that the frequency of molecules interacting with each other match the Larmor frequency of the excited nucleus. The result of all this is that the energy loss due to spin-lattice interactions is more rapid and $T_1$ will be correspondingly shorter. Different biological tissues exhibit different $T_1$s.

In addition to spin-lattice interactions, the nuclei immediately start undergoing spin-spin interactions. These involve individual nuclear spins interacting with other nuclear spins in their immediate neighborhood. In this process, energy is transferred back and forth between nuclei, speeding up some and slowing down others. As a result, the initial phase coherence (i.e., vectors precessing in phase) that existed immediately after excitation is degraded. This dephasing drives the MR signal to zero since the individual vectors revert to their random dephased orientations with subsequent cancellation of each other, and as a result the transverse magnetization goes to zero independently of longitudinal recovery. The rate at which the vectors dephase, and thus the rate at which the signal decays, is given by a second time constant, the $T_2$ relaxation time. Figure 2-4$B$ shows the signal diminishing to zero as dephasing progresses. $T_2$ is defined in a manner similar to but not exactly like that of $T_1$. $T_2$ represents the time necessary for signal to be reduced to 36.8 percent of its original value. The choice of 36.8 percent signal remaining is not entirely arbitrary—36.8 percent is merely the reciprocal of the exponential number (2.718). This particular percentage (and its complement, 63.2 percent) is chosen since it simplifies the mathematical equations related to exponential phenomena. In general, $T_2$ values are roughly one-tenth the values of $T_1$ for biological tissues, $T_1$ being in hundreds of milliseconds and $T_2$ in tens of milliseconds. What this means is that immediately after excitation the vectors commence dephasing rapidly, $M_t$ decays, and the signal approaches zero rapidly. This all occurs before the $M_l$ hardly begins to recover due to its long $T_1$ time.

One more level of complication beyond the two relaxation mechanisms given by $T_1$ and $T_2$ must be described. An additional mechanism that contributes to spin-spin interactions is due to the external magnetic field not being totally uniform. It does have local nonhomogeneities. In general, these local nonhomogeneities enhance spin-spin interactions and speed the dephasing process and consequently the signal decay. Thus in a simple MR experiment what one would principally measure after excitation is usually the loss of signal due to dephasing as a result of local magnetic

field nonhomogeneities. This dephasing is so rapid that it may mask all the $T_2$ and $T_1$ signal information. This relaxation time is referred to as $T_2^*$ and, as mentioned previously, is related to the quality of the magnets and its homogeneity. The conversion from a relaxed state to an excited state and then back to the relaxed state can be depicted as follows:

$$
\begin{array}{ccc}
M_l = \max & \underset{T_1}{\overset{+RF}{\rightleftarrows}} & M_l = 0 \\
\text{(Relaxed)} & & \text{(Excited)}
\end{array}
$$

$$
\begin{array}{ccc}
M_t = 0 & \underset{T_2}{\overset{+RF}{\rightleftarrows}} & M_t = \max \\
\text{(Relaxed)} & & \text{(Excited)}
\end{array}
$$

For the usual MR procedures, the influence of $T_2^*$ must be eliminated, to get at the more interesting $T_1$ and $T_2$ rates.

The simplest of MR experiments, referred to as the *free induction decay* (FID) process (Fig. 2-5$A$), can now be illustrated. The FID process also illustrates the $T_2$ behavior just discussed and is described as follows: A 90° RF pulse is given. This tips the magnetization entirely onto the transverse plane, with a correspondingly large signal detected. Notice that the initial magnitude of this signal is dependent on the number of nuclei (spin density) participating in this process and will be characteristic of the tissue properties at a given point. After cessation of the excitation pulse, all the individual nuclei are in phase with each other. But these rapidly lose their phase coherence owing to spin-spin interactions induced by local magnetic field nonhomogeneities as well as to a lesser extent the true $T_2$ interactions, and $m_t$ rapidly goes to zero. This loss occurs because individual vectors again revert to their random precessional motion and start to cancel in the transverse plane. Figure 2-4$C$ shows the resulting loss of signal that occurs. The $T_2^*$ relaxation dominates the signal in that it quickly drives it to zero. If $T_2^*$ were absent, the signal would follow the $T_2$ curve. However, $T_2$ in turn masks the relatively long $T_1$ relaxation signal. How to unravel $T_1$ from $T_2$ from $T_2^*$ is the subject of the next section. Notice in Fig. 2-5$A$ that longitudinal magnetization continues to grow and eventually reaches maximum value. If the original tip angle is 180° instead of 90°, an inversion occurs and longitudinal magnetization is maximum in the negative direction (Fig. 2-5$B$). After the cessation of the pulse, as was true of the FID, dephasing proceeds and $m_t$ goes to zero. However, $m_l$ steadily diminishes to zero and then continues growing (recovering) until it becomes a maximum in the positive direction.

In the preceding discussion, a classic description was invoked. The quantum mechanical approach views the excitation process as individual nuclei absorbing quanta of RF energy. Each nucleus reverts

**A**

RELAXATION FOR 90° TIP (FID)

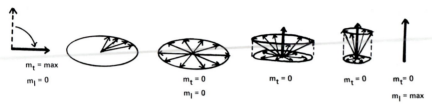

$m_t$ = max
$m_l$ = 0

$m_t$ = 0
$m_l$ = 0

$m_t$ = 0

$m_t$ = 0

$m_t$ = 0

$m_t$ = 0
$m_l$ = max

**B**

RELAXATION FOR 180° TIP

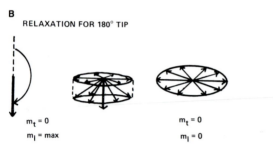

$m_t$ = 0
$m_l$ = max

$m_t$ = 0
$m_l$ = 0

*Figure 2-5* Dephasing of vectors. **A.** After a 90° tip angle, the vector rapidly dephases (FID) until $m_t$ = 0 and $m_l$ = 0. No signal is possible after this; however, longitudinal magnetization continues to recover until equilibrium is attained ($m_t$ = 0, $m_l$ = max). **B.** If a 180° tip angle is used, the longitudinal magnetization is maximum but negative. No signal is possible since $m_t$ = 0. As time goes on the vectors dephase and $m_l$ assumes smaller negative values. Since vectors are dephased, no signal is possible. When vectors arrive at the transverse plane, $m_l$ = 0, $m_t$ = 0. Progress after this is the same as for the FID response.

from the low-energy, parallel-alignment state to the higher-energy antiparallel state. A 90° flip, for instance, corresponds to half the nuclei inverting, as seen in Fig. 2-6A. As a consequence, no net longitudinal magnetization exists. As flip angle increases, more magnetization is continuously inverted to a point where it is all aligned at 180°. Notice in Fig. 2-6B that an intermediate $m_l$ corresponds to the classic description using tilted vectors. For instance, intermediate $m_l$ at position 1 corresponds to tilted vector 1', which in turn corresponds to some intermediate $m_t$. On relaxation, the individual nuclei emit RF energy and each reverts to the original low-energy state. Though the quantum mechanical description is the more rigorous one, the classic description is used here because of its simplicity.

**A.**

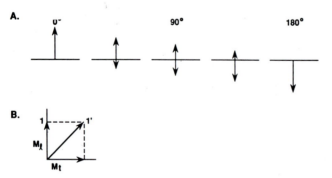

u⁻        90°        180°

**B.**

1 ---- 1'

$M_l$

$M_t$

*Figure 2-6* **A.** In the quantum mechanical description, an individual nucleus can be either in the low-energy or high-energy state. Therefore, individual nuclei invert from the low-energy parallel state to the higher-energy antiparallel state upon absorbing a quantum of RF energy. For a 90° flip half the nuclei have been inverted, while at 180° they all have. In the relaxation process, events are exactly reversed. **B.** Correlation with the classical description is seen by the fact that $m_l$ at some particular height (1) and at some particular angle corresponds to a particular transverse component $m_t$.

## Saturation Recovery

To determine $T_1$ or $T_2$, $T_2^*$ effects must be suppressed. Various pulse sequences have been designed to accomplish this. One of these is the saturation recovery pulse sequence. This sequence, though not generally used, illustrates nicely the MR process at its simplest and is discussed now.

The saturation recovery pulse sequence is merely a repeated FID sequence; that is, a series of 90° RF pulses is given separated by a repetition time TR, as shown in Fig. 2-7A. The number of times the sequence is repeated depends on the matrix size. For a 256 × 256 matrix, the sequence is normally repeated 256 times. This is true for all pulse sequences. Remember that after each 90° pulse, all the magnetic vectors are in phase and immediately start to dephase as well as spiraling back to the longitudinal position. (The ensemble of dephased vectors is indicated as dashed and the in-phase signal-producing vectors as solid throughout this chapter.) Since the 90° pulses are repeated, the second 90°, for instance, will catch the vectors at some intermediate position before they have completely recovered to their longitudinal alignment and will project them 90° into the next quadrant, as seen in Fig. 2-7B. Here there is a net vector projection onto the transverse axis, and a signal results. The magnitude of this signal depends, for each image pixel, on the degree of longitudinal recovery of $T_1$ relaxation that had occurred within each pixel. Therefore, we have a way of distinguishing between different $T_1$s and the different tissue they represent. For instance, if the longitudinal magnetization has recovered to position 1 and the second 90° pulse is given, these dephased (dashed)

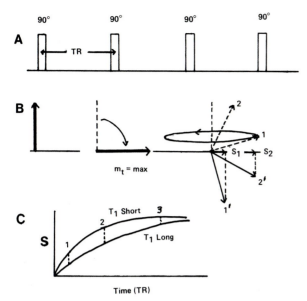

**Figure 2-7** **A.** Saturation recovery. Saturation recovery pulse sequence consisting of a series of 90° pulses separated by some repetition time (TR). A signal whose magnitude correlates with spin density and whose fall-off is governed mainly by $T_2^*$ is detectable after each pulse. **B.** $T_1$ can be determined from the saturation recovery sequence by repeating the sequence so that only partial longitudinal recovery has occurred for subsequent pulses. For instance, dephased vectors (dashed) at position 1 yield no signal; however, when they are projected 90° to position 1′ they once again are coherent (all add up) and yield a signal ($S_1$). A shorter $T_1$ tissue would have recovered to position 2 and be projected 90° so that signal $S_2$ is higher. **C.** Plot of signal magnitude as a function of TR. Contrast is given by the relative $T_1$ differences between the differing tissues. At long TR (point 3), relatively little contrast results. Higher contrast is found at intermediate and lower TR values (points 1 and 2).

vectors are rephased and are projected 90° into position 1′ in the next quadrant, yielding a signal corresponding to the transverse magnetization signal $S_1$. If $T_1$ is short, vectors have recovered to position 2 which is closer to the relaxed state and will project to a larger signal $S_2$ after the 90° pulse. If a period of time greater than the $T_1$ values of the tissues in question elapses before the 90° pulse is repeated, the spin system recovers closer to the full longitudinal magnetization value and subsequent pulses will not distinguish between the different $T_1$ values as well (point 3 in Fig. 2-7C). In all cases, however, the initial signal measured is devoid of $T_2^*$ influence.

If repetition times are short relative to $T_1$, longitudinal magnetization has only partially recovered and subsequent 90° pulses will yield relatively low signals yet yield relatively high signal differences and consequently better $T_1$ contrast. The degree of contrast between tissues will be dependent on the recovery rate $T_1$ of each tissue. This is seen in Fig. 2-7C where level 1 will have greater image contrast then at level 3. Note that the image contrast is always the

relative difference between the two recovery curves. Sometimes the above pulse sequence is referred to as partial saturation in the sense that usually TR is sufficiently short that the system recovers only partially before the next pulse is applied. Equation (2) shows the magnitude of the signal as a function of the various timing parameters

$$S_{sr} = N\left[1 - \exp\left(\frac{TR}{T_1}\right)\right] \qquad (2)$$

where $N$ is a constant dependent on the number of protons present (spin density) and exp represents the exponential function that all MR signal decay processes follow. From Equation (2) it is seen that the signal depends on the ratio $TR/T_1$ or the fraction that TR represents relative to $T_1$. It is this fraction that determines the degree of longitudinal recovery occurring between the different tissues (or $T_1$ weighting) and thus the contrast between them. Notice also that signal strength is greater at long TR since protons have more completely recovered and can return a greater signal.

The saturation recovery sequence is also applicable in determining proton-weighted images. In Equation (2), if TR is sufficiently long to allow full recovery, the exponential term goes to zero and the initial signal is related only to proton density. A more intuitive description of proton weighting is based on the fact that different tissues have different proton densities. When a 90° flip is applied, there will be different signals from each tissue. The larger the proton density, the larger the signal since more protons have been flipped and are participating in the MR process (Fig. 2-8A,B). At very long repetition times (TR′), essentially all protons have recovered so that new excitation will yield signal devoid of $T_1$ and weighting the proton density. Various possibilities exist. For instance, white matter has a short $T_1$ but lower proton density as compared with CSF (Figure 2-8C). At short TR, the signal will be $T_1$-weighted and white matter, owing to its short $T_1$, will appear brighter on image than CSF. At long repetition times, however, where proton weighting occurs CSF will be brighter owing to its greater proton density. This is an example of a gray scale inversion. The following rules can be postulated.

As TR ↑
$T_1$ weighting ↓
Proton weighting ↑
Signal strength ↑

The saturation recovery sequence is quite sensitive to irregularities in tip angle accuracy and consistency as well as having a relatively low contrast scale available

applied for each value of $G_y$. This process essentially goes through the selected slice, interrogating each line defined by the $x$-$y$ gradient combination until MR signals from the entire slice are accumulated. Figure 2-14 illustrates the process of gradient application in the specific case of a spin-echo pulse sequence.

It is also interesting that the only noise heard by the patient during an MRI scan is from the electric current flowing through the gradient coils, where it experiences a force in the presence of the external magnetic field. As a result, the gradient coils "thump" back and forth as they are turned on and off. The magnitude of this noise is proportional to the square of the external field strength. See Table 2-8 for a summary of MR image generation.

The possibilities of three-dimensional FT techniques are much discussed. In this approach, rather than a narrow (slice-selective) bandwidth range of frequencies, a broad (nonselective) band of frequencies is beamed into the patient. This broad frequency range essentially excites the entire volume. Then two variable-phase encoding gradients are applied simultaneously. The data are collected after the readout gradient. Three Fourier transformations must be performed, first along the readout gradient and then along the other two directions. These data can be reformatted to yield any combination of planes, including oblique ones. Optimal resolution is achieved in 3DFT reformatted images if all the gradient slopes are the same, yielding isotropic resolution voxel elements. Anisotropic imaging results if resolution elements are not the same (i.e., if the voxel shape is not a cube).

There is a distinct signal-to-noise ratio advantage from the three-dimensional approach in that signals are collected from a larger volume. On the other hand, the penalty paid is increased scan times, especially for isotropic imaging. Compromises can be made to speed up the three-dimensional approach, such as anisotropic imaging, less than 90° flip angles, and shorter TR times. The former affects resolution and the latter two affect signal strength and contrast.

## MULTIPLANAR AND MULTIECHO IMAGING ACQUISITION

In general, $T_1$ relaxation time is relatively long (in hundreds of milliseconds) and determines how short a TR can be used. Additionally, the required interpulse delay times ($T_1$ or TE) can add up in repeating sequences for each point. To efficiently use the inherent TR and delay times, a multiplanar approach can be used. Here

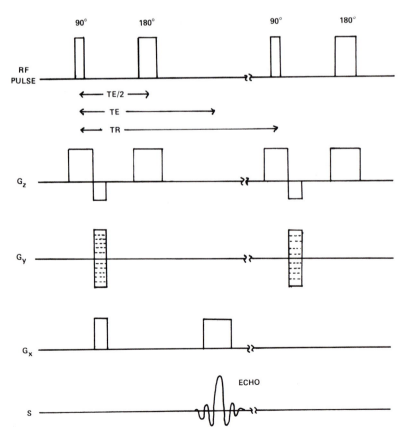

**Figure 2-14** Depiction of events occurring in a two-dimensional FT spin-echo pulse sequence. The initial 90° pulse is given in the presence of a slice selection gradient $G_z$. (Only those spins within this particular slice will be flipped 90°.) The $G_z$ gradient is followed by the phase encoding gradient $G_y$ and a frequency encoded gradient $G_x$. $G_s$ defines the spatial position of each row in terms of frequency, and $G_y$ defines the position along each column in terms of phase. These are followed by a reapplication of $G_z$ when the 180° pulse is given. (This will flip 180° those spins within the slice that had been defined originally by $G_z$.) Finally $G_x$ is applied as a readout gradient, and the spin-echo signal is collected. The whole sequence is repeated for a different value of the phase encoding gradient $G_y$ (dashed lines) for the number of times equal to the matrix size (e.g., 256 times for a 256 × 256 matrix).

## Table 2-8   Summary of MR Image Generation

1. Signals detected must be localized in space. Gradients in three directions are utilized for this task. Gradient strengths vary up to 25 to 30 mT/m.
2. A gradient is a linear variation of the magnetic field such that each point in space is defined by a unique frequency (or phase) given by the Larmor equation ($F = KB_0$).
3. Detected signals, even though spatially localized, still have contributions from $T_2^*$, $T_2$, and $T_1$ processes. $T_2^*$ is due to both tissue $T_2$ and the presence of local nonhomogeneities, which drive the signal to zero very rapidly.
4. To unfold $T_2$, $T_1$, and spin density from $T_2^*$, special pulse sequences are needed: saturation recovery, inversion recovery, and the spin-echo sequence.
5. For a given pulse sequence, the image can be weighted for protons (spin density), $T_1$, or $T_2$ by varying the time parameters TR, TE, and TI.
6. Image contrast between tissues depends critically on the time parameters selected. Gray scale inversions are possible.
7. Special fast scan sequences are possible which can drastically reduce scan times.

the TR interval can be used to excite other planes. The result is the acquisition of a multiple number of planar images at the end of the pulse sequence. Looking at acquisition times will illustrate the timing considerations in MR.

Equation (4) can be used to calculate the image acquisition time for a single slice:

$$\text{Time} = \text{matrix size} \times \text{number of excitations} \times \text{TR} \quad (4)$$

Notice that this includes not only matrix size and TR but also the number of times the sequence or excitation is repeated (number of data acquisitions) for purposes of signal averaging to gain an improvement in the signal-to-noise ratio. For a simple example, consider a matrix size of $256 \times 256$ (implies 256 phase steps), the number of acquisitions = 2, and TR = 1000 milliseconds (1 second). Then acquisition time is 512 seconds ($256 \times 2 \times 1$), or 8.53 minutes. A 10-slice procedure, for instance, would require $10 \times 8.53$, or 85.3 minutes. This would be an inordinately long time, and the multiplanar approach becomes very attractive in that rather than repeat time necessary for each individual slice, multiple slices are acquired, utilizing the waiting times between pulses. The maximum number of slices is approximately TR/TE. The multiplanar technique allows not only for the acquisition of multiple planes but also for different pulse timing sequences.

Thus, in a particular sequence, two separate and different TE-weighted images can be obtained. This then can provide additional clinical information to differentiate between different disease states, as illustrated in Fig. 2-11C.

Another consideration relative to slices is the fact that the thickness of each slice produced is not rectangular but rather trails off in a gaussian manner (similar to CT slices). This means that if a slice is excited with a 90° pulse, then part of the adjacent slice is also excited. Going immediately to that adjacent slice with another 90° pulse, that slice has then suffered a double excitation summing up to 180° and signal is significantly reduced. It is necessary to be careful how each plane is excited. The planes are usually acquired in interleaved fashion to avoid cross-talk effects between planes. With interleaving, immediately adjacent slices are not excited one after another but rather interspersed. This essentially allows more recovery time before exciting any particular slice level which might have been cross-excited previously. Gaussian tail-off of the slice can also be minimized by custom tailoring the frequency distribution of the RF pulse such that slice profile is more rectangular in shape. Finally, a space can always be left between slices if desired anatomical coverage needs allows it.

## Fast Imaging

As in any imaging technique, it is desirable to reduce the imaging time and therefore reduce image-degrading patient motion as well as optimizing patient throughput. In addition, faster scan times reduce patient discomfort as well as allowing for new imaging possibilities such as dynamic scanning, MR angiography, and three-dimensional imaging. Table 2-9 describes various approaches in fast scanning. Equation (4) specified the three major factors determining imaging time. Specifically, it is the product of the number of acquisitions, matrix array size, and repetition time TR. To reduce scan time, one or more of these must be reduced.

## Number of Excitations

Many times, if the signal-to-noise ratio for a particular image is relatively low, that particular image acquisition process is repeated and the separate images are added pixel by pixel. This has the effect of increasing the number of quanta contributing to each image point, and noise levels are reduced. One can repeat this process as many times as is necessary. Repeating the scans, however, obviously extends the overall scan time. Improvements in instrumentation and magnetic field uniformity over the years have allowed a reduction in the number of acquisitions necessary to achieve

## Table 2-9    Fast-Scan Techniques

| TECHNIQUE | IMPLEMENTATION |
|---|---|
| 1. Multi-planar acquisition | Obtain additional slices during TR wait time. |
| 2. Limit matrix size | Obtain fewer phase exciting steps. Penalty = loss resolution. |
| 3. Lower NEX | Obtain fewer repeat images. Penalty = enhanced noise. |
| 4. Partial Fourier | Sample half of K space; calculate other half. Penalty = enhanced noise. |
| 5. Fractional echo | Sample half of echo; shorter TE is possible; calculate other half. Penalty = enhanced noise. |
| 6. Fast spin echo (turbo spin echo) | Obtain multiple K-space lines per 90° excitation. Use effective $T_2$. |
| 7. Gradient echo | Perform small angle excitation and gradient reversals to reduce TR. Penalty = enhanced noise and susceptibility artifacts. |
| 8. Echo planar | Obtain all K-space lines in one 90° RF pulse excitation. Penalty = enhanced noise. |

current levels of 1 or 2. To go even lower, one approach is referred to as half the number of excitations (NEX) acquisition (Feinberg 1986). To understand this approach, it is necessary to remember that normally one steps through the full range of phase encoding steps once for each array step (256 times for a $256 \times 256$ array). However, there is a certain symmetry here in that half these steps are complex conjugates of the other half. This means that it is possible to sample only half the field (or K space, as will be discussed later) and mathematically calculate the other half. For instance, an image can be obtained with 128 phase steps in half the time that 256 would have required. In practice, rather than half the data, about 60 percent is sampled. Notice also that half NEX acquisition results in lower signal to noise since less signal is actually being sampled. Theory predicts a reduction to $1/\sqrt{2}$ of SNR if 50 percent of phase space is sampled. Rather than calling this approach half-NEX, it is more appropriate to call it *partial Fourier sampling*. Partial Fourier sampling results in fractional phase encoding information and is not to be confused with fractional echo sampling that results in fractional frequency encoding information. Fractional echo sampling is directed toward reducing susceptibility artifacts common in gradient-echo imaging, where echo times have to be as

short as possible to reduce phase dispersion effects (Wehrli 1990). When fractional echo imaging is invoked, symmetry properties of data are also capitalized on to synthesize the unsampled part of the echo. Like partial Fourier, a noisier image results. Unfortunately, fractional echo and partial Fourier are not possible at the same time. This is to be expected, since only a small fraction of total signal would be collected, and signal-to-noise ratio would suffer significantly.

## Matrix Array Size

Matrix array size ultimately determines the possible resolution available in the system. Reduction here would not be totally productive. More specifically, the matrix array refers to the number of phase encoding and frequency encoding steps. There is no time penalty in keeping the number of frequency encoding steps high, whereas the opposite is true for the phase encoding steps. Accordingly, time reductions are accomplished by using fewer phase encoding steps. Anisotropic matrices (in which vertical and horizontal matrix sizes are not equal) of $128 \times 256$ would cut the scan time by 50 percent compared with a $256 \times 256$ matrix. This, however, results in loss of resolution in the phase-encoding direction unless complex conjugate symmetry interpolation is invoked as in half-NEX acquisition.

## Reduced Repetition Time (Gradient Echoes)

The remaining parameter is TR. TR in fact is the longest period of time in the pulse sequence, and it is here that the greatest time saving can be obtained. Of course, one can take advantage of the TR interval to excite additional slices to accomplish multislice acquisition. The real reason, however, that TR is relatively long is that it is necessary to reestablish longitudinal magnetization after the 90° flip in spin-echo imaging. This full, or near-full, magnetization assures high signal strength on subsequent excitations. Remember also that reduction of TR in a standard spin-echo sequence introduces $T_1$ weighting and less $T_2$ weighting, as seen in Table 2-5. Also, there would be a decrease in the number of tissue slices that could be imaged during multislice acquisition schemes. When using a partial flip angle, however the time for the longitudinal magnetization to recover is less and a net reduction of scan time is possible (Fig. 2-15).

As seen in Fig. 2-15*A,* a normal spin-echo sequence flips $m_1$ (vector 1) to the transverse plane (vector 2). A partial flip angle is seen to reduce the longitudinal magnetization only minimally (vector 3 versus full height vector 1). Yet the transverse magnetization vector 4, though not at full possible magnitude as vector 2, is still appreciable. This means that a relatively large

**A**

**B**

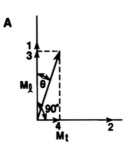

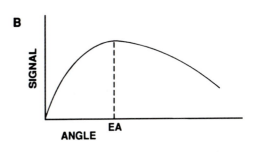

*Figure 2-15* **A.** A 90° flip of the longitudinal magnetization (vector 1) yields full signal along $m_t$ (vector 2). Partial flip, however, hardly affects $m_t$ (vector 3 is almost the same as the original $m_t$ vector). There is, however, still an appreciable signal along $m_t$ (vector 4). **B.** Signal obtainable as a function of flip angle will vary with tissue $T_1$ and TR set. Shown here is maximum response at the flip angle referred to as the Ernst angle (EA).

gain in transverse magnetization (signal) is possible at a relatively small loss in longitudinal magnetization at small flip angles. Though subsequent excitations will yield less signal and signal to noise will not be optimal, this is the mechanism for reducing scan times significantly. This is true since a small flip angle has not appreciably moved the system away from the full recovery position.

The actual signal obtainable as a function of the flip angle is depicted in Fig. 2-15*B*. Signal magnitude will depend on tissue $T_1$ and TR. The angle at which maximum signal is obtained is called the Ernst angle. It should be noted that the Ernst angle need not give the maximum contrast between any two tissues. Distinction between high contrast-to-noise ratio (CNR), yielding large signal differences between tissues, and high signal-to-noise ratio must be made, the latter yields a larger signal from any given tissue.

One major problem immediately comes into play when reduced flip angles are used: the normal 180° RF flip inverts $m_1$. This inverted $m_1$ yields an unstable situation in that vectors proceed to recover back to the longitudinal position and subsequent excitations yield much lower signal strengths. This problem is avoided by not using RF to rephase spins. Instead, the gradients can be reversed to recover a gradient echo.

This requires further explanation. Remember that the purpose of the 180° pulse is to null the effects of magnetic inhomogeneities. These inhomogeneities are not only due to the $B_0$ main field but also to the presence

of the gradients. Gradients after all also represent a fixed inhomogeneity. An additional possible source of inhomogeneity is due to the presence in the patient of magnetic materials like microscopic iron loads, such as in liver and clotted blood (susceptibility effects). In a gradient-recalled pulse sequence instead of following up the initial 90° RF pulse with a 180° RF pulse, a negative gradient in the readout direction is applied instead. This is immediately followed by a positive gradient. This gradient reversal undoes the dephasing because of the presence of the gradient and provides an echo for signal detection. Gradient-echo techniques have been dubbed with acronyms such as GRASS, FISP, and FLASH (Haase 1986). These techniques are particularly advantageous for short-TR, small-angle techniques because of the shorter time necessary for gradient reversals compared with 180° magnetization flips.

Gradient echoes represent the rephasing of spins that were dephased by the presence of the gradient. This does not, however, reverse the dephasing caused by magnetic inhomogeneities nor susceptibility effects. As a result, the signal returned is $T_2^*$-weighted. Current magnet technology and the ability to achieve very uniform fields by shimming* have reduced magnetic inhomogeneity dephasing contributions considerably.

*Shimming is accomplished by incorporating various coils (called shim coils) within the gantry. These coils produce small magnetic fields that can be adjusted to make the overall magnetic field distribution more uniform.

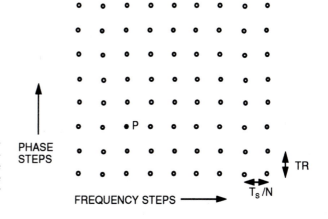

*Figure 2-16* K space consists of the collection of all the phase and frequency sampling measurements obtained which define the image. A two-dimensional Fourier transform of this data yields the desired image. Space between measurements along the phase direction is TR, whereas space along the frequency direction is the readout sampling time ($T_s$) divided by the number of sampling points $N(x)$.

In fact, gradient-echo techniques were proposed much earlier but were not implemented until recently, owing in part to their high sensitivity to $B_0$ magnetic field inhomogeneities. This limitation has been relaxed owing to advances in magnetic field shimming technique. The gradient-echo approach is also very sensitive to RF field nonhomogeneities. One important consideration when using gradient echoes is the associated sensitivity to magnetic susceptibility and flow artifacts. This is particularly apparent in the vicinity of air cavities (sinuses, mastoids, bowel) and near ferromagnetic implants. Another problem is that water and fat signals are not rephased, as occurs with RF pulses. This results in the possibility of imaging low-intensity borders at fat-water interfaces (chemical shift artifact). This would also suppress tumor contrast in the fatty liver and bone marrow tumor imaging. The fat-water cancellation disadvantages of the gradient-echo approach are much reduced for lower magnetic field strength units. As in spin-echo imaging, gradient-echo imaging allows for multiecho acquisition. This is accomplished by reversing the readout gradient repeatedly.

Concerning weighting strategies with partial flip angles, as is similar to spin echo, the longer the TE the greater the $T_2^*$ weighting. The TR effects are also the same as in previous pulse sequences. The flip angle, however, also affects weighting. Small angles correspond to relatively large TR, for example, vectors are almost all recovered and proton weighting occurs. Larger angles correspond to situation where vectors are still close to the transverse plane with little recovery having occurred. This latter condition corresponds to $T_1$ weighting. The following summarizes these findings.

As flip angle ↓
        Proton weighting ↑
        $T_1$ weighting ↓
        TR ↓
        Scan times ↓

An additional advantage of gradient echoes is that much less overall RF power is deposited in the patient by eliminating the 180° RF rephasing flip. There is no RF power deposition for gradient reversals, whereas 180° rephasing pulses deposit up to four times more energy in patients compared with the initial 90° excitation pulses. Additionally, if partial flips are employed, there is an additional reduction in RF power. This reduction factor is $(\theta/90)^2$. Thus, at 45° the RF power is reduced by $(45/90)^2$, or one-fourth. This has particular importance in scanning at high magnetic field strengths, where RF power deposition becomes limiting (Winkler 1988).

In summary, scan times and RF power deposition are significantly reduced using a combination of partial flip and gradient echoes. TRs of 10 to 50 milliseconds, TEs less than 10 milliseconds and overall scanning times of a few seconds per image are now possible.

One way to avoid shortcomings of the gradient-echo technique (high noise, susceptibility and flow artifacts, nonrephasing of $B_0$ main field inhomogeneities) is to do a fast spin echo (FSE). In FSE (also called turbo spin echo), the usual 90°, TE/2, 180° sequence is still used; however, multiple echoes are collected for each 90° excitation such as in Fig. 2-11C. In FSE, however, each echo, rather than being allocated to separate images, is used to fill in one line within the same image. For instance, if there are 20 echoes, then 20 lines will be collected for one 90° pulse and for one TR line interval. Scan times would therefore be ½₀ the normal scan times. This is a very significant reduction in scan time. However, each echo that is collected has a different $T_2$ weighting. What would $T_2$ weighting of the overall image then be? To answer this question and to further understand FSE, it is necessary to analyze how data is collected in MRI. Figure 2-16 shows what is referred to as K space. K space is the collection of all the frequency and phase data points which are collected. For instance, point P in Fig. 2-16 represents a particular data point having a particular frequency and a particular phase. The lines are separated along the phase direction by the TR times. Each point in the frequency direction is separated by the sampling time divided by the number of frequency encodings. To obtain an image, a particular phase encoding gradient is applied and all the frequency data corresponding to that row are collected. The sequence is repeated at a higher pulse encoding gradient after a time TR and the next line collected. This is repeated until all lines are collected (256 lines for a 256 matrix etc.). It is characteristic of K space that the greatest signal intensity is found in the center. Additionally, it is the center that provides the contrast while the periphery of K space provides the resolution. K space is quite different from intuition. For instance, each point in K space does not correspond to a unique point in the image. Rather, each point in K space contributes to every point in the final image.

In the normal spin-echo process, one 90° pulse with its associated 180° rephasing pulse produces one line of K space, and the excitation has to be repeated for each line of the matrix allowing for the relatively long TR delay between lines.

In FSE, the 180° flip is repeatedly applied, generating repeated echoes and multiple lines of K space for each 90° initial pulse. Scan times are reduced by the number of echoes obtained for each 90° initial pulse. The number of such echoes are referred to as the echo train length (ETL). Equation (4) is thus modified as shown below, where $N(y)$ is the number of phase encoding steps (the matrix size):

$$\text{Scan time} = \frac{N(y) \times \text{TR} \times \text{NEX}}{\text{ETL}}$$

Therefore, if 20 echoes are collected (ETL = 20) then 20 lines in K space have been obtained and the overall scan time is reduced by a factor of 20.

In FSE, the question of weighting remains. Recall that long TE yields enhanced $T_2$ weighting. In FSE, sampling is done at a wide variety of TEs. $T_2$ weighting is accomplished by starting out assigning to the center of K space those echoes gathered at a time corresponding to the TE which is desired. It is at the center of K space where the most signal and contrast is generated. An effective TE and a corresponding effective $T_2$ can then be stated. This approach sometimes is referred to as centric ordering of K space.

Echoplanar imaging (EPI) is another approach that can drastically reduce scan times. Here the entire K space is sampled after just one 90° excitation. This has the potential for producing images within milliseconds and therefore opens the door for MR fluoroscopy. In EPI, however, very accurate and fast-switching gradient amplifiers and circuits are imperative.

## FLOW EFFECTS

In the previous discussions, the protons being excited were assumed to be stationary. If, in fact, the protons are moving, one can easily see that signals may be altered significantly. For instance, moving protons may not receive both the 90 and 180° pulses in a spin-echo sequence and thus cannot be rephased. Flow effects lead to signals that can be either enhanced or suppressed. Signal suppression resulting in a flow void can result from losses due to time-of-flight (TOF) effects, turbulence loss, and odd echo dephasing effects. Signal enhancement can come about from even echo rephasing, flow-related enhancement, and diastolic pseudogating (Table 2-10).

### Time-of-Flight Effects

In TOF high-velocity losses, the protons acquire an initial 90° pulse in the standard spin-echo sequence, then flow out of slice before acquiring the 180° rephasing pulse. A subsequent signal loss will thus occur, since protons need to experience both the 90 and 180° pulses to return an echo signal. The degree of TOF losses depends wholly on flow velocity, thickness of the slice, and timing sequence. The faster the flow, the greater the reduction in protons able to participate in

### Table 2-10   MR Flow Effects

Flow signal suppressed via
  Time-of-flight (TOF) losses
  Turbulence losses
  Odd echo dephasing
Flow signal enhanced via
  Even echo rephasing
  Flow-related enhancement
Diastolic pseudogating

both the 90 and 180° pulses. This is a linear function governed by the ratio of protons receiving both pulses and thus also depends on slice thickness and timing sequence. In a similar manner, view-to-view velocity variations during the cardiac cycle also affect the flow signal (Bradley 1984; Axel 1984).

It is interesting to note that velocity profiles across a vessel tend to be parabolic, with the highest velocity at the center. This is referred to as *laminar flow,* which is just the opposite of plug flow, where the entire fluid volume moves at the same velocity. In the presence of laminar flow, a flow void may be observed in the center of a vessel that will suffer the greater TOF loss since flow velocity is greater there, along with a stronger signal from the outer rim of the vessel, where velocity flow is lower and fewer TOF effects occur. Laminar flow, that is, undisturbed flow but with a velocity gradient, tends to occur at higher flow velocities and smaller vessel diameters.

### Turbulence

Turbulence loss occurs whenever flow is disturbed, for instance, slower protons moving over rough atherosclerotic vessel walls, at points of vascular branching, at stenotic constrictions, and for acceleration and deceleration associated with arterial flow. Flow disturbance tends to induce random fluctuations in velocity components, which in turn induce phase loss in spins that finally result in signal loss. Under laminar flow conditions, there will be no signal loss resulting from turbulence. There will, however, still be TOF loss effects.

The velocity at which turbulence occurs is directly proportional to the product of the vessel diameter, fluid velocity, and fluid density and inversely proportional to fluid viscosity (Bradley 1984).

In general, turbulence losses are more severe for slow flow in large vessels and may be present in vessels at any diameter at regions of transition between a high flow center and the slow flow region near the vessel wall.

## Odd Echo Dephasing

The third flow mechanism by which the MR signal is suppressed is odd echo dephasing (Valk 1981; Waluch 1984). This effect and its companion even echo rephasing, yielding an enhanced signal, occur for laminar flow, and are due to flowing protons experiencing different magnetic field gradients as they flow into the plane (weaker gradients are used for slice selection) or flow within the plane (readout and phase encoding gradients are stronger). Additionally, the flow velocity profile across the vessel is important. The greater this profile, the greater the dephasing that will occur. To understand this dephasing mechanism, remember that in a spin-echo sequence, the spins, after experiencing the 90° pulse, dephase relative to each other. When the 180° pulse is given at TE/2 time, these same spins rephase until they zero out at time TE. However, if these spins, for instance, are moving into a magnetic gradient, they experience a phase advance; to the extent to which they are out of phase at the time of the spin echo the echo signal will be reduced. A similar effect occurs if spins are moving into a lesser gradient, in which case spin phases are retarded; this also yields a relative dephasing effect.

The degree of dephasing depends on both the magnetic field gradient strength and its flow velocity. It can be shown (Bradley 1988) that the net result will be a signal loss in echo in every other (odd) slice in a multi-echo sequence. However, dephasing is totally rephased on every other (even) echo. Such rephasing returns an enhanced image signal. TE is important as well, since it determines the time given the spins to interact with the gradients. As TE increases, dephasing increases and greater signal loss occurs.

There are three modes by which signals can be enhanced: even echo rephasing, flow-related enhancement, and diastolic pseudogating.

## Even Echo Rephasing

Even echo rephasing results from the fact that the dephasing that occurred for the entry first slice (odd echo) cyclically rephases to reestablish coherence at the time of the second echo (even echo). This rephasing, however, occurs only for uniform velocity into linear gradients with no acceleration or deceleration effects (Waluch 1984). Additionally, this phenomenon holds only for symmetric echoes. The reader is referred to the literature for clinical examples of this flow phenomenon (Bradley 1988).

## Flow-Related Enhancement

Flow-related enhancement (FRE) occurs under conditions of slow laminar flow when fully magnetized spins move into a slice and displace saturated spins (spins that have experienced an initial 90° pulse but have not yet fully recovered). These fully magnetized spins return a higher signal when applying a 90° pulse if a saturation recovery pulse sequence is used. In the more usual spin-echo case, the signal depends on whether spins experience both the 90 and 180° pulses, in which case FRE competes with TOF signal suppression effects. For sufficiently low velocities, enhancement may still occur, since signal loss due to TOF effects is then offset by signal gain from unsaturated spins that experience both the 90 and 180° pulses. Even echo rephasing depends on flow characteristics, being much more prominent for laminar than for more random turbulent flow. Maximum signal in the entry slice occurs when the flow rate is such that all the blood in the slice is replaced in the time interval TR (true for venous flow for 1 cm/sec for a 1-cm slice and a TR of 1000 msec). For higher velocities, inflowing spins can avoid the 90° pulse until arriving at an inner slice, in which case enhanced signals can arise from these inner slices. In general, flow-related enhancement increases for longer $T_1$ (as is characteristic of unclotted blood) and shorter TR (less longitudinal recovery of the spins) as well as for higher magnetic field systems. The latter is true since field strength determines the degree of magnetization that spins begin with. The position of the slice is important when utilizing multislice acquisitions. Enhancement is greatest in the first slice, where the inflow of fully magnetized spins is greatest. Notice that FRE can be eliminated by applying a presaturation pulse to tissue volume just outside the imaging volume. Spins flowing into the first slice would therefore be just as saturated as stationary spins within that slice.

FRE is more prominent at high magnetic field strength, since the degree of magnetization is greater. Also, it is more prominent for short TR, since this determines the fraction of the stationary spins relative to inflowing spins. Likewise, stationary tissues with longer $T_1$ relaxation times will be more saturated and will return lower signal than will inflowing spins.

With the exception of the entry slices, signals in general are suppressed within tissue volume owing to flow effects. FRE can be exploited to visualize lesions by using single-slice acquisitions with the anatomy of interest at the entry slice (Kucharczyk 1986). This aids in determining vascularity and allows more confident separation of tumor from surrounding edema.

## Diastolic Pseudogating

Diastolic pseudogating can occur whenever the cardiac and MRI cycles become synchronized. If synchronization occurs in diastole, the signal is enhanced since flow is slower. If synchronization occurs in systole, the signal is suppressed owing to faster, more turbulent flow. Synchronization in fact is more likely during diastole, since this phase occupies the major time of the heartbeat cycle. Whenever diastolic pseudogating occurs, the resulting enhanced signal can be erroneously mistaken for a thrombus or tumor. In this case, a gating technique may be needed to eliminate the possibility of pseudogating. Note that the enhanced signal character of slow flow could be exploited by purposely gating to the R wave and therefore introducing enhanced flow signals.

All the above effects work in combination and may or may not compete with each other. At very low flow velocities, FRE dominates at entry slices. As velocities increase, FRE will be noticed for the inner slices as a function of distance from the entry slice. Concurrently, signal begins to diminish at the entry slice as TOF and odd echo dephasing begin. Likewise, to the extent that there is odd echo dephasing, even echo rephasing will also kick in, and as a result, the second echo as well as succeeding even echoes will begin to show enhanced signals. This signal, however, will be offset by the losses due to TOF effects, since higher velocity allows more spins to flow out of the slice before it receives the second 180° pulse. Simultaneously, there is the possibility of pseudogating effects.

Finally, it should be mentioned that the flow effects described are also associated with CSF flow. The reader is referred to the literature (Thomas 1989; Bradley 1988; Enzmann 1986) for more on this, as well as for applications in angiography (Edelman 1990; Nishimura 1990).

# OTHER IMAGING FEATURES

Like CT scanning, MR allows for a number of additional imaging features.

1. *Projected scanning:* A projected scan is merely a quick scan similar to a "scoutview" or "topogram." That is, it is a two-dimensional image in which all structures are superimposed one on the other. To accomplish this, a broadband RF (non-slice-selective) input is used.
2. *True zoom imaging:* A true zoom image can be produced by supplying the full gradient not over the entire patient but rather over a limited region of the patient. This has the effect of increasing the gradient over the region of interest. Furthermore, the operator then applies the full number of available pixels to the desired region. The result is that image is magnified and spatial resolution improves (since each pixel now corresponds to a smaller region of space). In the zoom approach, the excitation pulses must be limited to the specific region of interest to avoid artifacts.
3. *Image manipulation:* As in CT scanning, a number of gray scale and image quality manipulations can

be performed. Examples are window width and window level selection. Also available are the usual range of different filtering kernels for such operations as image smoothing and edge enhancement. Essentially, all software functions available to CT can be made available for MRI (distance and angle calculations, histogram analysis, etc.).

## Suppression Techniques

There are a number of instances where suppression of certain tissue signals is necessary to enhance the image of structures desired to be visualized. Suppression could be performed either by removing an interfering dominant signal or by suppressing artifactual ghosts produced by motion. Examples of these are given in Table 2-11 and are now discussed.

### PRESATURATION TECHNIQUES

Moving structures such as produced by involuntary motion, blood flow, and other phenomena, produce artifactual ghost signals. There are a number of methods available for suppressing these effects, including respiratory and cardiac gating techniques as well as gradient reordering. One very simple technique, however, is known as *presaturation*. A tissue volume is saturated if its longitudinal magnetization has been flipped into the transverse plane. The idea is to merely presaturate region where the source of motion is originating from with a 90° so-called presat pulse, just before giving the normal 90° spin-echo pulse. This has the effect that the motion source will then experience two 90° pulses and be flipped 180° and therefore will yield no projection on the transverse plane where desired signals are being collected.

Presat pulses may be applied, for instance, to the plane just before or after the plane of interest to suppress flowing blood into and through the plane. Likewise, any part within the plane being scanned can be presaturated. Examples of the latter approach include

## Table 2-11   Suppression Techniques

| TECHNIQUE | APPROACH |
| --- | --- |
| Presaturation | Saturate source of motion and suppress motion ghosts. |
| Chemical (spectral) saturation | Selectively saturate specific tissues. |
| Null point suppression | Rule out specific tissues in an inversion recovery sequence (STIR, FLAIR). |
| Magnetization transfer | Transfer protein bound water saturation to bulk phase water. |

sagittal views where CSF motion is desired to be suppressed; likewise, the region anterior to the spine can be suppressed to remove the motion effects of the heart and great vessels. Another application is to suppress venous flow for MR arteriography or arterial flow to enhance MR venography.

## CHEMICAL (SPECTRAL) SATURATION

Rather than suppress a tissue volume source of motion, it may be advantageous to selectively suppress the signal from one particular tissue. This is true when strong signals from a particular tissue are masking the visualization of the more desired but much weaker tissue signals. The gray scale in an MR image is apportioned between the strongest and the weakest signals. If a very strong signal is present, then available gray scale for small and subtle differences is drastically reduced.

In chemical saturation, 90° RF pulses with frequencies corresponding to the Larmor frequency of tissue being suppressed are given just before the normal 90° spin-echo pulse. For instance, fat protons precess 220 hertz slower than water protons. When a selective frequency pulse corresponding to fat protons is given then as in the presaturation approach, such a tissue will experience two 90° pulses and will be flipped 180°, again yielding no signal. One disadvantage of this technique is that it usually requires longer TR and increased scan times. Also, there is additional RF heating in the patient from the additional RF pulses.

## NULL POINT TECHNIQUES

Advantage can be taken of null points in the inversion recovery pulse sequence. As seen in Fig. 2-10C, such null (or bounce) points yield zero signal at the appropriate $T_1$ time. The required $T_1$ time to produce a null is merely 0.693 multiplied by the tissue $T_1$ to be suppressed. Example of this is the short time inversion recovery (STIR) and fluid attenuated inversion recovery (FLAIR) pulse sequence. The STIR sequence is designed to null fat with a $T_1$ of ≈200 milliseconds at 1.5 tesla. The appropriate $T_1$ would then be $0.693 \times 200 \approx 140$ milliseconds. The FLAIR pulse sequence is also an inversion recovery null point technique. This, however, is directed to nulling other nonfat tissues, an example of the latter being suppression of CSF to bring out periventricular hyperintense lesions such as MS plaques.

Some of the advantages of inversion recovery null technique other than nulling tissues desired is that no extra RF heating occurs such as in spectral presaturation. Neither is it as sensitive to magnetic field inhomogeneities as is spectral presaturation. Disadvantages, however, include long TR times and thus long scan times, low signal-to-noise ratio, and suppression of other tissues with similar $T_1$ values as that which is being nulled.

## MAGNETIZATION TRANSFER

Magnetization transfer is a technique to suppress protein-bound water. It is actually another example of frequency-selective chemical saturation. The effect, however, is more indirect. The basis for this technique is that bulk water (free water) is in rapid exchange with protein-bound water. If a frequency-selective pulse centered on protein-bound water is given, these bound water protons selectively transfer saturation to the bulk water protons and signals from these are suppressed, as these would then have experienced two 90° flips. An example of this technique includes suppression of background brain tissue to improve visualization of the smaller more peripheral vessels (Hashemi 1997). Magnetization transfer technique can also be used to study exchange dynamics between protein-bound and bulk water protons.

# INSTRUMENTATION

Figure 2-17 shows a block diagram of a typical MRI system. The major components consist of a large magnet providing the strong magnetic field, the radio-frequency generator and coil, a set of gradient coils with its power supply, and finally the computer, which serves as the control center along with its peripherals. As in CT, there is also a facility for image storage and multiformat or laser printing filming. Given these features, excitational RF energy is generated and made incident on the patient, the signal is detected, and the MR image is finally generated. The analog-to-digital converter (ADC) converts the analog RF signal to a digital form for computer processing. Since the video display is analog, the final image data must go through the digital-to-analogue converter (DAC). It is important to look closely at some of these instrument components.

## MAGNETS

Magnets are of three general types as currently configured for magnetic resonance imaging: permanent, resistive, and superconducting. They are quite distinct in their features (Table 2-12) and result in significant differences in possible field strengths, stability, and uniformity, as well as expense in their purchase and operation. In all cases, however, a relatively strong, uniform, and temporally stable magnetic field must be produced. To help establish magnetic field uniformity within the gantry and counteract the presence of magnetic field warping due to ferrous structures in the environment, a number of small coils (called shim coils) are usually incorporated at various spots within the gantry. Electric current is passed through these coils to create a series of small magnetic fields to balance any magnetic nonuniformities present.

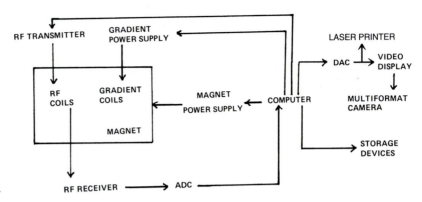

***Figure 2-17***  Block diagram of MRI imager.

The direction of the magnetic field, $B_0$, can be aligned either across the bore (transverse), as in the permanent as well as iron core resistive magnet types, or parallel to the bore (longitudinal), that is, from head to foot on the patient, as in superconducting magnets and certain earlier designs of air resistive magnets. These magnet types are now discussed.

## PERMANENT MAGNETS

Permanent magnets usually consist of two opposing north and south poles within which the patient may be placed. Two possible configurations are shown in Fig. 2-18*A*; these are the C and H types. The magnetic field in such configurations is confined between the two poles. These north and south poles are connected via the body of the magnet, creating a return path for the magnetic field lines. Because the magnetic field is directed and confined between the poles, the permanent magnet configuration will result in only minimal magnetic field levels outside and around the magnet. These stray magnetic fields are referred to as *fringe fields*. The lack of fringe fields greatly facilitates the operation of the MR scanner and the expenses related to its installation. This is true since the presence of fringe fields not only affects nearby instrumentation but can also pose a hazard, for instance, to persons wearing cardiac pacemakers. In addition, the interaction of the fringe fields with stationary ferrous structures (structural girders, ducts, etc.) and moving ferrous structures (vehicular traffic, elevators, etc.) warp the magnetic field within the magnet gantry. This results in detrimental effects on MR image quality. The continuing upkeep costs for permanent magnets, however, are expected to be relatively low since no field driving electrical power is necessary as in electromagnets nor are cryogen replacement costs necessary; as is true for superconducting systems.

One possible disadvantage of the permanent magnet approach is its relatively large weight (up to and beyond 100,000 pounds). One saving grace, however, concerning weight is that these magnets can usually be shipped and installed in smaller pieces. Another factor is temperature sensitivity; the magnet must be kept under controlled temperature conditions.

## Table 2-12   Major Advantages and Disadvantages of Various Magnet Types

| TYPE | ADVANTAGES | DISADVANTAGES |
|---|---|---|
| Permanent | Low fringe fields<br>Relatively inexpensive upkeep<br>No cryogens<br>Transverse field (enhanced SNR coils) | Limited field strength<br>Relatively heavy<br>Temperature-sensitive |
| Resistive (iron core) | Good field uniformity<br>Relatively inexpensive<br>No cryogens<br>Transverse field possible | Limited field strength (up to 0.6 T)<br>Field not as stable<br>Electrical costs higher |
| Superconducting | Very high fields possible<br>High field uniformity<br>Very stable field | Expensive to buy and maintain<br>Expensive site preparation<br>Cryogens needed<br>Quenchable<br>Fringe field problem |

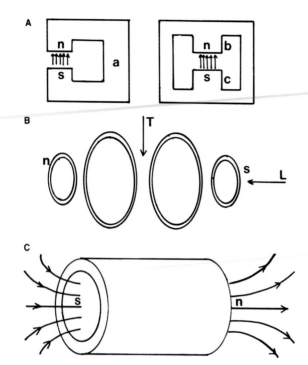

**Figure 2-18** **A.** Permanent magnet of either the C (*left*) or H (*right*) type of pole configurations. These confine the magnetic field between the pole faces. The return path for the magnetic flux is through the body of the magnet, and very little fringe magnetic field is produced. To obtain an iron-core resistive magnet a coil of wire is placed either at **a** or at **b** and **c** for nonpermanent magnet poles. **B.** Air-resistive magnets are configured with air core Helmholtz coils (two central coils) or a four-coil arrangement as seen above. These coils are arranged around the gantry, and flowing current through these coils generates the desired magnetic field. If the patient is placed along T, a transverse field results. If the patient is placed along L, a longitudinal field results. **C.** Fringe fields produced by air-core resistive and superconducting systems. There is no internal magnetic field line return path. Such a path must be established outside the gantry. Superconducting magnets have coil configured solenoidally around gantry. Magnetic field is maintained without need for continuing electrical current or power. Patient is placed within bore of magnet, and magnetic field is longitudinal (along long axis of patient). Significant fringe fields are produced in both superconducting and air-core resistive magnets.

Permanent magnets can be made from ceramic materials or rare earth materials. The latter, however, tend to be more costly and weigh more. Alnico magnets are not used because of possible gradual loss of their field strength. Using permanent magnets means that magnetic field quenching is not a problem. The quenching phenomenon possibility is characteristic of superconducting systems whereby the superconducting state suddenly ceases and there is a sudden reduction and collapse of the magnetic field. Quenching may result in damage to the magnet as well as significant amounts of down time. A very serious drawback of permanent magnet systems is the limitation on magnetic fields possible. Such systems at present operate at a maximum of 0.3 to 0.4 T.

One additional very important feature of permanent magnets is the fact that since the magnetic field is confined within and directed between the pole faces, simple cylindrical RF coils can be designed that provide greater inherent signal-to-noise characteristics (two to three times better) and correspondingly better image quality. This serves to offset somewhat the inherent advantages in signal-to-noise ratio obtainable at higher field strengths characteristic of superconducting systems.

## RESISTIVE MAGNETS

Air-core resistive magnets are configured with a series of wire coils. These coils are referred to as Helmholtz coils. They are arranged as seen in Fig. 2-18*B*. As an electric current flows through the coils, a magnetic field is produced whose direction is perpendicular to the plane of the coils. For optimal field uniformity, the coils should be arranged such that their diameters fall on the surfaces of a sphere. At least four coils in air (air core) are used as a sufficient approximation to produce a homogeneous field. These four coils consist of two large-diameter coils and two of smaller diameter. For clinical scanning, the complete spherical coil arrangement cannot be utilized, as there must be at least an opening for the patient. Magnets produced by passing electrical current through wire coils are referred to as resistive, since copper from which the coil wires are made provides for a small but not insignificant amount of electrical resistance and therefore power consumption. The magnitude of the magnetic field is proportional to the magnitude of the current. The electric power consumption, however, varies as the square of the current. Thus doubling the magnetic field strength would require quadrupling the electric power needed to drive the magnets. In addition, considerable heat is produced. The wire coils may in fact be made of hollow copper tubing that allows cooling water to run through to carry off the heat generated. Because of the electrical and heat production problems, air-core resistive magnets are typically limited to field strengths of only up to 0.15 to 0.20 T.

Resistive magnets can be configured such that the magnetic field can be either longitudinal (along the length of the patient) or transverse (perpendicular to the patient). The transverse arrangement is obtained by placing the patient at the center of the coils perpendicular to the field lines. To obtain the longitudinal arrangement, the patient is placed down through the bore of the coils parallel to the field lines.

One important concern with air-core magnets is that fringe fields are produced. There is no internal path for magnetic field lines, and such a path is established outside the gantry.

Air-core resistive magnets are no longer used and have been supplanted entirely by other designs. Iron-core systems, on the other hand, have become more and more popular because of their lower costs and relatively good imaging performance.

Iron-core resistive magnets are accomplished by placing solenoidal coils at region **a** for a C arrangement and at regions **b** and **c** for an H arrangement, as seen in Fig. 2-18A. These iron-core resistive magnets have the advantage of providing a return path for the magnetic field lines and thus have minimal fringe fields beyond the gantry. Additionally, the advantages of these are relatively uniform and stable fields. At present, though, these features are not as optimal as is found in superconducting systems. The magnetic field alignment between the pole faces provides for greater signal-to-noise RF coil design, as is true for permanent magnets.

## SUPERCONDUCTING MAGNETS

Superconducting magnet systems operate at very low temperature (near absolute zero). At these temperatures, some metals lose all electrical resistance and flow without additional energy being expended. Under these conditions, very large currents can flow and therefore very large magnetic fields can be produced. Typical units can operate between 0.5 and 2.0 T, but there are prototype imaging units operating up to 4.0 T. The fringe field problem is present in superconductive systems and is even more critical as these systems operate at much higher magnetic field levels. Fringe fields come right out of magnet bore and out into the environment (Fig. 2-18C). Unlike air-core Helmholtz coil pair resistive systems, the main field coils are configured in the much simpler solenoidal fashion. This is necessary because of the considerable forces which individual coils would experience. This could result in warping of the coils and the magnetic field. In any case, because of the high current possible with superconducting systems, the efficiency of Helmholtz coil pairs is not needed. Additionally, for human lengths and for large bores, the solenoidal configuration is sufficient (Crooks 1984; Kaufman 1981). Superconducting systems must be provided with a cryogenic environment to maintain the low temperatures necessary. The coils are thus immersed in liquid helium and surrounded by a vacuum and then a bath of liquid nitrogen. Nitrogen serves to absorb the heat from the environment and maintain the necessary low temperatures for helium. If there is a loss of helium or loss of the vacuum, the system rises in temperature and the superconducting state is eventually lost, with a resultant collapse of the magnetic field. This is referred to as a *quench,* and large electric currents can flow through the conductor, which would then revert to operating in the resistive temperature producing mode. Meltdown of the conductor is then possible and must be prevented. The material used for the superconductor is NbTi embedded in a copper matrix. In the superconductor state, the copper serves as a heat conductor and the current flow is through the NbTi. When superconductivity is lost, the excess currents flow through the copper and damage to NbTi is avoided. An even more serious possible consequence of a field quench is the possibility of electrocuting the patient. This is possible since large electrical currents will be induced in tissues by rapidly changing magnetic fields. To avoid such consequences of a quench, a soft quench feature is engineered into MRI systems. Under these conditions the loss of the magnetic field is gradual rather than rapid.

In addition to high field strengths, another advantage of superconducting systems is the high stability and very high uniformity of the field.

Among the disadvantages is the relatively high cost of purchase and the continuing high cost of operating the system due to cryogen replacement expenses. Because of the large fringe fields produced, siting is also a problem, though this has been minimized recently by using magnetic field containment systems around the magnet gantry or around the room. These field containment systems consist of steel structures that soak up the magnetic fields and greatly reduce the fringe field beyond the containment area. The need for magnetic field steel shielding should not be confused with the need for RF field shielding. Because of the high sensitivity to RF fields necessary in MR scanning, it is necessary to shield the gantry from external RF energy such as from radio and TV broadcasts and power lines. RF shielding is simply accomplished by incorporating copper within the iron shield around the magnet. An older approach was to place copper plates around walls (similar to lead shielding for x-ray rooms).

## Gradient Coils

As previously discussed, three gradients, one in each of three directions, must be available to perform MR imaging. These gradients are produced with special additional coils that produce a linearly varying magnetic field superimposed on the uniform main magnetic field. The magnitude of this gradient field is relatively low and is usually between 0.5 and 1 G/cm (5 to 20 mT/m). A linear gradient can be sufficiently approximated in the magnetic field direction with a Maxwell coil pair. This coil pair is similar to a Helmholtz coil arrangement except that the electric current is flowing in opposite directions. The other two gradients are produced using two Golay coils (Golay 1971). Golay coils consist of opposing coil loops with parallel sides wrapped around the gantry. These coils are displaced

field gradients; psychological effects such as claustrophobia, anxiety, and panic disorders; the potential risks of scanning pregnant women; and monitoring physiologic parameters during MR procedures (Shellock 1994a).

Four areas relating to the use of MR systems have been identified by the FDA. The safety guidelines from the FDA Safety Parameter Action Levels include the static magnetic field, the gradient magnetic fields, the RF power of the examination, and the acoustic considerations (FDA 1998).

## BIOEFFECTS OF STATIC MAGNETIC FIELDS

Data are scarce concerning the effects of high-intensity static magnetic (SM) fields on humans. SM fields have no effect on human *skin and body temperatures* up to 1.5 T (Shellock 1989). Electric induction and *cardiac* effects are caused by the flow of blood through a magnetic field. The induced biopotential is exhibited by an augmentation of T-wave amplitude, as well as by other nonspecific waveform changes that are apparent on the ECG and have been observed at SM field strengths as low as 0.1 T (Keltner 1990). The increase in T-wave amplitude is directly related to intensity of the SM fields. Also, these ECG voltage abnormalities revert to normal once the patient is no longer exposed to the SM fields. No circulatory alterations appear to coincide with these ECG changes in fields up to 2.0 T (Mezrich 1985). Theoretically, electrical impulse conduction in *nerve tissue* may be affected by exposure to SM fields. At present, exposures to SM fields of up to 2.0 T do not appear to significantly influence bioelectrical properties of neurons in humans (Hong 1990; Muller 1990; Vogel 1991). There is no evidence of neuropsychiatric, cognitive function, acute or chronic behavioral changes, or memory alterations. In summary, there is no conclusive evidence of irreversible or hazardous biologic effects related to acute, short-term exposures of humans to SM field strengths up to 2.0 T. However, possible bioeffects on 3.0- to 4.0-T whole-body MR systems need further research (Schenk 1991).

## BIOEFFECTS OF GRADIENT MAGNETIC FIELDS

According to Faraday's law of induction a gradient magnetic (GM) field can induce electrical fields and currents in conductive media (i.e., biologic tissue) during transient application of magnetic field gradients in MR imaging sequences. The induced current between GM fields and biological tissue in human subjects is proportional to the conductivity of the biological tissue and the rate of change of the magnetic flux density. Bioeffects can be due to the power deposited by induced currents (thermal effects) or to direct effects of the current (nonthermal effects). Thermal effects due to switched gradients used in MR procedures are negligible and are not believed to be clinically significant (Bottomley 1981; Schaefer 1988; Persson 1989). Possible nonthermal effects, including nerve stimulation and ventricular fibrillation, are known to have much higher threshold currents than those with routine clinical MR procedures. Seizure induction threshold and reversible nerve damage seem to require significantly higher current densities (Budinger 1979, 1981, 1983). The production of magnetophosphenes is considered to be one of the most sensitive physiologic responses to GM fields. These visual sensations supposedly caused by electrical stimulation of the retina and are completely reversible with no associated health effects. Although no reported cases of magnetophosphenes for fields of 1.95 T or less are known, they have been reported in volunteers working in and around a 4.0 T system (Redington 1988). Additional metallic taste and vertigo seem to be reproducible in these 4.0-T systems.

Echoplanar techniques expose patients to considerably increased levels of induced voltages. Sensory and direct skeletal muscle stimulation has been induced from echoplanar imaging sequences (Budinger 1991; Ehrhardt 1993).

## BIOEFFECTS OF RADIO-FREQUENCY ELECTROMAGNETIC FIELDS

General bioeffects of radio-frequency (RF) electromagnetic fields are related to the thermogenic and athermal field-specific alterations in biologic systems (NCRP 1986; Erwin 1988, Gordon 1984, 1987, 1988). With regard to RF power deposit concerns, specific absorption rate (SAR) determines quantified exposure to RF radiation in units of watts per kilogram. RF power used during an MR procedure is typically expressed as both "whole-body averages" and "local" SAR (Gordon 1987). During MR procedures, tissue heating results primarily from magnetic induction with a negligible contribution from the electrical fields, so that ohmic heating is greatest at the surface of the body and approaches zero at the center of the body (Shellock 1986, 1989, 1994).

Thermoregulatory response due to RF power absorption during MR procedures reveals that conscious adults are different from sedated and anesthetized pediatric patients. This is also quite dissimilar to laboratory animals (Gordon 1988). Physiologic responses of patients with conditions that may impair thermoregulatory function may require additional studies prior to subjection to higher SAR.

The testes and the eye are temperature-sensitive organs because of their reduced capabilities of heat dissipation. Scrotal skin and corneal temperature changes are below the threshold known to impair testicular-function (Berman 1984) or cause thermal damage in ocular tissue, including cataractogenic effect (NCRP 1986; Gordon 1984).

RF radiation hot spots are caused by the uneven distribution of RF power and RF radiation absorption mainly by peripheral tissues. Thermoregulatory systems apparently disturb the thermal load, producing a "smearing" effect of the surface temperatures. No evidence of surface thermal hot spots related to MR procedures is demonstrated in humans (Shellock 1986, Schaefer 1986).

## MR PROCEDURES AND ACOUSTIC NOISE

The repetitive sound produced by the activation and deactivation of electric current induces vibrations of the gradient coils. This is enhanced by higher gradient duty cycles and sharper pulse transitions, and is increased with thinner section thickness, decreased fields of view, repetition times and echo times. The sound levels varied from 82 to 93 dB on the A-weighted scale and from 84 to 103 dB on the linear scale (Hurwitz 1989).

Other acoustic noise associated with the MR system are related to the cryogen reclamation systems and pulsed radiation i.e., "RF hearing," "RF sound," or "microwave hearing" (Elder 1984; Roschmann 1991). Since the GM field-induced noise is primarily responsible for acoustic noise in the MR environment, the safest and least expensive means of providing a sufficient decrease in acoustic noise during MR procedures is to use routinely the disposable ear plugs, which can abate noise by 10 to 20 dB and prevent the potential temporary loss associated with MR procedures (Brummett 1988). MR-compatible headphones are also available for routine use. "Antinoise" or destructive interference technique is an acceptable alternative with a reduction of noise as much as 50 to 70% in the sound level perceived by the ear (Goldman 1989).

## IMPLANTS, DEVICES, AND FOREIGN BODIES

The FDA also requires labeling of MR systems to show that the device is contraindicated for patients who have electrically, magnetically activated implants, because electromagnetic fields produced by the system may interfere with the operation of these devices (FDA 1988). MR compatibility of metallic implants, materials, foreign bodies, and various biomedical devices should be carefully evaluated prior to the MR procedures. Table 3-1 provides a summary of pertinent information.

Only the fragment measuring $3.0 \times 1.0 \times 1.0$ mm rotated, but it did not cause any discernible damage to the ocular tissue in laboratory animals during exposure to a 2.0 T MR system (Williams 1988). Intraocular metallic fragments as small as $0.1 \times 0.1 \times 0.1$ mm are detected using standard plain film radiographs. Therefore, screening patients with possible intraocular metallic foreign bodies using plain film radiography may be an acceptable technique with minimal, if any, risks (Shellock 1991, 1994; Williamson 1994). Any patients with occupational, educational, recreational, or known accidental orbital exposure to metallic fragments should be evaluated with radiographs of the orbits. Psychotic, demented, or unreliable patients should also continue to undergo screening studies (Murphy 1996).

## USE OF MRI IN PREGNANCY

No definite association has been demonstrated between SM fields and any deleterious biological effects in human embryo (Baker 1994), although studies have shown some teratologic effects of high-field-strength MR imaging in the developing chick and mouse embryo (YIP 1994). MR imaging has been performed in normal human fetuses without deleterious effects (Baker 1994; Hubbard 1997). However, the maternal-fetal safety of MR imaging during pregnancy has not been established by the FDA (1988). MR imaging may be used cautiously in pregnant women after a critical assessment of the relative, perhaps theoretical, risks versus the indications and benefits of the examination, as well as an alternative to other procedures requiring ionizing radiation exposure (Shellock 1991). Complete disclosure of the limited evidence and experience in this area and the patient's consent are required prior to MR imaging.

It is well known that a fetus in the first trimester is highly susceptible to damage from different types of physical agents. Therefore, in Great Britain, the National Radiological Protection Board has specified that "It might be prudent to exclude pregnant women during the first three months of pregnancy" (NCRP 1986; Erwin 1988). Particular care should be exercised with the use of MR procedures in this period because of potential medicolegal implications related to spontaneous abortions in the first trimester, the rate of which is also high in the general population (Wilcox 1988).

## Table 3-1    List of Implants, Materials, Devices, and Objects Tested **Positive** for Attraction/Deflection Forces During Exposure to Static Magnetic Fields

| IMPLANT, MATERIAL, DEVICE, OR OBJECT | HIGHEST FIELD STRENGTH (T) |
| --- | --- |
| **Aneurysm and hemostatic clips** | |
| Downs multi-positional (15-7PH) | 1.39 |
| Drake (DR 14, DR 21) (Edward Weck, Triangle Park, NJ) | 1.39 |
| Drake (DR 16) (Edward Weck) | 0.147 |
| Drake (301 SS) (Edward Weck) | 1.5 |
| Heifetz (17-7PH) (Edward Weck) | 1.89 |
| Housepian | 0.147 |
| Kapp (405 SS) (V. Mueller) | 1.89 |
| Kapp, curved (404 SS) (V. Mueller) | 1.39 |
| Kapp, straight (404 SS) (V. Mueller) | 1.39 |
| Mayfield (301 SS) (Codman, Randolf, MA) | 1.5 |
| Mayfield (304 SS) (Codman) | 1.89 |
| McFadden (301 SS) (Codman) | 1.5 |
| Pivot (17-7PH) | 1.89 |
| Scoville (EN58J) (Downs Surgical, Inc., Decatur, GA) | 1.89 |
| Sundt-Kees (301 SS) (Downs Surgical, Inc.) | 1.5 |
| Sundt-Kees Multi-Angle (17-7PH) (Downs Surgical, Inc.) | 1.89 |
| Vari-Angle (17-7PH) (Codman) | 1.89 |
| Vari-Angle Micro (17-7PM SS) (Codman) | 0.15 |
| Vari-Angle Spring (17-7PM SS) (Codman) | 0.15 |
| | |
| **Biopsy needles and devices** | |
| Adjustable, Automated Biopsy Gun—6, 13, and 19 mm (304 SS) (MD Tech, Watertown, MA) | 1.5 |
| Adjustable, Automated Aspiration Biopsy Gun—10, 15, and 20 mm (304 SS) (MD Tech) | 1.5 |
| ASAP 16, Automatic 16 G Core Biopsy System—19 cm length (304 SS) | 1.5 |
| Automatic Cutting Needle with Depth Markings—14 G, 10 cm length (304 SS) (Manan, Northbrook, IL) | 1.5 |
| Automatic Cutting Needle with Ultrasound Tip & Depth Markings—18 G, 16 cm length (304 SS) (Manan) | 1.5 |
| Automatic Cutting Needle with Ultrasound Tip & Depth Markings—18 G, 20 cm length (304 SS) (Manan) | 1.5 |
| Basic II Hookwire Breast Localization Needle (304 SS) (MD Tech) | 1.5 |
| Beaded Breast Localization Wire Set—20 G, 2 inch needle with 5-7/8 inch wire (304 SS) (Inrad, Grand Rapids, MI) | 1.5 |
| Beaded Breast Localization Wire Set—19 G, 3-1/2 inch needle with 7-7/8 inch wire (304 SS) (Inrad) | 1.5 |
| Biopsy Gun—13 mm (Meadox, Oakland, NJ) | 1.5 |
| Biopsy Gun—25 mm (Meadox) | 1.5 |
| Biopsy Needle—17 G, 10 cm length (Meadox) | 1.5 |
| Biopsy Needle—20 G, 15 cm length (Meadox) | 1.5 |
| Biopsy Needle—22 G, 15 cm length (Meadox) | 1.5 |
| Biopsy Needle—22 G, 15 cm (Cook, Inc., Bloomington, IN) | 1.5 |
| Biopsy-Cut Biopsy Needle—14 G, 10 cm length (304 SS) (C.R. Bard, Inc., Covington, GA) | 1.5 |
| Biopsy-Cut Biopsy Needle—16 G, 16 cm length (304 SS) (C.R. Bard, Inc.) | 1.5 |
| Biopsy-Cut Biopsy Needle—18 G, 18 cm length (304 SS) (C.R. Bard, Inc.) | 1.5 |
| Biopsy-Cut Biopsy Needle with centimeter markings—18 G, 20 cm length (304 SS) (C.R. Bard, Inc.) | 1.5 |
| Breast Localization Needle—20 G, 5 cm length (304 SS) (Manan) | 1.5 |
| Breast Localization Needle—20 G, 7 cm length (304 SS) (Manan) | 1.5 |
| Chiba Needle with HiLiter Ultrasound Enhancement—22 G, 3-7/8 inch needle (304 SS) (Inrad) | 1.5 |
| Coaxial Needle Set Chiba-type needle—22 G, 5-7/8 inch needle (304 SS) (Inrad) | 1.5 |
| Coaxial Needle Set Introducer Needle—19G, 2-15/16 inch needle (304 SS) (Inrad) | 1.5 |
| Cutting Needle—14 G, 9 cm length (West Coast Medical, Laguna Beach, CA) | 1.5 |

## Table 3-1 *Continued.*

| IMPLANT, MATERIAL, DEVICE, OR OBJECT | HIGHEST FIELD STRENGTH (T) |
|---|---|
| **Biopsy needles and devices (continued)** | |
| Cutting Needle—16 G, 17 mm length (304 SS) (BIP USA, Inc., Niagara Falls, NY) | 1.5 |
| Cutting Needle—16 G, 19 mm length (304 SS) (BIP USA, Inc.) | 1.5 |
| Cutting Needle—18 G, 100 mm length (Meadox) | 1.5 |
| Cutting Needle—18 G, 150 mm length (Meadox) | 1.5 |
| Cutting Needle—18 G, 9 cm length (West Coast Medical) | 1.5 |
| Cutting Needle—18 G, 15 cm length (West Coast Medical) | 1.5 |
| Cutting Needle—19 G, 6 cm length (West Coast Medical) | 1.5 |
| Cutting Needle—19 G, 9 cm length (West Coast Medical) | 1.5 |
| Cutting Needle—19 G, 15 cm length (West Coast Medical) | 1.5 |
| Cutting Needle—20 G, 9 cm length (West Coast Medical) | 1.5 |
| Cutting Needle—20 G, 15 cm length (West Coast Medical) | 1.5 |
| Cutting Needle—20 G, 20 cm length (West Coast Medical) | 1.5 |
| Cutting Needle & Gun — 18 G, 155 mm length (Meadox) | 1.5 |
| Hawkins Blunt Needle (304 SS) (MD Tech) | 1.5 |
| Hawkins III Breast Localization Needle (MD Tech) | 1.5 |
| Percucut Biopsy Needle and Stylet—19.5 gauge 3 10 cm (316L SS) (E-Z-Em, Inc.) | 1.5 |
| Percucut Biopsy Needle and Stylet—21 gauge 3 10 cm (316L SS) (E-Z-Em, Inc.) | 1.5 |
| Sadowsky Breast Marking System—20 G, 5 cm length needle and 7 inch hook wire (316L SS) (Ranfac Corportion Avon, MA) | 1.5 |
| Soft Tissue Biopsy Needle Gun & Needle (304 SS) (Anchor Products Co. Addison, IL) | 1.5 |
| Trocar Needle (304 SS) (BIP USA, Inc.) | 1.5 |
| Trocar·Needle, Disposable (SS) Cook, Inc.) | 1.5 |
| Ultra-Core, biopsy needle 16 G, 16 cm length (304 SS) (MD Tech, Gainesville, FL) | 1.5 |
| **Breast tissue expanders and implants** | |
| Infall, breast implant (inflatable) (magnetic port) 3101198 Model (Heyerschultzz) | 1.5 |
| Tissue expander with magnetic port (McGhan Medical Corporation) | 1.5 |
| **Carotid artery vascular clamps** | |
| Crutchfield (SS)* (Codman) | 1.5 |
| Kindt (SS)* (V. Mueller) | 1.5 |
| Poppen-Blaylock (SS)* (Codman) | 1.5 |
| Salibi (SS)* (Codman) | 1.5 |
| Selverstone (SS)* (Codman) | 1.5 |
| **Dental devices and materials** | |
| Brace band (SS)* (American Dental, Missoula, MT) | 1.5 |
| Brace wire (chrome alloy)* (Ormco Corp., San Marcos, CA) | 1.5 |
| Castable alloy* (Golden Dental Products, Inc., Golden, CO) | 1.5 |
| Cement-in keeper* (Solid State Innovations, Inc., Mt. Airy, NC) | 1.5 |
| GDP Direct Keeper, Pre-formed post* (Golden Dental Products, Inc.) | 1.5 |
| Keeper, pre-formed post* (Parkell Products, Inc., Farmingdale, NY) | 1.5 |
| Magna-Dent, large indirect keeper* (Dental Ventures of America, Yorba Linda, CA) | 1.5 |
| Palladium clad magnet* (Parkell Products, Inc., Farmingdale, NY) | 1.5 |
| Palladium/palladium keeper* (Parkell Products, Inc.) | 1.5 |
| Palladium/platinum casting alloy* (Parkell Products, Inc.) | 1.5 |
| Stainless steel clad magnet (Parkell Products, Inc.) | 1.5 |

*(continued on next page)*

## Table 3-1　*Continued.*

| IMPLANT, MATERIAL, DEVICE, OR OBJECT | HIGHEST FIELD STRENGTH (T) |
|---|---|
| **Dental devices and materials** *(continued)* | |
| Stainless steel keeper* (Parkell Products, Inc.) | 1.5 |
| Titanium clad magnet (Parkell Products, Inc.) | 1.5 |
| | |
| **Halo vests and cervical fixation devices** | |
| Ambulatory Halo System[a] (AOA Co., Greenwood, SC) | 1.5 |
| EXO adjustable collar[a] (Florida Manufacturing Co., Daytona, FL) | 1.0 |
| Guilford cervical orthosis[a] (Guilford & Son, Ltd., Cleveland, OH) | 1.0 |
| S.O.M.I. cervical orthosis[a] (U.S. Manufacturing Co., Pasadena, CA) | 1.0 |
| | |
| **Heart valve prostheses** | |
| Beall* (Coratomic Inc., Indiana, PA) | 2.35 |
| Bjork-Shiley (universal/spherical)* (Shiley Inc.) | 1.5 |
| Bjork-Shiley, Model MBC* (Shiley Inc.) | 2.35 |
| Bjork-Shiley Model 22 MBRC 11030* (Shiley Inc.) | 2.35 |
| Carpentier-Edwards, Model 2650* (American Edwards Laboratories, Santa Ana, CA) | 2.35 |
| Carpentier-Edwards (porcine)* (American Edwards Laboratories, Baxter Healthcare Corporation) | 2.35 |
| Hall-Kaster, Model A7700* (Medtronic, Minneapolis, MN) | 1.5 |
| Hancock I (porcine)* (Johnson & Johnson, Anaheim, CA) | 1.5 |
| Hancock II (porcine)* (Johnson & Johnson) | 1.5 |
| Hancock extracorporeal Model 242R* (Johnson & Johnson) | 2.35 |
| Hancock extracorporeal Model M 4365-33* (Johnson & Johnson) | 2.35 |
| Inonescu-Shiley, Universal ISM* | 2.35 |
| Lillehi-Kaster, Model 300S (Medical Inc., Inver Grove Heights, MN) | 2.35 |
| Lillehi-Kaster, Model 5009* (Medical Inc.) | 2.35 |
| Medtronic Hall* (Medtronic Inc.) | 2.35 |
| Medtronic Hall Model A7700-D-16* (Medtronic Inc.) | 2.35 |
| Omnicarbon, Model 35231029* (Medical Inc.) | 2.35 |
| Omniscience, Model 6522* (Medical Inc.) | 2.35 |
| Smeloff-Cutter* (Cutter Laboratories, Berkeley, CA) | 2.35 |
| Sorin, No. 23* | 1.5 |
| Starr-Edwards, Model 1000* (Baxter Healthcare Corporation) | 1.5 |
| Starr-Edwards, Model 1200* (Baxter Healthcare Corporation) | 1.5 |
| Starr-Edwards, Model 1260* (American Edwards Laboratories, Baxter Healthcare Corporation) | 2.35 |
| Starr-Edwards, Model 2300* (Baxter Healthcare Corporation) | 1.5 |
| Starr-Edwards, Model 2310* (Baxter Healthcare Corporation) | 1.5 |
| Starr-Edwards, Model 2320* (American Edwards Laboratories, Baxter Healthcare Corporation) | 2.35 |
| Starr-Edwards, Model Pre 6000* (American Edwards Laboratories, Baxter Healthcare Corporation) | 2.35 |
| Starr-Edwards, Model 6000* (Baxter Healthcare Corporation) | 1.5 |
| Starr-Edwards, Model 6120* (Baxter Healthcare  Corporation) | 1.5 |
| Starr-Edwards, Model 6300* (Baxter Healthcare Corporation) | 1.5 |
| Starr-Edwards, Model 6310* (Baxter Healthcare Corporation) | 1.5 |
| Starr-Edwards, Model 6320* (Baxter Healthcare Corporation) | 1.5 |
| Starr-Edwards, Model 6400* (Baxter Healthcare Corporation) | 1.5 |
| Starr-Edwards, Model 6520* (Baxter Healthcare Corporation) | 2.35 |
| St. Jude, Model A 101* (St. Jude (Medical Inc.) | 2.35 |
| St. Jude, Model M 101* (St. Jude (Medical Inc.) | 2.35 |

## Table 3-1   *Continued.*

| IMPLANT, MATERIAL, DEVICE, OR OBJECT | HIGHEST FIELD STRENGTH (T) |
|---|---|
| **Intravascular coils, filters, and stents** | |
| Cook occluding spring embolization coil, MWCE-338-5-10*† | 1.5 |
| Cook-Z Stent Gianturco-Rosch Biliary Design 10 mm × 3 cm*† (Cook, Inc.) | 1.5 |
| Cook-Z Stent Gianturco-Rosch Tracheobronchial Design 20 mm × 5 cm*† (Cook, Inc.) | 1.5 |
| Gianturco embolization coil*† (Cook, Inc.) | 1.5 |
| Gianturco bird nest IVC filter*† (Cook, Inc.) | 1.5 |
| Gianturco zig-zag stent*† (Cook, Inc.) | 1.5 |
| Greenfield vena cava filter, Stainless steel*† (MD Tech) | 1.5 |
| Gunther IVC filter*† (William Cook, Europe) | 1.5 |
| New retrievable IVC filter*† (Thomas Jefferson University, Philadelphia, PA) | 1.5 |
| Palmaz endovascular stent*† (Ethicon) | 1.5 |
| Palmaz-Shatz balloon-expandable stent*† (Johnson & Johnson Interventional) | 1.5 |
| **Ocular implants and devices** | |
| Fatio eyelid spring/wire | 1.5 |
| Retinal tack (SS-martensitic) (Western European) | 1.5 |
| Troutman magnetic ocular implant | 1.5 |
| Unitech round wire eye spring | 1.5 |
| **Orthopedic implants, materials, and devices** | |
| Perfix interence screw (17-4stainless steel, A 630-Cr17) (Instrument Makar, Okemos, MI) | 1.5 |
| **Otologic implants** | |
| Cochlear implant 3M/House | 0.6 |
| Cochlear implant 3M/Vienna | 0.6 |
| Cochlear implant Nucleus Mini 20-channel Cochlear Corporation Englewood, CO | 1.5 |
| McGee piston stapes prosthesis (platinum/Cr17-Ni4, SS) (Richards Medical Co.) | 1.5 |
| **Patent ductus arteriosus (PDA), atrial septal defect (ASD), and ventricular septal defect (VSD) occluders** | |
| Rashkind PDA Occlusion Implant 12 mm, lot n. 07IC1391, (304V SS)† (C.R. Bard, Inc., Billerica, MA) | 1.5 |
| Rashkind PDA Occlusion Implant 17 mm, lot no. 514486, (304V SS)† (C.R. Bard, Inc.) | 1.5 |
| Lock Clamshell Septal Occlusion Implant 17 mm, lot no. 07BCO321, (304 V SS)† (C.R. Bard, Inc.) | 1.5 |
| Lock Clamshell Septal Occlusion Implant 23 mm, lot no. 07CC1903, (304 V SS)† (C.R. Bard, Inc.) | 1.5 |
| Lock Clamshell Septal Occlusion Implant 28 mm, lot no. 07BC1557, (304 V SS)† (C.R. Bard, Inc.) | 1.5 |
| Lock Clamshell Septal Occlusion Implant 33 mm, lot no. 07AC1785, (304 V SS)† (C.R. Bard, Inc.) | 1.5 |
| Lock Clamshell Septal Occlusion Implant 40 mm, lot no. 07AC1785, (304 V SS)† (C.R. Bard, Inc.) | 1.5 |
| **Pellets and bullets** | |
| BB's (Daisy) | 1.5 |
| BB's (Crosman) | 1.5 |
| Bullet, 7.62 × 39 mm (copper, steel) (Norinco) | 1.5 |
| Bullet, .380 inch (copper, nickel, lead) (Remington) | 1.5 |
| Bullet, .45 inch (steel, lead) (Evansville Ordinance) | 1.5 |
| Bullet, 9 mm (copper, lead) (Norma) | 1.5 |

*(continued on next page)*

## Table 3-1   *Continued.*

| IMPLANT, MATERIAL, DEVICE, OR OBJECT | HIGHEST FIELD STRENGTH (T) |
|---|---|
| **Penile implants** | |
| Penile implant, Duraphase | 1.5 |
| Penile implant, OmniPhase (Dacomed Corp.) | 1.5 |
| | |
| **Vascular access ports and catheters** | |
| A Port Implantable Access System (titanium) (Therex Corporation, Walpole, MA) | 1.5 |
| Groshung Catheter* | 1.5 |
| Hickman Port (316L SS)* (Davol Inc.) | 1.5 |
| Q-Port (316L SS)* (Quinton Instrument Co., Seattle, WA) | 1.5 |
| | |
| **Miscellaneous** | |
| Cerebral ventricular shunt tube connector, (type unknown) | 0.147 |
| Contraceptive diaphragm All Flex* (Ortho Pharmaceutical, Raritan, NJ) | 1.5 |
| Contraceptive diaphragm Flat Spring* (Ortho Pharmaceutical) | 1.5 |
| Contraceptive diaphragm Koroflex* (Young Drug Products, Piscataway, NJ) | 1.5 |
| Flex-tip Plus Epidural catheter (304V SS)†† (Arrow International Inc., Reading, PA) | 1.5 |
| Scalpel (SS) | 1.5 |
| Shunt valve, Holtertype* (The Holter Co., Bridgeport, PA) | 1.5 |
| Sophy adjustable pressure valve | 1.5T |
| Super ArrowFlex PSI 9 Fr × 11 cm (304V SS)†† (Arrow International Inc.) | 1.5 |
| Super ArrowFlex PSI 10 Fr × 65 cm (304V SS)†† (Arrow International Inc.) | 1.5 |
| TheraCath (304V SS)†† (Arrow International Inc., Reading, PA) | 1.5 |
| Vascular marker, O-ring washer (302 SS)* (PIC Design, Middlebury, CT) | 1.5 |

*"Highest field strength" refers to the highest intensity of the static magnetic field that was used for the evaluation of deflection force, or magnetic field attraction of the various metallic implant materials, devices, or objects tested.*

*\*Denotes the metallic implants, materials, devices, or objects that were considered to be safe for patients undergoing MR procedures despite being attracted by static magnetic fields. For example, certain prosthetic heart valves were attracted to the magnetic fields but the attractive forces were considered to be less than the forces exerted on the prosthetic heart valves by the beating heart.*

*†Ferromagnetic coils, filters, stents, and cardiac occluders typically become firmly incorporated into the vessel wall several weeks following placement. Therefore, it is unlikely that they will be moved or dislodged by attraction to magnetic fields. Patients with coils, filters, and stents marked "*†" should wait a minimum 6 weeks prior to an MR procedure to assure firm implantation of the implant into the vessel wall.*

*††These devices are attracted to the static magnetic field of the MR system, however, because of the relative amount of attractive force and their in vivo use, these devices are unlikely to pose a hazard associated with dislodgement. The potential risk to performing MR procedures in patients with these devices is related to induced current and excessive heating. Therefore, it is inadvisable to perform MR procedures patients with these devices.*

*ª These halo vests are known to have ferromagnetic components. However, the relative amount of attraction to the magnetic field was not determined.*

*Manufacturer information was provided if known.*

*SS, Stainless steel.*

*SOURCE: From Shellock FG & Kanal E 1994 and 1996.*

*For complete list of all tested implants, materials, devices, and objects, please see source articles.*

A survey of female MR operators of child-bearing age did not show any deleterious effects from exposure to the SM field component of an MR system (Kanal 1993). The questionnaire addressed menstral and reproductive experiences as well as work activities. Therefore, it is recommended for a pregnant health care worker to enter the MR room but not to remain within the room or magnet bore during the actual operation of the device (Kanal 1993.).

## PSYCHOLOGICAL EFFECTS

A variety of psychological reactions, including claustrophobia and anxiety and panic disorders, may be encoun-

# Ref

BAKER PN, JC
follow-up o
magnetic res

BERMAN E: Re
diofrequency
Printing Offi
publication E

BORE PJ, GALL
gerous? Magi

BOTTOMLEY P,
body NMR im

BRUMMETT RE,
loss resulting f

BUDINGER T, C
health hazard:
A, Higgins C,
resonance im
and Education

BUDINGER T, FI
SCHMITT F: Pl
field gradients.

BUDINGER T, N
studies: known
sist Tomogr 5:8

BUDINGER T, Th
and magnetic
Nucl Sci NS-26

Committee on D
Guidelines for
patients during
peutic procedur

EHRHARDT J, LIN
Neural stimulati
system. In: Boc
nance in Medici
onance in Medic

ELDER JA. Special
Agency, Health I
fects of Radiofre
search Triangle P

ERWIN DN: Mech
quency electrom:
Environ Med 59(s

FDA: Magnetic res
mendation and re
Fed Regist 53:7575

tered in as many as 5 to 10 percent of patients undergoing MR procedures because of the nature of the MR system, the gradient-induced noises, and the restrictive conditions within the bore of the scanner (Scott 1996). An "open magnet" MR system may be of some help in this respect. Fortunately, adverse psychological responses to MR procedures are usually transient, although the rare report of two patients with persistent claustrophobia requiring long-term psychiatric treatment is noted (Fishbain 1988).

Several techniques have been developed to reduce the incidence of delay and cancellation of MR examination (Shellock 1991): (1) Brief the patient appropriately on the specific nature of the examination. If necessary, a preliminary visit to the site and the scanner may be of help. (2) Allow patients to have a friend or relative present in the scan room. (3) Have the technologist speak with the patient (through an intercom) after the completion of each series. (4) Make the patient as comfortable as possible because of the requirement to lie motionless for extended periods of time. (5) Suggest relaxation techniques to the patient. Such techniques could rely on controlled breathing or mental imagery (desensitization technique). (6) Use mirrors or a blindfold to help alleviate the feelings of "closed-in" surroundings. (7) Use headphones with music to decrease the noise created by the gradient coils and to serve as a distraction. Also, back projected video system has become commercially available recently. (8) Consider the use of short-acting sedation or anesthesia.

## PATIENT MONITORING DURING THE MR PROCEDURE

Frequently, monitoring of physiological parameters is required in patients who are sedated, anesthetized, comatose, critically ill, or otherwise unable to communicate with the system operator. Monitoring patients during MR procedures should be done by using MR-compatible monitors and should include heart rate, systemic blood pressure, respiratory rate, oxygen saturation, cutaneous blood flow, and temperature. MR-compatible monitoring devices including pulse oxemeter and ventilators are also available (Shellock 1996).

Monitors that contain ferromagnetic components can be attracted to the mid- and high-field MR systems, which may become potential projectiles. Since the intensity of standard static magnetic fields falls off as the third power of the distance from the magnet, placing the monitor at a suitable distance from the system should sufficiently prevent any possible hazards.

Electromagnetic noise from certain monitors can result in imaging artifacts, and looping of conductive leads, wires, and cables from various devices may induce potential burns, particularly in patients with decreased sensorium (Shellock 1994b).

## PEDIATRIC SEDATION

The elimination of patient motion is fundamental to optimal imaging of CT and MR. In general, all patients under 5 years of age and older, uncooperative patients require sedation. Three levels of sedation can be considered: (1) conscious sedation, (2) deep sedation, and (3) general anesthesia. Conscious sedation is most commonly utilized by nonanesthesiologists.

Following careful preparation of the child and family, documentation of risks, benefits, and alternatives, evaluation of clinical status (Table 3-2), selection of a sedative agent (Table 3-3) should be done with the safety of the patient as the primary consideration (Frush 1996). Despite the variety of acceptable options, no single sedative regimen is perfect. Currently, however, chloral hydrate is most frequently recommended in children up to 24 months old.

Preprocedural preparation, administration of selective agents, monitoring during sedation, and postprocedure care and discharge should be performed according to the guidelines of American Academy of Pediatrics' Committee on Drugs (AAPCOD) (1992) and the Joint Commission on Accreditation of Health Care Organizations (1995).

**Table 3-2    Risk Factors for Sedation**

| SYSTEM | RISK FACTOR |
|---|---|
| Respiratory | Pneumonia, chronic lung disease (asthma, bronchopulmonary dysplasia, aspiration), tracheal or bronchial narrowing |
| Cardiovascular | Cyanotic heart disease, congestive heart failure, hypotension |
| Neurologic | Central respiratory depression/apnea, seizures, increased intracranial pressure |
| Gastrointestinal | Gastrointestinal reflux, hepatic dysfunction |
| Genitourinary | Renal dysfunction, dehydration, electrolyte disturbance |
| Systemic/other | Sepsis, allergies, medications |
| Syndromic | Airway impairment (macroglossia, micrognathia); Restrictive lung disease: chest wall deformity, scoliosis |

SOURCE: Frush 1996.

Table 3

AGEN

Chloral
hydratec
Pentobarbit
sodium

Fentanyl
citrate

Midazolam

Diazepam

Methohexital
Morphine

Meperidine

Naloxone
hydrochlori

Flumazenil

*Note.—IM = in.*
a*Preferred rout*
b*Duration of se*
*istration.*
c*Thioridazine [*
SOURCE: *Frush 1*

## CRYOGI
## OF MR

*Liquid heli*
ical MR sys
perconducti
stat rises p
state at ap
1983). Gase
ably lighter
conductivity
sociated wit
helium gas
sure within t
cility. Also, p
to an increa
and frostbite

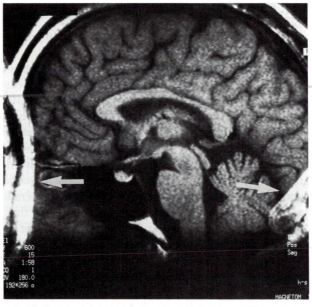

**Figure 3-4** Wrap-around (arrows) in the phase-encoding direction resulting from the use of an FOV smaller than the size of the head.

## PHASE-ENCODING DIRECTION

Aliasing in the phase-encoding direction (Fig. 3-4) is somewhat more difficult to comprehend. In the second on spatial frequency representation, Equations (4) through (6), it was shown that the signals as a function of the phase- and frequency-encoding directions are both representations of the imaged object in spatial frequency. in Equation (4) the $x$ direction information is encoded for each phase-encoding value $g_y$ by using $t$ as the independent variable and $k_x$ as the dependent variable ($k_x = \gamma g_x t$), while $g_x$ remains constant. That is, as time increases, a range of spatial frequencies is swept through. For the phase-encoding direction, $g_y$ is the independent variable which has discrete values $G_x/(N/2)$ (for a square pixel) and $T$ is a constant. However, as only the product $g_y T$ is used, the phase-encoding information can be thought of as time variable with the same aliasing problems that occur in the $x$ direction. It is more difficult to suppress the aliased information in the $y$ direction, since there is no equivalent receiver low-pass filter for data which are gathered discretely and since oversampling adds time to the scan.

To get a more intuitive feel for aliasing in the phase-encoding direction, consider a distribution of spins (Fig. 3-5) to which no gradient has been applied. Next, consider the spins' transverse orientation after the increment $\gamma g_y T$ has been applied. $g_y$ is chosen so that the variation in phase angle [Equation (3)] across the FOV is $2\pi$, causing a $\pm\pi$ rotation at the two extremes and intermediate values for $|y| < L/2$. The next time $2\gamma g_y T$ is applied, causing a $4\pi$ rotation across the FOV. Note that the spins at $\pm L/2$ are changing their sign every step; that is, $M_{xy}$ is oscillating at a frequency one-half

**Figure 3-5** Schematic representation of incremental applications of the phase-encoding gradient. *Top.* Spins are initially aligned after an FR pulse and no phase encoding. *Middle.* The smallest phase-encoding increment is applied, causing a $2\pi$ variation in the phase angle across the FOV, L. *Bottom.* Two units of the phase-encoding gradient have been applied, causing a $4\pi$ rotation across L. Note that the spins outside L mimic the behavior of those inside. This effect gives rise to aliasing, or wrap-around.

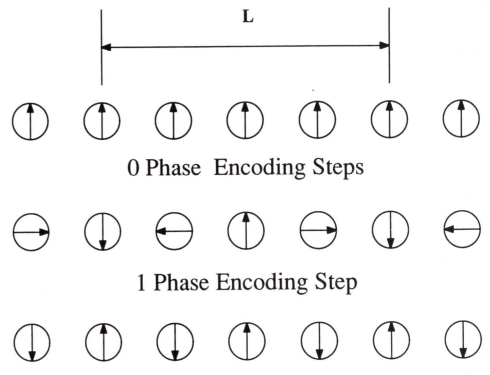

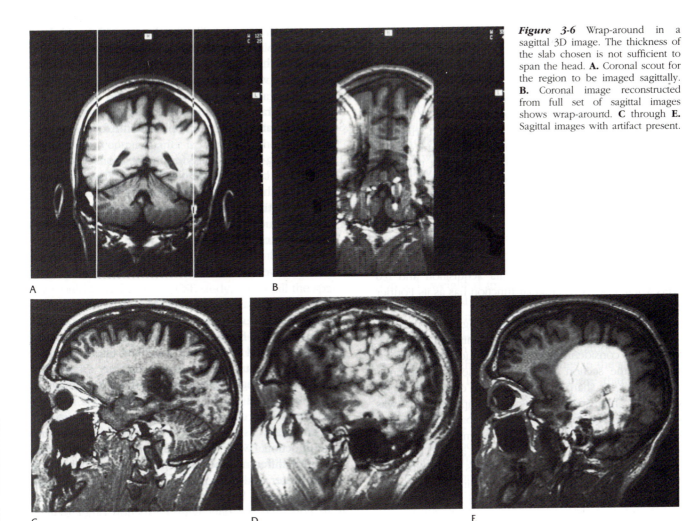

A    B    C    D    E

**Figure 3-6** Wrap-around in a sagittal 3D image. The thickness of the slab chosen is not sufficient to span the head. **A.** Coronal scout for the region to be imaged sagittally. **B.** Coronal image reconstructed from full set of sagittal images shows wrap-around. **C** through **E.** Sagittal images with artifact present.

that of the sampling rate. This is the highest frequency allowed by the Nyquist sampling theorem. However, the physical extent of the body may exceed $\pm L/2$. Note that these spins are indistinguishable from spins inside the FOV. That is, they oscillate at the same frequency and with the same phase and give rise to the familiar wraparound in the phase-encoding direction if the FOV in the $y$ direction is not great enough.

How can this be avoided? The simplest technique is to choose the FOV to be larger than the object or to eliminate the signal from those spins which are causing the aliasing. The latter is accomplished through the application of *presaturation pulses* to regions outside the FOV (Edelman 1988). Presaturation pulses are slice-selective 90° pulses that are followed by strong gradients which crush, or scramble, the transverse magnetization so that its net value within a voxel is approximately zero. The imaging sequence immediately follows these pulses.

An additional tehnique, sometimes referred to as *no-phase wrap* doubles the FOV and the number of phase-encoding steps and uses a half-Fourier method

to acquire the data and reconstruct the image. In this case only the top or bottom half of $k$ space is covered, so the scan time is unchanged, and mathematical methods are used to fill in the missing data.

## SLICE-SELECTION DIRECTION

In three-dimensional (3D) data acquisition, phase encoding is applied in the slice-selection direction. Thin contiguous slices are reconstructed by Fourier transformation in this direction. The use of a non-slice-selective RF pulse, which excites the whole volume, will lead to wrap-around if the dimension as determined by the 3D phase-encoding gradient is less than the physical extent of the object being imaged. It will appear (Fig. 3-6) as if two anatomic regions were superimposed in the same image.

This artifact can be eliminated by means of a careful choice of the slab thickness or minimized by using a slice-selective RF pulse to excite only the volume of interest. In the latter case some wrap-around may occur as a result of imperfect slice profiles (see the section

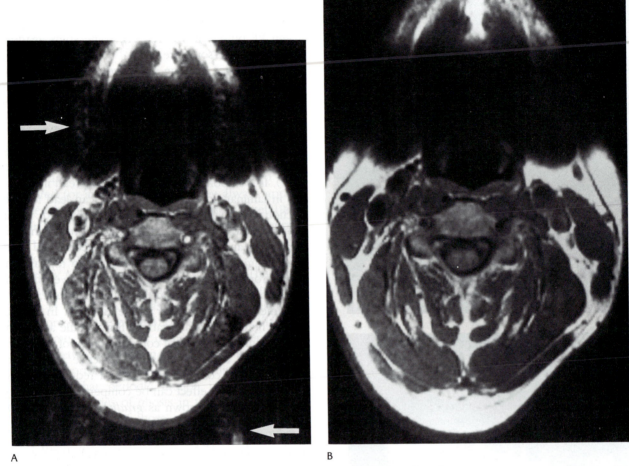

A                                                                        B

***Figure 3-10***   $T_1$-weighted spin-echo images of the cervical spine. **A.** Note the ghost artifacts due to blood flow (arrows). **B.** Application of presaturation regions superiorly and inferiorly has eliminated the blood signal and the accompanying ghosts.

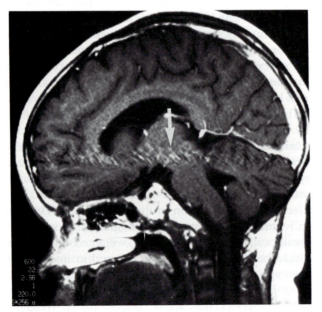

***Figure 3-11***   Flow artifact (arrow) due to CSF motion in a $T_1$-weighted spin-echo image after the administration of Gd-DTPA.

of little consequence, as static spins are generally not reduced in intensity.

To remove the effects of flow on MR images, three techniques are useful.

1. *ECG or pulse triggering.* Imaging is synchronized with the cardiac cycle so that blood or CSF motion is nearly identical form one phase-encoding step to the next and ghosts are eliminated. The limitation is that one has less control over the effective TR, which can vary through the image acquisition and is limited to being a multiple of the R-R interval.

2. *Presaturation of blood.* The effect of presaturation (a slice-selective 90° pulse followed by strong gradients to dephase the transverse magnetization) is to eliminate the signal from the blood. That is, if there is no blood signal, there is no ghost artifact. The elimination of ghosts and the blood signal are shown in Figs. 3-10 and 3-12.

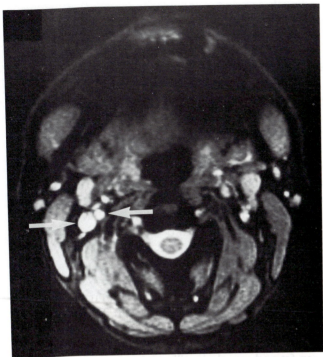

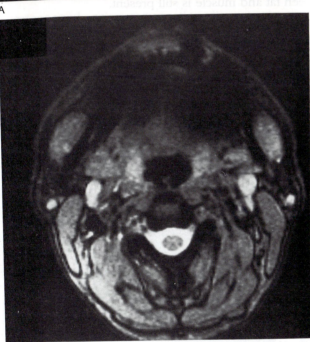

***Figure 3-12*** Gradient moment refocused FLASH images of the cervical spine (TR = 500, TE = 12, 15° flip angle). **A.** Note the bright appearance of the blood (arrows). **B.** Application of presaturation regions superiorly and inferiorly has eliminated the blood signal.

3. *Dephasing of moving spins.* This is the opposite of GMR. Instead of choosing the gradient amplitudes to rephase the transverse magnetization of the flowing spins, deliberately choose the amplitudes to dephase the magnetization of those spins. This tech-

nique is also used in MRA. Rephased and dephased images are acquired and subtracted from one another.

### EVEN ECHO REPHASING

There has been much discussion (Axel 1984; Waluch 1984; Katz 1987*a,b*) of the phenomenon known as *even echo rephasing*, which is related to GMR. It has been reported that in some circumstances of spin-echo imaging, the intensity of blood in the second echo of a double echo sequence is greater than it is in the first. It was necessary to have slow flow and for the second echo time to be equal to twice the first. Slow flow, or in-plane flow, is also necessary to avoid the wash-out effect.

The analyses done by Waluch (1984) and Axel (1984) do not represent the actual gradients used in an imaging sequence. Waluch analyzed the case of a constant magnetic field gradient. Axel considered this case as well as two 180° pulses with a slice-selection gradient applied. However, imaging is not done with gradients applied constantly, nor is it proper to ignore the gradients applied to the slice-selective 90° pulse. A more complete theoretical analysis of even-echo rephasing has been done by Katz (1987*a,b*) for both constant velocity and pulsatile flow, showing that the conditions under which flow is rephased for the second echo are quite limited. There may be less dephasing in the second echo than in the first, but it does not follow a priori that flow will appear brighter in the second echo than it does in the first. Thus, the radiologist should be aware that this phenomenon may occur in some cases, but reduced intensity of blood in spin-echo imaging (Fig. 3-13) versus bright blood in gradient-echo imaging (Fig. 3-12*A*) is generally the rule.

## Chemical Shift

The *chemical shift artifact* appears as a displacement of the fat signal along the frequency-encoding direction relative to other tissues. This occurs because the protons in fatty acids have a resonant frequency slightly different from that of protons in the water molecule. This difference is referred to as a chemical shift (Brateman 1986).

In NMR spectroscopy, this effect is represented by including an additional factor $\sigma$, which is known as the shielding constant (Harris 1986). It represents the shielding of the nucleus from the magnetic field and replaces the magnetic field $B_0$ with the effective field $B_0 (1 - \sigma)$. When this factor is carried through to Equation (2), the frequency at a given position is changed. When a Fourier transform of the data is performed, this difference in frequency is transformed to a difference in spatial location by $\Delta x = -\sigma B_0/g$. For a given imaging sequence, the appearance of this shift depends on the readout gradient amplitude. As the read-

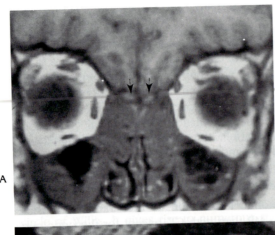

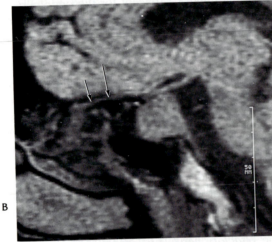

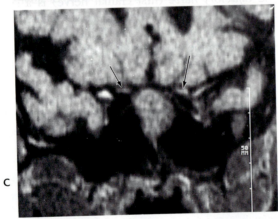

*Figure 4-9* **The olfactory nerve. A.** T$_1$-weighted coronal MR demonstrates the **olfactory bulb** (small arrows) in a child. Sagittal (**B**) and coronal (**C**) T$_1$-weighted MR in an adult demonstrating the **olfactory nerve** (small arrows).

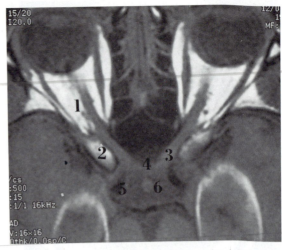

*Figure 4-10* **The optic nerve.** Axial T$_1$-weighted MR. 1 = orbital segment of optic nerve; 2 = intracanalicular segment; 3 = cisternal segment; 4 = optic chiasm; 5 = optic tract; 6 = pituitary stalk.

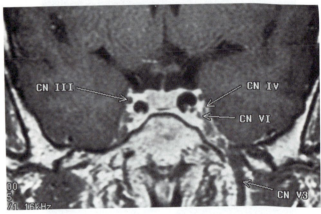

*Figure 4-11* Coronal T$_1$-weighted CEMR. The **cranial nerves 3, 4, and 6** within the enhancing cavernous sinus.

its meningeal sheath, to proceed to the apex of the orbit. It exits the orbit after passing through the optic canal. Within the cranium, the two optic nerves run for a short distance within the suprasellar cistern in a superior and medial direction to form the optic chiasm. Within the chiasm nerve fibers from the medial or nasal half of the retinal surface decussate. The optic pathway continues posterolaterally as the optic tract. Within the brain, the majority of the visual fibers enter the lateral geniculate body, whereas a few fibers end in the Edinger-Westphal nuclei (pretectal midbrain) forming the afferent limb of the pupillary light reflex. From the geniculate body, the visual fibers diverge in a fan-shaped pattern—the optic radiation, which eventually ends in the visual center located in the occipital lobe. The various segments of the optic nerve are best imaged with MR (Fig. 4-10).

In the majority of cases the pituitary stalk is located behind the optic chiasm (prefixed chiasm), although in 10 percent of individuals the pituitary stalk may be in front of the chiasm (postfixed chiasm).

The optic radiation fibers are myelinated and merge with the white matter tracts in adults; however, during

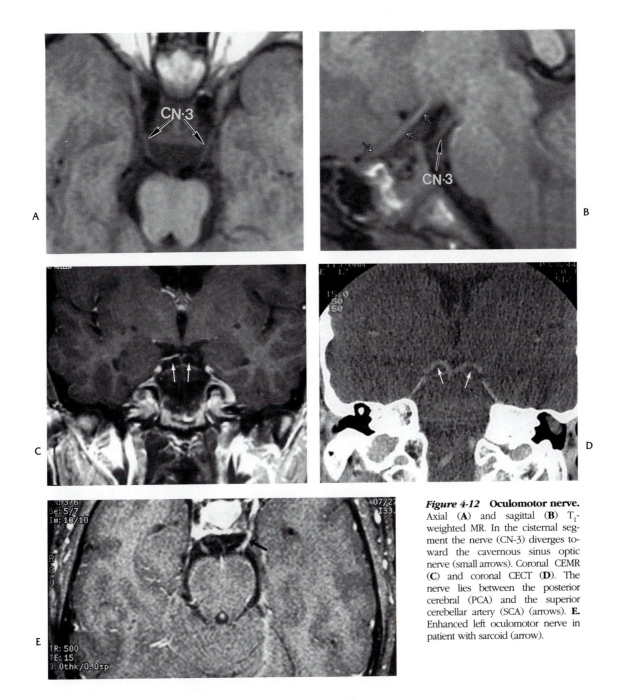

***Figure 4-12*** **Oculomotor nerve.** Axial (**A**) and sagittal (**B**) $T_1$-weighted MR. In the cisternal segment the nerve (CN-3) diverges toward the cavernous sinus optic nerve (small arrows). Coronal CEMR (**C**) and coronal CECT (**D**). The nerve lies between the posterior cerebral (PCA) and the superior cerebellar artery (SCA) (arrows). **E.** Enhanced left oculomotor nerve in patient with sarcoid (arrow).

the process of myelination, this can be identified on MR in infants below the age of 12 months as a hyperintense signal on $T_1$WI (Fig. 4-32).

The oculomotor (CN III), trochlear (CN IV), abducens (CN VI), and ophthalmic division of trigeminal (CN V3) nerves are often seen within the cavernous sinus, on contrast-enhanced coronal $T_1$-weighted MR (Fig. 4-11).

The *oculomotor* (third cranial nerve), *trochlear* (fourth cranial nerve), and *abducens* (sixth cranial nerve) are the nerves which innervate the extraocular muscles of the eye. The trochlear nerve innervates the

superior oblique muscle, and the abducens innervates the lateral rectus muscle; the remaining extraocular muscles and the levator palpebrae superioris are innervated by the oculomotor nerve.

All three of these nerves are difficult to identify on CT. On MR, the cisternal segment of the third cranial nerve can be identified in most instances in the axial plane and occasionally in the sagittal and coronal planes (Fig. 4-12). The oculomotor nerve emerges from the pontomedullary junction in the midline and diverges toward the cavernous sinus. The nerve is situated between the posterior cerebral and superior cerebellar arteries. In the cavernous sinus, it is located along the superior lateral wall of the sinus, adjacent to the trochlear nerve, but above the abducent nerve and ophthalmic division of the trigeminal nerve (Fig. 4-11).

Because of the thin nerve bundle, the trochlear nerve is difficult to demonstrate. Its nucleus is situated in the tegmentum of the midbrain at the level of the inferior colliculus. The nerve enters the cisternal segment from the dorsal aspect of the brainstem and winds around the brainstem. It then follows slightly caudal to the oculomotor and above the trigeminal nerve (Fig. 4-14D). It enters the cavernous sinus and superior orbital fissure to innervate the superior oblique muscle.

The abducens nerve innervates the lateral rectus muscle. Its nucleus is situated in the dorsal tegmentum, close to the surface forming the floor of the fourth ventricle. The location of its nuclei can be suspected from the location of the facial colliculus projecting into the fourth ventricle. The nerve courses anteriorly through the corticospinal tract emerging at the pontomedullary junction and proceeds anterolaterally and upward toward the clivus. The nerve may be identified in the sagittal section in the mesencephalic cistern between the anterior belly of the pons and the posterolateral aspect of the dorsum sellae, and in the axial section where the inferior petrosal sinus joins the cavernous sinus (Fig. 4-13).

The *trigeminal nerve* (fifth cranial nerve) is associated with motor, sensory, and proprioceptive functions. Its sensory fibers innervate the scalp and face and the mucous membrane of the sinuses, nasal cavity, and mouth. Its motor fibers innervate the muscles of mastication, the tensor muscles (palatine and tympani), and the digastric and mylohyoid muscles. It is one of the largest cranial nerves.

The nuclei of the trigeminal nerve extend in a longitudinal plane between the inferior colliculi and the second cervical segment of the spinal cord.

The cisternal segment of the trigeminal nerve extends from the anterolateral surface of the brainstem to the Meckels cave (Fig. 4-14). Within Meckel's cave the three divisions of the trigeminal nerve—the ophthalmic (V1), maxillary (V2), and mandibular (V3) divisions—leave the skull base after piercing the dural attachments through the superior orbital fissure (ophthalmic division), the foramen rotundum (maxillary division), and the foramen ovale (mandibular division), respectively. The sensory and proprioceptive fibers join the nerve roots near the gasserian or semilunar ganglion, which is located within the trigeminal cistern, a CSF space within the dural folds also known as Meckel's cave. Meckel's cave is posterolateral to the sella and cavernous sinus, in close proximity to exit foramina of the trigeminal nerve branches.

In high-resolution thin-section CECT, Meckel's cave is seen as an oval hypodense region (Kapila 1984; Chui 1985). CT density within Meckel's cave depends on the amounts of CSF and fat. It is defined laterally by the dural attachment and the contained venous sinus, and medially by the petrous tip and the dural fold (Fig. 4-14). On MR the Meckel's cave is hypointense or isointense on $T_1$WI and hyperintense on $T_2$WI. The trigeminal nerve is best seen in $T_1$WI MR studies in axial sections at the level of the upper pons and can also be seen in the coronal and sagittal sections. CEMR in the axial and coronal planes often demonstrates the

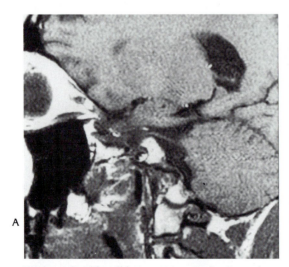
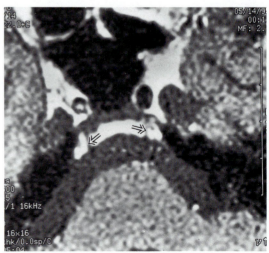

*Figure 4-13*  **The abducens nerve:** In the cisternal segment on $T_1$-weighted MR (arrow). Sagittal (**A**) and axial (**B**) views.

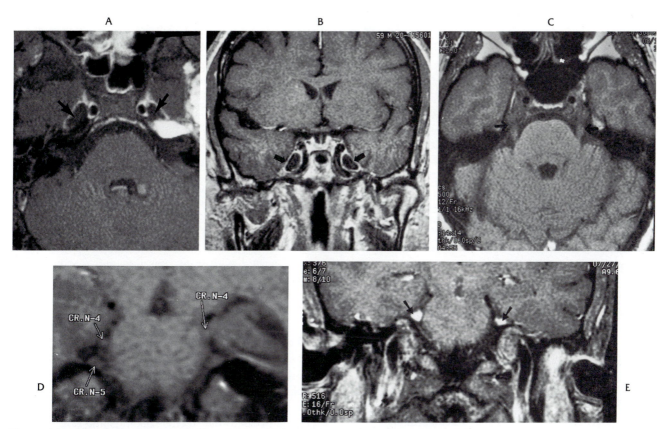

*Figure 4-14 Trigeminal nerve.*   Axial (**A**) and coronal (**B**) CEMR T$_1$-WI, demonstrates the Meckel's cave (arrows). **C.** Axial T$_1$-WI demonstrates the cisternal segment of the trigeminal nerve (arrow), as it enters the Meckel's cave. (**D**) Coronal T$_1$-W MR demonstrates the relationship of the trochlear nerve (1) to the trigeminal nerve (2) in the cisternal space. (**E**) Coronal CEMR. Enhancing trigeminal nerve (arrow) in a patient with sarcoidosis.

maxillary and mandibular divisions of the trigeminal nerve as it exits through the foramen ovale and foramen rotundum.

The *facial nerve* (seventh cranial nerve) is a mixed nerve consisting of motor, sensory, and special-function fibers. Its nuclei are situated anterolaterally within the pons, in front of the floor of the fourth ventricle. The nerve emerges at the lateral margin of the pons. A short segment runs in the cerebellopontine (CP) angle cistern between the brainstem and the internal auditory canal. In the internal auditory canal, the nerve is located in the superior outer quadrant. At the lateral end of the canal, the nerve makes a loop, with the anterior end of the loop forming the labyrinthine segment and the posterior end forming the tympanic segment. The labyrinthine segment is connected to the geniculate ganglion. The tympanic segment passes under the lateral semicircular canal to form the vertical, or mastoid, portion of the facial nerve. The facial nerve leaves the cranial base through the stylomastoid foramen.

The nerve is isointense in both T$_1$WI and T$_2$WI. Within the internal auditory canal, the facial nerve is separated from the acoustic nerve by the crista falciformis. On CT the seventh and eighth nerves are difficult to separate within the internal auditory canal unless the crista falciformis can be identified (Fig. 4-15) (Teresi 1987; Daniels 1984*a*).

The *acoustic nerve* (eighth cranial nerve) consists of the cochlear component, which is associated with hearing, and the vestibular component, which is associated with the sense of position in space.

The cochlear nucleus is located in the lateral aspect of the inferior cerebellar peduncle. The vestibular nucleus is between the cerebellum and the inferior cerebellar peduncle.

The intratemporal and intracanalicular segments of the nerve are visualized on CT and MR in similar planes and pulse sequences as for the seventh cranial nerve (Fig. 4-15). The brainstem nuclei and connections are located in sections through the levels of the inferior cerebellar peduncles.

The *glossopharyngeal nerve* (ninth cranial nerve) innervates the stylopharyngeal muscle. Its sensory component receives sensation from the posterior oropharynx and the soft palate. It has special sense fibers that

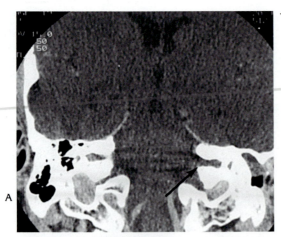

A

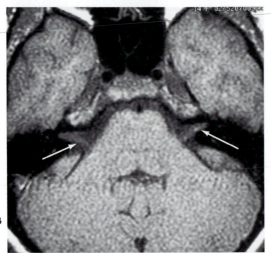

B

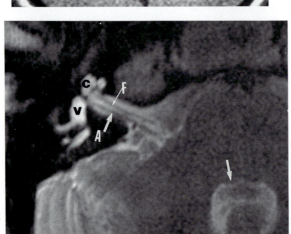

C

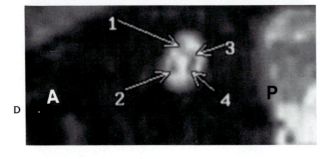

D

*Figure 4-15 Seventh and eighth cranial nerves.* **A.** Coronal CECT of internal auditory canal (arrow). **B.** Axial T₁-W MR demonstrates the bony canal and the seventh and eighth cranial nerve complex within the cerebellopontine angle cistern and the internal auditory canal (arrow). **C.** Axial CISS image. c = cochlea, v = vestibule and semicircular canal, a = acoustic nerve, f = facial nerve, facial nerve colliculus (arrow). **D.** Sagittal oblique CISS image demonstrates relationship of the seventh and eighth cranial nerves within the internal auditory canal. 1 = facial nerve, 2 = cochlear division of acoustic nerve, 3 = superior and 4 = inferior division of the vestibular nerve.

are associated with taste sensation and discrimination in the posterior third of the tongue. It also has fibers that subserve parasympathetic functions and Jacobson's nerve, which is the sensory nerve to the middle ear.

The *vagus nerve* (tenth cranial nerve) is a mixed nerve that enters the skull base in the posterior compartment, along with the accessory nerve (eleventh cranial nerve). The vagus nerve carries motor fibers from the nucleus ambiguus and sensory and parasympathetic fibers to the tractus solitarius and dorsal motor nucleus.

The *accessory-spinal nerve* (eleventh cranial nerve), as the name suggests, has a spinal component. The spinal component of the eleventh cranial nerve enters the cranial cavity along the anterolateral portion of the foramen magnum and joins with the cranial component. These three cranial nerves run a short course in the medullary cistern to enter the posterolateral compartment of the jugular foramen.

In the jugular foramen the ninth cranial nerve is located in the anterior compartment, along with the inferior petrosal sinus. A fibrous band separates the anterior compartment from the posterolateral compartment (Daniels 1985; Han 1984). The posterior compartment of the jugular foramen (pars vascularis) contains the internal jugular vein. The vagus (CN X), the accessory (CN XI), and the glossopharyngael (CN IX) nerves are anteromedial to the jugular vein. The nuclei of the three nerves are close to each other.

The cisternal segment is difficult to visualize on CT but can be identified occasionally in axial and coronal MR studies (Fig. 4-16) (Remly 1987).

The *hypoglossal nerve* (twelfth cranial nerve) is a pure motor nerve that primarily supplies the muscles of the tongue, both intrinsic and extrinsic. The nucleus of the nerve has a bulbar and spinal extension. The bulbar nuclei lie in a paramedia location in the floor of the fourth ventricle. The fibers exit as rootlets between the inferior olivary nucleus and the pyramid (corticospinal tract). In the medullary cistern they fuse to

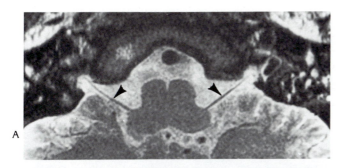

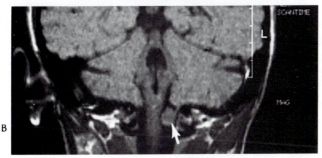

**Figure 4-16** **A.** Fast spin-echo T$_2$-weighted axial MR demonstrating the glossopharyngeal nerve (arrow). **B.** Coronal enhanced MR in a patient with XI CN schwanomma (arrow).

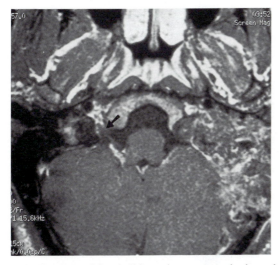

**Figure 4-17** CEMR of the skull base demonstrates the hypoglossal nerve within the canal (arrow). Note tumor invasion on the left side.

form the hypoglossal nerve. The nerve has a very short cisternal segment, directed anterolaterally and downward, in which it enters the hypoglossal canal (anterior condylar foramen) of the occipital bone. The canal is posteromedial and inferior to the jugular foramen (Fig. 4-17).

The cisternal and canalicular segments of the hypoglossal nerve are demonstrated on MRI in both the axial and coronal planes (Smoker 1987). In the axial

plane the nerve is seen in section parallel to the foramen magnum (Fig. 4-17).

Pathological processes that affect the cranial nerves in the cisternal or extracranial pathways are best evaluated with MRI after paramagnetic contrast (Barakos 1991).

## Brain Parenchyma

The brain parenchyma consists of three major components, each of which is composed of several parts: (1) the forebrain (prosencephalon), which consists of the telencephalon and the diencephalon; (2) the midbrain, or the mesencephalon; and (3) the hindbrain, consisting of the pons and medulla.

## COMPONENTS OF THE BRAIN

The forebrain, or prosencephalon, consists of the two cerebral hemispheres (telencephalon), which are connected to the midbrain by several structures consisting of fiber tracts (diencephalon). The anatomy of the cerebral hemisphere and midbrain is evaluated in sagittal and coronal T$_1$WI (Figs. 4-18 and 4-19). The internal gray and white matter are best evaluated on T$_2$WI (Figs. 4-20 to 4-23).

## Cerebral Hemispheres

The two cerebral hemispheres occupy the cranial cavity above the tentorium. They are separated from each other in the midline by the interhemispheric fissure, which extends anteriorly to the floor of the anterior cranial fossa. In its middle part the interhemispheric fissure stops at the corpus callosum, which connects the two cerebral hemispheres. Posteriorly, the interhemispheric fissure separates the two occipital lobes. The posterior inferior surfaces of the cerebral hemispheres are separated from the cerebellum by the tentorium cerebelli.

Each cerebral hemisphere consists of outer gray matter (the cerebral cortex and underlying white matter (the centrum semiovale), and white matter extending within the gyri (subcortical white matter). Deeper in the white matter is the diencephalon (Figs. 4-18 and 4-19).

The cerebral cortex covers the surface of the cerebral hemisphere. There are three surfaces for each hemisphere, separated by three borders. The superior border separates the medial and lateral surfaces, the inferolateral border separates the inferior and lateral surfaces, and the inferomedial border separates the medial and inferior surfaces. The three surfaces of the cerebral hemisphere contain numerous sulci that separate the cerebral gyri. Four of these sulci are helpful in dividing the cerebral hemispheres into their constituent

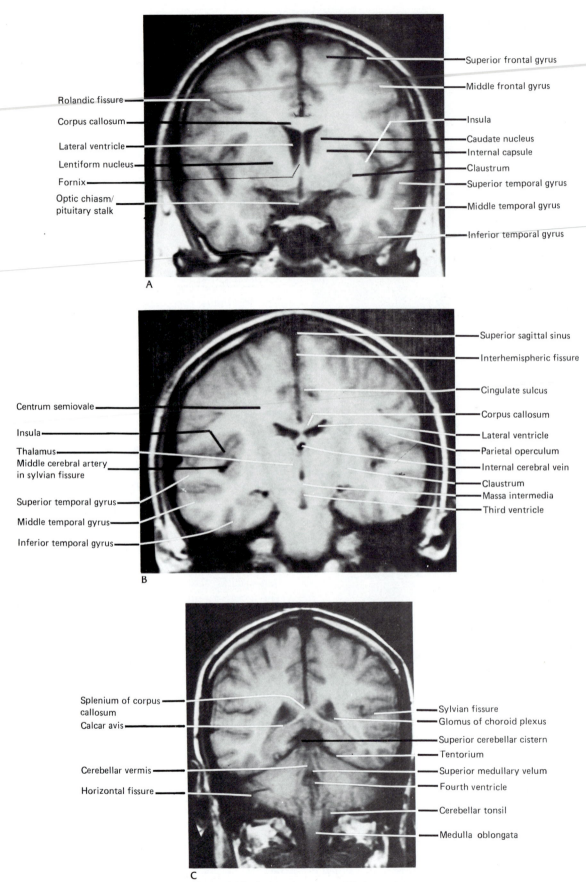

Rolandic fissure

Corpus callosum

Lateral ventricle

Lentiform nucleus

Fornix

Optic chiasm/
pituitary stalk

Superior frontal gyrus

Middle frontal gyrus

Insula

Caudate nucleus

Internal capsule

Claustrum

Superior temporal gyrus

Middle temporal gyrus

Inferior temporal gyrus

A

Centrum semiovale

Insula

Thalamus

Middle cerebral artery
in sylvian fissure

Superior temporal gyrus

Middle temporal gyrus

Inferior temporal gyrus

Superior sagittal sinus

Interhemispheric fissure

Cingulate sulcus

Corpus callosum

Lateral ventricle

Parietal operculum

Internal cerebral vein

Claustrum

Massa intermedia

Third ventricle

B

Splenium of corpus
callosum

Calcar avis

Cerebellar vermis

Horizontal fissure

Sylvian fissure

Glomus of choroid plexus

Superior cerebellar cistern

Tentorium

Superior medullary velum

Fourth ventricle

Cerebellar tonsil

Medulla oblongata

C

*Figure 4-18*  See caption at top of facing page.

**Figure 4-18** Coronal T1-weighted MR. At level of foramen of Monro (**A**), level of posterior third ventricle (**B**), level of fourth ventricle (**C**), and behind fourth ventricle (**D**).

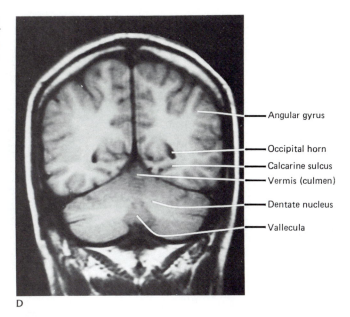

— Angular gyrus

— Occipital horn
— Calcarine sulcus
— Vermis (culmen)
— Dentate nucleus
— Vallecula

D

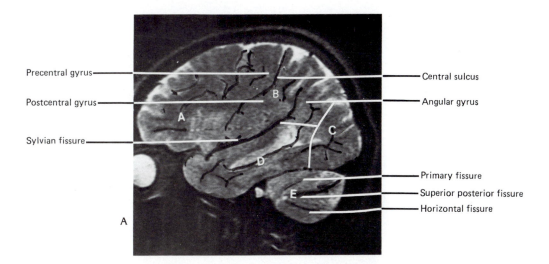

Precentral gyrus——
Postcentral gyrus——
Sylvian fissure——

————Central sulcus
————Angular gyrus

————Primary fissure
————Superior posterior fissure
————Horizontal fissure

A

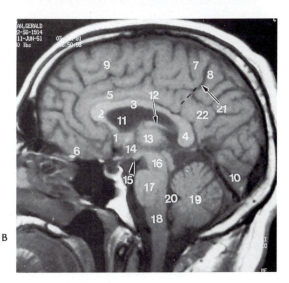

B

**Figure 4-19 A.** Extreme lateral section demonstrating the different lobes of the brain. a = frontal; b = parietal; c = occipital; d = temporal; and e = cerebellum. **B.** Midsagittal T$_1$-weighted MR. 1 = rostrum of corpus callosum, 2 = genu of corpus callosum, 3 = body, 4 = splenium, 5 = cingulate gyrus, 6 = gyrus rectus, 7 = precentral gyrus, 8 = postcentral gyrus, 9 = frontal lobe, 10 = occipital lobe, 11 = lateral ventricle, 12 = fornix, 13 = thalamus, 14 = third ventricle, 15 = mamillary body, 16 = cerebral peduncle, 17 = pons, 18 = medulla, 19 = vermis of cerebellum, 20 = fourth ventricle, 21 = rolandic fissure, 22 = parietal lobe. Dashed lines represent the imaginary boundary between the frontal and parietal lobes.

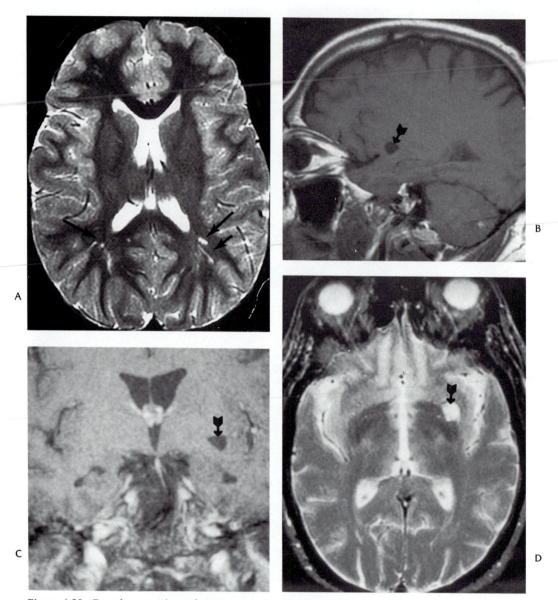

*Figure 4-20*  **Prominent perivascular spaces. A.** Axial T2-weighted MR in an infant, with prominent perivascular spaces (arrows). **B.** Sagittal $T_1$-WI. **C.** Coronal $T_1$-WI. **D.** Axial $T_2$-WI. MR demonstrating a large perivascular space (arrow) in an adult.

lobes (Figs. 4-18 and 4-19). The lateral sulcus (sylvian fissure) separates the greater part of the temporal lobe from the frontal lobe and the anterior part of the parietal lobe above. The central sulcus (rolandic fissure) begins on the medial surface of the hemisphere at about the middle of the superior border. It runs on the lateral surface of the hemisphere downward and forward and stops short of the lateral sulcus.

The parietooccipital sulcus lies on the medial surface of the cerebral hemisphere (Fig. 4-19). It starts at the superior margin about 5 cm from the occipital pole and extends downward and forward, where it meets the calcarine sulcus near the splenium of the corpus

callosum. The calcarine sulcus extends from this point backward on the medial surface of the occipital lobe and ends at the occipital pole (Figs. 4-18 and 4-19).

Each cerebral hemisphere is divided into five lobes, demarcated by the sulci described above and in part by imaginary lines (Fig. 4-19). The frontal lobe is the anterior part of the hemisphere, limited posteriorly by the central sulcus (rolandic fissure) and inferiorly by the lateral sulcus (sylvian fissure). On the medial surface, it is limited posteriorly by a line drawn downward and anteriorly from the end of the central sulcus to the corpus callosum. The occipital lobe is the small posterior part of the hemisphere. On the medial surface it is limited anteriorly by the parietooccipital sulcus. Its anterior border on the lateral surface is an imaginary line extending from the upper end of the parietooccipital sulcus at the superior border of the hemisphere to the preoccipital notch on the inferolateral border. The parietal lobe lies between the frontal lobe anteriorly and the occipital lobe posteriorly. The inferior border of the parietal lobe on the lateral surface is formed by the posterior part of the lateral sulcus and by an arbitrary line extending from the lateral

sulcus toward the arbitrary line which forms the anterior border of the occipital lobe. The separation between the parietal, temporal, and occipital lobes on the lateral surface is formed by arbitrary lines and thus is ill defined. On the medial surface, the posterior border of the parietal lobe is formed by the parietooccipital sulcus, which separates the parietal lobe from the occipital lobe. The insula (central lobe), which is formed by portions of the frontal, parietal, and temporal lobes, is hidden in the depth of the lateral sulcus.

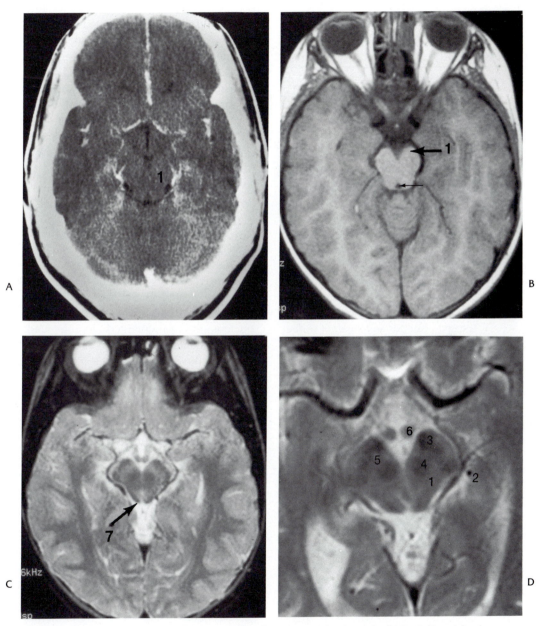

***Figure 4-21 Midbrain.***    Axial section at level of midbrain. **A.** CT. **B.** T₁-weighted MR. **C.** T₂-weighted MR. **D.** More detailed view of the midbrain. 1 = cerebral peduncle; 2 = medial surface of the temporal lobe (uncus, hippocampus, amygdala); 3 = substantia nigra; 4 = red nucleus; 5 = pars compacta; 6 = mamillary bodies; 7 = superior colliculi.

The centrum semiovale constitutes the white matter of the internal portion of the cerebral hemisphere. Prominent perivascular spaces in infants and especially in adults may occasionally be mistaken for ischemic changes (Table 4-2). Perivascular spaces are isointense to CSF, whereas ischemic foci are usually bright, on spin-density images (Fig. 4-20).

The corpus callosum is a thick band of white matter which connects the two cerebral hemispheres (Figs. 4-18 and 4-19). It is divided into four parts: rostrum, genu, body, and splenium. The corpus callosum develops in an anterior to posterior manner from genu to splenium, with the rostral part of the callosal fibers developing last. The most anterior part of the genu and the rostrum are less bright than the rest of the corpus callosum. The rostrum of the corpus callosum continues inferiorly to join the lamina terminalis. The body of the corpus callosum overlies the roof of the lateral ventricle but continues in the midline posteriorly in a thick rounded free edge—the splenium—that overhangs the pineal body and the colliculi. The roof of the lateral ventricles in the midline is formed by the corpus callosum. The corpus callosum connects the axonal fibers of the two cerebral hemispheres. In developmental anomalies associated with dysgenesis of the corpus callosum, the disrupted axonal fibers form longitudinal callosal fibers (Probst bundles). The frontal horns and the body of the two lateral ventricles are separated by the septum pellucidum. The two layers of the septum pellucidum containing CSF are consistently seen in infants. In the majority of instances they fuse. Nonfusion of the two layers results in the CSF-containing spaces identified as the cavum septum pellucidum and its posterior extension, the cavum vergae. The septum pellucidum has neural connections with the cerebral hemispheres (Sarwar 1989).

The basal ganglia represent the central gray matter of the telencephalon in the lower parts of each cerebral hemisphere. The basal ganglia consist of the corpus striatum (caudate nucleus and lentiform nucleus); the claustrum, a thin strip of gray matter lateral to the lentiform nucleus and separated by a band of white matter (Figs. 4-18, 4-21, and 4-22); and the amygdala, which is located in the roof of the temporal horn and represents the tail of the caudate nucleus. The caudate nucleus has an enlarged anterior end, the head of which indents the lateral wall of the anterior horn of the lateral ventricle. It has a narrow posterior portion—the tail—that follows the superolateral border of the thalamus. The lentiform nucleus has a wedge-shaped appearance in the axial and coronal planes (Figs. 4-18 and 4-22). It consists of the globus pallidus medially and the putamen laterally.

White matter tracts consisting of the corona radiata, association fibers, and the corpus callosum cover the superior surface of the lentiform nucleus. The inferior surface of the lentiform nucleus is above the anterior perforated substance and the anterior commissure. The perforated substance is the site of entry zones of the striate vessels. The perivascular (Robin-Virchow) spaces surrounding the strait vessels appear as oval areas of bright signal intensity adjacent to the anterior commissure (Jungreis 1988).

The internal capsule is a boomerang-shaped thick white matter bounded anteromedially by the caudate nucleus, posteromedially by the thalamus, and laterally by the lentiform nuclei (Figs. 4-21 and 4-22). Adjacent

## Table 4-2    Anatomic Regions of Normal Hyperintense Signal on $T_2$-Weighted MRI

| LOCATION | ANATOMIC/PATHOLOGICAL CORRELATION |
|---|---|
| Tips of frontal horns | Anterolateral aspects of frontal horns. Triangle-shaped. Related to decreased myelin. Fissures in ependymal lining with extracellular fluid. Astrocytic gliosis. |
| Posterior internal capsule | 3 to 4 mm in size. Medial to distal putamen and anterolateral to thalamus. Usually seen beyond age 10. Probably related to decreased myelination or absent iron. Bilateral, symmetrical, not seen on $T_1$ WI or in low-field-strength magnets. |
| Paratrigonal region | Located posterior and superior to the trigone. Usually seen before the second decade, often in high-field MR systems. Probably represents delayed myelination in associated fiber tracts. |
| Anterior-posterior commissural regions | Perivascular spaces: seen on axial and coronal planes; represents perivascular CSF spaces around the striatal vessels. More prominent with aging. |
| Choroidal fissure | Perivascular spaces: seen on axial sections in medial temporal pole, adjacent to the quadrigeminal cistern. These focal bright regions represent entry zones of choroidal vessels. |
| Centrum semiovale | Perivascular spaces: small punctate foci, isointense to CSF, related to perivascular extracellular fluid. Becomes more visible with aging. |

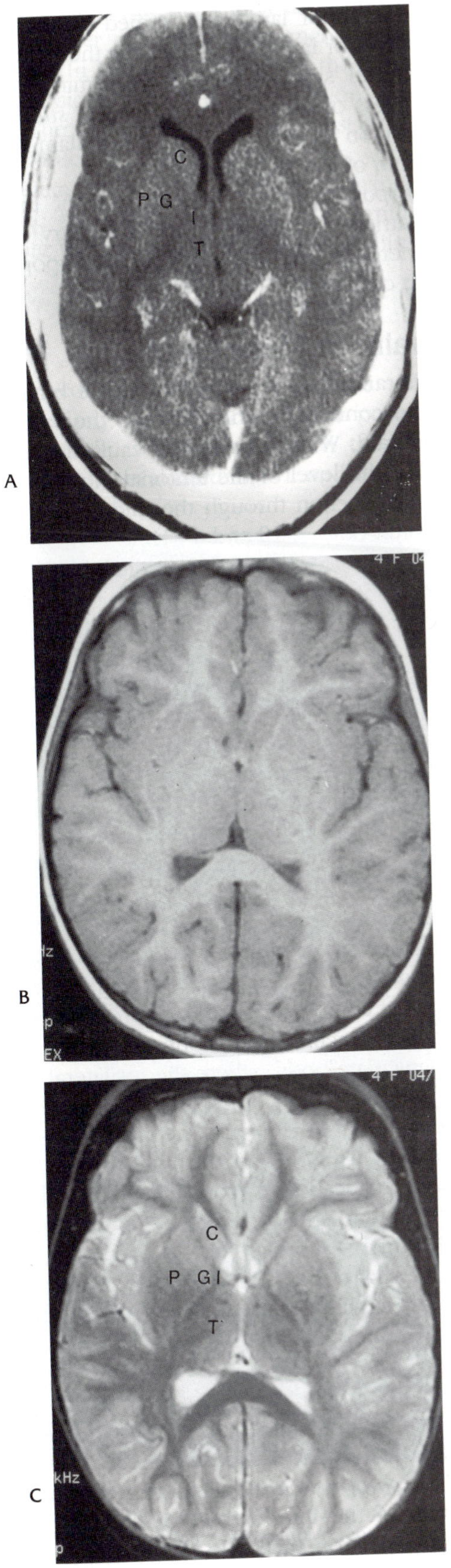

*Figure 4-22 Basal ganglia.* **A.** CT. **B.** $T_1$-weighted MR. **C.** $T_2$-weighted MR. C = caudate nucleus; P = putamen; G = globus pallidus; I = internal capsule; T = thalamus.

to the posterior limb of the internal capsule bright foci are often seen on $T_2WI$ axial images (Fig. 4-23). The bright signal foci represents the paracentral corticospinal tract.

## Diencephalon

The diencephalon is made up of several structures around the third ventricle, consisting of fiber tracts that connect the midbrain on one side to the cerebral hemispheres on the other side. It includes the thalami, the geniculate bodies, the epithalamus, the subthalamus, and the hypothalamus (Figs. 4-18, 4-21, and 4-22).

The *thalami* are two large ovoid masses that are small anteriorly and more voluminous posteriorly. Each thalamus is 4 cm long. Its medial surface forms the lateral wall of the third ventricle. Each thalamus is covered with ependyma and is separated from the opposite thalamus by the third ventricle (Figs. 4-18 to 4-23). The superior surface forms part of the floor of the lateral ventricle on each side. The posteromedial part of the superior surface of the thalamus is covered with the fold of pia called the tela choroidea, which forms the velum interpositum in the roof of the third ventricle. The fornix lies on the superior surface of the thalamus, separating the lateral part from the medial part. The anterior end of the thalamus forms the posterior boundary of the foramen of Monro, whereas the column of the fornix that overlies the thalamus forms the anterior border of this foramen. Each foramen of Monro forms the passageway between the third and lateral ventricles.

The voluminous posterior end of the thalamus is called the pulvinar. The pulvinar on each side extends beyond the posterior end of the third ventricle so that each pulvinar overlies a superior colliculus. The pineal gland lies in the midline, between the two pulvinars and above the superior colliculus. The inferior surface of the thalamus is continuous with the upper end of the tegmentum of the midbrain. The lateral surface forms the posteromedial boundary of the internal capsule. The massa intermedia in the middle (Fig. 4-18) connect the two thalami.

The *geniculate bodies* constitute the metathalamus. On each side there are the lateral and medial geniculate bodies, which serve as relay stations. The lateral geniculate body is connected by the superior brachium to the superior colliculus and serves as part of the visual pathways that end in the visual cortex of the occipital lobe. The medial geniculate body on each side is connected by the inferior brachium to the inferior colliculus and serves as part of the auditory pathways that end in the auditory cortex of the superior temporal gyrus.

The habenula, the pineal body, and the posterior commissure constitute the *epithalamus* (Fig. 4-19). The pineal stalk has a superior lamina and an inferior lam-

A

B

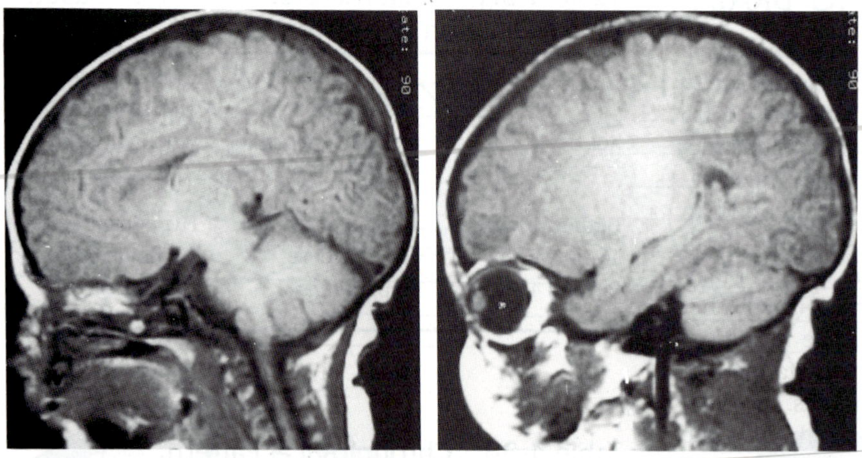

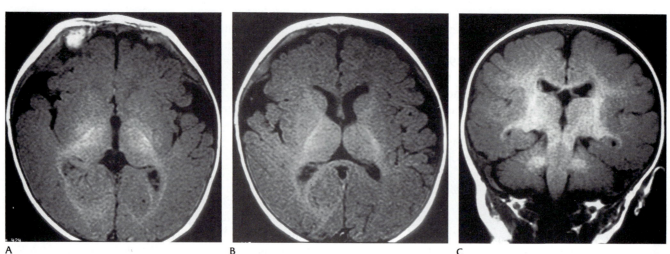

*Figure 4-30*   **Three-week-old infant. A, B.** Sagittal T₁WI. **C–E.** Axial images. Hyperintense signal in the cerebellar peduncles, brainstem, optic radiation and precentral cortical gyri.

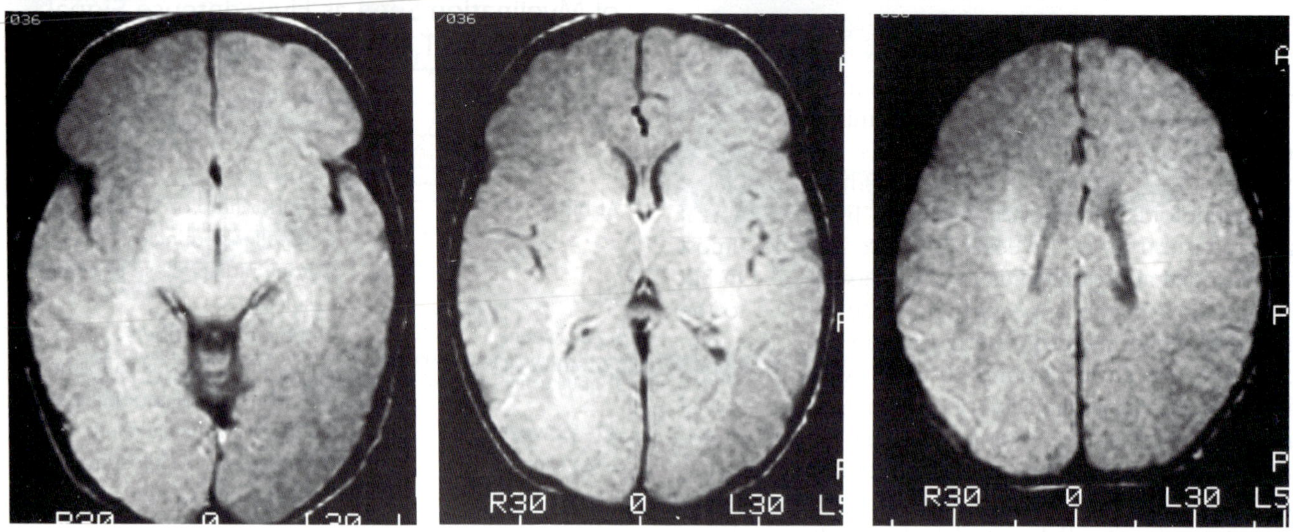

C

D

E

A

B

C

*Figure 4-31*   **Twelve-week-old child.** Axial (**A, B**) and coronal (**C**) T₁-weighted MR. Note the decrease in the water content with a fairly well defined pattern of myelination.

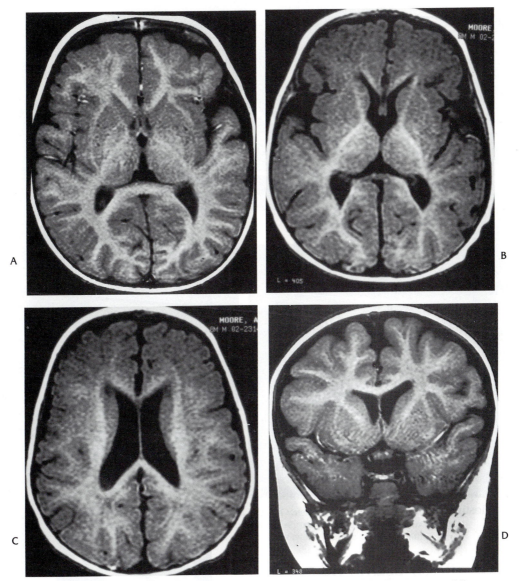

***Figure 4-32*** **Eight-month-old infant.** Axial (**A–C**) and coronal (**C**) T$_1$-weighted MR. Better differentiation of gray and white matter. Persistent hyperintense signal along the forceps major, the frontal region, and the postcentral gyrus.

Between 3 and 6 months, there is a progressive decrease in signal intensity in the basal ganglia, the centrum semiovale, and the splenium of the corpus callosum (Fig. 4-32).

Between 6 and 12 months, the white matter signal changes toward the adult type, progressing from the subcortical white matter of the occipital lobe to the frontal lobe (Fig. 4-33).

Hyperintensity on T$_2$WI (long TR/TE), particularly in the periventricular region adjacent to the occipital horns and trigone of the lateral ventricle, may persist beyond 12 to 24 months. These should not be confused with periventricular leukomalacia (PVL). The hyperintense signal of PVL is seen in both spin density and T$_2$WI, and are separated from the walls of the ventricles by a thin layer of white matter.

Prominent perivascular spaces adjacent to the trigone are often present as hypointense or isointense signal on T$_1$WI, isointense in spin density, and hyperintense on T$_2$WI (Fig. 4-34). These should not be confused with dysmyelinating disorders.

Hyperintense signal on T$_1$WI of the adenohypophysis of the pituitary gland is normal in the first 2 to 3 months. Beyond this period the adenohypophysis becomes isointense and the neurohypophysis is hyperintense on T$_1$WI.

# References

ATLAS SW, ZIMMERMAN RA, BILANIUK LT, et al: Corpus callosum and limbic system: Neuroanatomic MR evaluation of developmental anomalies. *Radiology* 160:355–358, 1986.

BARAKOS JA, DILLON WP, CHEW WM: Orbit, skull base and pharynx: Contrast enhanced fat suppression MR imaging. *Radiology* 179:191–198, 1991.

BARKOVICH AJ, KJOS BO, JACKSON DE, et al: Normal maturation of the neonatal and infant brain: MR imaging at 1.5 T. *Radiology* 166:173–180, 1988.

BARKOVICH AJ: Analyzing the corpus callosum: commentary. *AJNR* 17:1643–1645, 1996.

BERMAN SA, HAYMAN LA, HINCK VC: Correlation of cerebral vascular territories with cerebral function by computed tomography: I. Anterior cerebral artery. *AJNR* 1:259–263, 1980.

BERMAN SA, HAYMAN LA, HINCK VC: Correlation of CT cerebral vascular territories with function: III. Middle cerebral arteries. *AJNR* 1:161–166, 1984.

BRADLEY WG, KORTMAN KE, BURGOYNE B: Flowing cerebrospinal fluid in normal and hydrocephalic states: Appearance on MR images. *Radiology* 159:611–616, 1986.

BRAFFMAN BH, ZIMMERMAN RA, RABISSCHONG P: Cranial nerves III, IV, VI: A clinical approach to the evaluation of their dysfunction. *Semin US CT MR* 8:185–213, 1987.

CHUI M, TUCKER W, HUDSON A, et al: High resolution CT of Meckel's cave. *Neuroradiology* 27:403–409, 1985.

DANIELS DL, WILLIAMS AL, HAUGHTON KVM: Jugular foramen: Anatomic and computed tomographic study. *AJR* 142:153–158, 1984a.

DANIELS DL, HERFKINS R, GAGER WE, et al: Magnetic resonance imaging of the optic nerves and chiasm. *Radiology* 152:79–83, 1984b.

DANIELS DL, HERFKINS R, GAGER WE, et al: Magnetic resonance imaging of the optic nerves and chiasm. *Radiology* 152:79–83, 1984c.

DANIELS DL, SCHENCK JF, FOSTER T, et al: Magnetic resonance imaging of the jugular foramen. *AJNR* 6:699–703, 1985.

DANIELS DL, PECH P, POJUNAS KW, et al: Magnetic resonance imaging of the trigeminal nerve. *Radiology* 159:577–583, 1986.

GADO M, HANAWAY J, FRANK R: Functional anatomy of the cerebral cortex by computed tomography. *J Comput Assist Tomogr* 3:1–19, 1979.

HAN JS, HUSS RG, BENSON JE, et al: MR imaging of the skull base. *J Comput Assist Tomgr* 8:944–952, 1984.

HAYMAN LA, BERMAN SA, HINCK VC: Correlation of CT cerebral vascular territories with function: II. Posterior cerebral artery. *AJNR* 2:219–225, 1981.

HINSHAW DB Jr, FAHMY JL, PECKHAM N, et al: The bright choroid plexus on MR: CT and pathologic correlation. *AJNR* 9:483–486, 1988.

HOLLAND BA, HAAS DK, NORMAN D, et al: MRI of normal brain maturation. *AJNR* 7:201–208, 1986.

JUNGREIS CA, KANAL E, HIRSCH WL, et al: Normal perivascular spaces mimicking lacunar infarction: MR imaging. *Radiology* 169:101–104, 1988.

KAPILA A, CHAKERAS DW, BLANCO E: The Meckel cave: Computed tomographic study. *Radiology* 152:425–433, 1984.

KEMP SS, ZIMMERMAN RA, BILANIUK IT, et al: Magnetic resonance imaging of the cerebral aqueduct. *Neuroradiology* 29:430–436, 1987.

KIEV L, TRUWIT CL: The normal and abnormal genu of the corpus callosum: An evolutionary, embryologic, anatomic, and MR analysis. *AJNR* 17:1631–1641, 1996.

KIMURA H, FUJII Y, ITOH S, et al: Metabolic alteration in the neonate and infant brain during development: Evaluation with proton MR spectroscopy. *Radiology* 194:483–489, 1995.

KREIS R, ERNST T, ROSS BD: Development of the human brain: In vivo quantification of metabolite and water content with proton magnetic spectroscopy. *J Mag Reson* 102:9–15, 1993.

LEE BCP, LIPPER E, NAAS R, et al: MRI of the central nervous system in neonates and young children. *AJNR* 7:605–616, 1986.

MCARDLE CB, RICHARDSON CJ, NICHOLAS DA, et al: Developmental features of the neonatal brain: MR imaging: I. Graywhite matter differentiation and myelination. *Radiology* 162:223–229, 1987.

NOWELL MA, HACKNEY DB, ZIMMERMAN RA, et al: Immature brain: Spin-echo pulse sequence parameters for high contrast MR imaging. *Radiology* 162:119–124, 1987.

PEDEN CJ, COWAN FM, BRYANT DJ, et al: Proton MR spectroscopy of the brain in infants. *J Comput Assist Tomgr* 14:886–894, 1990.

REMLEY K, HARNSBERGER HR, SMOKER WRK, et al: CT and MR in the evaluation of glossopharyngeal, vagal and spinal accessory neuropathy. *Semin US CT MR* 8:284–300, 1987.

RUTLEDGE JN, HILAL SK, SILVER AJ, et al: Study of movement disorders and brain iron by MR. *AJNR* 8:397–411, 1987.

SARWAR M: The septum pellucidum: Normal and abnormal. *AJNR* 10:989–1006, 1989.

SHERMAN JL, CITRIN CM, BOWEN BJ, et al: MR demonstration of normal CSF flow. *AJNR* 7:3–6, 1986.

SMOKER WRK, HARNESBERGER HR, OSBORN AG: The hypoglossal nerve. *Semin US CT MR* 8:301–312, 1987.

SUZUKI M, TAKASHIMA T, KADOYA M, et al: MR imaging of olfactory bulbs and tracts. *AJNR* 10:955–957, 1989.

TERESI L, LUFKIN R, NITTA K, et al: MRI of the facial nerve: Normal anatomy and pathology. *Semin US CT MR* 8:240–255, 1987.

YAKOVLEV PL, LECOUR AR: The myelogenic cycles of regional maturation of the brain, in Mankowski A (ed): *Regional Development of the Brain in Early Life*. Philadelphia, W A Davis, 1967, pp 3–69.

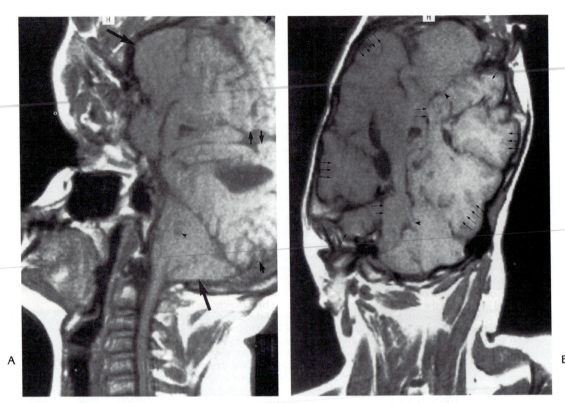

A    B

***Figure 5-2***   **Twins conjoined at the lateral aspect of the forehead (craniopagus). A.** Sagittal T₁WI
(600/15) demonstrates posterior fossa structures (large arrows) and portions of the occipital and parietal
lobes (small arrows) of both twins. Posterior fossa structures are crowded in both twins; note virtual effacement of the fourth ventricle (arrowhead) in the larger twin (located more inferiorly). **B.** Coronal
T₁WI (600/15) through the posterior aspects of the brains of both twins demonstrates contiguity and
some interdigitation of structures of the two somewhat dysmorphic brains (arrowheads); no dural plane
is identified between them. Portions of the twins' respective cerebellums (single arrows), brainstems
(two arrows), temporal lobes (three arrows), and parietal lobes (four arrows) are seen.

anomaly as an elongation of the cerebellar tonsils and
the medial part of the inferior aspects of the cerebellar
hemispheres into the cervical canal. He defined the
type II anomaly as a displacement of part of the inferior vermis, the pons, and the medulla into the cervical
canal and elongation of the fourth ventricle into the
cervical canal. The rare type III anomaly has been described as a more severe variant of the type II anomaly, with an associated low occipital or high cervical
(C1–C2) encephalocele. The relatively common type I
malformation and type II (or Arnold-Chiari) malformation differ significantly in their clinical manifestations;
this is consistent with their differences in regard to
morphological abnormalities. These differences also
suggest that the type I and type II anomalies are developmentally unrelated.

## CHIARI I MALFORMATION

The type I malformation consists of a chronic tonsillar
displacement below the foramen magnum (Fig. 5-3).
The malformation needs to be distinguished from acute

tonsillar herniation secondary to increased intracranial
pressure (pressure cones). The level to which the tonsils must descend to constitute the malformation has
been debated. It has been suggested that more than 3
mm below a line joining the basion to the opisthion is
sufficient (Barkovich 1986). Patients with tonsillar ectopia of this or a greater degree may or may not be
symptomatic; it may be discovered incidentally at autopsy or on an MR scan obtained for unrelated reasons
(Elster 1992). When patients do present clinically, it is
usually because of symptoms related to either brainstem compression at the foramen magnum or, more
commonly, an associated syringohydromyelia. Most of
these patients develop symptoms in the teenage or
adult years, though symptomatic children as young as 2
years of age have been reported (Dauser 1988). The incidence of associated syringohydromyelia has been
suggested to be as low as 20 percent (Banarji 1974)
and, since the advent of MR, as high as 75 to 80 percent (Naidich 1987). There is no association of other
brain anomalies with the type I malformation. Although

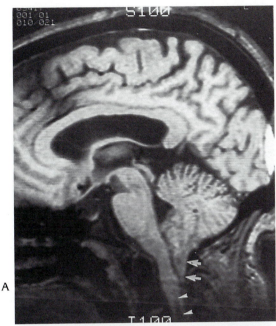

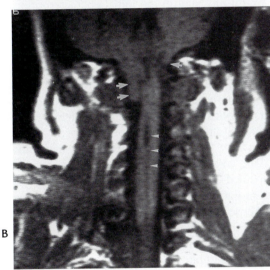

Some patients have craniocervical dysgenesis consisting of the Klippel-Feil anomaly, occipitalization of C1 (Fig. 5-4A), or other anomalies, such as partial fusion of the cervical vertebrae. Others may have basilar invagination, either congenital, as from anomalies of the clivus (Fig. 5-4B), or acquired. In many patients, no intrinsic bony abnormality is identified. Often the cerebellar tonsils themselves appear to be intrinsically abnormal,

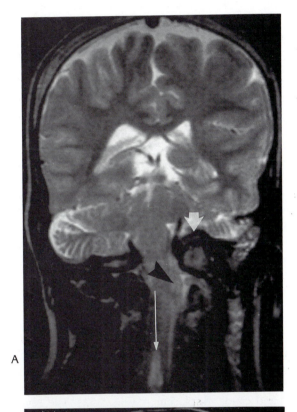

*Figure 5-3*  **Chiari I malformation. A.** Sagittal T₁WI (600/20) image reveals downward extension of peglike cerebellar tonsils through the foramen magnum to the level of C2 (arrows). The fourth ventricle is normally positioned. There is a hint of a syrinx in the cervical cord on this image (arrowheads). **B.** Coronal T₁WI (600/15) confirms the small syrinx cavity (arrowheads). There is asymmetry of the tonsillar displacement, with the right tonsil located more inferiorly than the left one (arrows).

the neural tissue involved in this anomaly is restricted to the cerebellum, the developmental origin appears to be variable. This is the case because associated pathology at the cervicomedullary junction, which in some cases appears fundamentally related to the anomaly, is variable. In fact, instances of reversible Chiari I malformation have been reported (Castillo 1995), suggesting that altered cerebrospinal fluid (CSF) dynamics or intracranial-intraspinal pressure relationships may be responsible for some cases of reversible tonsillar ectopia.

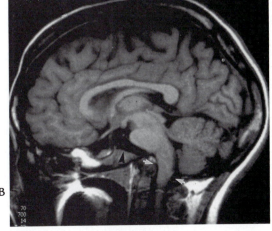

*Figure 5-4*  **Chiari I malformations. A.** Coronal T₂WI shows occipitalization of the lateral mass of C1 (arrow), cerebellar tonsil herniation (arrowhead) and a syringohydromyelic cavity in the cervical cord (long white arrow). **B.** Sagittal T₁WI shows caudalization of the medulla oblongata into the upper cervical canal (arrows). The clivus is short and horizontal (arrowhead).

enlarged, and peglike (Fig. 5-3A). The tonsils may be asymmetrical, with one extending more caudally than the other (Fig. 5-3B).

It is difficult to diagnose this malformation with certainty with plain CT. It may be suspected when images just below the level of the foramen magnum fail to demonstrate CSF density around the upper cervical cord. Before the advent of MR, confirmation depended on a demonstration of caudalization of the tonsils by myelography. An associated syringohydromyelia could be suggested when the spinal cord appeared widened and delayed postmyelogram CT demonstrated intramedullary high density resulting from entry of dye into the syrinx cavity within the widened cord. This means of diagnostic evaluation is no longer indicated unless the patient has a contraindication to obtaining an MR. MR is now the method of choice for evaluating abnormalities at the craniocervical junction and associated spinal cord pathology. Sagittal and coronal $T_1WI$ most clearly demonstrate the normal to small posterior fossa and cerebellar tonsils that are low-lying relative to the foramen magnum. Syringohydromyelia is most commonly seen as a smoothly marginated elongated area of low intensity within the central portion of the cord (which may contain septations), beginning at the C2 level (Fig. 5-3A) and extending for a variable distance inferiorly (Fig. 5-3B); occasionally the upper margin of the syrinx cavity appears at a lower cervical level (Fig. 5-4A).

## CHIARI II MALFORMATION

The Chiari II (or Arnold-Chiari) malformation is a morphologically more complex anomaly than the Chiari I malformation. By definition, it is characterized by cerebellar, brainstem, and fourth ventricular dysplasia (deformity) and caudal displacement (Fig. 5-5A). The severity of the characteristic hindbrain deformity covers a wide range so that in its milder forms in some patients, it may be difficult to distinguish radiographically from the Chiari I deformity (Fig. 5-5B). However, the greater spectrum of anomalies typically associated with the Chiari II malformation permits its proper identification in these cases. These other anomalies involve different elements of the neural axis, i.e., the midbrain, cerebral hemispheres, commissures, and ventricles, as well as mesodermal derivatives, i.e., the skull, intracranial dural partitions, and the spine, particularly in the lumbosacral and cervical regions (McClone 1992). Several hypotheses have been proffered regarding the pathogenesis of the malformation (Barry 1957; Daniel 1958; Gardner 1959; Gilbert 1986; McClone 1989). The tissue elements involved, however, suggest that the inciting influence and initiating maldevelopmental events occur during the phase of dorsal induction (3 to 4 weeks' gestation). Whether, for example, there is a primary dysgenetic

process involving the hindbrain with faulty secondary bony development or a primary maldevelopment of bony structures (e.g., a small posterior fossa or a spinal dysraphic state) with secondary effects on the compartmentalization of the hindbrain structures is not yet known; nonetheless, maldevelopmental interaction at an early embryonic stage is apparent.

The Chiari II malformation is nearly always associated with a myelomeningocele (Ingraham 1943; Naidich 1983b); thus, all these patients present at birth, though not all are symptomatic in terms of the Chiari malformation at this time. Virtually all these patients develop hydrocephalus, the etiology of which has been speculated to be attributable to either aqueductal stenosis (primary or secondary to a hydrodynamic consequence of the repair of the myelomeningocele) or occlusion of CSF spaces at the level of the foramen magnum and upper cervical canal. In contrast to the Chiari I malformation, because of the frequently associated anomalies in the Chiari II malformation, CT is often a useful modality in the initial characterization and follow-up of these chronically shunted patients. The CT signs of the Chiari II malformations have been described in detail (Zimmerman 1979; Naidich 1980a–c, 1983b). MR, however, demonstrates the parenchymal anomalies in greater detail and the craniocervical pathology more definitively.

Characteristically, there is a small posterior fossa and low tentorial attachment. In more severe cases, the attachment may approximate the foramen magnum (Fig. 5-5A). The cerebellar vermis, which may or may not be accompanied by the tonsils, impacts with the lower brainstem into the foramen magnum and upper cervical canal. These hindbrain structures appear variably elongated and dysplastic. The displaced pons is narrowed in its anteroposterior dimension, with the belly of the pons being imperceptible in some cases. The medulla extends below the foramen magnum; frequently a posterior kinking occurs at the cervicomedullary junction. As the spinal cord may also be displaced downward, cervical and upper thoracic nerve roots commonly are angulated, ascending within the canal to exit at their intervertebral foramina. Scarring, gliosis, and parenchymal loss can affect the cerebellum so that folia may be poorly visualized and little cerebellar tissue may be present (Fig. 5-5A). Rather than gliosis, histologically the brainstem typically manifests distortion of its nuclei and fiber tracts. It has been postulated that this distortion, rather than the degree of brainstem herniation or the nature of the cervicomedullary deformity, accounts for the difficulties in breathing and swallowing experienced by some of these children (Wolpert 1988). The cerebellar hemisphere tissue that is present tends to crowd anterolaterally around the margins of the brainstem and may nearly encircle it (Fig. 5-5C). The inferiorly elongated

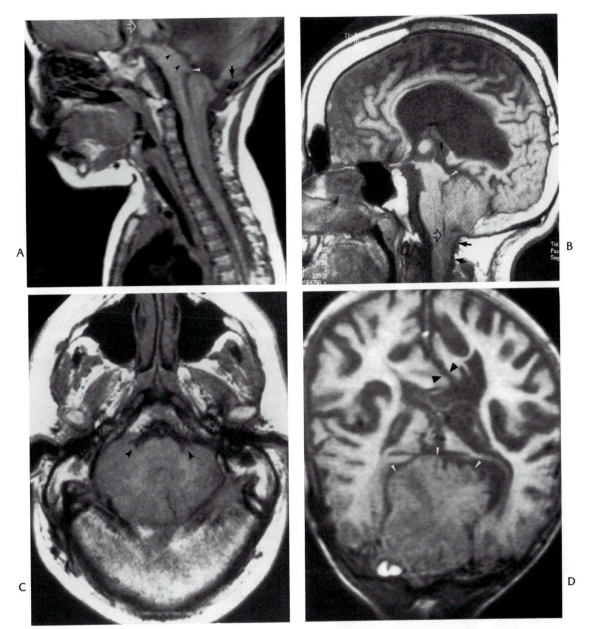

***Figure 5-5***  **Chiari II malformation. A.** Sagittal $T_1WI$ (600/20) demonstrates the extremely small posterior fossa: note that the flow void of the torcula (black arrow) is nearly at the posterior lip of the foramen magnum. Deformed cerebellar vermis, cerebellar tonsils, and fourth ventricle extend downward into the spinal canal behind the cervical spinal cord to the T1 level. Other features of the malformation—the beaked tectum (white arrowhead), prominent massa intermedia (open white arrow), lack of flow void in the aqueduct (double black arrowheads) secondary to aqueductal stenosis, and the associated hydrocephalus—are evident. **B.** Sagittal $T_1WI$ (600/15) demonstrates a less severe variant of the Chiari II malformation. In this case, more cerebellar tissue occupies the posterior fossa. Inferior vermis and cerebellar tonsils extend inferiorly only to the level of C2 (black arrows). Note, however, that the fourth ventricle extends below the foramen magnum (open black arrow). The midbrain appears somewhat elongated. The tectum is stubbier than in the previous case but is still beaked (white arrowhead). There is partial absence of the corpus callosum; there is thinning of the portion of the corpus callosum that formed secondary to hydrocephalus. Aqueductal stenosis is evident. The calvarium is thickened in this patient, who has been chronically shunted. **C.** Axial $T_1WI$ (600/15) in the same patient at the level of the foramen magnum, which appears large, shows portions of the cerebellar hemispheres extending anteriorly, partially encircling the lower brainstem (arrowheads). Note the concavity of the clivus. **D.** Coronal $T_1WI$ (600/20) demonstrates the "towering cerebellum" (white arrowheads) extending superiorly through the deficient tentorial incisura consequent to the small posterior fossa. Note the absence of crossing commissural fibers in the expected location of the splenium of the corpus callosum (black arrowheads) as a result of partial agenesis of the corpus callosum. Also note the inferior parasagittal portions of the cerebral hemispheres in this region interdigitating and wandering off the midline as a result of falx hypoplasia. Cortical sulci are prominent in this shunted patient.

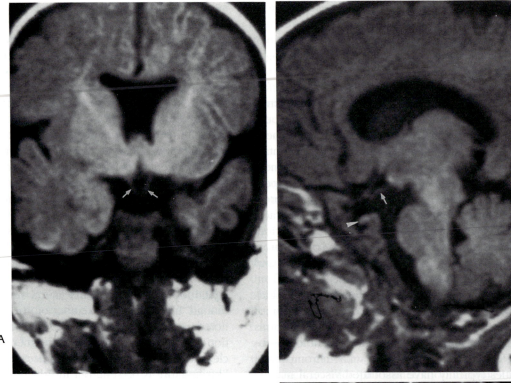

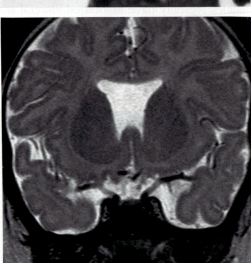

facial anomalies characterized by hypotelorism and cleft lip and palate.

While the alobar type and several of the features of the semilobar type of holoprosencephaly may be recognizable on CT (Fitz 1983; Altman 1984), more subtle manifestations of the anomaly may be appreciated only with the greater detail and multiplanar capability of MR. Lobar holoprosencephaly, for example, may have only a few features which distinguish it from a normal brain, such as the necessarily absent septum pellucidum and incomplete separation of the frontal lobes (Fig. 5-8B); in this case MR may actually be necessary for diagnosis.

## Septo-Optic Dysplasia

Septo-optic dysplasia (DeMorsier's syndrome) is an anomaly of midline structures which in its fullest extent is characterized by the triad of (1) absence or hypoplasia of the septum pellucidum, (2) hypoplasia of the optic nerves, and (3) hypothalamic-pituitary dysfunction of a varying degree (DeMorsier 1956; Hoyt 1970). The clinical manifestations are variable, but hypoplasia of the optic disks on ophthalmologic examination and growth retardation suggest the diagnosis (Standhope 1984). The findings on imaging studies may in fact be subtle. Small optic nerves and canals may be visible on CT (Manelfe 1979; O'Dwyer 1980), whereas small

*Figure 5-10* **Septo-optic dysplasia. A.** Coronal $T_1WI$ (600/15) demonstrates absence of the septum pellucidum and the relatively "boxlike" configuration of the frontal horns. The optic chiasm and tracts appear threadlike (arrows). **B.** Sagittal $T_1WI$ (600/15) reveals a hypoplastic optic chiasm (arrow). The pituitary gland (arrowhead) may also be somewhat hypoplastic. **C.** Coronal $T_2WI$ shows absence of the septum pellucidum.

nerves and a small chiasm may be seen on MR (Fig. 5-10A,B), but determining whether these structures are hypoplastic is often difficult. Frequently, the more obvious finding is an absence of the septum pellucidum, which is associated with a boxlike appearance of the frontal horns on CT and MR (Fig. 5-10A,C). The anterior recesses of the third ventricle and the suprasellar cistern may appear prominent, whereas the hypothalamus appears diminutive. Schizencephaly has been reported to be associated in approximately half these cases (Barkovich 1988*d*).

## Dysgenesis of the Corpus Callosum

Near the end of the phase of ventral induction, the dorsal portion of the thin rostral wall of the newly formed telencephalon—the lamina reuniens—thickens and then invaginates and begins to elongate posteriorly along the midline cleft between the rudimentary cerebral hemispheres. Over the next 2 months this process leads to the formation of the massa commissuralis—the cellular framework for ingrowth of the commissural fibers of the corpus callosum. After the formation of the massa commissuralis there is immediate development of the corresponding portion of the corpus callosum. That is, the corpus callosum develops as neurons in the cerebral hemispheres and are induced to send their axons into the massa commissuralis (Rakic 1968) through the genu, then the body, then the splenium, and finally the rostrum. The rostrum, which is the short segment posteroinferior to the genu, is the exception to the otherwise anteroposterior trend in the development of the corpus callosum. When an insult interferes with the process of formation of the corpus callosum, it may lead to complete or partial absence of this structure. When there is only a partial absence, however, a predictable pattern results. The regions that normally form first are present, whereas those that form last are absent. Thus, with partial agenesis, the genu is always present. It may be present alone or may be associated with some portion of the body, with only the splenium and rostrum being absent (Rubenstein 1994).

Lack of formation of all or a portion of the corpus callosum is invariably accompanied by other alterations in brain morphology. These characteristic deformities may be useful signs in the identification of the callosal anomaly. However, on axial CT, incomplete forms of agenesis may be difficult to recognize. By contrast, multiplanar MR permits ready identification of the anomaly and the segments of the corpus callosum which are involved (Fig. 5-7) (Davidson 1985; Barkovich 1988*c*). In the absence of the corpus callosum, axons that otherwise would have crossed between the two hemispheres do reach the medial aspect of their respective cerebral hemispheres but then turn to run posteriorly, parallel to the interhemispheric fissure. These axonal fibers (Probst bundles) course longitudinally between the bodies of the lateral ventricles laterally and the cingulate gyri medially (Fig. 5-11C,D). These fiber bundles impress the medial walls of the ventricles, giving the frontal horns a

characteristic crescent-shaped deformity on coronal images (Fig. 5-11A,C,D). There is a characteristic "straightening" or "paralleling" of the bodies of the lateral ventricles posteriorly, which is evident on axial images (Fig. 5-11B,E). The cingulate sulci do not form; consequently, the cingulate gyri do not become inverted but remain everted (Fig. 5-11A,C,D). Gyri dorsal to the cingulate gyri along the medial aspect of the hemispheres thus do not abut a cingulate sulcus but radiate unimpeded ventrally toward the third ventricle. This can be appreciated on sagittal MR images (Figs. 5-7F, 5-11A). In the absence of the capping effect of the corpus callosum, the third ventricle often protrudes superiorly between the two cerebral hemispheres, giving the impression that the interhemispheric fissure has been focally widened (Fig. 5-11C,D). An interhemispheric cyst, which may or may not communicate with the third ventricle, may be present in this location; it is usually distinguished by its larger size and mass effect. There is a characteristic irregular and often asymmetrical dilatation of the posterior portions of the bodies and trigones of the lateral ventricles. In the absence of the splenium of the corpus callosum, it is hypothesized that there is disorganization of the white matter that would have constituted crossing fibers in the parietooccipital regions, resulting in this altered ventricular appearance, which is known as *colpocephaly* (Fig. 5-11E,F).

In addition to malformation of the cingulate gyri, other limbic lobe anomalies are typically present (Atlas 1986). The cingulate gyri are continuous, via the cingulate isthmus, with the parahippocampal gyri. With dysgenesis of the corpus callosum, the parahippocampal gyri and more medial hippocampal formations often appear underdeveloped, giving a patulous appearance to the temporal horns; this finding is best demonstrated on coronal images (Fig. 5-11C,D). The fornices are fiber bundles that normally arc posterosuperiorly from the hippocampal formations, run along the undersurface of the corpus callosum, pass anteriorly along the roof of the third ventricle, and subsequently run downward in the region of the foramina of Monro, terminating in the mamillary bodies. With complete agenesis of the corpus callosum, they appear to be widely separated anteriorly. They may appear to be hypoplastic, and their commissure (the hippocampal commissure) may be absent. With complete agenesis, the leaves of the septum pellucidum are divergent.

Other anomalies, though not typically associated with agenesis of the corpus callosum, occur more often with this anomaly than would be expected in a random association (Parrish 1979). These anomalies include interhemispheric lipomas, Chiari II malformations, Dandy-Walker malformations, basal encephaloceles, and heterotopias (Rao 1990). Lipomas are

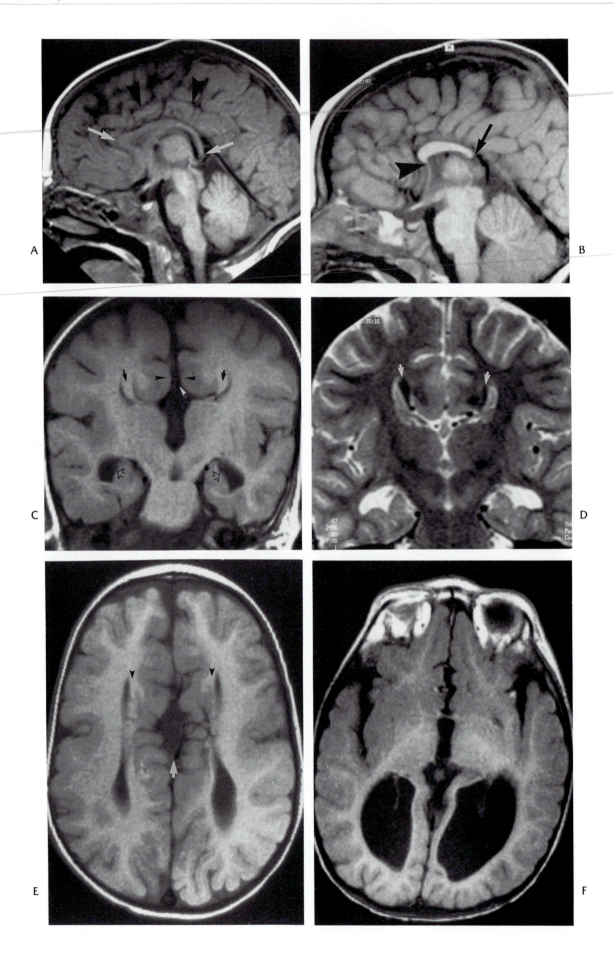

*Figure 5-11* **Agenesis of the corpus callosum. A.** Sagittal $T_1$WI in an infant under age 4 months, shows a complete normal, but thin corpus callosum (arrows). The premyelinated thin corpus callosum should not be mistaken for agenesis. Note that there is a normal cingulate gyrus (arrowheads). **B.** Sagittal $T_1$WI shows parietal agenesis of the corpus callosum, involving the posterior body and splenium (arrow) and the rostrum (arrowhead). **C.** Coronal $T_1$WI (600/20) demonstrates the persistently everted cingulate gyri (black arrowheads) and upward extension of the third ventricle (white arrowhead) above the level of the bodies of the lateral ventricles in continuity with the interhemispheric fissure. The frontal horns manifest a crescentic shape in this plane because of the impressions on their medial aspects made by the bundles of Probst (black arrows), which are white matter tracts normally destined to become crossing callosal fibers. Note the prominence (keyhole configuration) of the tips of the temporal horns as a result of underdeveloped Ammon's horns (open arrows). **D.** Coronal $T_2$WI shows the steer-horned shaped bodies of the lateral ventricles and the dilated temporal horns. Bundles of Probst (arrows) can be seen as myelinated tracks. **E.** Axial $T_1$WI (600/20) demonstrates the high-riding third ventricle (white arrow) and characteristic parallel configuration of the bodies of the lateral ventricles, with the bundles of Probst running medially (black arrowheads). The flaring of the atria and occipital horns (referred to as *colpocephaly*) is due to the thinning of the Probst bundles posteriorly and associated disorganization of white matter tracts consequent to the absence of the corpus callosum. **F.** Axial $T_1$WI at a lower level shows dilatation of the occipital horns, colpocephaly.

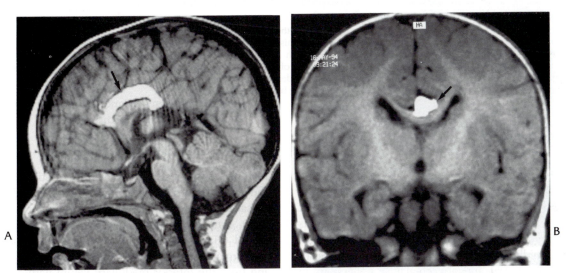

*Figure 5-12* **Partial agenesis of the corpus callosum with lipoma. A.** Sagittal $T_1$WI shows a lipoma superior to the remaining anterior body and genu of the corpus callosum. The lipoma is of increased signal intensity (arrow). The posterior body and splenium are absent. **B.** Coronal $T_1$WI shows the lipoma (arrow) lying on top of the body of the corpus callosum.

relatively rare anomalies that may occur along the interhemispheric fissure in the presence, partial absence (Fig. 5-12), or complete absence (Fig. 5-13) of the corpus callosum (Dean 1988). In its absence, interhemispheric lipomas are more commonly bulky midline masses, portions of which may insinuate into the bodies of the lateral ventricles on either side (Fig. 5-13A,B). On MR, these masses have the signal intensity of fat, appearing hyperintense on $T_1$WI and hypointense on $T_2$WI. Their characteristic fatty density is also readily detectable on CT (Figs. 5-12, 5-13C); dystrophic calcification may appear along the margins of the lipoma. Traditionally, their pathogenesis has been ascribed to a faulty disjunction of cutaneous ectoderm from overlying mesoderm during the formation of the neural tube. More recently, faulty regression and mal-

differentiation of the "meninx primitiva" (a neural crest derivative related in part to the primitive lamina reuniens, a source for the normal development of the subarachnoid cisterns) has been proposed (Truwit 1990). Agenesis of the corpus callosum is also a component of several syndromes, including Aicardi's syndrome (females with infantile spasms, mental retardation, and ocular and vertebral abnormalities as well as agenesis of the corpus callosum).

Patients with isolated agenesis of the corpus callosum may be asymptomatic. Careful neuropsychological testing may reveal a deficit in integrative capacities related to perceptual and language capabilities. Patients with other associated anomalies frequently have severe neurological disability, including mental retardation and seizures.

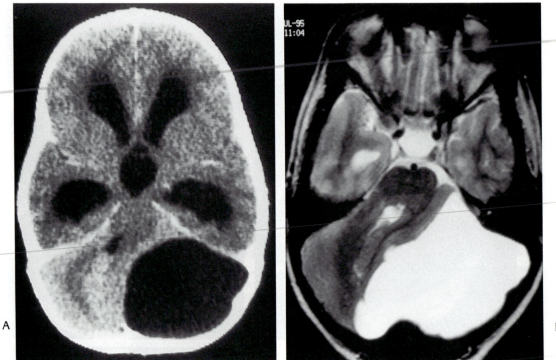

***Figure 5-16*** **Arachnoid cyst. A.** On this CECT image, a large posterolaterally located cyst is seen displacing and severely compressing the cerebellum and fourth ventricle. There is obstructive hydrocephalus. **B.** Axial $T_2WI$ shows marked displacement of the left cerebellar hemisphere, brain stem and fourth ventricle from left to right.

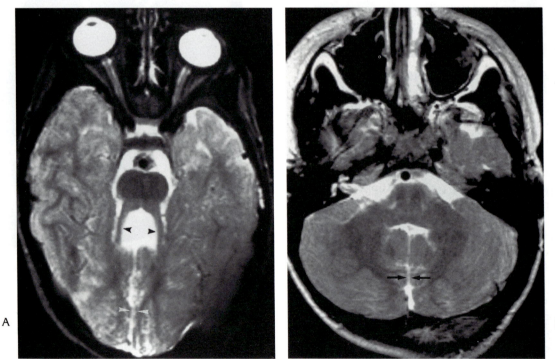

***Figure 5-17*** **Joubert's syndrome. A.** Axial $T_2WI$ (2500/80) near the pontomesencephalic junction demonstrates the batwing configuration of the fourth ventricle and the unusual definition of the superior cerebellar peduncles (black arrowheads) at this level. The vermis is not seen, and the two cerebellar hemispheres (white arrowheads) appose each other in the midline. **B.** Axial $T_2WI$ at a lower level in a different patient shows absence of the vermis. The two cerebellar hemispheres are separated by a cleft of CSF (arrows). *(Continued on next page)*

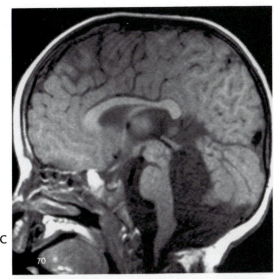

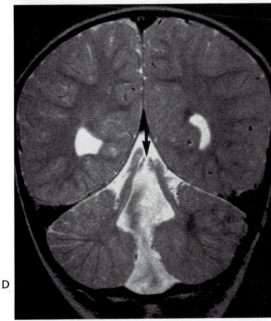

*Figure 5-17* **(continued) C.** Sagittal T$_1$WI shows dilated fourth ventricle, absent vermis, and malformed cerebellum. **D.** Coronal T$_2$WI (same patient as **C**) shows enlarged fourth ventricle, absent inferior vermis, and a split (arrow) hypoplastic superior vermis.

patient is symptomatic. Arachnoid cysts that are located elsewhere in the posterior fossa and have sufficient mass effect (Fig. 5-16) are commonly symptomatic, necessitating shunting and/or direct surgical decompression.

Finally, it is important to distinguish degenerative disorders involving posterior fossa structures from posterior fossa cystic malformations, as the prognosis is much different and shunting is not warranted. Enlargement of posterior fossa CSF spaces is only relative when there is a loss of hindbrain tissue (prominent cerebellar folia and/or small brainstem). No mass effect is seen.

## Joubert's Syndrome

This is a rare familial disorder characterized by nearly total aplasia of the cerebellar vermis. Microscopically, it is associated with cerebellar heterotopias and dysplasias of the cerebellar nuclei, inferior olives, trigeminal tract, and dorsal column nuclei as well as incomplete pyramidal decussation (Joubert 1969). Males are more commonly affected. Children with this disorder have abnormal eye movements, abnormal breathing patterns, and ataxia and are mentally retarded. They may have associated anomalies, including occipital encephaloceles, retinal dysplasia, syndactyly, and renal cystic disease (King 1984).

The CT and MR findings are characteristic (Kendall 1990). With absence of the cerebellar vermis, the cerebellar hemispheres appose each other directly in the midline (Fig. 5-17). There is a distinctive "batwing" configuration to the fourth ventricle at the level of the upper pons and midbrain, and the superior cerebellar peduncles are unusually apparent (Fig. 5-17) (Shen 1994).

## Lhermitte-Duclos Disease

Lhermitte-Duclos dysplasia, also described as dysplastic gangliocytoma is a form of cerebellar dysplasia. The essential pathological features consists of hypertrophic disorganized granular cells within neurons, hypermyelination of axons within the molecular layer of the cerebellum, and areas of necrosis or gliosis. There is gross thickening of cerebellar folia with or without mass effect. There is no sex prediction, often identified beyond the fourth decade. The lesion may mimic the appearance suggestive of an area of subacute or chronic infarction, or a neoplasm. On CT the mass is hypodense and does not enhance on CECT. Punctate hyperdensity within the lesion may represent calcification or hemorrhage. On MR the lesion has an ill defined margin, usually focal or involving the entire cerebellar hemisphere on one side, with some mass effect. It is hypointense signal on T$_1$ and hyperintense signal on T$_2$-weighted imaging. Lamellated or punctate hyperintense signal within the lesion may represent calcification or hemosiderine. It is rare to see enhancement on contrast-enhanced MR (Fig. 5-18) (Ashley 1990). The MR characteristic may be confused with tumor, venous, or arterial infarcs.

## Anomalies of Neuronal Proliferation and Migration

### DISTURBANCES OF BULK GROWTH

*Micrencephaly* refers to a primary hypoplasia of the brain and should be distinguished from *microcephaly,* which refers to a small cranial vault that may be due to a variety of causes (e.g., micrencephaly as well as a cavitated or atrophic brain secondary to vascular, infectious, or metabolic insults). Micrencephaly may manifest as an isolated phenomenon. That is, in some patients with micrencephaly, MR scanning reveals small cerebral hemispheres which appear to have nearly normal gross structural and relative gray-white matter proportions; commonly the convolutional pattern appears to be somewhat underdeveloped, however. The cerebellum is less affected, and so it appears relatively large. On the basis of experimental data (Dambska 1982; Hicks 1953), the anomaly is thought to be attributable to an interference with cellular proliferation of the germinal matrix (Dobbing 1973). Patients are typically moderately to severely retarded. Micrencephaly may also accompany other pathological conditions, such as agyria, pachygyria, and holoprosencephaly.

*Megalencephaly* refers to a focal or diffuse enlargement of the cerebral hemispheres. It may be primary, occurring in isolation, or may be associated with a syndrome (e.g., achrondroplasia, Soto's syndrome) (DeMeyer 1972). Generally, the gross morphology of the cerebrum is unremarkable, with all the portions of the cerebrum enlarged in proportion to each other (Friede 1989). The pathogenesis of diffuse primary megalencephaly is uncertain. Although it is known that in normal brain development neurons are initially overproduced and that neurons which are unable to form synaptic connections are eliminated, the mechanisms which regulate this process and may be disturbed in megalencephaly are unknown.

Megalencephaly may also be secondary to an abnormal accumulation of metabolic products in brain tissue,

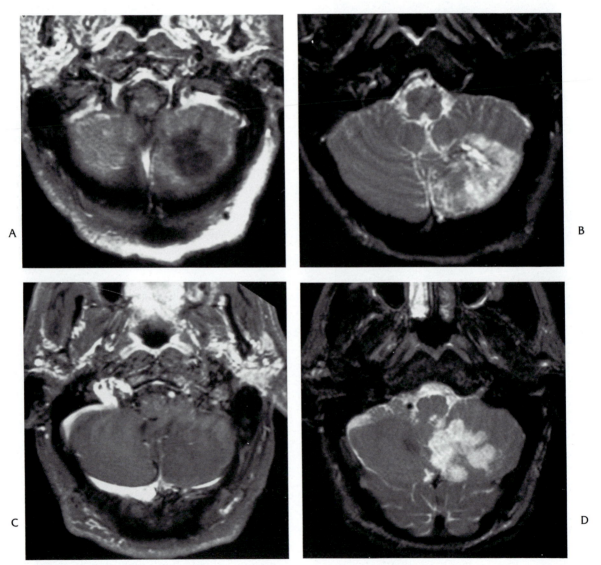

*Figure 5-18  Lhermitte-Duclos disease.* NCMR (T$_1$WI) shows hypodense lesion in the left cerebellum (**A**) and thick gyral and punctate hyperintense lesions on T$_2$WI (**B,C**). Minimal mass effect and no contrast enhancement is noted on axial CEMR (**D**).

A                                    B                                    C

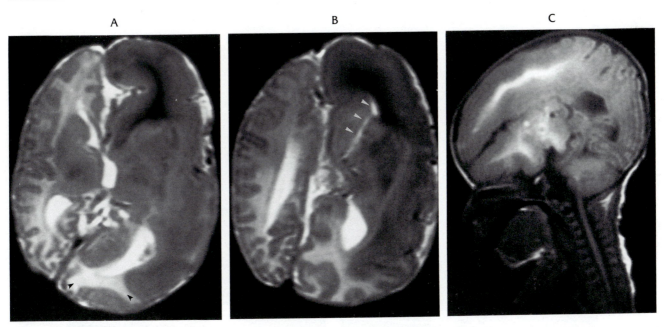

***Figure 5-19*** **Hemimegalencephaly. A,B.** Axial T₂WI (3000/120) in this newborn reveal marked asymmetry of the two cerebral hemispheres, with the right hemisphere appearing relatively normal. The left hemisphere is enlarged. There is thickening and disorganization of the cortical mantle, most marked in the frontal and temporal regions, associated with an abnormally smooth (lissencephalic/pachygyric) cortical surface. Almost no radiographically normal white matter is identifiable in the left hemisphere except in the occipital region (black arrowheads). Characteristically, the body (atria) of the ipsilateral ventricle is enlarged and the frontal horn is narrowed and pointed (white arrowheads). **C.** Sagittal T₁WI (600/15) shows the pachygyric cortex, anomalous sulcation in the midfrontal region, and abnormal signal intensity for age in the expected location of white matter in the frontal and temporal lobes. Posterior fossa structures are normal.

as in the mucopolysaccharidoses, Alexander's disease, and Canavan's disease. These disorders typically demonstrate abnormalities of the brain parenchyma, particularly in the white matter.

Unilateral megalencephaly (hemimegalencephaly) is a rarer anomaly. There is significant variability in its manifestations. There may be enlargement of all brain structures on one side (cerebral hemisphere, ipsilateral brainstem, and cerebellar hemisphere) or, more commonly, enlargement of all or a part of one cerebral hemisphere alone (Fitz 1978). It may occur as an isolated lesion or occasionally with somatic ipsilateral hemihypertrophy. Radiographically and pathologically, at least two subtypes of anomaly have been suggested (Townsend 1975; Friede 1989; Barkovich 1990). In some cases, the overgrowth of the hemisphere is accompanied by signs of anomalous neuronal migration (e.g., pachygyria and/or polymicrogyria) (Barkovich 1992*d*). Characteristically, the trigone of the ipsilateral lateral ventricle is enlarged; the frontal horn may appear narrowed and straightened. The relative proportion of white matter may be less than or much greater than normal, a finding which may depend on the severity of the migrational anomaly (Friede 1989). Its signal intensity on MR (density on CT) is often like that of the white matter in the contralateral hemisphere;

however, heterotopic gray matter and foci of gliosis may be present. In other cases (Fig. 5-19A–C), the MR appearance of the affected hemisphere is more bizarre. In addition to a dysmorphic appearance which is not easily characterized in accordance with known forms of migration anomaly, the signal intensity of the parenchyma, particularly the white matter, appears to be grossly abnormal. Pathologically, these lesions may show signs suggestive of hamartomatous overgrowth (disorganized misshapen neurons and glial cells). Patients with unilateral megalencephaly typically have a severe seizure disorder which may require hemispherectomy (Vigevano 1989).

## SCHIZENCEPHALY

*Schizencephaly* refers to gray-matter-lined full-thickness clefts involving one or both cerebral hemispheres. The gray matter bordering these clefts is abnormal, consisting of polymicrogyria which may be associated with underlying heterotopias. The pial covering over the adjacent brain surface extends inward along the margins of the cleft, fusing in its depths with the ventricular ependyma (pial-ependymal seam). The current terminology is intended to distinguish *schizencephaly* from *porencephaly,* which refers to parenchymal de-

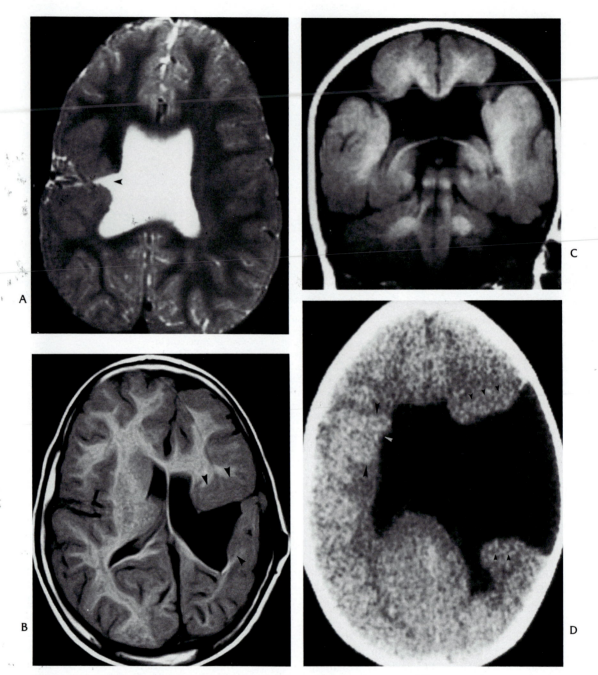

***Figure 5-20***  **Schizencephaly. A.** MRI. The excellent gray-white matter contrast definition on this T$_2$WI (2500/80) clearly distinguishes a closed-lip schizencephalic cleft. A ventricular "diverticulum" (arrowhead) characteristically defines the meeting of the closed-lip portion of the cleft with the margin of the ventricle. **B.** Axial T$_1$WI shows a closed-lip schizencephaly, lined by heterotopic gray matter (arrowheads). Note the deformity of the lateral ventricle, with the CSF pointing to the site of the closed-lip schizencephalic defect. **C.** Coronal T$_1$WI (600/15) clearly depicts large bilateral schizencephalic clefts in this 8 month old, who in addition to having seizures was severely delayed developmentally. **D.** Axial CT reveals a large CSF-filled cleft extending from the ventricle to the cortical surface. The parenchyma marginating the cleft (small black arrowheads) appears to have a relatively high density, like that of gray matter, consistent with a schizencephaly (open-lip type). There is the suggestion of a closed-lip schizencephaly on the contralateral side: irregularity along the edge of the body of the ventricle (white arrowhead) associated with apparent gray matter (large black arrowheads) extending inward to the ventricular margin at this point.

fects continuous with the ventricle that are not lined by gray matter and are thought to be due to an in utero insult that destroys nearly fully formed brain tissue. By contrast, it has been postulated that schizencephalic clefts result from an insult to the germinal matrix at around the seventh week of gestation, resulting in the loss of cells that otherwise would have migrated outward along glial cell processes to populate the overlying targeted portion of cortical mantle (Barkovich 1988b). Most schizencephalic clefts are located laterally, involving the region of the pre- and postcentral gyri. Occasionally they are located elsewhere in the hemispheres, including parasagittally. A cleft may be very narrow, with its gray-matter-lined edges directly apposing each other (closed-lip type) (Fig. 5-20A,B), or it may be very wide (open-lip type) (Fig. 5-20C) (Yakovlev 1946a,b).

On CT, it is sometimes difficult to diagnose schizencephaly (Fig. 5-20D) (Byrd 1989). The pathognomonic gray matter lining the cleft may or may not be discernible, compromising the distinction of this condition from porencephaly. The closed-lip type also may be difficult to distinguish from a focal irregularity along the margin of the ventricle, such as an irregularity due to periventricular leukomalacia. A thorough MR examination is usually definitive. Both $T_1WI$ and $T_2WI$ provide the necessary contrast resolution for discerning the anomalous gray matter along the cleft as well as the associated heterotopias (Barkovich 1988b; Osborne 1988). However, scanning along the plane of the cleft, particularly in instances of closed-lip schizencephaly, may obscure its relationship to the ventricular margin, confounding the diagnosis; thus, scanning is necessary in at least two planes. A helpful sign that aids in the detection of closed-lip schizencephaly is the focal ventricular irregularity that "points to" the cleft (Fig. 5-20A,B). The septum pellucidum is absent in the majority of patients with schizencephaly (Barkovich 1988b). Schizencephaly may coexist with septo-optic dysplasia .

Patients with schizencephaly typically have a seizure disorder. The accompanying neurological symptoms may, however, range from minimal to severe depending on the amount of brain tissue which is absent as a consequence of the cleft(s). Thus, patients with unilateral closed-lip clefts are generally the least disabled, whereas those with bilateral open-lip clefts are the most severely disabled (Barkovich 1992a).

## AGYRIA-PACHYGYRIA

The terms *agyria* and *pachygyria* refer to a range of severity in the manifestations of a particular type of neuronal migrational anomaly. Agyria, or lissencephaly, is the most severe, implying a complete absence of cor-

tical gyri. Pachygyria implies at least some gyral formation, although the gyri formed are abnormally broad and flat and are accompanied by shallow sulci. Complete agyria, or lissencephaly, is rare; the brains of most patients have regions of both agyria and pachygyria. In these cases, there is typically a frontotemporal predominance to the pachygyria and a parietooccipital localization of the agyria (Byrd 1988; Titelbaum 1989). In other instances pachygyria is a very focal abnormality that affects only a small region of cortex that may be located anywhere in the cerebral hemispheres. The underlying pathology in all cases reflects an arrest in the radial migration of waves of neuroblasts from the germinal matrix to their cortical locations (Smith 1989). This failure of migration is believed to occur between 8 and 16 weeks of gestation; there is then a subsequent lack of induction of formation of normal gyri, a process which begins after the fifth to sixth month of gestation. Microscopically, there is a derangement of the normal cortical architecture, with four abnormal layers instead of the normal six (Stewart 1975). The deepest of these four layers of neurons is the thickest and has been postulated to represent the region of halted neuronal migration. This abnormal cortex is actually broader in toto than is normal cortex, while the underlying white matter is thinned.

The more severe manifestations of the agyria-pachygyria complex can be appreciated on CT (Zimmerman 1983; Dobyns 1985b; Byrd 1988; Titelbaum 1989). In some cases, CT may in fact provide unique information, for example, when it reveals periventricular calcification in cases of cytomegalovirus (CMV) or toxoplasmosis-related malformations. In general, however, MR is the modality of choice for imaging these patients (Byrd 1988; Titelbaum 1989). Focal pachygyria frequently is discernible only with MR. In the most severe cases, the brain demonstrates a nearly completely smooth surface with an hourglass configuration as a result of shallow vertically oriented sylvian fissures (Fig. 5-21A–C). Less severe forms manifest some gyral formation (Fig. 5-21D–F). Pachygyria in the absence of agyria may be seen involving small or large areas anywhere, and so the multiplanar capability of MR is frequently useful in their detection. In all instances, the areas of involvement show thickening of the cortical mantle and a paucity of underlying white matter. The portions of the ventricular system that underlie regions of involvement typically are dilated, presumably secondary to the lack of formation of many white matter tracts. This also probably accounts for the small-appearing corpus callosum and brainstem in more severe cases. Pachygyria may also be seen in the brains of patients with other anomalies, such as hemimegalencephaly. The white matter that is present in the brains of more severely affected children may or may not ap-

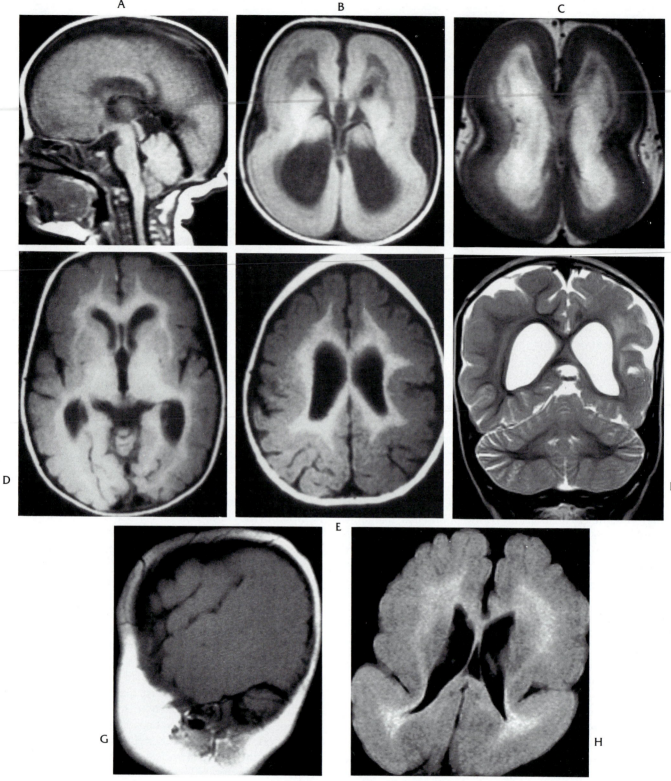

***Figure 5-21* Agyria-pachygyria. A.** Sagittal T$_1$WI (600/20) demonstrates the diffusely smooth cortical surface of the cerebrum in this infant with lissencephaly. Posterior fossa structures appear normal. **B,C.** Axial T$_1$WI (600/20) and T$_2$WI (3000/120) at different levels show the classic hourglass or figure-eight configuration of the cerebral hemispheres characterized by a smooth cortical surface and shallow, vertically oriented sylvian fissures. The cortical mantle is thick, while the rim of underlying white matter (seen as a band of intermediate signal intensity between the cortex and ventricles) is extremely thin. There is ex vacuo ventriculomegaly. **D,E.** Axial T$_1$WI (600/20) reveal a milder case in the spectrum of agyria/pachygyria than that shown in **A–C.** The cortex is diffusely thick, and myelinated white matter is scanty. In this patient, some gyri have developed, but most of those which have appeared are abnormally broad and flat. **F.** Coronal T$_2$WI shows bilateral, flat, thick gyri in both parietal regions, consistent with pachygyria. Note that the white matter is decreased in thickness. **G.** Sagittal T$_1$WI shows virtual absence of sulci in temporal lobe. **H.** Axial FLAIR image (same patient as **G**) shows bilateral thick cortex and decreased white matter involving all of the brain except for the frontal poles.

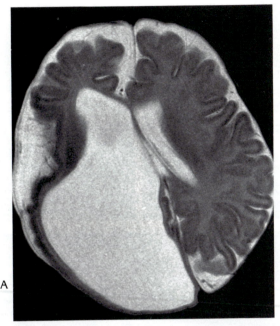
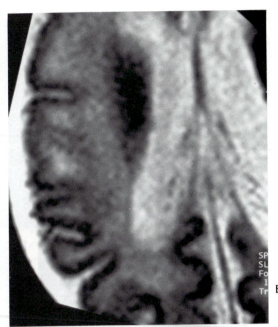
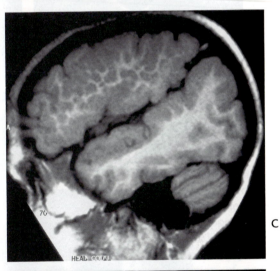
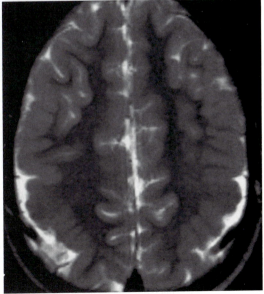

*Figure 5-22*  **Polymicrogyria. A.** Axial T₂WI shows marked dilatation of the right lateral ventricle and marked thinning of the overlying cortex. Notice that the surface of the cortex is finely irregular, indicating polymicrogyria. **B.** Axial T₂WI shows fine irregularity of overlying cortex. **C.** Sagittal T₁WI shows both finely nodular cortex of frontal and parietal lobes with an elongated sylvian fissure and thick cortex of the superior temporal gyrus. **D.** Axial T₂WI (same patient as **C**), cortex is thickened, but with irregular nodular surface. Gyral pattern is malformed.

pear normally myelinated; abnormal signal intensity in the white matter is frequently seen in patients with documented in utero infection (e.g., CMV) (Hayward 1991).

Patients with the more severe forms of agyria-pachygyria have small brains (micrencephaly). They are frequently hypotonic and severely delayed developmentally. Those with agyria have a dismal prognosis; most do not survive beyond 2 years of age. Patients with pachygyria are less severely retarded. A seizure disorder is common. Some patients have agyria as a component of a syndrome (e.g., Miller-Dieker and Walker-Warburg syndromes); others have cardiac or ocular anomalies (Dobyns 1984, 1985a). Some patients are reported to have had in utero infections (CMV more commonly than toxoplasmosis) (Titelbaum 1989).

## POLYMICROGYRIA

Polymicrogyria consists of an anomalous region of cerebral cortex characterized by multiple small gyri with an abnormal cytoarchitecture. It represents a disturbance in neuronal migration that appears to date to between the fourth and sixth months of gestation, which is the time of the onset of cortical gyral formation (Barkovich 1995; Gomez-Anson 1994). Some au-

LAING FC, FRATES MC, BROWN DL, et al: Sonography of the fetal posterior fossa: False appearance of mega-cisterna magna and Dandy-Walker variant. *Radiology* 192:247, 1994.

LIPSKI S, BRUNELLE F, AICARDI J, HIRSCH JF, LALLEMAND D: Gd-DOTA-enhanced MR imaging in two cases of Sturge-Weber syndrome. *AJNR* 11:690–692, 1990.

MANELFE C, ROCHICCIOLI P: CT of septo-optic dysplasia. *AJR* 133:1157–1160, 1979.

MARIA BL, ZINREICH SJ, CARSON BC, ROSENBAUM AE, FREEMAN JM: Dandy-Walker syndrome revisited. *Pediatr Neurosci* 13:45–51, 1987.

MASDEU JC, DOBBEN GD, AZAR-KIA B: Dandy-Walker syndrome studied by computed tomography and pneumoencephalography. *Radiology* 147:109–114, 1983.

MCCLONE DG, KNEPPER PA: The cause of Chiari II malformation: A unified theory. *Pediatr Neurosci* 15:1–12, 1989.

MCCLONE DG, NAIDICH TP: Developmental morphology of the subarachnoid space, brain vasculature, and contiguous structure, and the cause of the Chiari II malformation. *AJNR* 13:463–482, 1992.

MIROWITZ SA, SARTOR K, GADO M: High-intensity basal ganglia lesions on T1-weighted MR images in neurofibromatosis. *AJNR* 10:1159–1163, 1989.

MYRIANTHOPOULOS NC: Concepts, definitions and classifications of congenital and developmental malformations of the central nervous system and related structures, in Vinken PI, Bruyn GW (eds): *Handbook of Clinical Neurology*, vol 30, Amsterdam, Elsevier/North-Holland Biomedical, 1977, pp 1–13.

NAIDICH TP, PUDLOWSKI RM, NAIDICH JB, GORNISH M, RODRIGUEZ FJ: Computed tomographic signs of the Chiari II malformation: I. Skull and dural partitions. *Radiology* 134:65–71, 1980a.

NAIDICH TP, PUDLOWSKI RM, NAIDICH JB: Computed tomographic signs of Chiari II malformation: II. Midbrain and cerebellum. *Radiology* 134:391–398, 1980b.

NAIDICH TP, PUDLOWSKI RM, NAIDICH JB: Computed tomographic signs of the Chiari II malformation: III. Ventricles and cisterns. *Radiology* 134:657–663, 1980c.

NAIDICH TP, MCLONE DG, BAUER BS, KERNAHAN DA, ZAPARACKAS ZG: Midline craniofacial dysraphism. *Concepts Pediatr Neurosurg* 4:186–207, 1983a.

NAIDICH TP, MCLONE DG, FULLING KH: The Chiari II malformation: IV. The hindbrain deformity. *Neuroradiology* 25:179–197, 1983b.

NAIDICH TP, RADKOWSKI MA, BERNSTEIN RA, et al: Congenital malformations of the posterior fossa, in Taveras JM, Ferrucci JT (eds): *Radiology*. Philadelphia, Lippincott, 1986, pp 1–17.

NAIDICH TP, ZIMMERMAN RA: Common congenital malformations of the brain, in Brant-Zawadski M, Norman D (eds): *Magnetic Resonance Imaging of the Central Nervous System,* New York, Raven Press, 1987, pp 131–150.

NAIDICH TP, ALTMAN NR, BRAFFMAN BH, et al: Cephaloceles and related malformation. *AJNR* 13:655–690, 1992.

NIELSEN SL, BARINGER JR: Reovirus-induced aqueductal stenosis in hamsters: Phase contrast electromicroscopic studies. *Lab Invest* 27:531–537, 1972.

NUGENT GR, AL-MEFTY O, CHOU S: Communicating hydrocephalus as a cause of aqueductal stenosis. *J Neurosurg* 51:812–818, 1979.

O'DWYER W, NEWTON TH, HOYT W: Radiologic features of septo-optic dysplasia: De Morsier syndrome. *AJNR* 1:443–447, 1980.

OSBORN RE, BYRD SE, NAIDICH TP, BOHAN TP, FRIEDMAN H: MR imaging of neuronal migrational disorders. *AJNR* 9:1101–1106, 1988.

PARRISH ML, ROESSMANN U, LEVINSOHN MW: Agenesis of the corpus callosum: A study of the frequency of associated malformations. *Ann Neurol* 6:349–354, 1979.

PILLAY P, BARRETT GH, LANZEIRI C, et al: Dandy-Walker cyst upward herniation: The role of magnetic resonance imaging and double shunts. *Pediatr Neurosci* 15:74–79, 1989.

POSWILLO D: Mechanisms and pathogenesis of malformations. *Br Med Bull* 32:59–64, 1976.

RAKIC P, YAKOVLEV PI: Development of the corpus callosum and cavum septi in man. *J Comp Neurol* 132:45–72, 1968.

RAO AS, RAO VR, MANDALAM KR, et al: Corpus callosum lipoma with frontal encephalocele. *Neuroradiology* 32(1): 50–52, 1990.

RAYBAUD C: Cystic malformations of the posterior fossa. *J Neuroradiol* 9:103–133, 1982.

ROACH E, DEMYER W, CONNEALLY P, et al: Holoprosencephaly: Birth data, genetic and demographic analyses of 30 families. *Birth Defects* 11:294–313, 1975.

ROACH ES, WILLIAMS DP, LASTER DW: Magnetic resonance imaging in tuberous sclerosis. *Arch Neurol* 44:301–303, 1982.

RUBINSTEIN D, YOUNGMAN V, HISE JH, et al: Partial development of the corpus callosum. *AJNR* 15(5):869–875, 1994.

RUSSELL DS: Observations on the pathology of hydrocephalus, in Medical Research Council Special Report Series, No. 265, London. His Majesty's Stationery Office, 1949, pp 1–138.

SHAW CM, ALVORD EC: "Congenital arachnoid" cysts and their differential diagnosis, in Vinken PI, Bruyn GW (eds): *Handbook of Clinical Neurology,* vol 31, Amsterdam, Elsevier/North-Holland Biomedical, 1977, pp 75–135.

SHEN W-C, SHIAN W-J, CHEN C-C, et al: MRI of Joubert's syndrome. *Eur J Radiol* 18:30, 1994.

SIMPSON DA, DAVID DJ, WHITE J: Cephaloceles: Treatment, outcome and antenatal diagnosis. *Neurosurgery* 15:14–21, 1984.

SMITH AS, ROSS JS, BLASER SI, et al: Magnetic resonance imaging of disturbances in neuronal migration: Illustration of an embryologic process. *Radiographics* 9(3):509–522, 1989.

SOVIC O, VAN DER HAGEN CB, LOKEN AC: X-linked aqueductal stenosis. *Clin Genet* 11:416–420, 1977.

STANDHOPE R, PREECE MA, BROOK CHD: Hypoplastic optic nerves and pituitary dysfunction. A spectrum of anatomical and endocrine abnormalities. *Arch Dis Childhood* 59:11–141, 1984.

STEWART RM, RICHMAN DP, CAVINESS VS Jr: Lissencephaly and pachygyria: An architectonic and topographical analysis. *Acta Neuropathol (Berl)* 31:1–12, 1975.

STRAND RD, BARNES PD, POUSSAINT TY, et al: Cystic retrocerebellar malformations: Unification of the Dandy-Walker complex and the Blake's pouch cyst. *Pediatr Radiol* 23:258, 1993.

TITELBAUM DS, HAYWARD JC, ZIMMERMAN RA: Pachygyriclike changes: Topographic appearance at MR imaging and CT and correlation with neurologic status. *Radiology* 173:663–667, 1989.

TOWNSEND JJ, NIELSEN SL, MALAMUD N: Unilateral megalencephaly: Hamartoma or neoplasm? *Neurology* 25:448–453, 1975.

TRUWIT CL, BARKOVICH AJ: Pathogenesis of intracranial lipoma: An MR study in 42 patients. *AJNR* 11:665–674, 1990.

TURKEWITSCH N: Die Entwicklung des Aquaeductus Cerebri des Menschen. *Morphol Jahrb* 76:421–477, 1935.

TURNBULL IM, DRAKE CG: Membranous occlusion of the aqueduct of Sylvius. *J Neurosurg* 24:24–33, 1966.

VAGHI M, VISCIANI A, TESTA D, BIVELLI S, PASSERNI A: Cerebral MR findings in tuberous sclerosis. *J Comput Assist Tomogr* 11:403–406, 1987.

VAN DER KNAAP MS, VALK J: Classification of congenital abnormalities of the CNS. *AJNR* 9:315–326, 1988.

VIGEVANO F, BERTINI E, BOLDRINI R, et al: Hemimegalencephaly and intractable epilepsy. Benefits of hemispherectomy. *Epilepsia* 30:833–843, 1989.

VOLPE JJ: Normal and abnormal human brain development. *Clin Perinatol* 4:3–30, 1977.

WASENKO JJ, ROSENBLOOM SA, DUCHESNEAU PM, LANZIERI CF, WEINSTEIN MA: The Sturge-Weber syndrome: Comparison of MR and CT characteristics. *AJNR* 11:131–134, 1990.

WILLIAMS B: Is aqueduct stenosis the result of hydrocephalus? *Brain* 96:399–412, 1973.

WOLPERT SM, SCOTT RM, PLATENBERG C, RUNGE VM: The clinical significance of hindbrain herniation and deformity as shown on MR images of patients with Chiari II malformation. *AJNR* 9:1075–1078, 1988.

YAKOVLEV PI, WADSWORTH RC: Schizencephalies: A study of the congenital clefts in the cerebral mantle: I. Clefts with fused lips. *J Neuropathol Exp Neurol* 5:116–130, 1946a.

YAKOVLEV PI, WADSWORTH RC: Schizencephalies: A study of the congenital clefts in the cerebral mantle: II. Clefts with hydrocephalus and lips separated. *J Neuropathol Exp Neurol* 5:169–206, 1946b.

YAKOVLEV PI: Pathoarchitectonic studies of cerebral malformations. *J Neuropathol Exp Neurol* 18:22–30, 1959.

YAKOVLEV PI, LECOURS AR: The myelogenetic cycles of regional maturation of the brain, in Minkowski A (ed): *Regional Development of the Brain in Early Life,* Philadelphia, Davis, 1967, pp 3–70.

ZIMMERMAN RA, BRECKBILL D, DENNIS MW, et al: Cranial CT findings in patients with meningomyelocele. *AJR* 132:623–629, 1979.

ZIMMERMAN RA, BILANIUK LT, GROSSMAN RI: Computed tomography in migratory disorders of human brain development. *Neuroradiology* 25:257–263, 1983.

ZIMMERMAN RA, BILANIUK LT: Pediatric central nervous system, in Stark DD, Bradley WG Jr (eds): *Magnetic Resonance Imaging,* St. Louis, Mosby, 1988, pp 683–714.

# 6 DEGENERATIVE DISEASES AND HYDROCEPHALUS

*Krishna C.V.G. Rao*

## CONTENTS

The relative volume of brain parenchyma and CSF within the cranium varies, with the brain parenchyma occupying nearly 85 to 90 percent of the cranial compartment. In imaging studies, a slight increase in the relative volume of CSF spaces is not unusual in the neonatal period and again beyond the fifth decade. In the former it is seen during the period of neuronal and glial cell proliferation, and in the latter it is due to gradual loss of neurons, decreased cerebral perfusion, and alteration in the cellular metabolites. These subtle changes become obvious in neurodegenerative disorders, often resulting in significant loss of the brain parenchyma, described as *atrophy*. Enlarged ventricles are also seen in *hydrocephalus*, where there is an increase in volume of CSF, associated with increased cerebrospinal fluid pressure.

CT is useful in demonstrating the appearance of the ventricles and extracerebral CSF spaces in the diagnosis of atrophy or hydrocephalus. It is also useful in demonstrating obstructive lesions in the ventricular CSF pathways. MR, however, is ideal in evaluation of abnormalities of the gray and white matter in normal ag-

## Table 6-3   Atrophy and Neurodegenerative Disorders

Associated with dementia
  Primary
    Alzheimer's disease
    Pick's disease
  Secondary
    Multi-infarct dementia
    Binswanger's disease
    Jakob-Creutzfeldt disease
    Normal-pressure hydrocephalus
    Posttraumatic
    Paraneoplastic
    Infection (AIDS-related)
Associated with movement disorders
  Extrapyramidal nuclei
    Primary
      Parkinson's disease
      Huntington's disease
      Hallervorden-Spatz disease
      Leigh's syndrome
    Secondary
      Wilson's disease
      Zellweger's syndrome
      Hypoxic-ischemic insult
      Mitochondrial encephalopathy
  Substantia nigra and related nuclei
    Primary
      Parkinson's disease
      Striatonigral degeneration
      Shy-Drager syndrome
      Progressive supranuclear palsy
    Secondary
      Infarction
      Infection
      Trauma
      Toxins
Associated with ataxia involving cerebellum, brainstem,
  spinal cord
  Primary
    Olivopontocerebellar degeneration
    Olivary-cerebellar degeneration
    Friedreich's ataxia
    Progressive bulbar palsy
    Amyotrophic lateral sclerosis
  Acquired
    Alcohol
    Drug toxicity
    Infection
    Toxins
  Related disorders
    Wallerian degeneration

*Source: Modified from Adams 1989. Only those neurodegenerative disorders that have been demonstrated on imaging studies are included. The majority of these disorders demonstrate focal or diffuse atrophy.*

The purpose of imaging studies in patients with dementia is not only to document the loss in volume of the parenchyma and white matter changes but, more importantly, to evaluate the severity and progression of the disease process. Imaging studies are useful in identifying patients who may benefit from medical (hypertensive disease) or surgical intervention (space occupying lesion) and in evaluating preventive measures from further progression of the disease process.

Owing to increased longevity, there has been a progressive increase in the number of patients with dementia; nearly 15 percent of the people in the United States suffer from dementia-related syndromes (Fazekas 1987; Drayer 1988b). The percentage of the population with severe dementia increases from 1.5 percent at 65 years to 15 percent by age 85 years (Drayer 1988b). A fair number of these patients may suffer from dementia as a consequence of other risk factors, such as cardiovascular-related or metabolic causes. Recognition of the effect of these factors on the brain parenchyma utilizing imaging can be important in developing preventive methods and improving the quality of life.

Imaging studies may demonstrate a neoplasm, other space-occupying mass, or chronic communicating hydrocephalus (NPH) as one of the curable causes of dementia. However, in a significant number of patients the memory loss is severe and is related to one of the following neurodegenerative pathological causes.

## Alzheimer's Disease

This disease, a form of dementia seen as part of the aging process, is known as senile dementia of the Alzheimer's type (SDAT) when it presents after the sixth decade and as presenile dementia when it presents before the sixth decade. Both present with rapidly progressive memory loss (especially for recent events), confusion, gait apraxia, agnosia, and aphasia. The pathological features consist of generalized, almost symmetrical gyral atrophy with enlargement of the cortical sulci and ventricles. The atrophic process predominantly involves the frontal and temporal lobes but may also involve the parietal and occipital lobes (Tomlinson 1970, 1984). The histological changes consist of an abundance of senile plaques, neurofibrillary tangles made up of thickened tortuous fibrils within neuronal cytoplasm, neuronal cell loss, loss of dendritic spines, and branching fibers. The exact cause of these changes has not been established. A combination of factors may be involved, including multiple infarcts, mass lesions, low-grade or slow viral infections, and toxic or metabolic factors.

As previously mentioned, given the wide range of sulcul width and ventricular enlargement, depending on the patient's age, race, and sex (Manolio 1994; Yue 1997), the value of imaging studies is to exclude (1) space-occupying lesions, (2) the presence of extensive infarcts, or (3) evidence of NPH. CT and MRI provide similar information, although MRI is more sensitive in demonstrating the associated white matter changes. CT findings consist of (1) dilated ventricles and sulci and (2) disproportionate enlargement of the third ventricle, often associated with an abnormal neuropsychological screening test indicative of Alzheimer's disease (Drayer 1988a). Loss of gray matter–white matter discrimination, as well as hyperintensity of the medial temporal lobe and hippocampal atrophy, have also been described on MR of patients with Alzheimer's disease (Kido 1989; George 1981). Hippocampal atrophy is associated with enlarged hippocampal fissure, a finding not seen with normal pressure hydrocephalus (Holodny 1998, Jack 1992.)

Hyperintense lesions in the white matter (PVH, SCL, PVS) are common findings. Several studies have shown an increased incidence of these hyperintense lesions in patients with a known clinical diagnosis of Alzheimer's disease compared with an age-matched normal population (Bowen 1990; Fazekas 1987; George 1988a,b; Drayer 1986a,b). However, there has not been a good correlation between the severity of the dementia and the extent of the white matter changes (Bowen 1990). In fact, the diagnosis of Alzheimer's disease as the cause of dementia is more likely in the absence of these changes. MR in the coronal plane is useful in demonstrating the enlarged third ventricle and focal temporal horn enlargement from hippocampal atrophy (Fig. 6-12). $T_2$-weighted MR may also demonstrate hyperintensity along the medial temporal region, which probably represents interstitial fluid or gliosis (Kido 1989).

Apart from enlarged sulci (greater than 3 mm in width), gyral bands of hypointense signal in axial sections through the convexity have been described on $T_2$WI (Drayer 1987). They are attributed to ferritin deposits and are seen in nearly 50 percent of patients with Alzheimer's disease. From the preceding discussion it is obvious that the imaging diagnosis of Alzheimer's disease can be difficult to differentiate from other neurodegenerative conditions presenting with dementia (Tables 6-4 and 6-5).

## Pick's Disease

Pick's disease (lobar atrophy, lobar sclerosis) is a form of primary dementia associated with severe frontal and temporal lobe atrophy. It is rare compared with Alzheimer's disease and is clinically difficult to distinguish from Alzheimer's disease. The clinical diagnosis is based on progressive relentless loss of memory and concentration, with periods of apathy, agitation, unusual behavior, disorientation, and gait disturbance (Adams 1989; LeMay 1986). The disease is familial and probably is inherited. It is more common in females.

## Table 6-4   CT and MRI in Dementia: Imaging Characteristics

| DISEASE ENTITY | CT FINDINGS | MRI FINDINGS |
|---|---|---|
| Alzheimer's disease | Atrophic pattern, predominantly frontal and temporal lobes; wide sulci; enlarged third ventricle; prominent mesencephalic cistern | Similar to CT; increased signal on $T_2$WI in medial temporal lobe; subcortical white matter, basal ganglia; hypointensity due to deposition in parietal gyri |
| Pick's disease | Similar to Alzheimer's disease but greater atrophy in caudate nucleus, frontal and inferior temporal gyrus | Similar to CT findings |
| Multi-infarct dementia | Atrophy with generalized widening of sulci and lateral ventricles; diffuse periventricular and subcortical hypodensity | Similar to CT; hyperintense signal foci throughout white matter, basal ganglia thalamus, and pons; residual small hemorrhages due to amyloid angiopathy |
| Binswanger's disease | Vascular ectasia (hypertension); prominent sulcus; moderate ventricular enlargement; periventricular hypodensity | Bilateral symmetrical confluent regions of hyperintensity; sparing of subcortical arcuate fibers |
| Parkinsonian syndromes | Similar to Alzheimer's disease | In addition to findings under Alzheimer's disease, iso- or hyperintense signal in putamen, substantia nigra, and red nucleus |
| Normal-pressure hydrocephalus | Ventricular dilatation out of proportion to sulcal widening; rounded frontal horn | In addition to CT findings may show periventricular hyperintensity; prominent aqueductal flow-void signal |

## Multi-Infarct Dementia

Arteriosclerotic changes in the arterioles with prominent perivascular spaces, referred to as *etat crible* (seivelike) or leukoariosis, is a common feature of the aging brain. Although this is a normal process of aging, when similar changes are seen at an early age with loss of memory and cognitive functions it is defined as multi-infarct dementia (MID). The degenerative changes in the microvasculature leads to decreased perfusion of the brain parenchyma. Decreased perfusion leads to loss of neurons from ischemia, gliosis, and demyelination. Multi-infarct dementia is often associated with systemic diseases such as hypertension, cardiovascular disease, and diabetes mellitus. As a result of the primary disease, or the medical therapy in

these diseases, episodes of hypotension further decrease the cerebral perfusion of the neuronal cells and microvasculature, leading to ischemic episodes or infarction.

CT often shows regions of low attenuation in the centrum semiovale and the subcortical white matter. There is generalized cerebral atrophy, which often involves both the gray and white matter, seen as enlarged ventricles and sulci. These findings however are not specific for multi-infarct dementia, since similar changes may be seen in other neurodegenerative diseases. On $T_1$-weighted MR there is enlargement of the ventricles and sulci. Small lacunar infarcts are seen as hypointense signal foci in the periventricular and deep white matter. Spin density and $T_2$-weighted MR is ideal

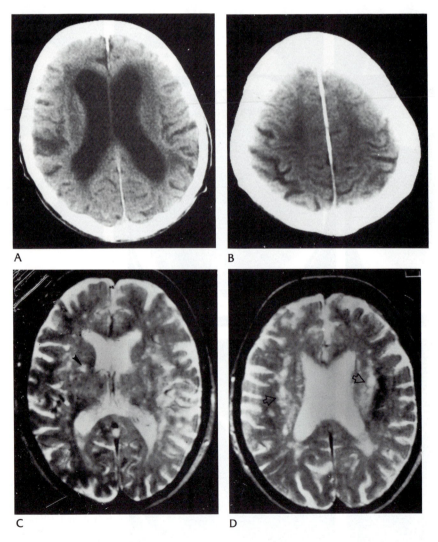

A

B

C

D

***Figure 6-14*** **Multi-infarct dementia** in a 62-year-old male with dementia and a history of hypertension controlled with medication. Axial CT **(A, B)** demonstrates moderate ventricular enlargement with periventricular hypodensity (arrows). **C, D.** $T_2$-weighted MR (SE 2700/80). Periventricular hyperintensity and multiple hyperintense signal foci of different sizes, with faded margins.

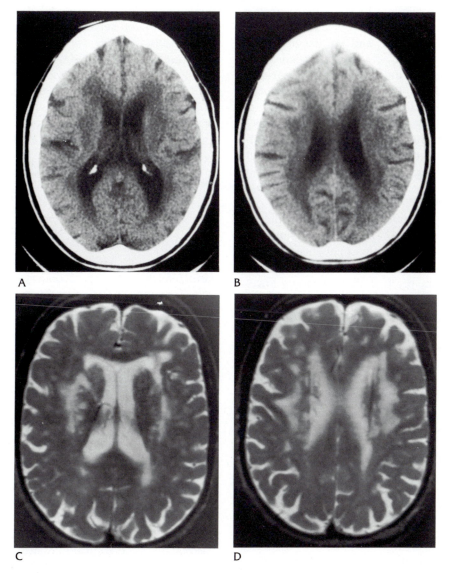

***Figure 6-15*** **Binswanger's disease** in a 59-year-old male with dementia. Axial CT. **A, B.** Mild ventricular enlargement with periventricular hypodensity and focal hypodensity in the centrum semiovale. **C, D.** MR demonstrates the typical linear hyperintense signal in the subcortical white matter, with sparing of the gray-white matter junction. In comparison to MID, there is more prominent PVH as well as mild ventricular enlargement.

and sensitive in demonstrating these regions as hyperintense signal in the periventricular region and the deep white matter. The majority of these hyperintense signal foci are usually subcortical, extensive, and asymmetrical (Fig. 6-14). The hyperintense signal foci may represent lacunar infarcts, gliosis, prominent perivascular spaces, or demyelination. Lacunar infarcts may also involve the basal ganglia. Unlike Alzheimer's disease, multi-infarct dementia is more common in the younger age group. They clinically present with progressive stepwise decline in mental function. A history of multiple focal neurologic deficits with recovery is suggestive of the etiology (LeMay 1986). In patients beyond the sixth decade in whom dementia could be due to com-

bination of Alzheimer's disease and degenerative microvascular disease it is difficult to correlate the severity of the dementia based on the extent of the ischemic changes (Kirkpatrick 1987; Braffman 1988 *a,b;* Kobari 1990; Bowen 1990).

*Binswanger's disease,* although initially described as a specific entity associated with dementia (Binswanger 1894), is now considered to represent a spectrum of multi-infarct dementia (Pantoni 1995; Caplan 1995). The disease is associated with progressive dementia, with periods of remission and exacerbation. Infarcts involve the subcortical arterioles, resulting in microangiopathic leukoencephalopathy with symmetrical involvement of both cerebral hemispheres (Burger 1976).

On imaging studies differentiation of Binswanger's disease from multi-infarct dementia is difficult, since they appear similar on both CT and MR imaging (Fig. 6-15). On CT there is patchy irregular hypodensity in the periventricular region and the deep white matter, dilated ventricles and loss in volume of the white matter (Zeumar 1980, Kinkel 1985, Lotz 1986, Rosenberg 1979). On MR they appear as hypointense signal foci in $T_1$-W images and bright signal in $T_2$-weighted images. Increased deposition of iron seen as abnormal hypointense signal in the putamen has been described (Drayer 1988*a*).

The clinical and imaging studies may mimic the dementia associated with normal pressure hydrocephalus (NPH). In certain percentage of cases the NPH may be associated with MID. In this group of patients the more extensive the subcortical and periventricular hyperintense foci, the lower the cerebral blood flow and lower the response to ventricular shunting (Bradley 1991*a*). It is conceivable that the availability of perfusion and diffusion imaging may be useful in the selection of patients suspected to have NPH, who may benefit from ventricular shunting.

## Jakob-Creutzfeldt Syndrome

Jakob-Creutzfeldt syndrome is a form of encephalopathy characterized by rapidly progressing dementia, presenting at an earlier age than other types of dementia. It is associated with altered perception, myoclonus, an increased response to startle stimulus, and cerebellar dysfunction. Initially believed to be caused by a specific viral strain similar to kuru (Gajdusek 1977), it is now thought to be caused by a slow infectious pathogen or prion, a transmissible protein substance. The disease may be familial in at least 15 percent of cases and has been explained on the basis of genetically inherited susceptibility (Kovanen 1985). The disease progresses to death, with an average course of less than 1 year from the time of diagnosis (LeMay 1986; Rao 1977). Pathological studies demonstrate atrophy of the gray matter with ventricular enlargement. Although rare, white matter changes have also been demonstrated (Macchi 1984). It is a form of encephalopathy with spongiform changes present in both the cerebral and cerebellar cortex, predominantly involving the temporal and occipital lobes (Masters 1978).

On imaging studies, the findings are nonspecific. Progressive atrophic changes have been described on sequential imaging studies (Rao 1977; Kovanen 1985; LeMay 1986, Tzeng 1997; DiRocco 1993). In some instances hyperintense signal foci on $T_2$WI have been demonstrated in the corpus striatum, thalamus, cerebral cortex (Gertz 1988), and caudate nucleus (Pearl 1989) in the early stages and with diffuse demyelination at the end stage of the disease. Diffuse demyelination can also be seen with Binswanger's MID or HIV encephalitis.

Diffuse hyperintense signal within the white matter and loss of gray matter, with rapid ventriculomegaly and dementia in a young person, is highly suggestive of this disease. Diagnosis usually requires an open brain biopsy.

## AIDS-Related Dementia

Dementia due to rapidly progressive diffuse cerebral atrophy in the younger age group is one of the manifestations of acquired immunodeficiency syndrome (AIDS) associated with HIV (Bursztyn 1984; Ekholm 1988; Chryskopoulos 1990; Flowers 1990). It probably represents quiescent or active encephalitis from the virus infection or from secondary infection, or as a result of immune suppression. The process results in cortical neuronal loss, gliosis, and vacuolation within the white matter. The pathological changes are the result of infection involving the microglia with toxic build-up of the intracellular $Ca^{++}$. Patients are also prone to infections such as toxoplasmosis and lesions of progressive multifocal leukoencephalopathy (PML), or lymphoma.

CT demonstrates extensive hypodense foci throughout the brain parenchyma, involving the white matter, the basal ganglia, pons, and cerebellum. CECT is essential to exclude the presence of lymphoma or toxoplasmosis. In patients with progressive HIV infection, MR often shows extensive areas of white matter involvement with hypointense signal on $T_2$WI and hyperintense signal foci on $T_1$WI, which are confluent. It also involves the cortical gray matter, the basal ganglia, and the pons (Fig. 6-16). Diffuse global atrophy with ventriculomegaly is a common feature. Gd-DTPA enhanced MR is sensitive and essential to exclude lymphoma, toxoplasmosis, or other infectious etiologies.

## Neoplasia and Metabolic Disorder

Diffuse brain atrophy is often present in patients with systemic neoplasia without metastatic brain involvement. The atrophic process is believed to be due to nutritional causes (Huckman 1975). A similar atrophic pattern is seen in patients (1) with anorexia nervosa (Enzmann 1977, Kohlmeyer 1983), (2) following the long-term use of adrenocorticotropic hormone (ACTH) or steroids (Bentson 1978; Okuno 1980) (Fig. 6-17), (3) in chronic alcoholics (Fox 1976; Schroth 1988) (Fig. 6-18), and (4) in patients with chronic renal failure who are on dialysis (Kretzschmar 1983; Savazzi 1986; Komatsu 1988). In all these conditions the atrophy is reversible after restoration of the proper nutrients or electrolytes.

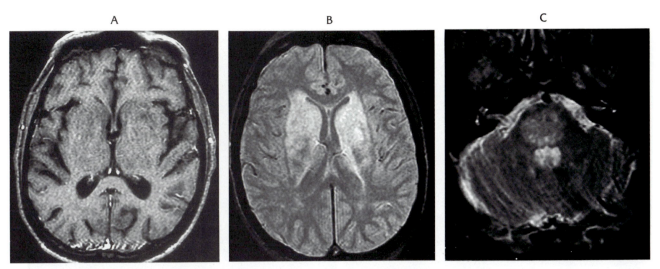

***Figure 6-16*** **AIDS-related dementia.** Axial $T_1$-weighted **(A)** and $T_2$-weighted **(B, C)** MR demonstrate extensive hyperintense signal within the basal ganglia, subcortical region, periventricular region, and pons due to AIDS-related chronic encephalomyelitis.

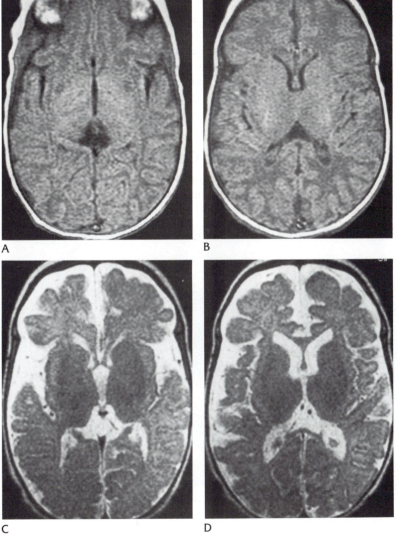

***Figure 6-17*** **Corticosteroid induced atrophy.** Axial $T_1$-weighted MR **(A, B)** before and **(C, D)** axial $T_2$-weighted MR 6 weeks later, demonstrating severe cerebral atrophy involving both gray and white matter. *(Continued on next page)*

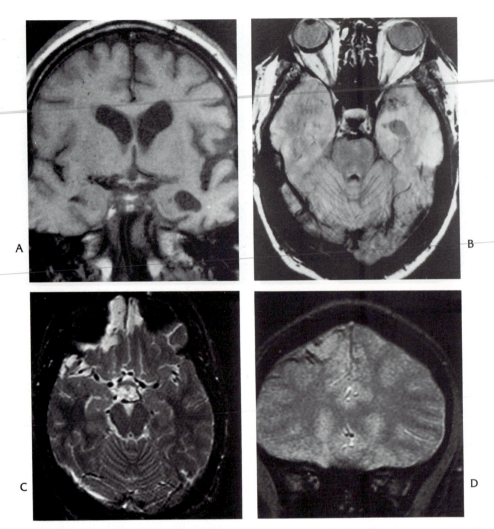

***Figure 6-21*** **Posttraumatic focal atrophy. A.** Coronal T$_1$-weighted MR demonstrates focal atrophy of the left temporal lobe with ipsilateral dilatation of the temporal horn and lateral ventricle. **B.** Axial T$_2$-weighted MR (2800/100) demonstrates focal dilatation of temporal horn and gliosis of the temporal lobe. Axial T$_2$-weighted **(C)** and coronal **(D)** gradient sequence MR in another patient demonstrates focal atrophy of the frontal lobes as well as hemosiderin deposition in another area of contusion (arrow).

metabolic factor. Depending on the age of the patient at the time of the insult and the duration of the anoxic episode, the end result of the atrophic patterns is different. Usually there is initial generalized edema followed over a period of weeks with neuronal loss and gliosis.

In infants and children the cerebral atrophy in those who survive anoxic or hypoxic insult depends on the gestational age when the anoxic episode occurred and the duration of the insult. The anoxic damage may be due to partial prolonged asphyxiation or insufficient perfusion of the developing brain due to cardiovascular insult (Barkovich 1990) (Fig. 6-22). Although CT or MR is useful in demonstrating the parenchymal damage in infants who survive these episodes (Flodmark 1980), they can be better evaluated with least amount of patient handling using sonography.

In the evaluation of children with a prior history of anoxic encephalopathy, clinical findings consisting of seizures, lethargy, hypotonia, or subtle neurologic deficits may not be helpful in assessing the extent or severity of the hypoxic or ischemic insult. MR is useful in demonstrating the pathological changes, which may be generalized or focal (Fig. 6-23). Hypoxemia or anoxia during the first two trimesters usually results in developmental anomalies such as loss of cortex, dysplastic gray matter, and smooth walled cyst formation (porencephaly), which may or may not communicate with the ventricles (Fig. 6-24). In hypoxic or ischemic changes during the perinatal period, imaging studies depend on the severity of the insult and whether the infant was premature or full term. In the premature infant immature periventricular blood supply and hypoxemia from poor lung capacity, in its mild form is seen

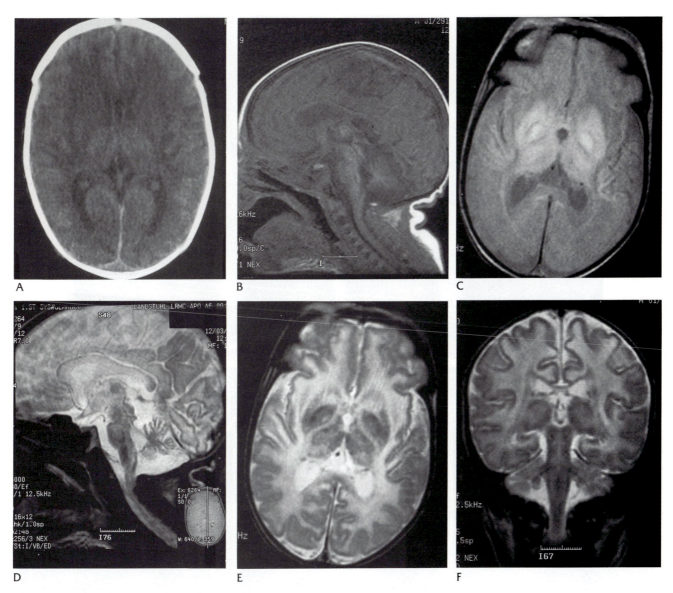

A

B

C

D

E

F

*Figure 6-22*  **Profound hypoxemia with circulatory arrest** in a 32-week infant following difficult delivery, initially presumed to have normal function that rapidly deteriorated clinically. **A.** CT performed on day 4 demonstrates diffuse cerebral edema. MR performed on day 10 **(B)** demonstrates diffuse hemispheric swelling, **(C)** with bright signal involving the basal ganglia and thalamus. $T_2$-weighted **(D)** sagittal, **(E)** axial, and **(F)** coronal images demonstrate bilateral white matter changes, loss of gray matter, and hypointense signal within the germinal matrix region.

as periventricular leukomalacia (PVL). Reperfusion of these ischemic regions, primarily the basal ganglia, results in germinal matrix hemorrhage, graded as to severity depending on whether the hemorrhage is confined to the germinal matrix (grade 1), extension into the ventricle or subependymal region (grade 2), or massive hemorrhage into the ventricle with hydrocephalus (grade 3). In those who survive, varying degrees of neurologic deficits are common. MR may be useful in determining the gestational age at the time of insult based on the pattern of atrophic changes as well as the extent of PVL (Baker 1988). PVL results from loss of white matter and gliosis. There is a higher inci-

dence of PVL in infants with birth weight less than 2000 g. It often involves the region of the germinal matrix and the periventricular region adjacent to the trigone of the lateral ventricles. PVL may also develop following hydrocephalus, certain metabolic disorders, and ventriculitis. On MRI, PVL is associated with a decrease in the amount of white matter, periventricular hyperintense signal, and irregular focal dilatation of the ventricle, as well as dilatation of the sulci in the involved region (Fig. 6-25).

Anoxic episodes occurring between 24 and 28 weeks of gestational age demonstrate an enlarged irregular trigone of the lateral ventricles without

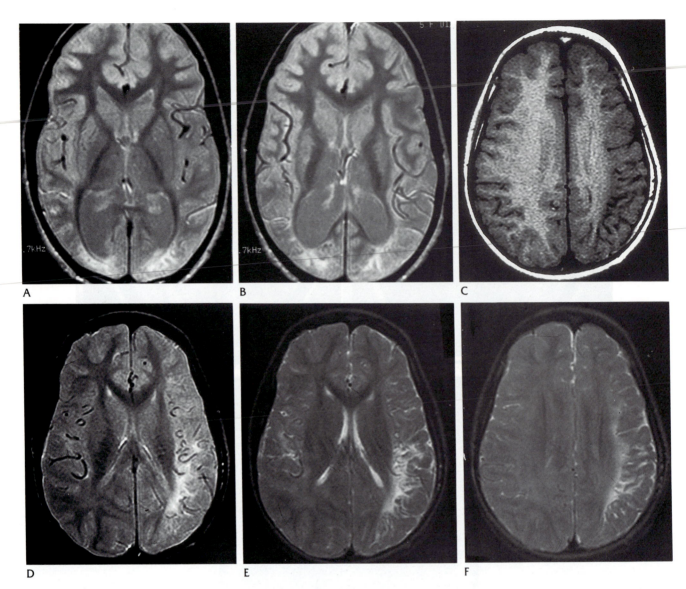

*Figure 6-26*  **Periventricular leukomalacia** in a 5-year-old infant with a history of perinatal asphyxia, with delayed developmental milestones and seizures. **A, B.** Axial spin-density-weighted MR demonstrates enlargement of the occipital horns of the lateral ventricle with periventricular gliosis and loss of white matter. **Ulegyria.**

**C.** Axial $T_1$-W MR **D.** Axial spin density MR. **E–F**. Axial $T_2$W. MR demonstrates loss of white matter and bright signal in spin density and $T_2$W MR. Note crowding of the gyral folds affecting the deeper portion of the gyri.

cumference is smaller than the standard deviation, occasionally patients may present with enlarging head. Both CT and MR demonstrate the cystic changes and the dilated ventricles (Fig. 6-27). Additionally MR demonstrates the septation as well as the glial changes surrounding the cysts.

## Porencephaly

Porencephaly is defined as a fluid-filled cavity (presumably CSF), usually secondary to infarction within the brain parenchyma, usually during the gestation pe-

riod. Porencephaly is often associated with other developmental anomalies such as corticle dysplasia. The cysts have smooth walls but not glial reaction. The cavity may communicate with the ventricle, in which case it is defined as porencephalic dilatation of the ventricle. When communicating with the ventricle it may have an ependymal lining similar to the rest of the ventricles. A porencephalic cyst may be noncommunicating either de novo or from secondary infection. The cyst can enlarge with time, necessitating decompression. Puncture porencephaly is the development of a cystic cavitation along the track of the ventricular nee-

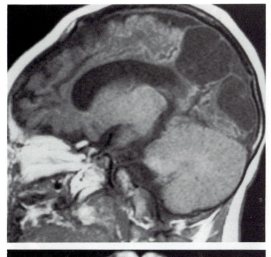

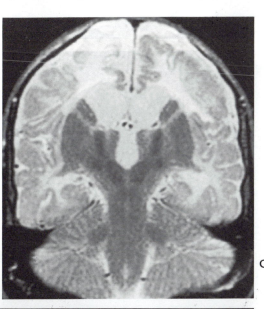

*Figure 6-27* **Multicystic encephalomalacia. A.** Sagittal T$_1$-weighted MR. **B.** Axial T$_2$-weighted MR. **C.** Coronal T$_2$-weighted (3000/40) MR. Extensive areas of encephalomalacic changes with loss of gray and white matter. Large cystic cavitation within the parenchyma is present. **D, E.** CT in another infant with multiple regions of focal destruction of the brain with cystic cavitation. In another infant (**E**) axial CT demonstrates extensive areas of infarct with a venous hemorrhagic component in the parietooccipital region in an infant. MR obtained 5 years later. Sagittal T$_1$-weighted (**F**) and coronal T$_1$-weighted (**G**) images show extensive encephalomalacic changes. **H.** Axial T$_2$-weighted MR shows the loss of gray and white matter with porencephalic dilatation of the right lateral ventricle and periventricular gliosis. *(Continued on next page)*

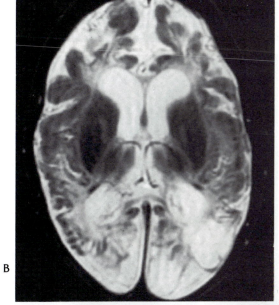

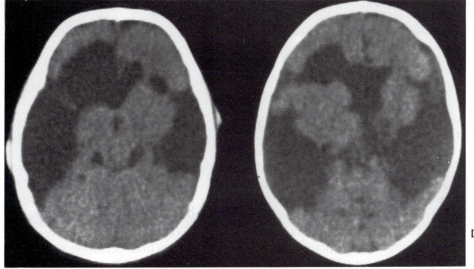

A

B

C

D

*Figure 6-29*   *(continued)*

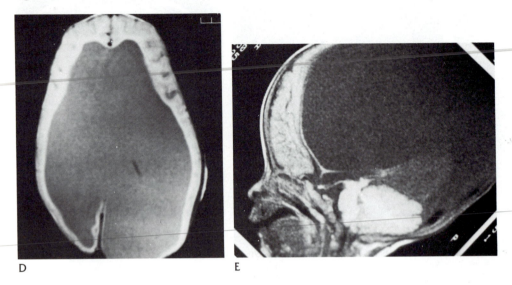

D                           E

# FOCAL ATROPHY

Unlike diffuse cerebral atrophy and dementia associated with neurodegenerative diseases and aging, focal atrophy may be seen at any age. The most common clinical presentation is that of a focal neurological deficit or seizures. Focal atrophy usually is secondary to trauma, infection, infarction, or dysgenesis, and usually follows surgery. Depending on the preceding cause, the focal atrophic process may manifest as early as few weeks following the event or years later. The pathogenesis of the atrophy is suggested by the location, although clinical history is necessary for correlation with the imaging findings.

Posttraumatic focal atrophy follows cerebral contusion or cerebral hematoma after surgical evacuation (Kishore 1980). Although atrophy may occur anywhere, the usual location is the frontal or temporal lobes. MR with gradient-echo sequence or FLAIR imaging is useful in demonstrating the micromolecular iron pigment within the myelin fibers or the focal gliosis (Fig. 6-30). Postinflammatory atrophy often follows brain abscess, herpes encephalitis, and TORCH infections (Fig. 6-31). Focal atrophy secondary to vascular anomalies follows hemorrhages or infarction. These infarcts are usually confined to the vascular distribution,

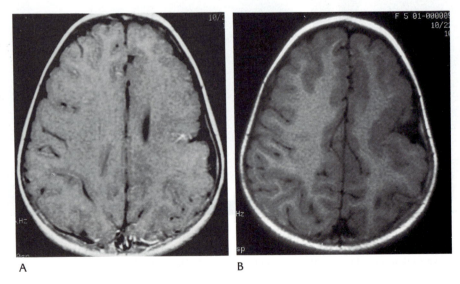

A                           B

***Figure 6-30***   $T_1$-weighted **(A, B)** axial and **(C)** coronal MR demonstrates **focal atrophy** involving the left cerebral hemisphere with minimal enlargement of the left lateral ventricle and cortical dysplasia (arrow).

often involving the watershed areas of the major vascular channels. In long-standing cases, focal prominence of the cortical sulci and/or ipsilateral ventricular enlargement may be the only findings.

# CEREBRAL HEMIATROPHY

Cerebral hemiatrophy is a pathological entity associated with focal or diffuse atrophy involving one cerebral hemisphere. It usually presents with hemiplegia, convulsions, and seizures. *Dyke-Davidoff-Masson syndrome* is a form of focal cerebral atrophy which involves the whole cerebral hemisphere on one side (Dyke 1933). It is presumably due to neonatal or gestational vascular occlusion, primarily involving the middle cerebral vascular territory with focal parenchymal destruction. It may also follow prolonged childhood febrile seizures. Usually it manifests during adolescence with seizures. Imaging studies demonstrate unilateral atrophy of the cerebral hemisphere with ipsilateral shift of the ventricles. The sulci on the involved side are wide and often are replaced by gliotic brain tissue. Since the initial description, recent studies have demonstrated in addition to the above constellation of findings, an associated contralateral atrophy of the cerebellar hemisphere. On CT the volume of the brain parenchyma on affected side is smaller, with thickening of the calvaria and marked enlargement of the air sinuses (Zilkha 1980) (Fig. 6-32). On MRI (T$_2$WI), the gliotic areas are seen as hyperintensity of both the gray matter and white matter, with a thin rim of cortical gray matter (Sener 1992). In addition to the thickening

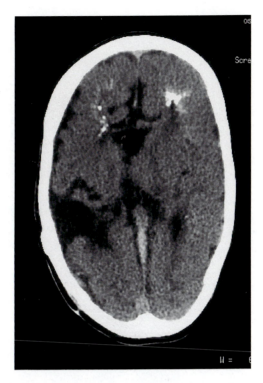

***Figure 6-31*** **Focal atrophy** in a child with cytomegalovirus infection.

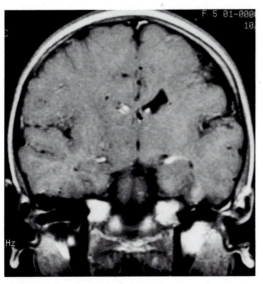

C

of the calvaria and hemispherical encephalomalacic changes, the roof of the orbit is elevated, and the adjacent air sinuses are prominent and enlarged.

*Sturge-Weber disease,* or encephalotrigeminal angiomatosis, is a condition associated with focal or hemispheric atrophy, facial nevus, and a vascular anomaly. The anomaly often presents with a facial nevus along the distribution of the trigeminal nerve, seizures, hemiparesis, and varying degrees of mental retardation. The intracranial pathologic lesion is a leptomeningeal angioma with abnormal venous drainage affecting the pial and outer layer of the cortex. Prominent arterial and venous channels are seen coursing along the undersurface of the cortex. Calcifications may be seen as gyral bands on the surface. Although commonly seen in the parietooccipital region, similar gyral bands of calcification having the appearance of a "tram track," may also be seen in the frontal and temporal region. This calcification usually is well seen beyond the age of 2 years. The choroid plexus on the affected side is often enlarged, either owing to hyperplasia or as part of the angiomatous malformation. Diagnosis is based on presence of facial nevus and cerebral hemiatrophy with leptomeningeal enhancement. On CT and MRI, enhancement of the surface of the brain may be the only finding (Fig. 6-33). Occasionally the enhancing vascular channels traversing the brain parenchyma may be seen on CT. MR is

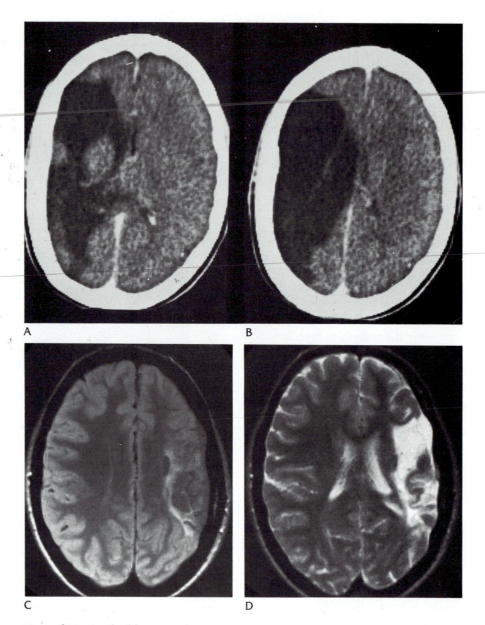

*Figure 6-32*  **Cerebral hemiatrophy. A, B.** Axial CECT. There is extensive loss of parenchyma of the right cerebral hemisphere with compensating thickness of the calvaria on the affected side. **C, D.** Similar finding on MR involving the left cerebral hemisphere.

ideal in demonstrating the enhancement of the leptomeninges, gyri, and choroid plexus. MR also demonstrates the enlarged deep medullary veins.

*Linear nevus sebaceous syndrome* is a dysplastic neurocutaneous syndrome associated with cerebral hemiatrophy, with some features similar to the Sturge-Weber syndrome (Chalhub 1975). Clinical presentation consists of intractable seizures and varying severity of mental retardation, usually in infancy or adolescence. The skin lesion consists of a linear patchy yellowish verrucous lesion involving the forehead, which may extend to a

*Figure 6-33 (right page)*  **Cerebral hemiatrophy in Sturge-Weber disease. A.** Axial CT in an adult demonstrates focal atrophy of left cerebral hemisphere, with extensive tram track calcification of the outer cortical layer. MR in a 15-month-old child with Sturge-Weber. **B.** $T_1$-weighted sagittal MR demonstrates large deep medullary vein. Axial **(C)**, coronal **(D)**, and sagittal **(E)** gadolinium-enhanced MR demonstrates extensive enlarged deep medullary veins (arrows) and enlarged choroid plexus. **Linear nevus sebaceous syndrome. F.** Axial CT demonstrates severe atrophy of the right cerebral hemisphere with gyral calcification. **G.** Coronal $T_2$-weighted MR demonstrates extensive atrophy with loss of white matter and thick gyral folds, and contralateral megaloencephaly. **H.** Gadolinium-enhanced MR demonstrates anomalous venous drainage and enhancement of the cortical surface.

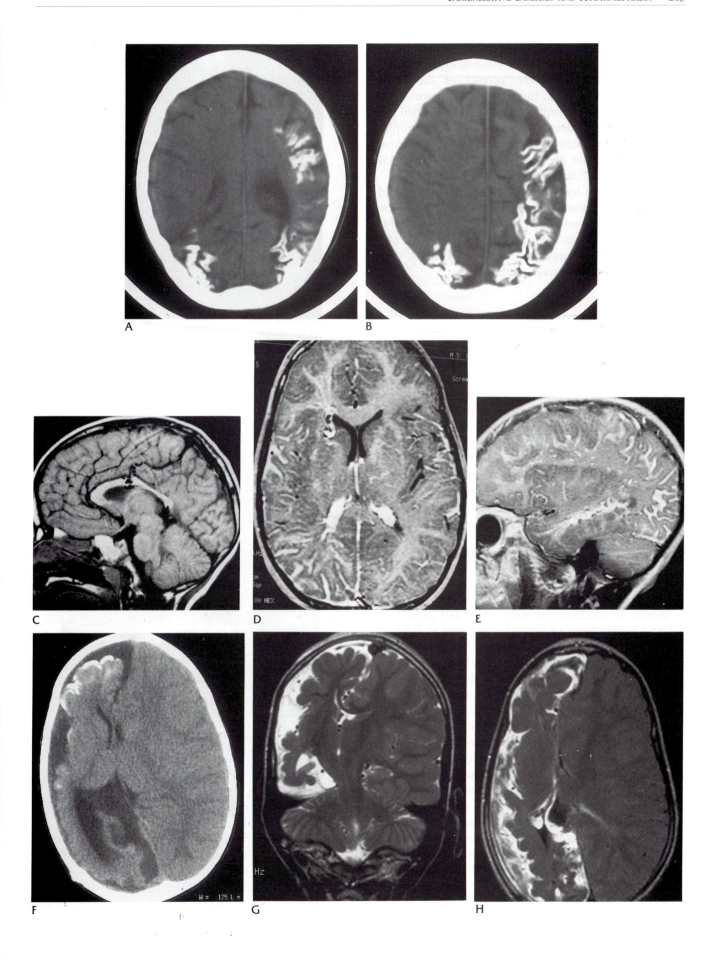

## Table 6-7    Imaging Features in Movement Disorders

| DISEASE ENTITY | CEREBRAL ATROPHY | HYPERINTENSE SIGNAL ON T$_2$WI | MIDBRAIN ATROPHY | HINDBRAIN ATROPHY | HYPOINTENSE SIGNAL ON T$_2$WI |
|---|---|---|---|---|---|
| Parkinson's disease (tremor, rigidity, akinesia) | Mild to moderate Beyond 5th decade | White matter; lesser extent, BG/pons and thalamus | Normal to mild Pars compacta of SN | None | Moderate to marked bright signal: SN/GP/RN/DN |
| Striatonigral degeneration (rigidity, akinesia) | Normal to mild Beyond 4th decade | On low and midfield MR: hyperintense putamen ? gliosis | Pars compacta Atrophy of putamen | Present when part of multisystem atrophy | Putamen/SN Lesser extent, caudate |
| Shy-Drager syndrome (orthostatic hypotension, urinary incontinence, inability to sweat) | Moderate Usually beyond 5th decade | Nonspecific, white matter | When associated with OPCA | When part of MSA | Primarily involves putamen |
| Progressive supranuclear palsy (rigidity, pseudobulbar palsy, ophthalmoplegia) | Mild to moderate Usually beyond 5th decade | Periaqueductal region | Moderate to severe of mesencephalon | Moderate to severe | SN/RN Tectum |
| Hallervorden-Spatz disease (dystonia, dysphasia dysarthria, rigidity, gait disturbance) | Normal to mild Usually 2d decade 50% familial Progressive course | Occasional GP/pars reticularis of SN | Mild to moderate Mesencephalon | Not common | SN/GP |
| Huntington's disease (choreoathetosis, dementia) | Mild to moderate Involves caudate Beyond 4th decade | Occasionally present Caudate, putamen May represent gliosis | Usually none | None | Caudate and putamen: may represent iron |

## Parkinson's Disease and Syndrome

Parkinson's disease (paralysis agitans) is a movement disorder associated with cogwheel-type rigidity (Parkinson 1817). The rigidity is followed by tremor, akinesia, and postural deformities. The onset of the disease usually occurs in the fourth or fifth decade, with progressive neurological deterioration and without remissions or exacerbations. The disease involves the cells and fibers of the substania nigra. In later stages, there is involvement of the corpus striatum and globus pallidus. There is a loss of neuromelanin-containing neurons in the pars compacta of the substantia nigra, the locus ceruleus, and the dorsal vagal nucleus, with resulting gliosis. Other subtypes of Parkinson's disease have been described, such as striatonigral degeneration (Adams 1983) and Shy-Drager syndrome. In striatonigral degeneration, rigidity is the predominant feature. There is involvement of the putamen, and patients respond poorly to antiparkinsonian medication (Adams 1983). In Shy-Drager syndrome, patients present with orthostatic hypotension, inability to sweat, and swallowing problems. This is due to a degenerative process not only in the substantia nigra but also the vagal nuclei. Parkinson's syndrome refers to rigidity and intentional tremor similar to Parkinson's disease but usually secondary to encephalitis. It is less common these days. Parkinson's syndrome can be seen following infection, trauma, or vascular insult. It also may be drug induced or related to toxins.

CT often demonstrates moderate to severe atrophy compared with age-matched groups. Focal hypodensity may be present within the basal ganglia. Dystrophic calcification may be present as punctate hyperdensity. There is, however, no correlation between the

## Table 6-7    continued

| DISEASE ENTITY | CEREBRAL ATROPHY | HYPERINTENSE SIGNAL ON $T_2$WI | MIDBRAIN ATROPHY | HINDBRAIN ATROPHY | HYPOINTENSE SIGNAL ON $T_2$WI |
|---|---|---|---|---|---|
| Wilson's disease (tremor, rigidity, dystonia, dysarthria, gait apraxia) | Mild to moderate Primarily lenticular nuclei Ceruloplasmin deficiency Between 1st and 5th decades | Putamen, GP On CT hypointense | Moderate | None | May be seen in putamen, GP |
| Leigh syndrome (SNE) (ataxia, dystonia, psychomotor regression, nystagmus) | Mild to moderate 1st and 2nd decades Progressive course | Extensive, patchy gray and white matter Putamen | Mild | None | Occasionally in thalamus, lentiform nuclei |
| Hypoxic-ischemic syndrome | Variable | GP | Mild | None | Occasionally May represent iron deposition |
| Olivopontocerebellar atrophy | Variable Beyond 3d decade | Normal unless part of MSA | Variable | Moderate to severe Pons, cerebellum, middle cerebellar peduncle | May be present in middle cerebellar peduncle, pons |

*Note: GP = globus pallidus; SN = substantia nigra; RN = red nucleus; DN = dentate nucleus; OPCA = olivopontocerebellar atrophy; MSA = multisystem atrophy.*
*Source: Rutledge 1987; Savoiardo 1983, 1989, 1990; Braffman 1988; Drayer 1988.*

severity of the atrophy seen on CT and the severity of the akinesia and tremor (Inzelberg 1987). In patients receiving L-dopa therapy, the presence of calcification in the basal ganglia has been associated with a poor medical response.

The characteristic MRI findings in Parkinson's disease and the parkinsonian syndrome consist of the following features, which are best evaluated on axial and coronal $T_2$-weighted spin-echo sequence and in gradient-echo sequence:

1. A decrease in the width of the pars compacta resulting from loss of neuromelanine-containing cells and possible iron deposition (Duguid 1986; Braffman 1988c). Linear hyperintensity adjacent to the hypointense region is probably related to gliosis (Fig. 6-45).

2. The globus pallidus shows increased hypointensity. However, in Parkinson's disease there is a loss of normal hypointensity, and more frequently there is hyperintensity within the substania nigra, possibly as a result of gliosis or neuronal loss (Braffman 1988c) or microvascular infarct. The putamen has a normal signal (Rutledge 1987).

3. In Shy-Drager syndrome and more often in striatonigral degeneration, the major change occurs in the putamen (Adams 1983). Compared with Parkinson's disease, apart from the atrophy of the striate nuclei, the putamen is markedly hypointense (Drayer 1988a; Pastakia 1986) (Fig. 6-46). The greater the severity of rigidity, the greater the hypointense signal of the putamen (Brown 1988; Rutledge 1987). This results from increased deposition of iron or other rare elements.

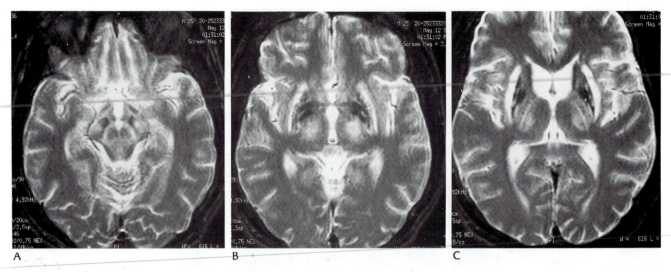

*Figure 6-48*   **Wilson's disease** in 25-year-old man. T$_2$-weighted axial MR **(A–C)** illustrates the classic appearance of hypointensity in the putamen and caudate nucleus from mineral (copper) deposition. Similar findings involve the substantia nigra. Hyperintense signal within the thalamus probably represents gliosis or edema.

sis and to determine the response to therapy and the prognosis. Since MRI is more sensitive, it probably should be utilized in the diagnosis and evaluation of patients with dystonia.

## Hepatolenticular Degeneration

Hepatolenticular degeneration is an acquired degenerative process, usually seen in liver failure and in immune-compromised patients following liver disease or liver transplants. Rapid progressive neurological deterioration over a period of days is present. In hepatic encephalopathy due to liver disease patients present in early stages with psychomotor and visual findings. They may present with disturbed consciousness or stupor and coma. Since the basal ganglia are involved they demonstrate choreiform movements, dysarthria, and tremors. CT may appear normal or show focal hypodensity in the basal ganglia. MR is sensitive in

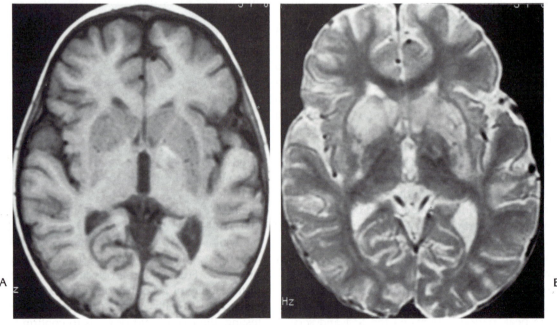

*Figure 6-49*   **Hepatolenticular degeneration. A.** Axial T$_1$-weighted MR. **B.** Axial T$_2$-weighted MR. Focal hypointense signal on T$_1$- and hyperintense signal on T$_2$-weighted MR involve the globus pallidus and the caudate nuclei in a patient following liver transplant.

demonstrating the bilateral foci of hyperintense signal within the globus pallidus (Fig. 6-49). The diagnosis can be established by the increased levels of ammonia. MR spectroscopy findings described in this condition include significant increase in myoinosital, creatin, and choline (Cho/Cr) ratio and an increase in glutamine and glutamate content (Ross 1994).

## Leigh's Disease

Leigh's disease is an uncommon neurodegenerative process due to a mitochondrial disorder that usually presents in infancy or childhood, although occasional cases may present at a later age. The clinical features and pathological changes are similar to those of Wernicke's encephalopathy associated with chronic ethanol use and nutritional encephalopathy, but without involvement of the mamillary bodies. The encephalopathy in Leigh's syndrome is a result of metabolic acidosis caused by a biochemical defect. The enzyme defect (pyruvate dehydrogenase, carboxylase, and cytochrome c oxidase) leads to excessive accumulation of lactate and pyruvates in the blood and CSF.

Patients with Leigh's disease present with behavioral disorders, ataxia, dystonia, nystagmus, and visual disturbance. Of these, nystagmus although not pathognomic, is one of the earliest findings in Leigh's disease. The disease runs a short clinical course, with death from respiratory failure occurring within a year. The pathological changes consist of subacute necrotizing encephalomyelitis characterized by necrosis with vascular proliferation in the gray and white matter, spongiform degeneration, and demyelination (Medina 1990; Geyer 1988). These findings are present in the brainstem (tegmentum), basal ganglia, optic pathways, and the spinal cord. Involvement of the dorsal pons in addition to the other lesions has been associated with cytochrome c oxidase deficiency (Medina 1990; Savoiardo 1991).

CT shows hypodense lesions that do not enhance. On MRI, the lesions are hypointense on $T_1WI$ and hyperintense on $T_2WI$ (Fig. 6-50) (Davis 1987). Bilateral symmetrical lesions within the midbrain are the most common presentation (Fig. 6-51). Occasional hypointensity in the putaminal region on $T_2WI$ probably represents iron deposition. Lesions often involves the deep gray matter and basal ganglia (putamen, globus pallidus, caudate nucleus), the cerebral peduncles, and the dentate nucleus in the cerebellum.

Characteristic changes are often seen on chemical shift imaging (MRS) (Krageloh-Mann 1993) (Fig. 6-52). MR spectroscopy imaging demonstrates a relative increase in Cho and Cr, and a small decrease in NAA. More important is the abnormal increase in the lactate peak. Even though the rest of the brain may appear normal in spin-echo images, metabolic alteration can be present (Fig. 6-52B).

Other causes of mitochondrial disorders primarily affecting the white matter are discussed in Chap. 14.

## Hallervorden-Spatz Disease

Hallervorden-Spatz disease is a rare debilitating neurological disorder associated with parkinsonian symptoms including progressive gait ataxia, choreiform movements, rigidity, torsion dystonia, dysarthria, and dysphasia with rapid mental deterioration. The disease usually presents between the second and early part of third decade, and rarely in younger and older age groups. The disease is autosomal recessive. It is more common in males than females. The degenerative changes usually involve the substania nigra, the red

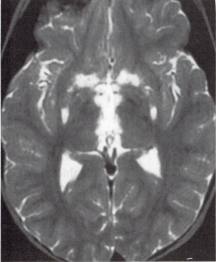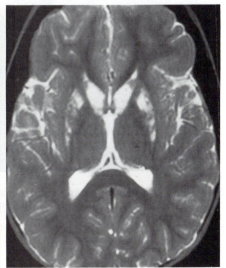

*Figure 6-50* Four-year-old child with **Leigh's disease. A–C.** Axial $T_2WI$, shows extensive hyperintense signal involving the putamen, caudate, and brainstem. **D.** Coronal $T_2$-weighted MR demonstrates similar findings. The child died 1 year following the diagnosis. (*Continued on next page*)

A                          B

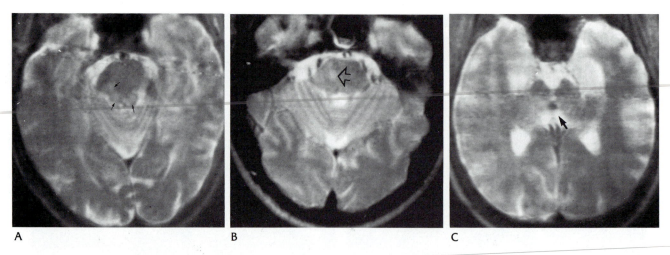

**Figure 6-54   Progressive supranuclear palsy (PSP).** Axial T$_2$-weighted MR (SE 4300/80). **A.** Patient with early progressive supranuclear palsy. Hyperintense signal (arrow) in tectum. **B.** Secondary parkinsonism due to midbrain infarct (arrow). **C.** Long-standing PSP with atrophy of the tectum (arrow).

# HINDBRAIN ATROPHY

Atrophy of the hindbrain (brainstem and cerebellar hemispheres) is associated with a variety of acquired and hereditary disorders (Table 6-8). The atrophic process, although predominantly involving the hindbrain structures, also involves in varying degrees the forebrain and midbrain. Although both CT and MRI are useful in evaluating the morphological changes Savoiardo 1983; Savoiardo 1990), the neurodegenerative changes involving the brainstem and the cerebellum are evaluated better with MRI than with CT because of a lack of bone artifact, the ability to image in all orthogonal planes, and better discrimination between gray and white matter.

Isolated atrophy of the cerebellum is associated with a variety of degenerative disorders (Abe 1983; Andreula 1984) and may be secondary to toxic or prolonged use of ethanol and drugs such as diphenylhydantoin. In chronic ethanol toxicity, the cerebellar atrophy primarily involves the vermis and to a lesser extent the cerebellar hemispheres (Allen 1979). Reversal of the atrophy has been reported after abstinence (Artmann 1981). Prolonged use of diphenylhydantoin results in degeneration of the Purkinje cells in animals. A similar mechanism is probably responsible for the cerebellar atrophy seen on CT, along with other systemic manifestations (McCrea 1980) (Fig. 6-55). Primary unilateral cerebellar atrophy associated with cerebellar type of seizures, although rare, usually demonstrates

## Table 6-8   CT and MR Features of Hindbrain Atrophy

| DISEASE ENTITY | BRAINSTEM | FOURTH VENTRICLE | VERMIS | CEREBELLUM | MR SIGNAL CHANGES |
|---|---|---|---|---|---|
| Olivopontocerebellar atrophy | 4 | 4 | 4 | 4 | Mild hyperintense signal middle cerebellar peduncle and pons |
| Cerebellar atrophy | 0 | 0–2 | 2–3 | 3–4 | |
| Friedreich's ataxia | 0 | 0 | 0 | 0–2 | Atrophic spinal cord |
| Chronic alcoholism | 0 | 0 | 2–4 Involves superior vermis | 0–2 | Associated cerebral atrophy |
| Phenytoin intoxication | 0 | 0–2 | 0–2 | 1–3 | |
| Occult neoplasm metabolic | 0 | 0–2 | 1–2 | 0–2 | Associated with cerebral atrophy |

*Note: 0 = normal; 1 = equivocal; 2 = mild; 3 = moderate; 4 = severe.*

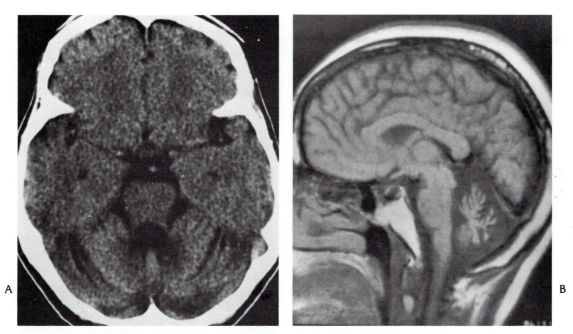

*Figure 6-55* **Cerebellar atrophy from alcohol abuse. A.** NCCT demonstrating prominent cerebellar folia, enlarged fourth ventricle, and prominent pericerebellar cisterns. **B.** $T_1$-weighted sagittal MR demonstrates vermian atrophy and normal brainstem.

atrophy primarily involving the cerebellar hemisphere (Fig.6-56). This could be confusing with an old infarct. In olivopontocerebellar atrophy (OPCA) the degenerative process involves the inferior olive, the pontine nuclei, the middle cerebellar peduncle, and the cerebellar hemisphere and vermis (Dejerine 1900). Depending on the subtype and the association with other regions of the brain, the clinical features and the age of onset

may differ. In general, patients with OPCA present with ataxia, which usually progresses in the extremities and the bulbar musculature in a caudocephalad direction. The degenerative process usually manifests between the second and fifth decades. The pathological changes associated with OPCA consist of neuronal loss and gliosis of the pontocerebellar fibers which run through the pons in a transverse course into the

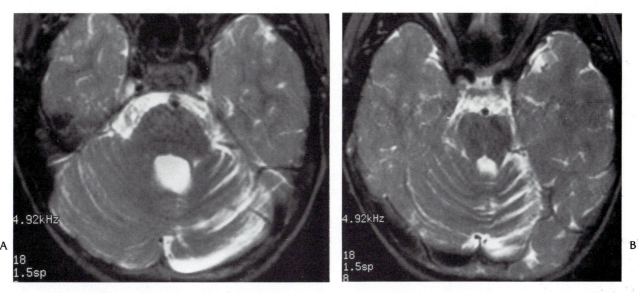

*Figure 6-56* **Unilateral cerebellar atrophy** in a 26-year-old female presenting with seizures. **A, B.** Axial $T_2$-weighted MR demonstrates left cerebellar atrophy. Subsequent MRA and angiography demonstrated absence of the left vertebral artery and atretic superior cerebellar artery.

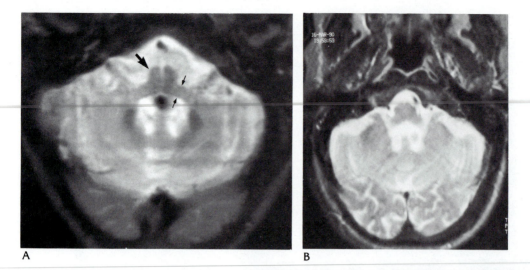

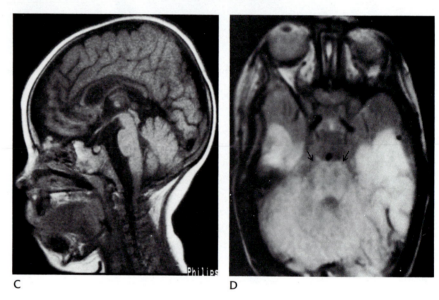

**Figure 6-57  Olivopontocerebellar atrophy (OPCA). A.** Axial T$_2$-weighted MR (SE 4300/80) in an adult with marked focal atrophy of the pons (large arrow) and brachium pontis (small arrow). Prominent CFVS within dilated fourth ventricle. **B.** Axial T$_2$-weighted MR (SE 2500/90) in another patient with OPCA. Hyperintense foci within pons (arrows) with atrophy of the medulla and the region of the olivary nuclei (arrowhead). Juvenile form of OPCA in a 3-year-old child. Sagittal **(C)** and axial **(D).** T$_1$-weighted MR demonstrates significant atrophy of the pons, medulla, and upper cervical cord.

middle cerebellar peduncle—resulting in atrophy of the pons and middle cerebellar peduncle. Degenerative changes in the Purkinje cells and fibers within the dentate nuclei explain the dilated fourth ventricle and vermian atrophy. Retrograde cell loss of the inferior olives as a result of cortical cerebellar lesions is associated with atrophy of the olive and cerebellar hemisphere.

These morphological changes can be appreciated in both CT and MRI (Fig. 6-57) (Nabatame 1988; Ramos 1987). In T$_2$WI, hyperintense signal within these areas of degeneration is common. MRI in the coronal and sagittal plane is useful in differentiating OPCA from other multisystem atrophy, where ataxia may be the common clinical presentation. In OPCA, the cells of the dentate nuclei are preserved, as are their projection fibers to the red nuclei and thalami through the supe-

rior cerebellar peduncle. Demonstration of a normal superior cerebellar peduncle (in coronal plane) excludes degenerative disorders associated with MSA such as Shy-Drager syndrome, striatonigral degeneration, and some cases of Leigh's disease. A combination of neurological examination with MR is useful in differentiating hindbrain atrophy (HBA) from MSA (Table 6-8).

## Atrophy of the Cervicomedullary Region

Evaluation of neurodegenerative changes involving the cervicomedullary region is best achieved with MR. Atrophy of the cervicomedullary region is often associated with atrophy of the pons and cerebellum (OPCA).

In motor neuron diseases the neurodegenerative process primarily involves the fiber tracts in the lower brainstem and cord. The motor neurons are the fiber tracts that constitute the corticospinal tract between its origin from the precentral gyrus and its passage through the brainstem to end in the anterior and lateral horn cells within the spinal cord. The neurodegenerative process may involve the upper or lower motor neuron, where synapse occurs either in the brainstem with the cranial nerve nuclei or in the spinal cord with the anterior horn cells.

## Amyotrophic Lateral Sclerosis

Amyotrophic lateral sclerosis is the most common of the motor neuron diseases. It is usually detected in patients beyond the fifth decade, and is usually sporadic. Although the exact pathogenesis is not known, the disease may be related to low-grade infection or toxic or vascular causes. The clinical presentation consists of atrophy and weakness of the forearm and spasticity in the lower limbs. There is generalized hyperreflexia. The degenerative process can extend between the pre-

central gyrus to the level of the lower brainstem and spinal cord. On MR imaging atrophy of the lower brainstem and cord involving the anterior and lateral portion of the medulla and spinal cord may be seen in $T_1WI$ (Fig. 6-58). $T_2WI$ may demonstrate bilateral symmetrical focal hyperintense signal in the lower brainstem, probably reflecting gliosis or myelin loss (Sherman 1987b; Biondi 1989). Occasionally the focal hyperintense signal may also be present at a higher level, such as the posterior aspect of the posterior limb of the internal capsule where the corticospinal tract fibers are located. In a majority of instances the hyperintense signal within the brainstem and the spinal cord is bilateral and symmetrical. This is a useful differential from the unilateral atrophy, seen in wallerian degeneration.

## Wallerian Degeneration

Wallerian degeneration represents anterograde degeneration of the axon and myelin sheath distal to the axonal cell injury, usually occurring months or years after the initial injury. Wallerian degeneration usually in-

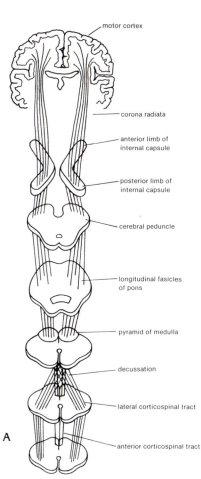

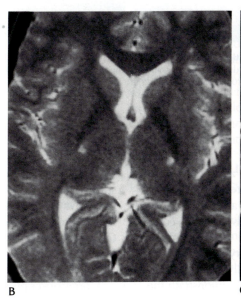

B

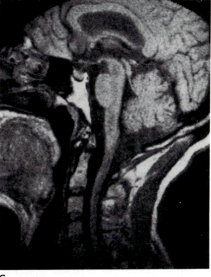

C

*Figure 6-58* **Amyotrophic lateral sclerosis. A.** Diagrammatic representation of the corticospinal tracts. In amyotrophic lateral sclerosis, focal symmetrical lesions are identified in posterior limb of internal capsule as well as varying degrees of atrophy in the brainstem and spinal cord. In wallerian degeneration, the atrophy is in an antegrade fashion and is always unilateral. **B.** Axial $T_2$-weighted MR (SE 3000/100). Bilateral hyperintense signal foci (arrowheads) in the posterior limb of internal capsule. These are anterior to the normal mildly hyperintense signal (arrow) normally seen in this region. **C.** Midsagittal MR demonstrating mild atrophy of the cervicomedullary region in another patient with a clinical diagnosis of ALS.

A

motor cortex

corona radiata

anterior limb of internal capsule

posterior limb of internal capsule

cerebral peduncle

longitudinal fasicles of pons

pyramid of medulla

decussation

lateral corticospinal tract

anterior corticospinal tract

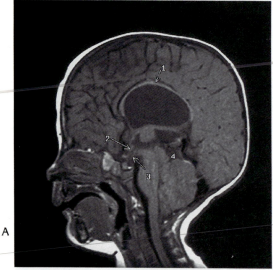

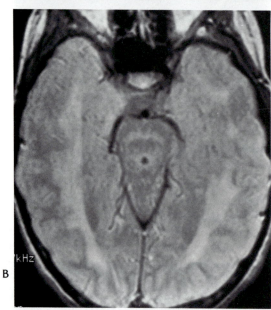

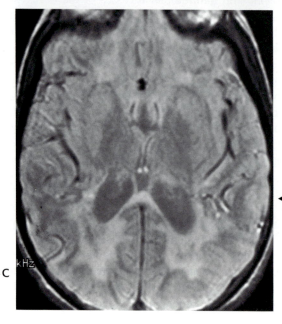

say 1977). The measurements are subject to variability caused by operator- and equipment-related factors.

It is probably more reliable to use an index system (Heinz 1980) (Fig. 6-64). The most commonly used indexes are the frontal horn ratio and the ventricular span ratio. The frontal horn ratio is obtained by dividing the maximum width of the frontal horns by the transverse diameter of the inner table of the calvarium at the same level. The normal ratio is about 35 percent. In atrophic ventricular enlargement the ratio is between 45 and 50 percent, and in hydrocephalus it is usually above 45 percent and often exceeds 55 percent. These ratios must be combined with other morphological features.

The distention of the ventricular system in hydrocephalus is symmetrical and is characterized by concentric expansion. The ventricles bulge as if multiple vectors of force radiating from a central axis result in a balloon-shaped appearance of the frontal horns. In cerebral atrophy all parts of the ventricles may be affected equally, whereas in hydrocephalus the larger parts of the ventricular system distend first (frontal and occipital horns), followed by a distention of the smaller parts (temporal horns and fourth and third ventricles). Hydrocephalus should be suspected when there is enlargement of the temporal horns and the sylvian and interhemispheric fissures are normal (Sjaastad 1969; LeMay 1970). These morphological changes are associated with changes in the parenchyma. On CT, periventricular hypodensity has been noted as a transient feature in the early stages of hydrocephalus (DiChiro 1979; Hiratsuka 1979; Mori 1980). This is often seen in acute noncommunicating hydrocephalus and in 40 percent of patients with communicating hydrocephalus. Periventricular hypodensity is best recognized along the dorsomedial and dorsolateral angle of the frontal horns of the lateral ventricles. Periventricular hypodensity is also seen in elderly patients with cerebral atrophy, in patients with leukoencephalopathies (Mori 1980), and in association with hypertensive diseases (Hatazawa 1984). The pattern and extent as well as density measurements have been utilized in differentiating the various causes of periventricular hypodensity (DiChiro 1979). MRI and CT demonstrate similar features in the general differentiation of hydrocephalus from atrophy. The periventric-

*Figure 6-63* **A.** Sagittal T$_1$-weighted MR demonstrating the features associated with **hydrocephalus**. (1) Elevated and thinning of the corpus collosum. Enlargement of (2) the optic and (3) infundibular recess. (4) Prominent pineal and suprapineal recess. Depending on the site of intraaxial lesion, the prepontine cistern may be narrowed. In communicating hydrocephalus the prepontine cistern is usually wider than normal. **B, C.** Axial spin-density images demonstrated the periventricular hyperintensity extending into the white matter from alternative pathway of CSF resorption or stasis. This finding is usually seen in the acute stage.

Ventricular
size
index

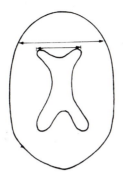

$$V.S.I. = \frac{\text{Bifrontal diameter}}{\text{Frontal horn diameter}}$$

| Normal | 30% |
| Mild enlargement | 30-39% |
| Moderate enlargement | 40-46% |
| Severe enlargement | 47% |

| | Atrophy | | Obstructive hydrocephalus | | Remarks |
|---|---|---|---|---|---|
| Angle of frontal horn | | Obtuse | | Acute | |
| Frontal horn ratio | | Small | | Wide | FHR: Measured at the widest part of the frontal horn perpendicular to the long axis of the frontal horn. |
| Temporal horn ratio | | Not visible or small | | Wide | Width of temporal horn measured at the genu. |
| Sulci and cistern | | Wide | | Obliterated | |

*Figure 6-64* **Differentiating features between atrophic and obstructive ventricular enlargement.** These measurements can also be applied utilizing the different plane of imaging on MRI. *(Modified from Heinz 1980.)*

ular hypodensity seen on CT appears as a periventricular hyperintense signal on T$_2$WI. In acute stages of hydrocephalus the periventricular hyperintense signal on T$_2$WI demonstrates a brighter signal along the ependymal surface which fades off along its lateral margin. This is probably indicative of relative acute change in the CSF flow between the brain parenchyma and the ependymal surface of the ventricles. In chronic hydrocephalus the width of the hyperintense signal may gradually decrease, probably as a result of a com-

*Figure 6-69   (continued)*

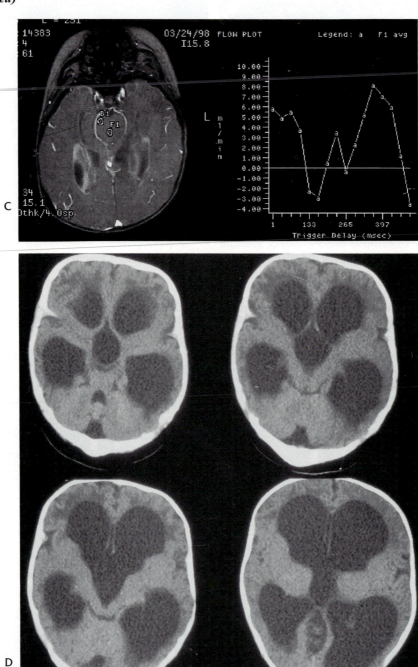

## Communicating Hydrocephalus

In communicating hydrocephalus, or extraventricular obstructive hydrocephalus (EVOH), there is symmetrical enlargement of the entire ventricular system. The obstruction usually involves the subarachnoid cistern, most often the basilar cisterns. Obstruction at a higher level may also involve the arachnoid villi along the parasagittal dural venous sinuses as well as following obstruction in the main venous drainage channels within the dural sinuses. Communicating hydrocephalus usually follows subarachnoid hemorrhage, meningeal carcinomatosis, meningeal infections, trauma, or intracranial surgery.

In the early or acute stage, the clinical presentation and the imaging features are similar to those of obstructive hydrocephalus. In addition, the aqueduct is dilated. On MRI ($T_2$WI), a prominent CFVS is seen not only within the aqueduct but also extending proxi-

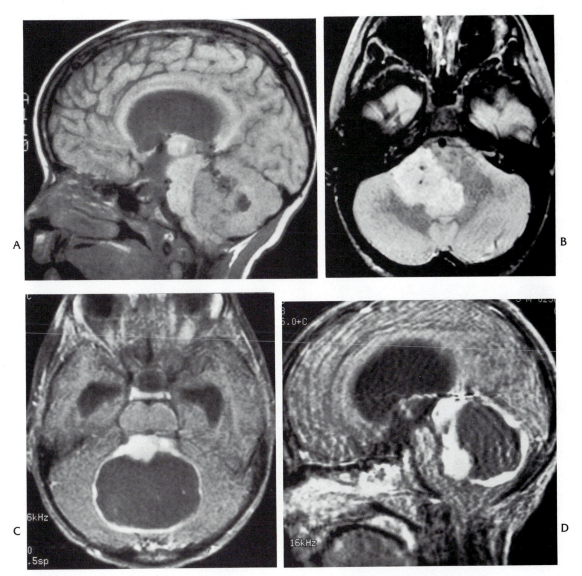

***Figure 6-70***   **Obstruction of the fourth ventricle and outlet foramen. A.** Sagittal T$_1$-weighted MR.
**B.** Axial spin-density MR in a patient with choroid plexus papilloma involving the fourth ventricle and
extending into the lateral recess of the ventricle on the right, with marked enlargement of the lateral
and third ventricles. Sagittal **(C)** and axial **(D)** gadolinium-enhanced T$_1$-weighted MR demonstrates a
large pilocytic astrocytoma compressing the fourth ventricle with proximal enlarged obstructive hydrocephalus.

mally into the third ventricle and distally within the dilated fourth ventricle (Fig. 6-71). Enhancement of the
cisternal space or pial surface is often seen on contrast-
enhanced MRI (CEMR) and sometimes on CECT (Fig.
6-72). Sometimes the granulomatous foci, inflammatory
adhesions, or nodular metastatic deposits can be well
demonstrated. In communicating hydrocephalus due to
a convexity block involving the arachnoid villi or the
dural venous sinuses, CT and MRI may demonstrate dilated ventricles as well as prominent sulci that suggest
an atrophic pattern. In these patients, increased CSF
pressure on lumbar puncture, and occasionally dural
enhancement along the convexity, may help in confirming the clinical diagnosis. In some cases magnetic
resonance angiography (MRA) or vascular studies may

be necessary to demonstrate the venous obstruction.
These distinctions are useful since the subsequent surgical or medical management depends on the exact
pathological process. In children, although hydrocephalus is the most common cause of an enlarging
head, other causes, such as megalencephaly, benign
subdural effusions (Maytal 1987), and dysmyelinating
disorders such as Canavan's disease or Alexander's disease should be excluded. These entities can be separated on the basis of CT and MR studies.

## Normal Pressure Hydrocephalus

Adams (1965) and Hakim (1965) described a group of
patients with the clinical features of dementia, gait
apraxia, and urinary incontinence who on imaging

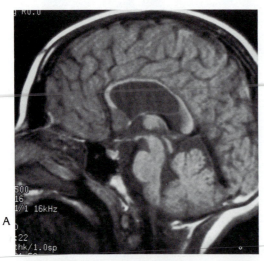

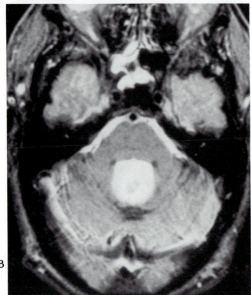

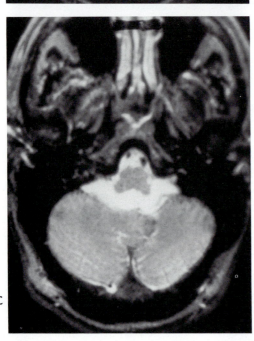

studies (pneumoencephalography) demonstrated enlarged ventricles with variable prominence of the cortical sulci and marked delay in the absorption of the air within the intracranial CSF spaces (Benson 1970). On isotope cisternography, there was delayed clearance of the isotope from the ventricles. Both studies indicated a delay in or a decreased rate of CSF absorption. In spite of the "normal" craniospinal CSF pressure, these authors described clinical improvement after shunting of the ventricular CSF space.

Since NPH is one of the treatable causes of dementia, there has been interest in defining the imaging characteristics and the clinical criteria for selecting patients who would benefit from the CSF diversionary procedure (Huckman 1981; Jensen 1979).

The causal relationship between the hydrocephalus and the clinical presentation has not been clearly established. NPH often presents in patients in the sixth decade.

It is presumed that the clinical manifestations result from (1) pressure on critical areas within the cerebrum from the hydrocephalus (Fisher 1982) and (2) decreased vascular perfusion further compromised as a result of increased CSF pressure. Both of these factors contribute to the decreased compliance of the cerebral parenchyma caused by aging.

Normal pressure hydrocephalus represents a combination of chronic communicating hydrocephalus and atrophic parenchymal changes. Although in some instances an earlier history of extraventricular obstructive hydrocephalus can be identified, in many cases such a history may not be available. Patients usually are in the sixth decade or beyond, with a history of worsening of the clinical triad of dementia, gait apraxia, and urinary incontinence. The exact pathogenesis of the dementia, gait disturbance, and urinary incontinence is not clear.

Pathological correlations have shown tangential shearing of the paracentral fibers of the corona radiata (Hakim 1965; Fisher 1982). These findings probably correspond to some of the hyperintense signal changes seen on MR.

Other pathological findings in patients with NPH consist of subcortical and periventricular lesions (Awad 1986b; Fazekas 1991). These are not specifically related to NPH but represent arteriosclerotic changes in the microvasculature of the brain caused by aging, or result from ischemia or infarcts. Many of these patients have a history of hypertension or other metabolic disorders such as diabetes and are prone to arteriosclerotic vascular disease affecting both the extracranial

◀ *Figure 6-71* **Communicating hydrocephalus. A.** Sagittal T₁-weighted MR demonstrates moderately enlarged lateral, third, and fourth ventricles in a 47-year-old male. Note the enlarged basal cisterns. **B, C.** Axial T₂-weighted MR demonstrates the enlarged fourth ventricle and the lateral outlet foramina.

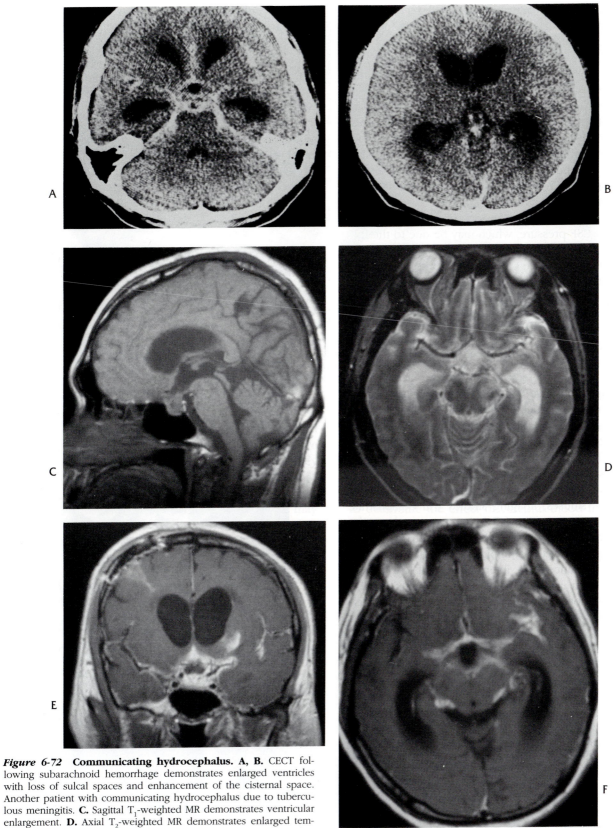

***Figure 6-72*** **Communicating hydrocephalus. A, B.** CECT following subarachnoid hemorrhage demonstrates enlarged ventricles with loss of sulcal spaces and enhancement of the cisternal space. Another patient with communicating hydrocephalus due to tuberculous meningitis. **C.** Sagittal T$_1$-weighted MR demonstrates ventricular enlargement. **D.** Axial T$_2$-weighted MR demonstrates enlarged temporal horns and absence of sulci indicative of communicating hydrocephalus. Coronal **(E)** and axial **(F)** T$_1$-weighted MR following contrast demonstrates communicating hydrocephalus with enhancing deposits throughout the cisternal spaces. Similar appearance may be seen in meningeal carcinomatosis.

# Communicating Hydrocephalus in Children

Communicating hydrocephalus in children is often seen following infection during the gestational period or during infancy. Less common causes are tumor (leukemia, medulloblastoma, neuroblastoma) and trauma. On imaging studies, the findings are similar to those of the adult type. CECT or CEMR is essential in demonstrating cisternal or dural enhancement.

A less common cause of communicating hydrocephalus described as external hydrocephalus is seen in children (Maytal 1987). In most of these children it is a benign process associated with macrocephaly and mild developmental delay during the first year. In some cases there may be a familial pattern. In other children the macrocephaly may be secondary to known genetic causes, including bone dysplasias resulting in obstruction of the dural venous sinuses (Yamada 1981; Allen 1982) and hypoplasia of the arachnoid granulation tissue (Gilles 1971).

On both CT and MR, the ventricles are mildly to moderately enlarged with a fluid collection over the surface of the brain, resulting in prominent sulci and a prominent interhemispheric fissure (Fig. 6-75). In most of these children it is a self-limiting condition, with normal development and head size occurring before age 2 years. If there is a progressive increase in head size with clinical signs of increased CSF pressure, the diagnosis must be confirmed by evaluating CSF or venous sinus pressure as well as performing vascular studies.

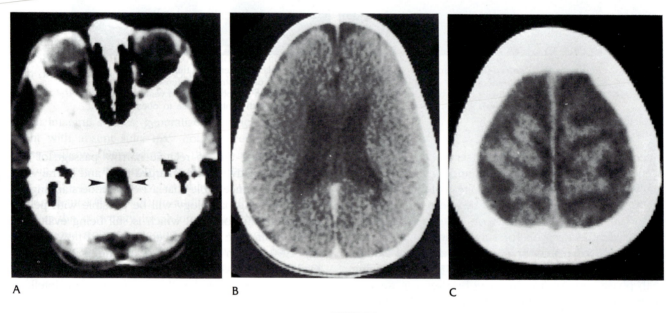

A          B          C

*Figure 6-75*  **External hydrocephalus.** Cranial CT in a child with craniometaphyseal dysplasia and enlarging head size due to external hydrocephalus. **A.** Thickening of the skull base (arrowheads). **B.** Moderately enlarged lateral ventricles. **C.** Prominent enlarged cortical sulci. **D.** Venous phase of the angiogram demonstrating severe narrowing of the jugular foramen (arrowhead).

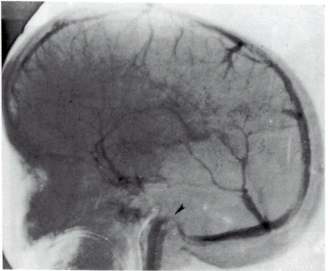

D

# Hydrocephalus Caused by Overproduction

Overproduction of CSF as a cause of hydrocephalus, although rare, is well recognized. This condition is often associated with benign or malignant neoplasms of the choroid plexus. The hydrocephalus is caused by the relative difference between the rate of CSF production and its absorption. In some cases the hydrocephalus is also related to a voluminous choroid plexus blocking the foramina (El Gammal 1987). In children the choroid plexus masses are often found in the lateral ventricles, whereas in adults they are often seen involving the choroid plexus of the fourth ventricle. Since the choroid plexus consists of fronds of vascular tissue, hemorrhage within the fronds may result in subsequent calcification. Choroid plexus papilloma or hemorrhage may even result in a trapped temporal horn or focal dilatation of the temporal horn proximal to the obstruction. This is more common in children. In adults, choroid plexus of the fourth ventricle or third ventricle may cause blockage of the outlet foramina of the fourth ventricle or the foramen of Monro (Schelahas 1988; Ford 1988; Hopper 1987). In diagnosing hydrocephalus due to choroid plexus papilloma in children, it is important to be aware that asymmetry in the size of the glomera of the choroid plexus is not unusual and that the normal glomera can be as large as 23 mm (Hinshaw 1988). Calcification within the tumor is best assessed with CT. On MRI, choroid plexus papilloma has a heterogeneous signal intensity as a result of small cysts, old hemorrhage, or lipid deposition (Zimmerman 1979; Hinshaw 1988) (Fig. 6-76). In patients of all ages but more often in adults, choroid plexus tumors must be differentiated from intraventricular meningioma. Meningiomas usually have denser calcification and demonstrate intense enhancement, and the hydrocephalus, if present, is less severe.

## Treated Hydrocephalus

Imaging studies are often necessary after the treatment of hydrocephalus to determine the position of the shunt catheter tip and to evaluate postsurgical complications, including improper placement of the shunt catheter tip and an intracerebral hematoma along the track of the shunt tubing. A subdural hematoma may be due to a torn subdural vein or to rapid decompression of the ventricles. In the later stages complications may result from infection, leading to isolated dilatation of the fourth ventricle, the slit ventricle syndrome, and porencephaly.

## Trapped Temporal Horn

Trapped temporal horn results from obstruction of CSF flow within the temporal horn of the lateral ventricle. It usually involves the atrial region of the lateral ventricle. Obstruction may be the result of intrinsic lesion, such as hemorrhage within the ependyma, tumors such as meningioma, choroid plexus papilloma, or extrinsic mass compressing the atrium of the lateral ventricle. Rapid increase in size of the temporal horn may lead to uncal herniation. Both CT and MR demonstrate the trapped temporal horn, and when combined with contrast-enhanced study the etiological cause for the obstruction (Fig. 6-77).

## Trapped Fourth Ventricle

One of the complications of repeated infection, most often associated with shunt revision, is isolation of the fourth ventricle. This involves the aqueduct above and the outlet foramina of the fourth ventricle below. The CSF formed within the fourth ventricle increases in volume and protein concentration. The obstruction results in progressive enlargement of the fourth ventricle with the maximum expansion along the superior and inferior medullary velum, resulting in transtentorial (upward) and tonsillar (downward) herniation. Both CT and MR can demonstrate the pathological cystic mass in the posterior fossa (Fig. 6-78). CT studies may require ventriculography to demonstrate the obstruction and to differentiate the cystic dilatation of the fourth ventricle from the extraaxial cyst. Because of the ex-

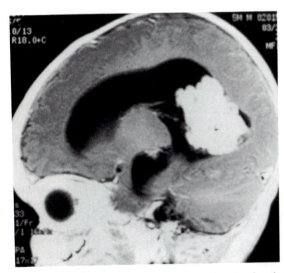

*Figure 6-76*  **Nine-month-old infant with enlarging head.** Sagittal gadolinium-enhanced T$_1$-weighted MR demonstrates a large enhancing choroid plexus papilloma in the trigone of the markedly dilated lateral ventricle.

## Table 7-10    Outline of Primary CNS Tumors and Tumorlike Masses (WHO-II, 1993)

I. Gliomas
  A. Astrocytomas
    1. Grade I gliomas, benign, well-circumscribed
       a. Pilocytic astrocytoma
       b. Subependymal giant cell astrocytoma
       c. Desmoplastic astrocytoma of infancy
    2. Grade II astrocytoma, low grade; diffuse, may progress
       a. Fibrillary
       b. Pleomorphic xanthoastrocytoma (grade is II–III per WHO-I)
       c. Gemistocytic (likely to progress to grade III rapidly)
    3. Grade III anaplastic astrocytoma
       a. Gemistocytic (likely to progress to GBM rapidly)
       b. Pleomorphic xanthoastrocytoma
       c. Gliomatosis cerebri
    4. Glioblastoma multiforme (GBM)
       a. Giant cell (monstrocellular sarcoma less aggressive)
       b. Small cell
       c. Gliosarcoma
       d. Typical
  B. Oligodendroglioma
    1. Typical, grade II
    2. Anaplastic or malignant, grade III
  C. Ependymoma
    1. Typical, grade II
    2. Anaplastic or malignant, grade III
    3. Subependymoma, low grade, probably grade I
    4. Ependymoblastoma (PNET)
  D. Choroid plexus papilloma and rarely carcinoma
II. Nonglial, Nonneural primary CNS tumors
  A. Pituitary region
    1. Pituitary adenoma
       a. Prolactin-secreting, most common, laterally located
       b. Other secreting adenomas include ACTH, TRH, GH
       c. Nonsecreting, null cell, frequently present as macroadenomas
    2. Pituitary carcinoma; evidence of metastasis
    3. Infundibuloma; pilocytic astrocytoma of stalk
    4. Choristoma; glial tumor of posterior pituitary
    5. Suprasellar neoplasms; germinoma, craniopharyngioma
    6. Rathke's cleft cyst, pars intermedia cyst
  B. Pineal tumors
    1. Seminoma
    2. Germinoma (may also be suprasellar)
    3. Teratoma, teratocarcinoma
    4. Endodermal sinus tumor (yolk sac tumor)
    5. Pineoblastoma (PNET)
    6. Pineocytoma
  C. Schwannoma
    1. Vestibular, superior division, most common
    2. Other cranial nerves, V, XII, X, IX, XI, VII by incidence
    3. Intracerebral, rare
  D. Meningioma
    1. Typical, many histological variants
    2. Anaplastic
    3. Papillary, may be synonymous with malignant
    4. Malignant, invasion of brain parenchyma
  E. Other
    1. Hemangiopericytoma (previously "angioblastic" meningioma)
    2. CNS Lymphoma, B-cell NHL
    3. Hemangioblastoma
III. Neuronal and mixed glioneuronal
  A. Ganglioglioma (grade II)
    1. Desmoplastic infantile ganglioglioma (DIG); (infants, grade I)
  B. Dysembryoplastic neuroepithelial tumor (DNET) (grade I)
  C. Primitive neuroectodermal tumors
    1. Medulloblastoma, midline in children, lateral in adults
    2. Pineo-, ependymo-, retino-, and neuroblastoma
    3. CNS rhabdoid tumors (PNET variant ?)
  E. Central neurocytoma (intraventricular, foramen of Monro)
IV. Nonneoplastic cysts and cyst like tumors
  A. Epidermoid (middle fossa, parasellar, CPA, calvarial)
  B. Dermoid (midline, suprasellar, may rupture with fat-fluid levels)
  C. Teratoma (midline or anywhere)
  D. Arachnoid cysts (intraarachnoid duplication cysts)
  E. Colloid cyst (foramina of Monro)
  F. Neuroepithelial cysts, (3rd, 4th ventricle)

## Table 7-11  WHO II Grading of Astrocytic Tumors, 1993

Grade I circumscribed astrocytomas
  Unique astrocytic tumors which are generally benign and
    well circumscribed. Specific histologic features are
    unique to each tumor. The most common example is the
    juvenile pilocytic astrocytoma.
Grade II astrocytoma
  Diffusely infiltrating
  Well-differentiated neoplastic astrocytes
  Minimal pleomorphism or nuclear atypia
  No vascular proliferation or necrosis
Grade III anaplastic astrocytoma
  Vascular proliferation and necrosis are absent (not a
    glioblastoma multiforme)
  Increased cellularity
  Pleomorphism and nuclear atypia
  Mitotic activity
Grade IV glioblastoma multiforme
  Increased cellularity
  Anaplasia and pleomorphism
  Cell type may be poorly differentiated, fusiform, round, or
    multinucleated
  Essential for the histological diagnosis is prominent
    vascular proliferation *and/or* necrosis. Mitotic activity is
    variable.

7-6). The dense enhancement is due to lack of a proper BBB in these neoplasms. However, the biological aggression of these tumors is low. When possible, surgical resection is curative.

### SUBEPENDYMAL GIANT CELL ASTROCYTOMA

Almost always seen in patients with other stigmata of tuberous sclerosis, these benign astrocytomas occur almost exclusively near the foramina of Monro and are attached to the ependymal surface under the caudate head. Obstructive hydrocephalus may be a presenting feature; however, as grade I lesions, surgical resection is generally curative. The imaging features are a rounded, well-circumscribed mass which may be heterogeneous, both before and after contrast administration on both CT and MRI (Fig. 7-9). Calcification is commonly seen on CT, and 90 percent of patients have other stigmata of tuberous sclerosis. It has been suggested that abnormal neuronal migration is part of the pathogenesis of these tumors (Steffanson 1989).

### Diffuse or Infiltrating Gliomas (Grades II to IV)

Other than the grade I circumscribed lesions, all astrocytomas are considered to be infiltrating tumors which cannot be completely resected for cure. More importantly, they tend to transform over time into more aggressive histologies. Current research has established a genetic basis for this transformation. There is a direct correlation between pathological grade and the num-

## Table 7-12  Neuroectodermal Cell Lines

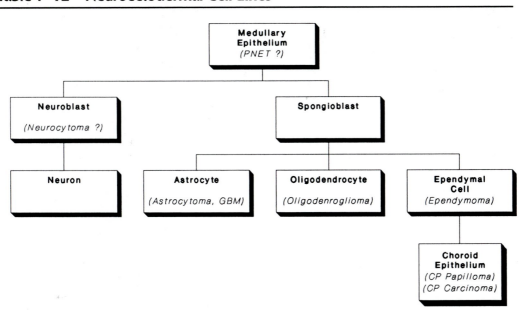

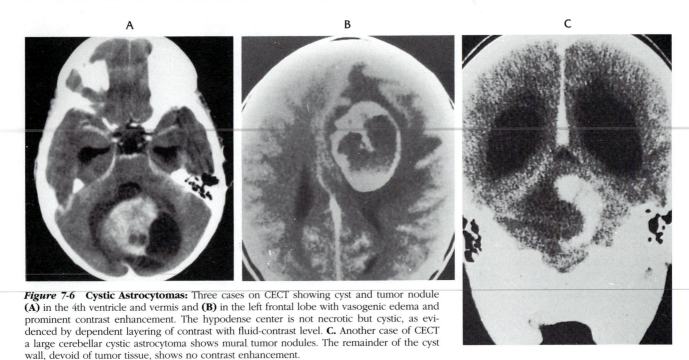

A                          B                          C

***Figure 7-6*** **Cystic Astrocytomas:** Three cases on CECT showing cyst and tumor nodule **(A)** in the 4th ventricle and vermis and **(B)** in the left frontal lobe with vasogenic edema and prominent contrast enhancement. The hypodense center is not necrotic but cystic, as evidenced by dependent layering of contrast with fluid-contrast level. **C.** Another case of CECT a large cerebellar cystic astrocytoma shows mural tumor nodules. The remainder of the cyst wall, devoid of tumor tissue, shows no contrast enhancement.

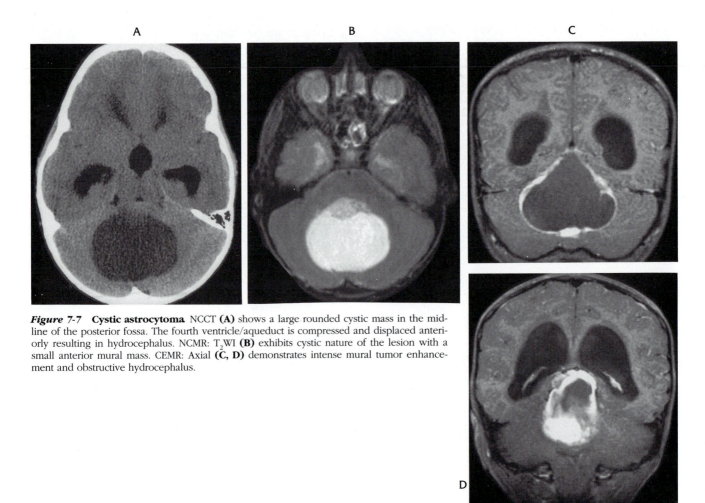

A                          B                          C

                                                      D

***Figure 7-7*** **Cystic astrocytoma** NCCT **(A)** shows a large rounded cystic mass in the midline of the posterior fossa. The fourth ventricle/aqueduct is compressed and displaced anteriorly resulting in hydrocephalus. NCMR: $T_2$WI **(B)** exhibits cystic nature of the lesion with a small anterior mural mass. CEMR: Axial **(C, D)** demonstrates intense mural tumor enhancement and obstructive hydrocephalus.

Table 7-13    Pattern Analysis
Neoplasm

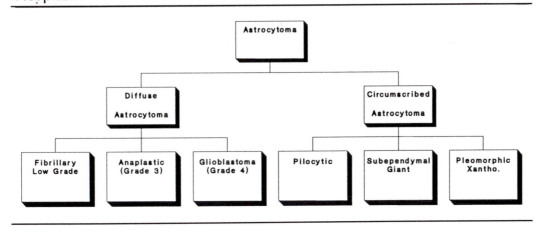

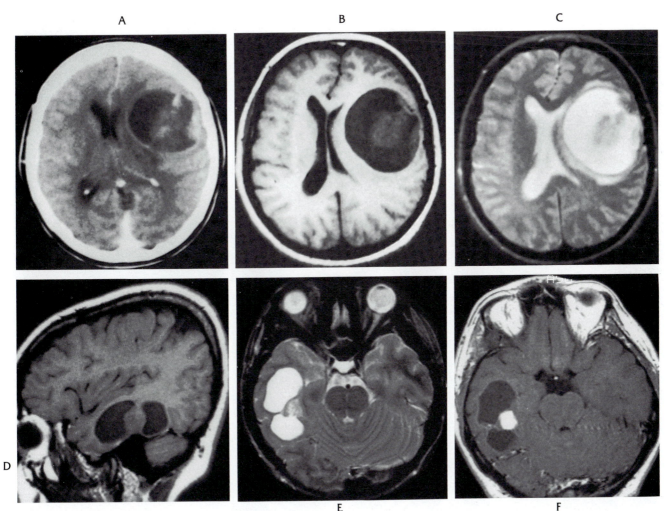

*Figure 7-8*  **Pilocytic astrocytomas.** CT: CECT **(A)** demonstrates a sharply demarcated cyst with central and marginal tumor nodules. Axial MR: $T_1$WI **(B)** and $T_2$WI **(C)** show the cyst filled with tumor debris. MR in another case: $T_1$WI **(D)**, $T_2$WI **(E)** and CEMR **(F)** show a well marginated cyst in the temporal lobe with a solid tumor nodule in a 25-year-old male.

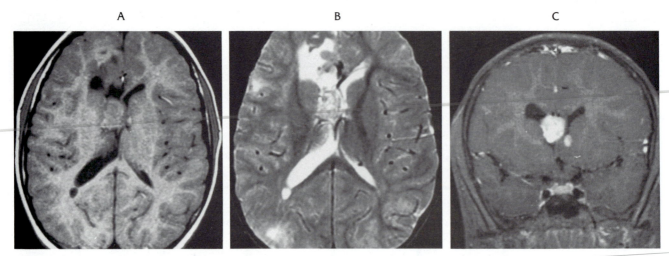

***Figure* 7-9  Subependymal giant cell astrocytoma** MR: Axial
T₁WI **(A)**, T₂WI **(B)**, and CEMR **(C)** show a well-circumscribed intraventricular mass near the foramen of Monro. Slightly heterogeneous
mass exhibits intense contrast enhancement. Subependymal nodules
are noted in the right frontal horn **(A, B)** and subcortical tubers are
presented as focal hyperintense lesions in the right hemisphere **(B)**.

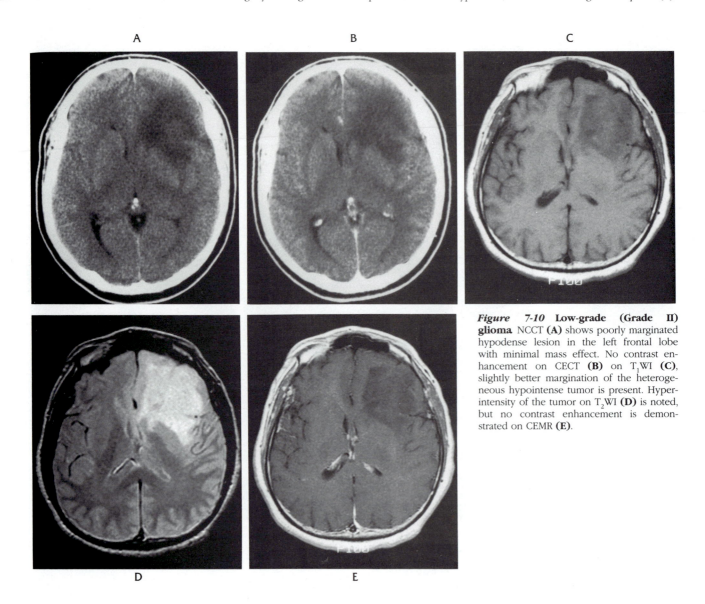

***Figure* 7-10 Low-grade (Grade II)
glioma** NCCT **(A)** shows poorly marginated
hypodense lesion in the left frontal lobe
with minimal mass effect. No contrast enhancement on CECT **(B)** on T₁WI **(C)**,
slightly better margination of the heterogeneous hypointense tumor is present. Hyperintensity of the tumor on T₂WI **(D)** is noted,
but no contrast enhancement is demonstrated on CEMR **(E)**.

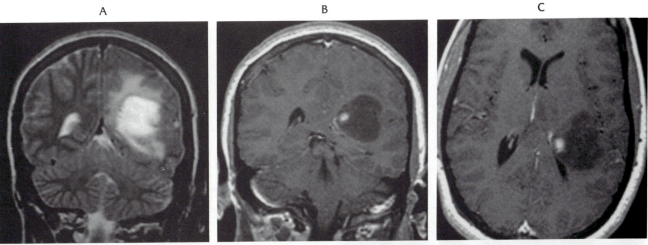

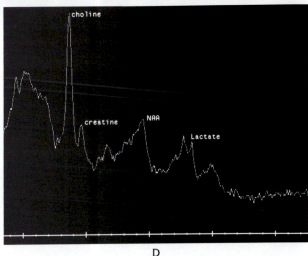

*Figure 7-11* **Grade II fibrillary astrocytoma** with focal anaplasia. Coronal $T_2WI$ **(A)** shows hyperintense rounded mass with focal contrast enhancing nodule on coronal **(B)** and axial **(C)** CEMR. MR spectroscopy (SV/PROBE) **(D)** in the center of the mass demonstrates low NAA peak with high choline concentration peak. Biopsy and surgery confirmed this diagnosis with a small mural anaplastic nodule.

ber and severity of chromosomal abnormalities of the neoplastic population of cells.

#### GRADE II ASTROCYTOMA

The most common histologies in this grade are *fibrillary astrocytomas*. Usually detected as an apparently focal abnormality in the brainstem or supratentorial white matter, they are widely infiltrating through adjacent white matter tracts. Although relatively benign in histological appearance, these tumors are prone to malignant transformation and progression to higher grades, particularly if a large number of gemistocytic astrocytes are present. The CT appearance of a fibrillary astrocytoma is a low-density mass with poorly defined borders (Fig. 7-10). On MRI, high signal intensity is seen on $T_2WI$ and low signal may be seen on $T_1WI$. However, conspicuity is low. On either CECT or CEMR, no significant contrast enhancement is seen (Fig. 7-10). If contrast enhancement is seen in a mass, the possibility of malignant progression should be suggested, (Fig. 7-11) even if previous biopsy has shown a low-grade glioma.

*Pleomorphic Xanthoastrocytoma* A less common type of grade II astrocytoma is the pleomorphic xanthoastrocytoma (PXA) (Kepes 1993). This tumor was previously considered to be a grade I, circumscribed astrocytoma, but cumulative clinical and pathological experience has led to its classification as a grade II or III in the WHO-II system (Kleihues 1993). This tumor is

believed to arise from the subpial population of astrocytes and is therefore generally found in a superficial location (Thomas 1993). CT and MR imaging features include many similarities to the pilocytic astrocytoma, including some densely enhancing tissue with clearly demarcated macroscopic borders and cystic components (Lipper 1993; Tien 1992). Occasionally a cyst with mural nodule appearance is seen. The tumor mass has a mixed SI on $T_1WI$, high or mixed SI on $T_2WI$, and minimal edema in the surrounding brain (Fig. 7-12). Unlike the pilocytic astrocytoma, which it resembles, and the superficial cerebral astrocytoma of infancy (also believed to be derived from subpial astrocytes), the PXA may be locally invasive and may display histological markers of a high-grade malignancy (Macaulay 1993). Progression of histological grade has also been reported in PXAs (Whittel 1989). Some PXAs of aggressive histology and biological activity, the less common variants, are considered to be grade III neoplasms (Kleihues 1993).

A          B          C

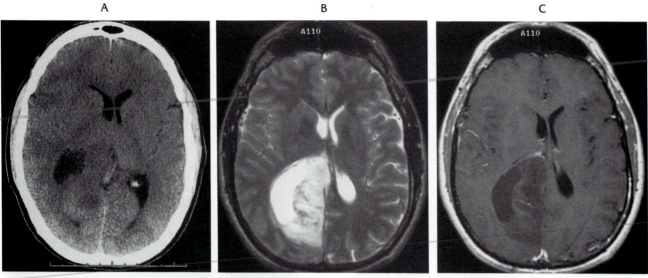

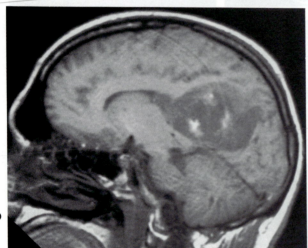

*Figure 7-14* **Anaplastic astrocytoma.** NCCT **(A)** shows a mixed density lesion in the deep right parietooccipital lobe involving the splenium and trigone of the right lateral ventricle. T₂WI **(B)** exhibits irregular hyperintense signal with adjacent trapped lateral ventricle and little edema. On CEMR **(C)**, minimal contrast enhancement is noted. Six months after biopsy and therapy, the tumor on the right side has decreased but contralateral extension to the left side is noted across the splenium on the axial CEMR **(D)**.

D

followed by seizure. First time seizure in adult onset should be thoroughly investigated for possible tumor.

Most commonly located in the deep supratentorial white matter, GBMs are distinctly uncommon in the posterior fossa and spinal cord locations. GBM is

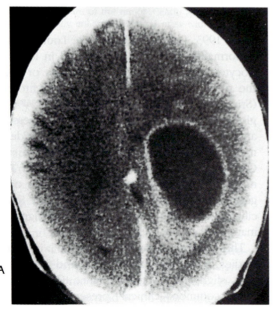

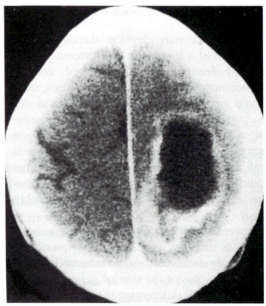

A          B

*Figure 7-15* **Glioblastoma multiforme.** CECT **(A, B)** demonstrates a large cavitary lesion with hypodense center and thin well- demarcated margins **(A)**. Thick, irregular ring of wall enhancement is better seen on slightly higher level **(B)**.

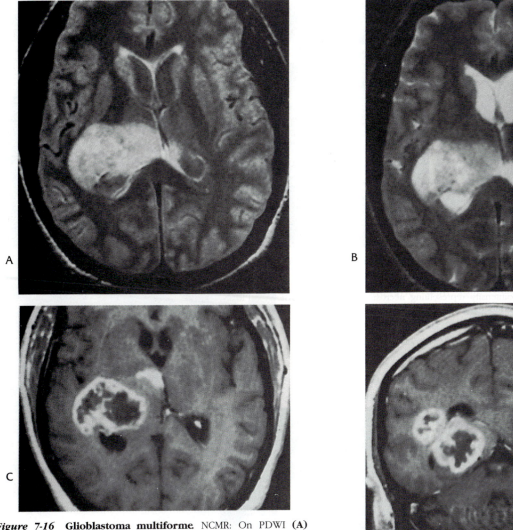

***Figure 7-16*** **Glioblastoma multiforme.** NCMR: On PDWI **(A)** and T$_2$WI **(B)** the tumor shows sharp margination and is relatively homogeneous. CEMR: On axial **(C)** and coronal **(D)** views, multiple contiguous foci of irregular ring enhancement with central necrosis are present.

usually identified on MR as a heterogeneous lesion that can be divided into four zones (Kelly 1987). The innermost region, central necrosis, is hypodense on CT and shows prolongation of both T$_1$ and T$_2$ relaxation times (more hypointense than brain on T$_1$WI and more hyperintense on T$_2$WI). The second zone is the solid, viable, fleshy, and hypercellular portion of the neoplasm. This is also the area of greatest tumor-induced neovascularity. This region shows contrast enhancement forming an irregular ring on both CT and MR (Figs. 7-15 and Fig. 7-16) and is often hypervascular on angiography (Fig. 7-17). Ring enhancement in glioblastomas usually has thick walls of varying width and a very shaggy inner margin—the interface between living tumor and necrotic debris. The solid ring of neo-

plastic tissue occasionally shows slight hyperdensity on NCCT and may display a corresponding decreased signal intensity on both PD- and T$_2$WI (Fig. 7-18). The exact mechanism for these changes is not established, but potential causes include the increased tissue density of the glial cells as well as the blood, connective tissue, and dense vascular proliferations characteristic of glioblastoma. Dean (1990) emphasized that one of the MR features that distinguishes the anaplastic (grade 3) astrocytoma from the glioblastoma (grade 4) is hemosiderin or other evidence of prior hemorrhage. It must be emphasized that routine MR, even with contrast enhancement, depicts only the gross macroscopic boundaries of the tumor. Neoplastic infiltration of malignant glial cells commonly extends well beyond the

D   E

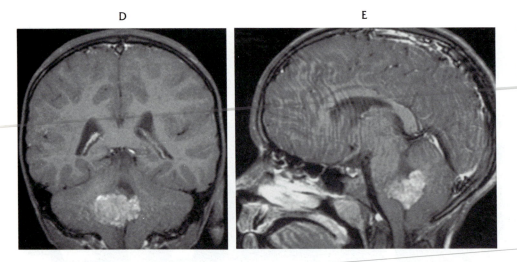

*Figure 7-26 (continued)* coronal **(D)**, and sagittal **(E)** images confirm the epicenter of the mottled contrast enhancing tumor in the fourth ventricle.

spectively (Jackson 1992). Grossly, these tumors are usually globular—sometimes rounded and smooth, sometimes lobulated. Despite gross appearances, close inspection reveals an irregular surface. Occasionally, a tumor may macroscopically or microscopically invade the adjacent brain to become choroid plexus carcinoma (Figs. 7-26, 7-27).

On NCCT, the choroid plexus tumor usually presents as a well-demarcated, smooth or lobulated mass of relatively homogeneous hyperdensity to normal gray matter. Mechanical effects of the tumor may cause local expansion of the surrounding ventricle. However, papillomas can produce hydrocephalus with panventricular enlargement. There are two mechanisms by which

A   B   C

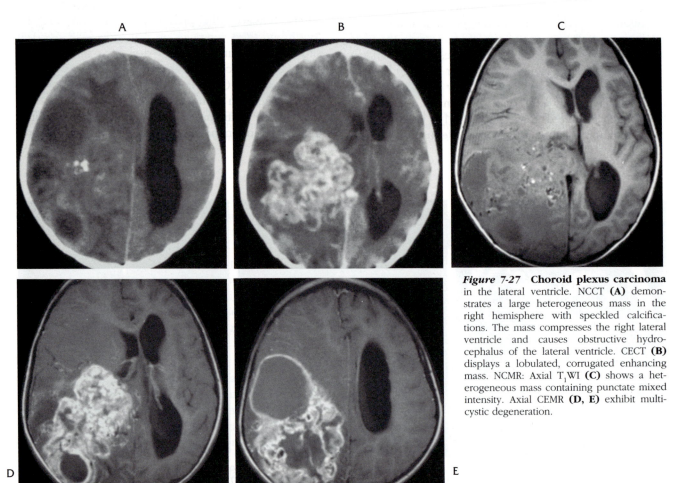

D   E

*Figure 7-27* **Choroid plexus carcinoma** in the lateral ventricle. NCCT **(A)** demonstrates a large heterogeneous mass in the right hemisphere with speckled calcifications. The mass compresses the right lateral ventricle and causes obstructive hydrocephalus of the lateral ventricle. CECT **(B)** displays a lobulated, corrugated enhancing mass. NCMR: Axial $T_1$WI **(C)** shows a heterogeneous mass containing punctate mixed intensity. Axial CEMR **(D, E)** exhibit multicystic degeneration.

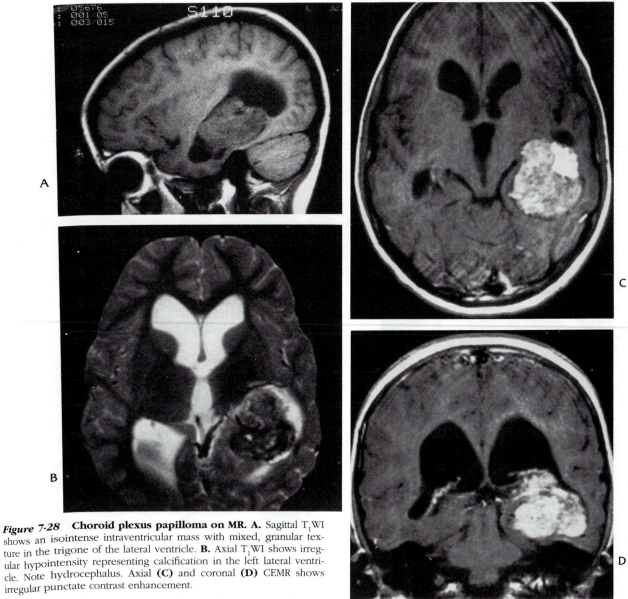

*Figure 7-28*  **Choroid plexus papilloma on MR. A.** Sagittal $T_1$WI shows an isointense intraventricular mass with mixed, granular texture in the trigone of the lateral ventricle. **B.** Axial $T_1$WI shows irregular hypointensity representing calcification in the left lateral ventricle. Note hydrocephalus. Axial **(C)** and coronal **(D)** CEMR shows irregular punctate contrast enhancement.

this may happen: (1) papillomas produce excessive quantities of CSF, duplicating normal choroid plexus function, and (2) these extremely vascular tumors are somewhat friable and thus especially prone to hemorrhage. Previous episodes of hemorrhage can lead to arachnoiditis in the skull base or obstructing the reabsorption pathway through the arachnoid granulation—both of which result in a communicating hydrocephalus. On CECT, there is dense and usually homogeneous enhancement (Fig. 7-27). Sometimes nonenhancing, hypodense areas are present either adjacent to, or occasionally inside, the tumor (Zimmerman 1979c). Although these hypodensities may represent degenerative changes in the tumor, they are often simply caused by entrapped lakes of CSF.

In children, choroid plexus papillomas are most of-

ten diagnosed by their characteristic location within the trigone of the lateral ventricle. On MR, these tumors are commonly hypo- to isointense to the brain at most pulse sequences; they are occasionally hyperintense on $T_1$WI (Fig. 7-27 and 7-28). The observed hypointensity may be due to a combination of microscopic calcifications and vascular signal voids from innumerable small vessels in these highly vascularized tumors. Serpentine signal voids from the large feeding and draining vessels are infrequently seen on MR. On $T_2$WI, the sequelae of hydrostatic edema are easily recognizable as regions of hyperintensity in the periventricular white matter. Choroid plexus tumors are attached to the normal choroid and invariably show intense contrast enhancement (Figs. 7-26, 7-27, 7-28, 7-29).

(Spagnoli 1986). In 1989 Elster and coworkers suggested that MR ability to predict histology could be improved by combining signal characteristics of the tumor with observations of secondary effects, such as edema. In their experience, syncytial and angioblastic meningiomas were markedly hyperintense on $T_2WI$, compared with hypointense fibroblastic and transitional meningiomas (Elster 1989). However, this may be a moot point, since within the group of typical meningiomas (see Table 7-14), which includes syncytial meningioma, there is no prognostic implication connected with any particular microscopic pattern. Demaerel (1991) investigated the histological bases of varying signal intensities on $T_1WI$, $T_2WI$, and PDWI or MR, and found great difficulty differentiating among various meningioma subtypes.

Many authors disagree about the etiology of the enhancing meningeal "tail sign" seen adjacent to some meningiomas on CEMR (see Fig. 7-41, 7-43). This dural tail sign is nonspecific and has been described in a wide variety of conditions, including postoperative states, radiation, sarcoidosis, lymphoma, chloroma, aspergillosis, metastasis, and schwannoma (Tien 1991). It is seen in 60 percent of all meningiomas (Goldsher 1990). The enhancing tail, seen with confirmed meningioma, is thought to represent a reactive (nonspecific) process in the meninges (Aoki 1990; Tokumaru 1990), but it may also be caused by the extension of neoplasm through dural infiltration (Wilms 1989; Tokumaru 1990; Goldsher 1990).

## SCHWANNOMAS

Schwannomas are benign tumors accounting for 6 to 8 percent of all primary intracranial tumors. They originate from schwann cells, a neural crest derivative. Most common location is the VIIIth nerve followed by Vth, VIIth and other cranial nerves (See Chap. 15).

## CONGENITAL INTRACRANIAL TUMORS

This group of tumors makes up less than 5 percent of all intracranial masses. Epidermoids are the most common within the group, followed closely by lipomas, dermoids and teratomas (Russell 1989). Embryologically, these epithelial tumors arise from the incorporation of ectoderm into the neural tube during closure, which occurs at 3 to 5 weeks of gestation. The location of the tumor is determined by the particular stage of fetal development during which incorporation takes place. If inclusion occurs early (at around 3 weeks), the lesion is usually located midline. Later inclusions place the tumor farther from the midline, and if inclusion takes place extremely late, the lesion becomes intradiploic (Toglia 1965).

## EPIDERMOIDS

The incidence of this tumor ranges from 0.2 to 1.8 percent of all intracranial neoplasms. The typical age range of the presenting patient is 25 to 60, with a male to female ratio of 2:1. Ectodermal inclusion during closure of the neural tube gives rise to this lesion, which occurs in the midline or, more commonly, laterally.

Epidermoids may take a multilobulated, grayish-white appearance, suggestive of a pearl. They may be intradiploic, extradiploic, or intraventricular, but are predominantly intradural and occur most commonly at the cerebellopontine angle (Gao 1992). Other sites, in order of reported frequency, include the parasellar region and the midposterior cranial fossa. Intradural lesions, which rarely calcify, were difficult to diagnose in the past owing to minimal neurological findings and normal skull radiographs. Extradural masses, which make up 25 percent of all epidermoids, are easier to recognize on plain films because they produce well-defined radiolucent defects and bone erosion of the adjacent skull. Their edges are sclerotic and may be scalloped (Chambers 1977) (Fig. 7-44). In addition, this radiographic appearance is nonspecific and should be differentiated from slowly erosive lesions, such as schwannoma, meningioma, aneurysm, chordoma and, rarely, metastatic lesions (Tadmor 1977).

Some epidermoids are found in the ventricles, with the fourth ventricle being the most common location, followed by the temporal horn of the lateral ventricles (Chambers 1977). Epidermoids may also rupture into the ventricular system, producing a lipid-CSF fluid level (Laster 1977; Zimmerman 1979$a$), although this is more commonly seen with dermoids. On CT, epidermoids frequently reveal low density, similar to that of CSF (Fig. 7-45). This tumor density reflects the composition of its two major components—keratin and cholesterin (Davis 1976$b$; Zimmerman 1979$a$). Most frequently, the density on CT is greater than the negative value of lipids, due to the presence of a large amount of non-lipid material (keratin), compared with the chief lipid (cholesterin). Less often, cholesterin is present in greater proportion than the keratin, such that tumor density falls into the minus range ($-16$ to $-80$ HU) (Cornell 1977; Laster 1977).

Epidermoid calcification is an inconsistent and uncommon finding. Very occasional increased density ($+80$ to $+120$ HU) and mural calcification (Fig. 7-45) are thought to be due to the calcification of keratinized debris, with saponification to calcification salts (Fawcitt 1976; Braun 1977). Enhancement on either CECT or CEMR is rarely seen due to the structureless, avascular nature of this tumor's central contents and its thin, avascular wall (Davis 1976$b$; Chambers 1977). Cerebral angiography merely confirms the avascular nature of this tumor. The rare occurrence of contrast enhance-

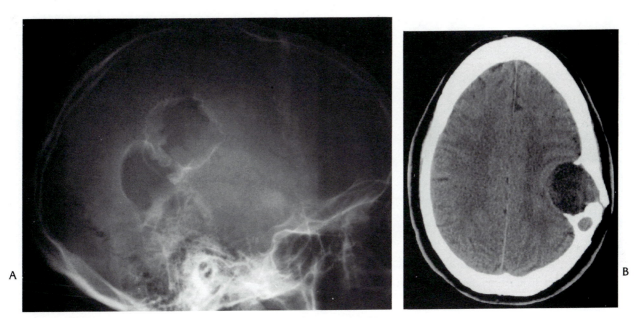

***Figure 7-44*** **Epidermoid. (A)** Lateral skull radiograph shows rounded radiolucent calvarial defects with sclerotic margins. **(B)**. Axial CT shows a sharp bony defect in the diploic space with parenchymal involvement.

ment at the periphery of the lesion is considered to be a result of the surrounding vascular connective tissue and/or dura mater (Tadmor 1977), the presence of gliosis (Mikhael 1978), and normal cerebral vessels stretched around the mass (Chambers 1977). Nosaka (1979) reported that a primary epidermoid carcinoma presents as an iso- or slightly hyperdensity which en-

hances homogeneously throughout the lesion on CECT.

The absence of hydrocephalus, the relative absence of a mass effect, and the lack of surrounding edema despite the size of these lesions are noteworthy. These features are due to soft consistency, slow rate of growth, and expansion of tumors into available spaces

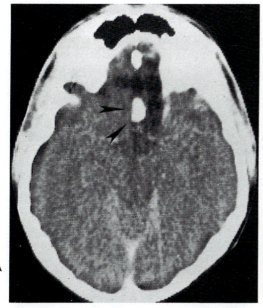
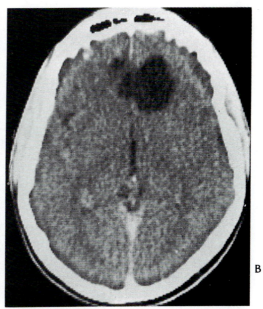

***Figure 7-45*** **Epidermoid calcification** on CT. Epidermoid tumors. **A** and **B.** Multiple areas of hypodensity in the basal frontal area, with the crista galli anteriorly and a calcification posteriorly (ar-

rowheads) within the tumor. Lobulated epidermoid crosses the midline. The absence of contrast enhancement of the wall and the absence of mass effect are noteworthy.

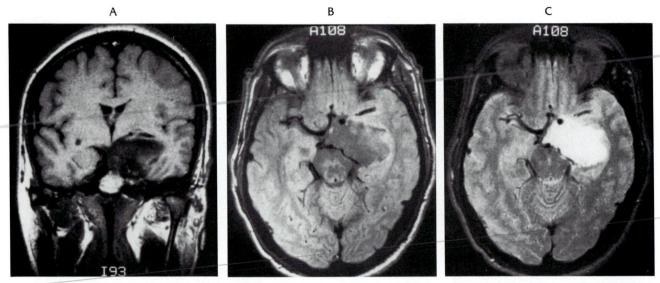

A          B          C

**Figure 7-46  Epidermoid** in the suprasellar and parasellar region. **A.** Coronal MR, $T_1WI$ (800/200) demonstrates a hypointense mass in the left suprasellar region with minimal mass effect on the medial temporal lobe. **B.** Axial MR: PDWI (2000/20) shows an isointense le-

sion encasing the patent internal carotid artery. **C.** Axial MR: $T_2WI$ (2000/20) exhibits a hyperintense lesion with minimal mass effect on the brainstem. *(Case courtesy of Dr. John Hesselink.)*

(Mikhael 1978). The tendency of these lesions to interdigitate with and insinuate themselves around adjacent structures is well known. Because intraventricular epidermoid density is similar to that of CSF, these epidermoids may not be readily detected or may be confused with arachnoid cysts. In some cases, diffusion-weighted MRI has been used to aid in the differentiation of epidermoids (Tsuruda 1990). Using diffusion MRI to distinguish solid from cystic lesions is more reliable than using $T_1$ or $T_2$ images because diffusion is insensitive to proteins or other paramagnetic substances in cystic fluid. (Le Biham 1992). In certain rare cases, intraventricular epidermoids have been described in association with focal ventricular dilatation or noncommunicating hydrocephalus (Issaragisil 1990).

The appearance of intracranial epidermoid tumors

varies widely, both on MR and on CT. Epidermoids are commonly homogeneous on CT but usually heterogeneous on MR, often associated with a lamellated or onion skin appearance (Steffey 1988). They also tend to have more irregular margins on MR than on CT. In 1990 Horowitz and colleagues describe two types of epidermoids on MR, both of which are hypodense on CT. The first type, the so-called "black" epidermoids, are relatively solid tumors of the pearly keratin type described earlier; chemically, they lack triglycerides. They typically exhibit water density (rather than fat) on CT, and are hypointense on $T_1WI$ (Fig. 7-46). The second type, "white" epidermoids, may have lower attenuation on CT, are usually more fluid or cystic, and are hyperintense on $T_1WI$. This epidermoid type contains mixed triglycerides, which probably accounts for both

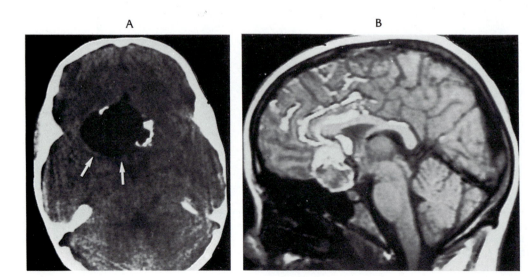

A          B

**Figure 7-47** Rupture of a **dermoid** into the subarachnoid space. Axial NCCT **(A)** demonstrates a parasellar fatty mass (arrows) with peripheral calcifications. A sagittal MRI, $T_1WI$ **(B)** discloses a hyperintense parasellar mass (dermoid) with hyperintense frontal sulci representing fatty tissue in the adjacent and distant subarachnoid spaces. Sulcal widening by fat is a characteristic MR finding in a ruptured intracranial dermoid. *(Courtesy of Dr. Francis J. Hahn, Omaha, Nebraska.)*

A

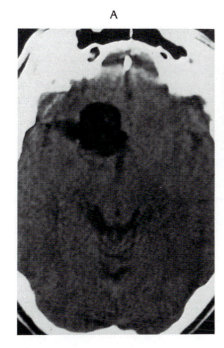

B

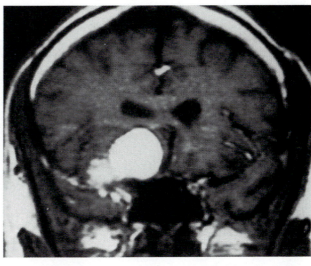

***Figure* 7-48**  Ruptured **dermoid.** On NCCT **(A)** a hypointense mass at the right basal frontal region extends into the sylvian fissure. MR, T₁WI **(B)** shows hyperintensity fatty tumor with multiple CSF seedings.

the T₁ shortening (increased signal intensity on T₁WI) and the lower attenuation on CT.

Epidermoids are usually hyperintense on T₂WI (Steffey 1988). Infrequently tumor rupture, with subsequent escape of keratin and cholesterin into the ventricular system, allows the less dense cholesterin to float, while the heavier keratin sinks (Laster 1977). As a result, a lipid-CSF level in the ventricles can be detected on both CT and MRI. Rupture of the tumor into the subarachnoid space may deposit cholesterin droplets into the adjoining cisterns and sulci. Contrast enhancement on CT or MR is not a usual feature of the epidermoids.

Early diagnosis may allow for curative surgery. Successful treatment involves surgical removal of the mass with its capsule intact. Unfortunately, the lesions may so insinuate themselves around adjacent structures that such removal is difficult. Iatrogenic liberation of contents into CSF compartments during surgery may initiate a chemical granulomatous meningitis and facilitate meningeal implantation, producing a "metastatic epidermoid."

### DERMOIDS

Dermoids are less common than epidermoids, representing roughly 1 percent of all intracranial tumors. Although dermoids, like epidermoids, are of congenital origin, their slow rate of growth often postpones clinical presentation until the third or fourth decade of life. Dermoids are derived entirely from ectoderm (Robbins 1979); the name *dermoid* itself means "skin-like," and the lesion has ectodermal glands, including sebaceous glands, apocrine sweat glands, and hair follicles. Even teeth which are highly unusual in intracranial lesions,

are ectodermal derivatives that have been reported in both dermoids and carniopharyngiomas (Burger 1982). True adipose tissue is not seen in dermoids; its presence may indicate another type of congenital tumor, such as teratoma or intracranial lipoma. It should be noted that most "dermoids" found outside the CNS are, in reality, benign cystic teratomas where the primary direction of differentiation has been into ectodermal tissues. Both epidermoid and dermoid are ectodermal inclusion cysts.

Dermoids are histologically more complex than epidermoids. They have thicker walls and are more likely to show calcification and may have recognizable contrast enhancement than epidermoids. In addition, the contents of dermoid cysts are almost invariably heterogeneous, with lighter lipid-containing debris forming a supernatant layer over the heavier, proteinaceous keratin material.

Dermoids are also much more likely than epidermoids to present as midline masses. It has been suggested that midline location is related to the embryologically earlier incorporation of ectodermal tissue into the neuraxis, an explanation consistent with the more complex nature of dermoids. Dermoids are commonly associated with other complex malformations, such as a dorsal or ventral dysraphism or a persistent cutaneous sinus tract (either patent or as a fibrous strand). Dermoids usually occur at the base of the brain, either in the posterior fossa (where they may invade the fourth ventricle), in the retroclival region, or in the suprasellar cistern. Peripheral ringlike or eggshell calcification is occasionally seen on plain film (Gross 1945; Lee 1977). Skull films may also reveal bony defects from an associated dysraphism or an in-

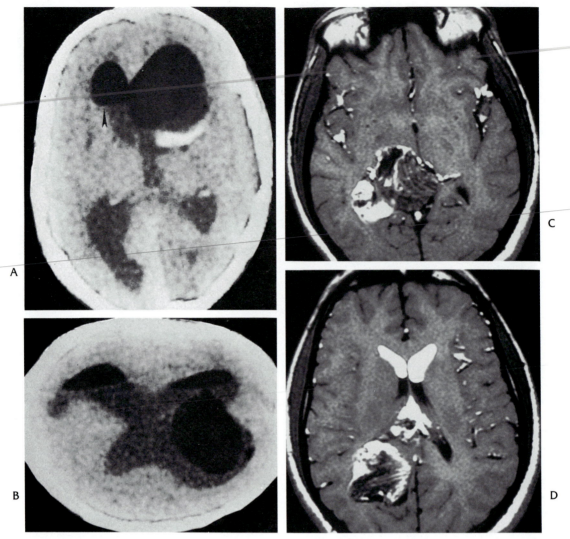

**Figure 7-49**   Frontal **dermoid** with intraventricular rupture. **A.** Axial CT in supine position demonstrates a large fat-containing mass projecting into the right frontal horn of the lateral ventricle. Calcification is present in the inferior wall of the mass. A fat-CSF level is present in the left front horn (arrowhead). **B.** Right lateral decubitus axial CT demonstrates multiple fat-CSF levels in the left lateral ventricle. Hydrocephalus and the right frontal dermoid are well visualized *(Zimmerman, 1979a.)*

MR in **ruptured dermoid** in the right lateral ventricle. T₁WI axial **(C, D)** *(Continued on next page)*

tradiploic component of the dermoid. Dermoids are usually avascular masses on angiography.

CT studies usually show dermoids as hypodense masses that are less dense than epidermoids, often in the range of attenuation for true fat ($-20$ or $-120$ HU) (Amendola 1978; Handa 1979) (Figs. 7-47, 7-48). However, the very negative absorption coefficients are not indicative of true fat, but rather of lipid material (sebum) that accumulates from the sebaceous and apocrine sweat glands, as well as cholesterol from the breakdown of squamous epithelium. In vitro, dermoid cyst fluid has shown measurements as low as $-80$ HU (Handa 1979). The thicker, more complex wall of a dermoid often develops dystrophic peripheral calcifications around the outside of the cyst (see Figs. 7-47, 7-49). In some cases, with appropriate windowing

techniques, a Rokitansky nodule or "hairball" can be seen floating in the lipid-protein interface (Lee 1977). The tissue contrast of modern third- and fourth-generation scanners allows visualization of the contrast enhancement in the dermoid wall. These tumors may be quite soft and pliable, molding themselves around the contours of adjacent structures. Dermoids are not, however, as insinuating as epidermoids, but tumor rupture is rather common in dermoids.

Spontaneous or iatrogenic rupture of dermoids may allow cystic contents to spread into the subarachnoid spaces or into the ventricular system, (Figs. 7-47, 7-48, 7-49) often with catastrophic consequences. Spillage of dermoid material initiates an acute and chronic reaction in the meninges. Acutely, there is a chemical meningitis, which may lead to severe vasospasm and

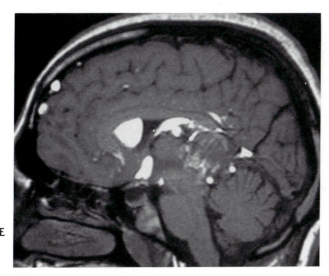

**Figure 7-49 (continued)** and sagittal **(E)** images show multiple fat-fluid of levels in the ventricles and the subarachnoid spaces.

even infarction. Later sequelae include granulomatous changes in the meninges and the potential for implantation of debris, causing "metastatic" dermoid tumors. Both CT and MR can clearly demonstrate the spread of lipid material into the subarachnoid spaces or the ventricular system, producing lipid-CSF levels (Zimmerman 1979a; Fawcitt 1976; Laster 1977; Amendola 1978; Smith 1991). (Fig. 7-49). Delayed hydrocephalus may accompany the rupture of a dermoid cyst. Surgery should be carefully performed to avoid spilling cyst contents and to effect complete and total removal. These tumors are not truly invasive but, like craniopharyngiomas, are often adherent to the adjacent brain, which can make complete resection difficult.

MR of dermoids shows a sharply demarcated, heterogeneous, extraaxial mass, typically in midline location. Although expansile, it appears soft, seemingly conforming to the shape of its surrounding structures. The mass is almost invariably heterogeneous, often demonstrating a characteristic fluid-fluid level. On $T_1WI$, the dependent portion tends to be dark, but slightly higher in signal than CSF. The supernatant usually has a short $T_1$ and is quite hyperintense on $T_1WI$. On $T_2WI$, the entire lesion may become hyperintense. If rupture has occurred, multiple droplets of lipid spreading throughout the subarachnoid spaces may exhibit focal areas of conspicuous hyperintensity on $T_1WI$ (Figs. 7-47, 7-48, 7-49). This can be pathognomonic when associated with a midline mass. However, residual droplets of the (old) oily, myelographic contrast material, iophendylate (Pantopaque), may also appear as bright droplets on $T_1WI$.

## LIPOMAS

Intracranial lipomas are rare tumors of developmental origin which may arise from an abnormal persistence

of the primitive surface layer of the neural tube, rather than through aberrant mesodermal inclusion (Truwit 1990). This tissue layer, the meninx primativa, subsequently undergoes differentiation into fat. Approximately half of all intracranial lipomas are asymptomatic, and they are usually found in the midsagittal plane or in or near the corpus callosum or quadrigeminal plate cistern. Another site of occurrence is at the base of the skull, including the cerebellopontine angle cistern. Some lipomas develop other elements, such as calcification, or become part of a more complex malformation, such as lipomeningocele, agenesis of the vermis, or cranium bifidum (Zettner 1960; Kushnet 1978). Some authors suggest that in the presence of an intracranial lipoma, abnormality of the adjacent brain, however slight, is likely (Atlas 1996). In practice, however, these lesions when small are usually considered to be incidental findings.

Lipoma of the corpus callosum is associated with agenesis of the corpus callosum in almost 50 percent of cases (Zettner 1960). Skull radiographs may show midline curvilinear or "eggshell" mural calcifications in the rim of the callosal lipoma surrounding the radiolucent fat. These findings are usually anterior, within the genu of the corpus callosum. Imaging studies, including pneumoencephalography and axial cross-sectional scans, demonstrate symmetrical separation of the frontal horns of the lateral ventricles, where they are

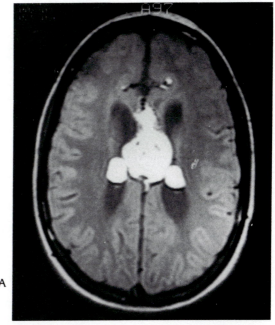

**Figure 7-50 Lipoma of corpus callosum and both choroid plexus.** Axial $T_1WI$ **(A)** demonstrates multiple contiguous rounded areas of hyperintensity. Semicircular (black) areas of chemical shift artifact from fat are noted along the posterior border of all these hyperintense masses. *(Continued on next page)*

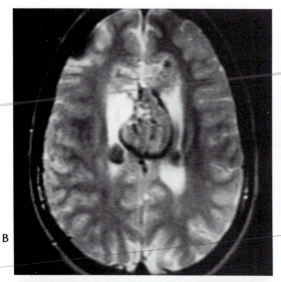

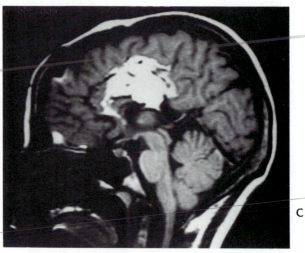

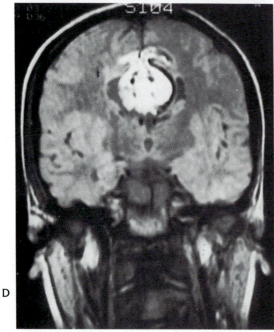

B

C

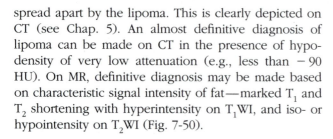

D

***Figure 7-50 (continued)*** Axial T$_2$WI **(B)** shows a marked decrease in signal from these fatty masses. T$_1$WI: Sagittal **(C)** and coronal **(D)** images show the midline location of the largest portion of the intracranial lipoma as well as the associated maldevelopment of the corpus callosum.

germ cell tumor is called *germinoma,* but its histology is identical with testicular seminoma. All histological types of germ cell neoplasms may also be seen, although less commonly, in the suprasellar or parasellar regions. Two prevailing theories attempt to explain the unusual origin of primary germ cell neoplasms deep within the CNS. One theory suggests that the fetal tissues of an aborted twin are absorbed by the viable fetus at the early stage of neural tube closure (3 to 5 weeks of gestation) and undergo partial metaplasia. The second theory suggests that at the time during which germ cells normally migrate to form the urogenital ridge, some cells become abnormally implanted within tissues in other regions, almost invariably in a midline location. These germ cell rests may later de-

spread apart by the lipoma. This is clearly depicted on CT (see Chap. 5). An almost definitive diagnosis of lipoma can be made on CT in the presence of hypodensity of very low attenuation (e.g., less than −90 HU). On MR, definitive diagnosis may be made based on characteristic signal intensity of fat—marked T$_1$ and T$_2$ shortening with hyperintensity on T$_1$WI, and iso- or hypointensity on T$_2$WI (Fig. 7-50).

## GERM CELL TUMORS

Germ cell tumors are the most common neoplasms found in the pineal region, (accounting for 60 percent), and the majority (80 percent) of intracranial germ cell neoplasms are related to the pineal gland (Smirniotopoulos 1992). The most common type of

## Table 7-15   Germ Cell Neoplasms

I. Germinoma (dysgerminoma, seminoma)

II. Embryonal carcinoma
   A. Extraembryonic type
      1. Endodermal sinus (yolk sac) tumor
      2. Choriocarcinoma
   B. Embryonic type
      1. Immature teratoma
      2. Mature teratoma

III. Mixed types
   A. Teratocarcinoma (teratoma and embryonal carcinoma)
   B. Other mixtures

velop into a wide variety of germ cell neoplasms, including tumors of fetal-type tissues.

Histologically, CNS germinomas are nearly identical with testicular seminomas. Different tumors with the same histology, occurring in the mediastinum or the ovary, are often called *dysgerminomas*. These tumors are marked by a "two-cell" pattern, where lobules of primitive germ cells are embedded in a matrix of lymphocytes (or lymphocyte-like cells). In addition to the typical germinoma histological types, other germ cell tumors that may arise include benign teratoma (mature), malignant teratoma (teratocarcinoma, immature

teratoma, teratoma with malignant change), embryonal carcinoma, choriocarcinoma, and endodermal sinus tumor (yolk sac tumor) (Table 7-15). Immature teratomas are composed of embryonic or fetal-type tissue; mature teratomas carry adult-type tissues. In both types, combinations of tissues are derived from more than one germ layer.

Germinomas tend to be isointense to gray matter on $T_1WI$ and isointense or slightly hyperintense on $T_2WI$. Although choriocarcinoma is prone to hemorrhage, dermoid, epidermoid, and teratoma tumors may contain lipid (cholesterol) or true fat. Thus, any of these

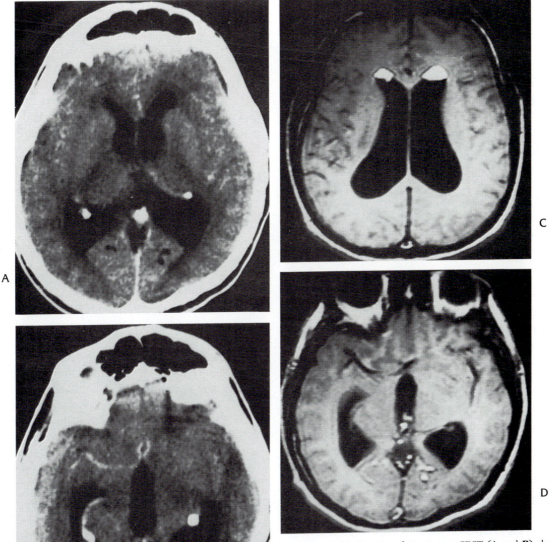

*Figure 7-51* **Ruptured teratoma.** CECT **(A** and **B)** shows a complex pineal region mass consisting of hyperdense foci of calcification and hypodense droplets of lipid. Because of rupture, lipid droplets are found in the subarachnoid spaces of the medial occipital sulci **(B)**. $T_1WI$ **(C)** shows the high intensity of the fat droplets in the sulci and in the ruptured teratoma itself. There is a fat-CSF level in the lateral ventricles on the adjacent section **(D).**

## Table 7-16    Pineal Region Masses

|  | CT | MRI |
|---|---|---|
| Germinoma | Dense, homogeneously enhancing, less commonly contain cysts, engulfs pineal calcification | Similar to CT, cystic components although less common, are better seen |
| Teratoma | Heterogeneous, may contain lipid and calcification | Heterogeneous, may identify fat |
| Yolk sac or endodermal sinus tumor sinus tumor | Heterogeneous | Heterogeneous, may contain blood |
| Pineal parenchymal tumors | Homogeneous, enhancing, may see "exploded" calcifications | Enhancement variable, may be heterogeneous |
| Tectal glioma | Variable, possibly cystic | Variable |
| Pineal cyst | Usually hypodense | May contain hemorrhage, ring enhancement possible |

## Table 7-17    Laboratory Tests for Pineal Neoplasms

| NEOPLASM | HCG | AFP |
|---|---|---|
| Germinoma | —* | — |
| Yolk sac | — | Increased |
| Choriocancer | Increased | — |
| Embryonal cancer | Increased | Increased |

*Occasionally positive.

four tumors may have hyperintense regions on $T_1WI$ (Fig. 7-51). Teratomas and epidermoids may also be hypointense (Tien 1990). Regions of hyperintensity on $T_1WI$ in a dermoid may show less intensity on the $T_2WI$ sequence when that signal is due mostly to lipid. However, hyperintense regions of epidermoids on $T_1WI$ may become even more hyperintense on $T_2WI$, because there is proteinaceous fluid in addition to cholesterol.

## Pineal Region Tumors

Tumors in the region of the pineal gland, which represents 0.5 to 1 percent of all intracranial neoplasms (Horowitz 1991), are of various histological types (Table 7-16). These tumors are colloquially referred to as *pinealomas*. However, the vast majority of tumors that are called pinealomas are not actually derived from pineal tissue, but instead arise from embryological rests of germ cells. Approximately 59 percent of pineal region masses are of such germ cell derivation

(Hoffman 1994), and most (39 percent) are typical germinomas. Many different lesions may present in the pineal region and within the germ cell group, and chemotherapeutic regimens are often quite specific for particular histologies. Because it is frequently not possible to accurately predict the actual tumor histology based on CT or MR alone, biopsy is usually required (Gouliamos 1994). Because of the high frequency of mixed germ cell tumors, neurosurgeons must be careful to obtain adequate samples. The identification of serum or CSF markers may also suggest a particular histology (Table 7-17).

### PINEAL GERMINOMAS

Germinomas may spread readily through the subarachnoid space and infiltrate the posterior third ventricle and thalamus. In some cases, however, they may be surprisingly well localized and demarcated. Eighty percent of intracranial germinomas are found in the pineal region; the remaining 20 percent are usually suprasellar. Germinomas tend to be homogeneous masses on both CT and MR and are almost always slightly more dense than normal brain on NCCT (Fujimaki 1994). On MR, germinomas tend to be isointense to gray matter on $T_1WI$ and isointense or slightly hyperintense on $T_2WI$ (Sumida 1995). Lesions may be rounded or slightly lobulated and can conform to the shape of the CSF-containing spaces that they fill, including anterior extension along the cistern of the velum interpositum (Fig. 7-52). However, lesions are also capable of CSF spread and direct invasion into the third ventricle and/or adjacent thalamus and brainstem tissues. The germinoma itself is usually not calcified, but there is a strong association between the presence of a germinoma and early dense calcification within the pineal

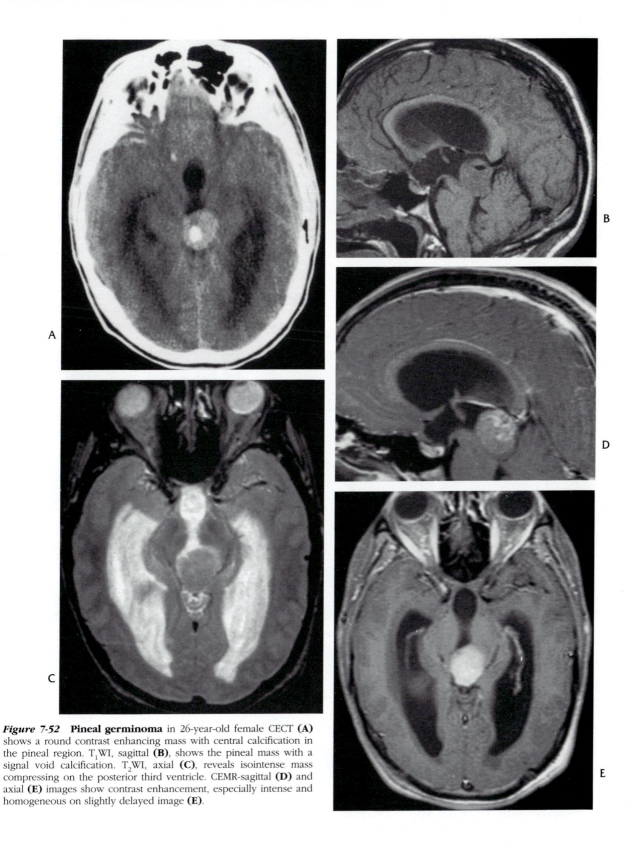

*Figure 7-52*  **Pineal germinoma** in 26-year-old female CECT **(A)** shows a round contrast enhancing mass with central calcification in the pineal region. $T_1$WI, sagittal **(B)**, shows the pineal mass with a signal void calcification. $T_2$WI, axial **(C)**, reveals isointense mass compressing on the posterior third ventricle. CEMR-sagittal **(D)** and axial **(E)** images show contrast enhancement, especially intense and homogeneous on slightly delayed image **(E)**.

gland itself (Chang 1989). As with many other masses that involve the subarachnoid space, the tumor may occasionally pinch off a "lake" of CSF and thus appear to be partially cystic. Since these tumors (and the nor-

mal pineal gland) lack a blood-brain barrier, contrast CT and MR invariably demonstrate some degree of enhancement that is usually very uniform (Fig. 7-52) (Chang 1989). CEMR typically demonstrates homoge-

A                              B                              C

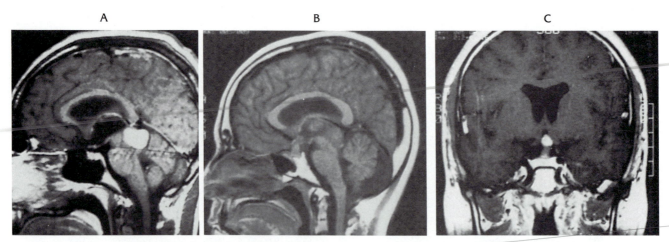

***Figure 7-53*** **Germinoma** with CSF metastasis. **(A)** NCMR: sagittal T₁WI **(A)** demonstrates an isointense mass in the pineal region which enhances homogeneously on CEMR **(B)**. Coronal CEMR **(C)** shows focal contrast enhancement in the sylvian fissures and suprasellar cistern representing seeding metastasis.

A                              B                              C

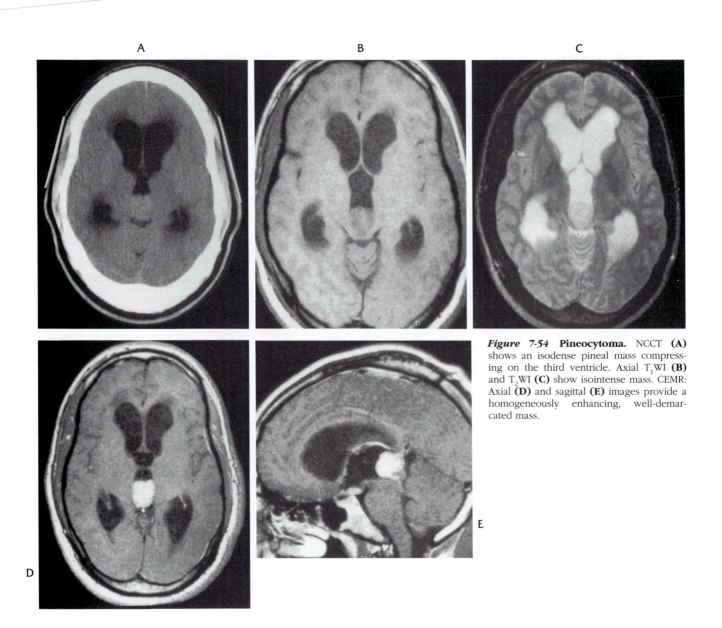

***Figure 7-54*** **Pineocytoma.** NCCT **(A)** shows an isodense pineal mass compressing on the third ventricle. Axial T₁WI **(B)** and T₂WI **(C)** show isointense mass. CEMR: Axial **(D)** and sagittal **(E)** images provide a homogeneously enhancing, well-demarcated mass.

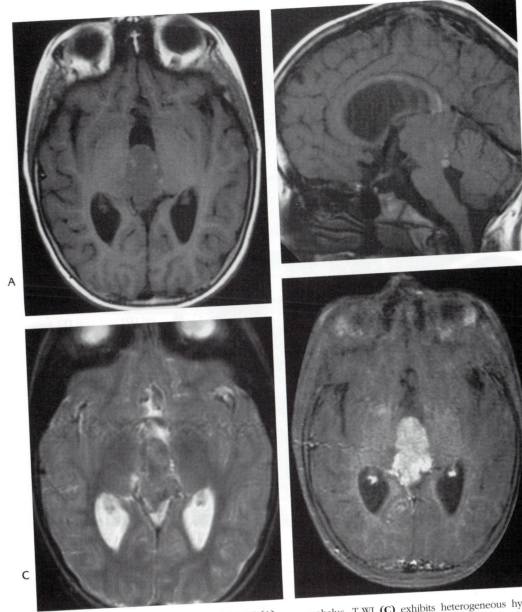

*Figure* 7-57
sion which exh

**Figure 7-55** **Pineoblastoma** in a 20-year-old male. Axial T₁WI **(A)** shows an isointense mass posterior to the third ventricle. On sagittal, T₁WI **(B)**, the mass is slightly irregular and infiltrates the aqueduct and the posterior third ventricle resulting in obstructive hydro-cephalus. T₂WI **(C)** exhibits heterogeneous hypo/isointense signal and CEMR **(D)** shows intense contrast enhancement with irregular margination.

the erroneou
neoplasm. Tl
be more e
(Smirniotopo

Tumors in
careful analys
nomas tend
rounding a
other lesions
cated by he
atoma), choles
cification, not
(teratoma). Pi
pineal gland fr
calcification to
are homogeneo
cytomas are h

neous enhancement and may reveal CSF seeding (Tien 1990) (Fig. 7-53).

## PINEOCYTOMAS AND PINEOBLASTOMAS

These uncommon neoplasms are the true intrinsic tumors of the pineal gland (Chiechi 1995). Malignant pineoblastomas, a subtype of primitive neuroectodermal tumors, are about twice as common as benign pineocytomas. They account for 15 to 25 percent of all pineal region masses, although statistics on these tumors vary widely in different series, possibly due to differences in classification systems. One distinguishing characteristic of potential differential value is that these

tumors usually contain intrinsic calcification and are located inside rather than around the pineal gland, unlike the germ cell tumors. Many intrinsic pineal "neoplasms are partially calcified and/or slightly hyperdense on NCCT; contrast enhancement usually occurs on CECT. These tumors may be slightly hypointense to white matter on T₁WI (Fig. 7-54) and have variable characteristics ranging from isointensity to hyperintensity on PDWI (Fig. 7-55).

Pineal region "retinoblastomas" may occur in patients with heritable retinoblastoma. This specific third primary location is the origin of the term *trilateral retinoblastoma*. Heritable retinoblastoma involves the

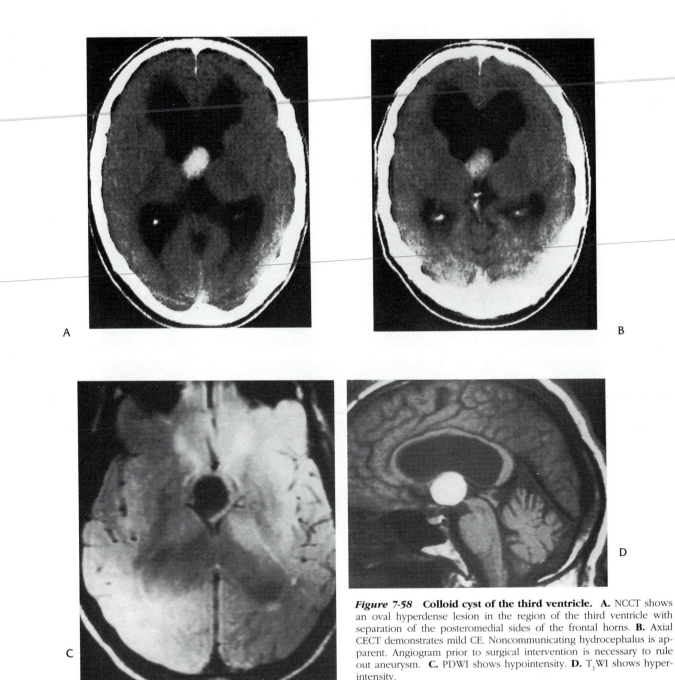

*Figure* 7-58  **Colloid cyst of the third ventricle. A.** NCCT shows an oval hyperdense lesion in the region of the third ventricle with separation of the posteromedial sides of the frontal horns. **B.** Axial CECT demonstrates mild CE. Noncommunicating hydrocephalus is apparent. Angiogram prior to surgical intervention is necessary to rule out aneurysm. **C.** PDWI shows hypointensity. **D.** $T_1$WI shows hyperintensity.

of these cysts, as with Rathke cleft cysts in the pituitary region, is composed of pseudostratified epithelium, with occasional ciliated epithelium. Goblet cells may also be seen. The similarity to bronchial epithelium has led to the idea that colloid cysts arise as a result of extreme upward displacement of primitive foregut elements during early embryology. The same embryological stage in which the Rathke pouch invaginates upward is suggested to occasionally result in even more extreme rostral displacement of cells intended for other locations (Itoh 1992). Although many plausible

theories exist, the exact origin of these and other endodermally lined cysts of the CNS remains speculative, that is, histological similarity does not guarantee etiological commonality.

The clinical importance of colloid cysts relates to their typical location, which is within the third ventricle at the foramina of Monro. Here, these benign cysts, which may be as large as 3 to 4 cm, can cause acute hydrocephalus and death if not quickly and correctly identified and treated. Intermittent obstruction of the cerebrospinal fluid is possible, particularly if the mass is somewhat pendulous and movable (Guner 1976), and patients may experience transient "drop attacks" or positional headaches that are relieved by a change in position.

In the more chronic setting, common symptoms and findings include headache, gait disturbance, and papilledema (Little 1974). These cysts are benign and can be completely removed early in their course, but Guner and coworkers (1976) reported a postoperative mortality rate as high as 53 percent in the 1970s, presumably due to the complex regional anatomy and proximity of vital structures. Current morbidity for complete resection by open craniotomy is believed to be 5 percent or less, and it is expected to become even lower with the advent of newer techniques for stereotactic aspiration.

NCCT shows a sharply marginated spherical or ovoid lesion, usually of homogeneously high density (45 to 75 HU) in the anterior third ventricle, in front of or behind the foramen of Monro (Fig. 7-58). Uncom-

monly, the lesion is isodense, and rarely, a central hypodensity within the lesion is noted (Ganu 1981). Surgical results indicate successful aspiration is more likely if the cyst is hypodense or isodense on NCCT, presumably indicating higher fluid composition of cyst contents (Kondziolka 1994). The high density noted on NCCT is probably due to desquamated secretory products of the cyst wall, hemosiderin, and possibly microscopic foci of calcification, not apparent on CT. Only mild enhancement has been shown on CECT (Osborn 1977; Ganti 1981) (see Fig. 7-58), but absence of contrast enhancement is not unusual. The presence of blood vessels in the wall or even inside the body of the cyst, as well as the diffusion of contrast media into the cavity, may account for enhancement. Hemorrhage is rare (Malik 1980). Although minimal to moderately severe hydrocephalus is present in most cases, the degree of severity is not always proportional to the size of the cyst. Frequently, the anterior portion of the third

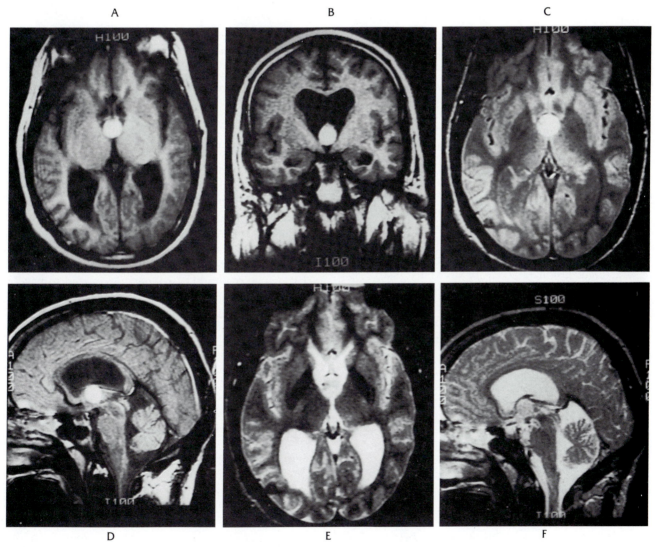

**A**  **B**  **C**

**D**  **E**  **F**

***Figure 7-59*** **Colloid cyst.** $T_1$WI: **A** (axial) and **B** (coronal) show a hyperintense lesion in the anterior third ventricle. PDWI: **C** and **D** show slight hyperintensity, which slightly decreases on $T_2$WI **(E)** and **(F).**

ventricle is not well visualized, and the posterior third ventricle is usually collapsed. Widening of the septum pellucidum and separation of the posteriomedial aspects of the frontal horns are demonstrated in most cases on axial and coronal sections (Ganti 1981) (Fig. 7-58). Intraventricular ependymoma, glioma, meningioma, choroid plexus papilloma, arteriovenous malformation, craniopharyngioma, teratomatous tumor, tuberous sclerosis, and cysticercosis should all be considered in the differential diagnosis. The need for additional invasive study such as contrast ventriculography or cisternography has greatly diminished because of the availability of high-resolution CT scanners and especially the multiplanar capability of MRI. However, when there is atypical and unusual contrast enhancement present, the possibility of aneurysm or ectatic vessels should be strongly considered and investigated promptly by MR or conventional cerebral angiography.

The appearance of colloid cysts on MR images is quite variable (Maeder 1990; Wilms 1990; Roosen 1987). Their appearance on MR is similar to their gross appearance on CT: they are sharply circumscribed lesions of the anterior superior third ventricle, usually in or near the foramen of Monro in symptomatic patients (Fig. 7-59). If the foramen is obstructed by a colloid cyst, MR may demonstrate periventricular signal abnormalities related to hydrostatic interstitial edema, as well as altered CSF flow dynamics within the ventricular system itself. Although they are usually homogeneous on CT, colloid cysts are heterogenous on MR in the majority of cases (Maeder 1990). Signal intensity of colloid cysts is an unreliable diagnostic criterion, since it may vary from hypointense to hyperintense on both $T_1WI$ and $T_2WI$ (Maeder 1990; Wilms 1990; Roosen 1987) (Figs. 7-58, 7-59). One unexpected MR finding, seen on $T_1WI$, is the presence of a hyperintense peripheral rim surrounding a hypo- to isointense center—a target lesion (Maeder 1990; Wilms 1990) (Fig. 7-45). This finding remains unexplained; it is not attributed to any pathologically visible process (Wilms 1990), nor has it been clarified by chemical analysis (Maeder 1990). Lack of contrast enhancement is usual except for occasional peripheral thin rim of enhancement. It may, however, represent hypointensity due to inspissated mucoid cyst contents. The most characteristic and suggestive features of colloid cysts are their sharp delineation and characteristic location within the third ventricle near the foramen of Monro.

## Miscellaneous Tumors

### HEMANGIOBLASTOMAS

Hemangioblastomas are histologically benign, true neoplasms of uncertain histogenesis. Although previously believed to be of vascular origin, immunohisto-

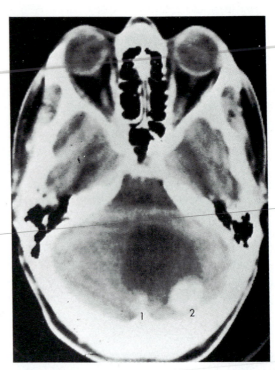

***Figure 7-60*** **Hemangioblastoma.** On CECT, a large cystic posterior fossa tumor is noted in the left cerebellum. Two round, homogeneously enhancing tumor nodules (1, 2) are present at the posterolateral wall of the cyst. Absence of enhancement of the cyst wall itself is characteristic.

chemical analysis has failed to establish that the stromal cells of these tumors are of endothelial origin (Lodrini 1991; Omulecka 1995). They constitute from 1.1 to 2.5 percent of all intracranial tumors; approximately 35 to 60 percent are cystic, usually with a mural nodule. These tumors may be associated with erythrocytosis and are the primary feature of von Hippel Lindau disease (Russell 1989; Choyke 1995). Approximately one-third of patients discovered to have a single hemangioblastoma are eventually found to have von Hippel-Lindau, although the odds are slightly greater for patients with an isolated spinal cord hemangioblastoma. These tumors are the most common primary intraaxial neoplasms of the posterior fossa in adults. Three main morphological patterns are seen. Most commonly, in about one-third of cases, hemangioblastomas present as cysts with enhancing mural nodules. A hemangioblastoma may also be seen as a solid enhancing mass without significant cystic component, or as a cystic mass with a relatively small amount of peripheral enhancing tissue. Mural nodules enhance homogeneously and may be single or multiple (Fig. 7-60) (Adair 1978). The central hypodense areas of the cyst fluid range from 4 to 23 HU and show no contrast enhancement. An isodense cyst margin with no demonstrable contrast enhancement represents gliosis and compressed cerebellum and is not neoplastic tissue. In contrast, areas that are hyperdense on NCCT and that show contrast enhancement correspond to richly vascular neoplastic tissue. Rarely, central hypodensity suggestive of a cyst may prove to be solid tumor tissue. Angiography not only confirms the presence of the hypervascular mural nodules but also increases the detection rate for multiple lesions (Seeger 1981). Rare cases of supratentorial hemangioblastomas have been recorded (Wylie 1973; Bachmann 1978).

MR of hemangioblastoma reveals the same gross characteristics noted on CT. The tumor may be solid, in which case differential diagnosis can be difficult (Fig. 7-61). However, MR may also reveal only a cyst or the classic cyst with mural nodule appearance (Fig. 7-62). Three additional features of hemangioblastoma have been identified on MR (Lee 1989; Katz 1989). First, the $T_1WI$ may show foci of signal hyperintensity within the solid portions of the hemangioblastoma (Fig. 7-61). These foci may contain blood breakdown products from a previous hemorrhage. Alternatively, $T_1$ shortening may come from the lipid-containing "stromal" cells that are an essential component of hemangioblastoma. Second, previous hemorrhage may deposit hemosiderin within or around the hemangioblastoma, which can cause hypointense curvilinear bands. The third unique MR feature of hemangioblastomas is a curvilinear or serpentine signal void representing the larger sinusoids within the tumor or the larger vessels supplying or draining the tumor. Thus there are two causes of arcs of hypointensity for hemangioblastoma; either may be noted around or leading to the tumor, as well as within it (Fig. 7-61). The presence of a serpentine

signal void related to a cystic mass, especially with a mural nodule, may be pathognomonic for hemangioblastoma (Lee 1989). The nodule or nodules in a hemangioblastoma will enhance after MR contrast injection (Fig. 7-62).

## PRIMARY INTRACRANIAL LYMPHOMA

CNS lymphoma has always been a confusing and controversial study in neoplasms. There have been numerous classifications of lymphoreticular proliferations in general and CNS lymphoma in particular. A variety of terms have been used to describe CNS lymphoma (Tadmor 1978; Kazner 1978; Hochberg 1988), including reticulum cell sarcoma, microglioma, histocytic lymphoma, perithelial sarcoma, and lymphosarcoma.

Tumors of the lymphoreticular system may be primary brain lesions or metastatic lesions that are part of a disseminated systemic lymphoma. Metastatic lymphoma involving the central nervous system is almost always extraaxial, usually presenting as a dural or calvarial mass. In the past, primary malignant lymphoma of the brain was a relatively rare tumor, with an incidence ranging from 0.8 (Jellinger 1975) to 1.5 percent (Zimmerman 1975) of all intracranial tumors. However, over the last two decades, its incidence has increased significantly owing to a number of factors, including the increased incidence of the acquired immune deficiency syndrome (AIDS), the increased number of patients who are iatrogenically immunosuppressed following chemotherapy or organ transplantation, the increased use of exogenous steroids for a variety of medical and nonmedical reasons including

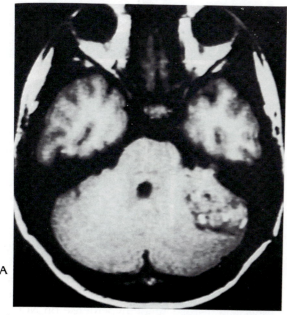

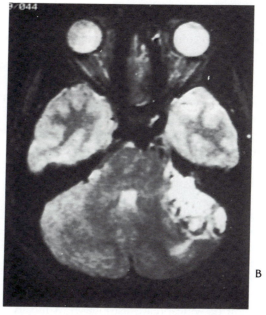

*Figure 7-61*  **Solid hemangioblastoma. A.** $T_1WI$ demonstrates multiple hyperintense foci in the left cerebellopontine angle. This can be caused by lipid-laden stromal cells and/or subacute hemorrhage. **B.** $T_2WI$ shows an overall increase in signal intensity but with persistence of the peripheral curvilinear dark bands, representing either previous hemorrhage or large sinusoids of vessels around the tumor.

MAIURI F, SPAZIANTE R, et al: Central neurocytoma: Clinico-pathological study of 5 cases and review of the literature. *Clin Neurol Neurosurg* 97(3):219–228, 1995.

MALIK GM, HOROUPIAN DS, BOULOS RS: Colloid cysts. *Surg Neurol* 13:73–77, 1980.

MENDONCA-DIAS MH, LAUTERBUR PC: Ferromagnetic particles as contrast agents for magnetic resonance imaging of liver and spleen. *Magn Reson Med* 3:328–330, 1986.

MIKHAEL MA, MATTAR AG: Intracranial pearly tumors: The role of CT, angiography and pneumoencephalography. *J Comput Assist Tomogr* 2:421–429, 1978.

MIKULIS DJ, ORLANDO D, EGGLIN TK et al: Variance of the position of the cerebellar tonsils with age: Preliminary report: *Radiology* 183:725–728, 1992.

MILHORAT TH: Classification of the cerebral edemas with reference to hydrocephalus and pseudotumor cerebri. *Childs Nerv Sys* 8(6):301–306, 1992.

MILLER DC, LANG FF, EPSTEIN FJ: Central nervous system gangliogliomas. Part 1: Pathology. *J Neurosurg* 79(6): 859–866, 1993.

MINEURA K, SAWATAISHI J, SASAJIMA T, et al: Primary central nervous system involvement of the so-called peripheral T-cell lymphoma. Report of a case and review of the literature. *Neurooncol* 16(3):235–242, 1993.

MODESTI LM, BINET EF, COLLINS GH: Meningiomas causing spontaneous intracranial hematomas. *J Neurosurg* 45:437–441, 1976.

MORK SJ, HALVORSEN TB, LINDEGARD KF, et al: Oligodendrogliomas, incidence and biologic behavior in a defined population. *J Neurosurg* 63:881–889, 1985.

NEW PFJ, SCOTT WR, SCHNUR JA, et al: Computed tomography with the EMI scanner in the diagnosis of primary and metastatic intracranial neoplasms. *Radiology* 114: 75–87, 1975.

NEW PFJ, ARONOW S, HESSELINK JR: National Cancer Institute Study: Evaluation of computed tomography in the diagnosis of intra-cranial neoplasms. IV: Meningiomas. *Radiology* 136:665–675, 1980.

NIIKAWA S, ITO T, MURAKAWA T, et al: Recurrence of choroid plexus papilloma with malignant transformation—Case report and lectin histochemistry study. *Neurol Med Chir (Tokyo)* 33(1):32, 1993.

NOSAKA Y, NAGAO S, TABUCHI K: Primary intracranial epidermoid carcinoma. *J Neurosurg* 50:830–833, 1979.

OKAZAKI H: *Fundamentals of Neuropathology.* New York, Igaku-Shoin, 1989.

OKAZAKI H, SCHEITHAUER BW: Neoplasms and related lesions, in *Atlas of Neuropathology.* New York, Gower, 1988, chap 3, pp 59–218.

OLSSON MBE, PERSSON BRB, SALFORD LG, et al: Ferromagnetic particles as contrast agent in T2 NMR imaging. *Magn Reson Imaging* 4:437–440, 1986.

OMULECKA A, LACH B, ALWASIAK J, GREGOR A: Immuno-histochemical and ultrastructural studies of stromal cells in hemangioblastoma. *Folia Neuropathol (Poland)* 33(1):41–50, 1995.

OOT RF, NEW PFJ, PILLE-SPELLMANN JT, et al: Detection of intracranial calcification by MR. *AJNR* 7:801–809, 1986.

OSBORN AG: Diagnosis of descending transtentorial herniation by cranial computed tomography. *Radiology* 123:93–96, 1977.

PASQUIER B, GASNIER F, PASQUIER D, et al: Papillary meningioma. Clinicopathologic study of seven cases and review of the literature. *Cancer* 58(2):299–305, 1986.

PAXTON R, AMBROSE J:The EMI scanner: A brief review of the first 650 patients. *Br J Radiol* 47:530–565, 1974.

PERROTT-APPLANAT M, GROYER-PICARD MTH, KUJAS M: Immunohistochemical study of progesterone receptors in human meningioma. *Acta Neurochir* 115:20–30, 1992.

PETERSON K, GORDON KB, HEINEMANN MH, DE ANGELIS LM: The clinical spectrum of ocular lymphoma. *Cancer* 72(3):843–849, 1993.

PULLICINO P, WILBUR DC, et al: Infarction in a meningioma after cardiac arrest. *Arch Neurol* 40:456–457, 1983.

RANKLIN JR, ROSENBLUM ML: Etiology and biology of meningiomas, in Mefty AL: *Meningioma,* New York, Raven, 1991, pp 27–35.

RASHEED BK, FULLER GN, FRIEDMAN AH, et al: Loss of heterozygosity for 10q loci in human gliomas. *Genes Chromosom Cancer* 5:75–82, 1992.

RAYMOND AA, FISH DR, SISODIYA SM, et al: Abnormalities of gyration, heterotopias, tuberous sclerosis, focal cortical dysplasia, microdysgenesis, dysembryoplastic neuroepithelial tumour and dysgenesis of the archicortex in epilepsy. Clinical, EEG and neuroimaging features in 100 adult patients. *Brain* 118(3):629–660, 1995.

RAYMOND AA, HALPIN SF, ALSANJARI N, et al: Dysembryoplastic neuroepithelial tumor. Features in 16 patients. *Brain* 117(3):461–475, 1994.

REES JH, SMIRNIOTOPOULOS JG: Oligodendroglioma, clinical and imaging features in 87 patients. Presented at 34th Annual Meeting of the American Society of Neuroradiology, June 23, 1996, Seattle, Washington.

RENGACHARY S, BATNITZKY S, KEPES JJ, et al: Cystic lesions associated with intracranial meningiomas. *Neurosurgery* 4:107–114, 1979.

RENSHAW PF, OWEN CS, McLAUGHLIN AC, et al: Ferromagnetic contrast agents: a new approach. *Magn Reson Med* 3:217–225, 1986.

REUBI JC, HORISBERGER U, LANG W, et al: Coincidence of somatistatin and EGF receptors in meningiomas. *Am J Pathol* 134:337–344, 1989.

ROBBINS SL, COTRAN RS: *Pathologic Basis of Disease.* Philadelphia, Saunders, 1979.

ROGERS LR, ESTES ML, ROSENBLOOM SA, HARROLD L: Primary leptomeningeal oligodendroglioma: Case report. *Neurosurgery* 36(1):166–168, discussion 169, 1995.

ROHRINGER M, SUTHERLAND GR, LOUW DF, et al: Incidence and clinicopathological features of meningioma. *J Neurosurg* 71:665–672, 1989.

ROMAN-GOLDSTEIN SM, GOLDMAN DL, HOWIESON J, et al: MR of primary CNS lymphoma in immunologically normal patients. *AJNR* 13(4):1207–1213, 1992.

ROOSEN N, GAHLEN D, STORK W, et al: Magnetic resonance imaging of colloid cysts of the third ventricle. *Neuroradiology* 29:10–14, 1987.

RUNGE VM, PRICE AC, WEHR CJ, et al: Contrast enhanced MRI: Evaluation of a canine model of osmotic blood-brain barrier disruption. *Invest Radiol* 20:830–844, 1985.

RUSSELL DS, RUBINSTEIN LJ: *Pathology of Tumors of the Nervous System*, 4th ed. Baltimore, Williams and Wilkins, 1989.

RUSSELL DS, RUBINSTEIN LJ: *Pathology of Tumours of the Nervous System,* 5th ed. Baltimore, Williams & Wilkins, 1989.

RUSSELL EG, GEORGE AJ, KRICHEFF II, et al: Atypical CT features of intracranial meningioma: Radiological-pathological correlation in a series of 131 consecutive cases. *Radiology* 134:409–414, 1980.

SAINI S, STARK DD, HAHN PE, et al: Ferrite particles: A superparamagnetic MR contrast agent for the reticuloendothelial system. *Radiology* 162:211–216, 1987.

SALIBI SS, NAUTA HJW, BREM H, et al: Lipomeningioma: Report of three cases and review of the literature. *Neurosurg* 25:122–126, 1989.

SATO N, BRONEN AB, SZE G, et al. Postoperative changes in the brain: MR imaging findings in patients without neoplasms. *Radiology* 204: 839-846, 1997.

SCHÖFNER W, LINIADO M, HIENDORF HP, et al: Time-dependent changes in image contrast in brain tumors after gadolinium-DTPA. *AJNR* 7:1013, 1986.

SCHRELL UMH, FAHLBUSH R, ADAMS EF, et al: Growth of cultured human meningiomas is inhibited by dopaminergic agents. *J Clin Endo Metab* 71:1669–1671, 1990.

SEEGER JF, BURKE DP, KNAKE JE, et al: CT and angiographic evaluation of hemangioblastomas. *Radiology* 138:65–73, 1981.

SHALLER CA, JACQUES DB, SHELDEN CH: The pathophysiology of stroke: A review with molecular considerations. *Surg Neurol* 14:433–443, 1980.

SHAPIR J, COBLENTZ C, MALANSON D, et al: New CT findings in aggressive meningioma. *Am J Neuroradiol* 6:101–102, 1985.

SHARMA R, ROUT D, GUPTA AK, RADHAKRISHNAN W: Choroid plexus papillomas. *Br J Neurosurg* 8(2):169–177, 1994.

SILVERSTEIN JE, LENCHIK L, STANCIU MG, SHIMKIN PM:

MRI of intracranial subependymomas. J Comput Assist Tomogr 19(2):264–267, 1995.

SMIRNIOTOPOULOS JG, RUSHING EJ, MENA H: Pineal region masses: Differential diagnosis. *Radiographics* 12(3):577–596, 1992.

SMITH AS, BENSON JE, BLASER SI, et al: Diagnosis of ruptured intracranial dermoid cyst: Value of MR over CT. *AJNR* 12:175–180, 1991.

SPAGNOLI MV, GOLDBERG HI, GROSSMAN RI, et al: Intracranial meningiomas: High-field MR imaging. *Radiology* 161:369–375, 1986.

SPOTO GP, PRESS GA, HESSELINK JR, SOLOMON M: Intracranial ependymoma and subependymoma: MR manifestations. *AJR* 154(4):837–845, 1990.

SRIVASTAVA S, ZOU Z, PIROLLO K, et al: Germ-line transmission of a mutated p53 gene in a cancer prone family with Li-Fraumeni syndrome. *Nature* 348:747–749, 1991.

STECK PA, BRUNER JM, PERSHOUSE MA, et al: Molecular, genetic, and biologic aspects of primary brain tumors. *Cancer Bull* 45:296–303, 1993.

STEFFANSON K, WOLLMANN R, HUTTENLOCKER P: Lineages of cells in the central nervous system, in Gomez MR, ed: *Tuberous Sclerosis*, 2d ed. New York, Raven, 1989, pp 75–87.

STEFFEY DJ, FILIPP GJ, SPERA T, et al: MR imaging of primary epidermoid tumors. J Comput Assist Tomogr 12:438–440, 1988.

SUMIDA M, UOZUMI T, KIYA K, et al: MRI of intracranial germ cell tumours. *Neuroradiology* 37(1):32–37, 1995.

TADMOR R, DAVIS K, ROBERSON G, et al: Computed tomography in primary malignant lymphoma of the brain. *J Comput Assist Tomogr* 2:135–140, 1978.

TADMOR R, TAVERAS JM: Computed tomography in extradural epidermoid and xanthoma. *Surg Neurol* 7:371–375, 1977.

TALLY PW, LAWS ER Jr, SCHEITHAUER BW: Metastases of central nervous system neoplasms: Case report. *Neurosurg* 68:811–816, 1988.

TAMPIERI D, MOUMDJIAN R, MELANSON D, ETHIER R: Intracerebral gangliogliomas in patients with partial complex seizures: CT and MR imaging findings. *AJNR* 12(4):749–755, 1991.

TANTTU JI, SEPPONEN RE, LIPTON MJ, et al: Synergistic enhancement of MRI with Gd-DTPA and magnetization transfer. *J Comput Assist Tomogr* 16:19–24, 1992.

THAPAR K, FUKUYAMA K, RUTKA JT: Neurogenetics and the molecular biology of human brain tumors, in Kaye, Laws: *Brain Tumors*, New York, Churchill Livingstone, 1995, chap 5, p 81.

THOMAS C, GOLDEN B: Pleomorphic xanthoastrocytoma: Report of two cases and brief review of the literature. *Clin Neuropathol* 12(2):97–101, 1993.

TICE H, BARNES PD, GOUMNEROVA L, et al: Pediatric and adolescent oligodendrogliomas. *AJNR* 14(6):1293–1300, 1993.

TIEN RD, BARKOVICH AJ, EDWARDS MSB: MR imaging of pineal tumors. *AJNR* 11:557–565, 1990.

TIEN RD, CARDENAS CA, RAJAGOPALAN S: Pleomorphic xanthoastrocytoma of the brain: MR findings in six patients. *AJR* 159(6):1287–1290, 1992.

TIEN RD, YANG PJ, CHU PK: "Dural tail sign": A specific MR sign for meningioma? *J Comput Assist Tomogr* 15:64–66, 1991.

TIEN RD: Fat-suppression MR imaging in neuroradiology. *AJR* 158:369–379, 1992.

TOGLIA JU, NETSKY MG, ALEXANDER E JR: Epithelial tumors of the cranium: Their common nature and pathogenesis. *Neurosurg* 23:384–393, 1965.

TOKUMARU A, O'UCHI T, EGUCHI T, et al: Prominent meningeal enhancement adjacent to meningioma on Gd-DTPA-enhanced MR images: Histopathologic correlation. *Radiology* 175:431–433, 1990.

TRUWIT CL, BARKOVICH AJ: Pathogenesis of intracranial lipoma: An MR study in 42 patients. *AJNR* 11:665–674, 1990.

TSURUDA JS, CHEW WM, MOSELEY ME, et al: Diffusion-weighted MR imaging of the brain-value of differentiating between extraxial cysts and epidermoid tumors. *AJNR* 11:925–931, 1990.

VALI AM, CLARKE MA, KELSEY A: Dysembryoplastic neuroepithelial tumour as a potentially treatable cause of intractable epilepsy in children. *Clin Radiol* 47(4):255–258, 1993.

VASSILOUTHIS J, AMBROSE J: Computerized tomography scanning appearance of intracranial meningiomas. *J Neurosurg* 50:320–327, 1979.

VONOFAKOS D, MARCU H, HACKER H: Oligodendrogliomas: CT patterns with emphasis on features indicating malignancy. *J Comput Assist Tomogr* 3:783–788, 1979.

WEHRLI FW, MacFALL JR, NEWTON TH: Parameters determining the appearance of NMR images, in Newton TH, Potts DG (eds): *Modern Neuroradiology, vol 2, Advanced Imaging Techniques*. San Anselmo, Clavadel Press, 1983, pp 81–117.

WEINSTEIN MA, MODIC MT, PAVLICEK W, et al: Nuclear magnetic resonance for the examination of brain tumors. *Semin Roentgenol* 19:139–147, 1984.

WHITTLE IR, GORDON A, MISRA BK, et al: Pleomorphic xanthoastrocytoma. Report of four cases. *J Neurosurg* 70(3):463–468, 1989.

WILMS G, LAMMENS M, MARCHAL G, et al: Thickening of dura surrounding meningiomas: MR features. *J Comput Assist Tomogr* 13:763–768, 1989.

WILMS G, MARCHAL G, VAN HECKE P, et al: Colloid cysts of the third ventricle: MR findings. *J Comput Assist Tomogr.* 14:527–531, 1990.

WOLF SD, BALABAN RS: Magnetization transfer imaging. Practical aspects and clinical correlation. *Radiology* 192:593–599, 1994.

WU JK, YE Z, DARRAS BT: Frequency of p53 tumor suppressor gene mutations in human primary brain tumors. *Neurosurgery* 33(5):824–830, 1993.

WYLIE IG, JEFFREYS R, MACLAINE GN: Cerebral hemangioblastoma. *Br J Radiol* 46:472–476, 1973.

YASARGIL MG, VON AMMON K, VON DEIMLING A, et al: Central neurocytoma: Histopathological variants and therapeutic approaches. *J Neurosurg* 76(1):32–37, 1992.

YUEN ST, FUNG CF, NG TH, LEUNG SY: Central neurocytoma: Its differentiation from intraventricular oligodendroglioma. *Childs Nerv Syst* 8(7):383–388, 1992.

YUH, WTC, ENGELKEN JD, MUHONEN MG et al: Experience with high dose gadolinium MR imaging in the evaluation of brain metastasis. *AJNR* 13:335–349, 1992.

YUH WTC, FISHER DJ, et al: MR evaluation of CNS tumors: Dose comparison study with gadopentetate dimeglumine and gadoteridol *Radiology* 180:485–491, 1991.

ZANKL H, ZANG KD: Correlations between clinical and cytogenetic data in 180 human meningiomas. *Cancer Gen Cytogen* 1:351–356, 1980.

ZEE CS, SEGALL H, APUZZO M, et al: MR imaging of pineal region neoplasms. *J Comput Assist Tomogr* 15:56–63, 1991.

ZEITNER A, NETSKY MG: Lipoma of the corpus callosum. *J Neuropathol Exp Neurol* 19:305–319, 1960.

ZIMMERMAN HM: Malignant lymphomas of the nervous system. *Acta Neuropathol* suppl VI: 69–74, 1975.

ZIMMERMAN RA, BILANIUK LT: Cranial computed tomography of epidermoid and congenital fatty tumors of maldevelopment origin. *J Comput Assist Tomogr* 3:40–50, 1979*a*.

ZIMMERMAN RA, BILANIUK LT: CT of choroid plexus lesions. *J Comput Assist Tomogr* 3:93–102, 1979*b*.

ZIMMERMAN RA: Central nervous system lymphoma. *Radiol Clin North Am* 28(4):697–721, 1990.

ZIMMERMAN RD, FLOEMING CA, SAINT-LOUIS LA, et al: Magnetic resonance imaging of meningiomas. *AJNR* 6:149–157, 1985.

ZULCH KJ: *Brain Tumors: Their Biology and Pathology.* New York, Springer-Verlag, 1986.

ZWETSLOOT CP, KROS JM, PAZ Y, GUEZE HD: Familial occurrence of tumours of the choroid plexus. *J Med Genet* 28(7):492–494, 1991.

# 8 PEDIATRIC BRAIN TUMORS

*Robert A. Zimmerman*

## CONTENTS

The most common site for the occurrence of solid tumors in childhood is the central nervous system (CNS) (Heideman 1989). More than one-half of the 2.4 brain tumors per 100,000 children that occur annually are found in the posterior fossa (Young 1975; Segall 1985);

the remainder arise in the supratentorial space. In childhood, primary neoplasms represent the vast majority of brain tumors, with metastatic lesions to the brain parenchyma being uncommon (Gusnard 1990).

The differential diagnosis of a brain tumor in a child is based on anatomic localization, clinical symptomatology, age, and changes in density with CT and signal intensity with MR (Zimmerman 1990b; 1992). Pediatric tumors in the CNS are of diverse histological origin and include tumors arising from primitive stem cells of the germinal matrix (e.g., primitive neuroectodermal tumors), from the supporting cell structure of the brain (e.g., astrocytomas and gliomas), from the choroid plexus (e.g., choroid plexus papillomas and carcinomas), from the ependymal lining of the ventricles or ependymal rests within the white matter (e.g., ependymomas), and from embryological rests within the pineal gland (e.g., germinomas) as well as tumors arising as inclusions (e.g., lipomas, dermoids, and teratomas) and tumors arising from malformative processes (e.g., hamartomas) (Zimmerman 1990b; Buetow 1990). Some of these tumors are highly aggressive in nature, with a propensity to spread into the subarachnoid and intraventricular spaces (Heideman 1989). The evaluation and treatment of these patients are made more difficult by their young age; in the infant, the brain is still undergoing active myelination and neuronal organization.

The purpose of an imaging evaluation is to determine if a tumor is present and, if this proves to be the case, to localize it and suggest the most likely histological diagnosis. After treatment, the goal is to detect response, persistence of tumor, regrowth of tumor, and tumor dissemination as well as to detect possible postoperative or posttherapeutic complications.

The two primary methods of evaluation are computed tomography (CT) and magnetic resonance imaging (MRI). The choice of technique first depends on availability and the patient's clinical stability (Zimmerman 1989). CT is relatively rapid but somewhat insensitive to small tumors

341

characterized by increased water content. MR is sensitive to tumors with increased water content, shows more obvious tumor enhancement, is more sensitive to the presence of old blood products, and is less sensitive to calcification. MR scans take longer than CT scans do, and so motion can be a problem; thus, sedation is generally required during the first 6 years of life and in older retarded or otherwise uncooperative patients (Zimmerman 1986). With MR, the use of a magnetic field requires special considerations. Unstable patients who require monitoring and support are more difficult to examine with MR than with CT. In general, the increased sensitivity of MR to the presence of a cerebral neoplasm justifies the greater difficulty in acquiring an MR study.

## POSTERIOR FOSSA TUMORS

The three most common tumors of the pediatric posterior fossa are brainstem gliomas, cerebellar astrocytomas, and primitive neuroectodermal tumors (medulloblastoma) (Heideman 1989). Ependymomas, choroid plexus papillomas, dermoids, epidural neuroblastoma metastases, and other neoplasms are much less common (Zimmerman 1992).

### Brainstem Gliomas

The peak age for the onset of symptoms of brainstem gliomas is around 5 years, with males slightly more frequently affected than females (Bilaniuk 1980; Mantravadi 1982). In up to 90 percent of patients, cranial nerve palsies are a significant form of presentation (Albright 1983). These palsies are most often bilateral and multiple, with the sixth and seventh nerves most often affected (Albright 1983). Long track signs, ataxia, paraparesis, sensory deficits, and gaze disorders also may be present. Hydrocephalus usually is not present at diagnosis but develops after later growth of the mass. In patients with midbrain tectal lesions, hydrocephalus may be the initial form of presentation (Robertson 1995). Hydrocephalus has been reported to be present at the time of diagnosis in up to 30 percent of these patients (Bilaniuk 1980). Brainstem gliomas most commonly arise within the pons, from which they may extend superiorly into the midbrain and thalamus, laterally into the cerebellar peduncle and cerebellum, and inferiorly into the medulla and upper cervical spinal cord. Subarachnoid spread is not present at the time of diagnosis but can be found in up to 20 percent of patients with malignant gliomas before death (Mantravadi 1982; Packer 1983a). Exophytic extension commonly occurs into the basilar subarachnoid space, often partially encompassing the basilar artery; less frequently, it impinges on the internal auditory canal.

Histologically, most pontine gliomas are fibrillary astrocytomas, a type of neoplasm that has a tendency to

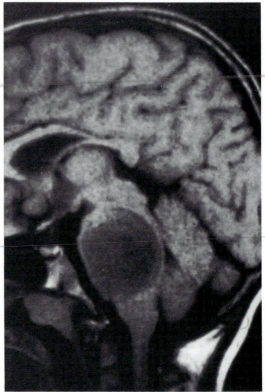

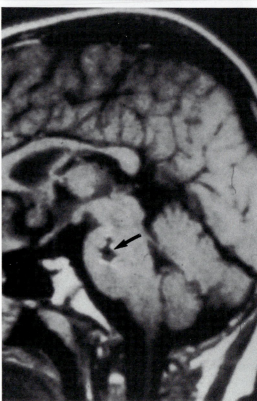

***Figure 8-1*** **Pontine glioma** before and after hyperfractionation. **A.** Sagittal $T_1$WI shows a hypointense mass expanding the pons and displacing and compressing the fourth ventricle. This examination was done before hyperfractionation radiotherapy. **B.** Sagittal $T_1$WI after hyperfractionation radiotherapy shows marked reduction in the size of the tumor. There is a focal area of low signal intensity (arrow) within the upper pons. Note that the fourth ventricle is no longer as compressed.

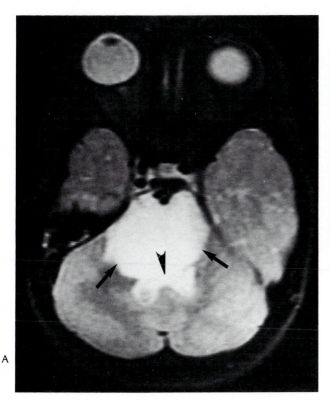

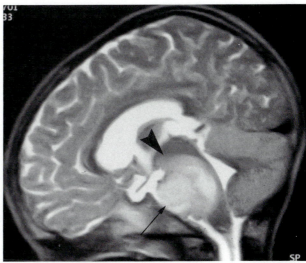

*Figure 8-2*  **A. Pontine glioma.** Axial T$_2$WI shows a high-signal-intensity mass (arrows) expanding the pons and compressing the fourth ventricle (arrowhead). **B.** Sagittal T$_2$WI performed with the half-Fourier turbo spin-echo technique is a single acquisition taking 1 sec, shows the increased signal intensity within the diffusely expanded pons. The mass extends forward exophytically into the prepontine space (arrow) and extends into the midbrain (arrowhead).

develop foci of anaplasia that undergo malignant degeneration, giving rise to an aggressive tumor that results in the patient's ultimate demise (Russell 1989). It is these foci of malignant degeneration that undergo cystic necrosis, hemorrhage, and contrast enhancement. Histologically, a fibrillary astrocytoma has little edema but enough interstitial fluid to appear high in signal intensity on proton density, T$_2$-weighted images (T$_2$WI), and fluid attenuated inversion recovery images (FLAIR). Fibrillary astrocytomas usually lack the microvasculature necessary for contrast enhancement. A smaller percentage of brainstem gliomas are pilocytic in nature, arising chiefly in the medulla and midbrain, often as exophytic masses (Smith 1990) but occasionally as a focal pontine mass (Edwards 1994). These tumors usually do not undergo malignant degeneration but may be associated with cysts, as is often seen with cystic cerebellar astrocytomas. These tumors have a microvasculature that usually produces contrast enhancement. Their slow growth rate appears to be responsible for the small incidence of long-term survivors with brainstem tumors.

Most brainstem gliomas are low in signal intensity on T$_1$-weighted images (T$_1$WI) (Fig. 8-1A) and high in signal intensity on long TR images (Fig. 8-2). On plain CT they are low in density, are isodense, or have a mixture of low-density and isodense components (Fig. 8-3). Calcification and hemorrhage in a brainstem glioma are un-

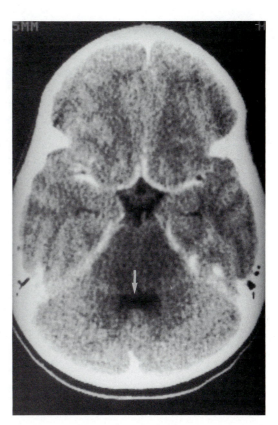

*Figure 8-3*  **Pontine glioma.** Axial CGCT shows a hypodense mass expanding the pons and compressing the fourth ventricle (arrow). The mass does not contrast-enhance.

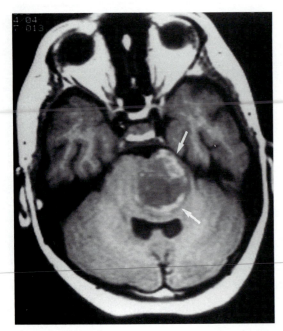

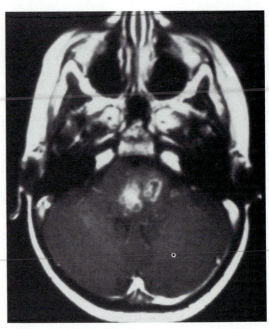

***Figure 8-4*** **Pontine glioma.** Axial T₁WI shows a hyperintense methemoglobin hemorrhage within portions of a pontine mass. The fourth ventricle is deformed, and most of the mass is of low signal intensity.

***Figure 8-5*** **Progressive pontine glioma.** Axial CEMR shows enhancement of the inferior portion of the pontine mass.

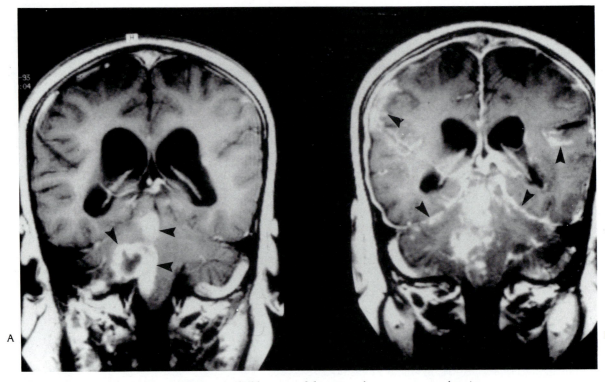

***Figure 8-6*** **A.** Coronal T₁WI in a patient with **glioblastoma of the pons,** shows a contrast enhancing necrotic tumor (arrowheads) after contrast administration. **B.** Follow-up CEMR, 3 weeks later, shows extension of the tumor into the subarachnoid space (arrowheads).

usual at diagnosis, but both may be seen in patients who have been treated with radiation. Hemorrhage seen on MR is not an uncommon finding with tumor progression (Fig. 8-4). With CT and MR, contrast enhancement is infrequent in malignant tumors at the time of diagnosis but occurs with increasing frequency with tumor progression (Fig. 8-5). Contrast enhancement is common on both CT and MR in low-grade pilocytic astrocytomas of the medulla and midbrain (Fig. 8-6).

Intrinsic pontine gliomas are diagnosed by imaging methods when the clinical findings are consistent and are not subjected to biopsy. Surgery is still performed when the tumor is largely exophytic, so that debulking and a histological diagnosis can be made; when the tumor is largely cystic, so that the cyst can be decompressed; and when the diagnosis of tumor is in doubt, so that therapy will not be instituted for a nonneoplastic disease process. Radiation is the only effective temporary therapy at present. Conventional doses up to 5400 cGy have been reported to result in a 5-year survival rate between 10 and 30 percent (Farwell 1977). Hyperfractionation radiotherapy with a twice-daily application of 100 cGy in doses of 6800 to 8200 cGy have led to some increase in survival, but the results so far are not encouraging (Packer 1987). The adjunctive use of chemotherapy has not resulted in improved survival. Follow-up studies of brainstem gliomas after hyperfractionation radiotherapy in some patients have indicated a significant reduction in tumor size (Fig. 8-1B). However, the course over the next 6 to 12 months is usually one of progressive growth and extension of the tumor from the pons through the cerebral peduncles into the cerebellum and from the pons superiorly and inferiorly into the adjacent brainstem structures (Smith 1990). These tumors are histologically malignant at this time and up to 20 percent of these diffuse pontine tumors disseminate into the subarachnoid and/or intraventricular space prior to death (Fig. 8-6).

Brainstem gliomas arising within the midbrain and medulla tend to have a more favorable prognosis than the diffuse pontine tumors. Midbrain tumors are found most often in the tectum where they produce obstructive hydrocephalus (Edwards 1994). MR with its multiplanar capability and increased signal intensity of the tumor on FLAIR, PDWI and $T_2$WI is ideal for demonstrating the mass within the midbrain (Figs. 8-7 and 8-8). On CT, the tumor may be difficult to see. The primary method of treatment is shunting for the hydrocephalus, and radiation and chemotherapy are reserved for tumors that are progressive clinically and by imaging.

Tumors of the medulla oblongata, in the lower brainstem, are particularly difficult to identify on CT because of artifacts, but are clearly shown on sagittal MR, especially with the use of PDWI, FLAIR, and $T_2$WI

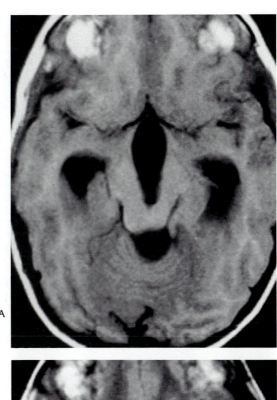

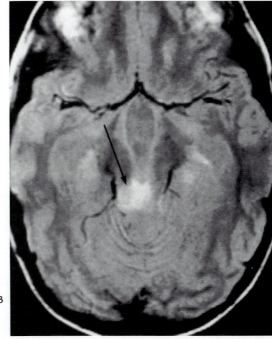

*Figure 8-7* **Tectal glioma. A.** Axial $T_1$WI shows obstructive hydrocephalus with expansion of the collicular plate. **B.** Axial PDWI shows increased signal intensity (arrow) at the site of the collicular mass.

images. They are often dorsally exophytic and contrast-enhanced (Figs. 8-9 and 8-10). The dorsally exophytic portion of the tumor can often be surgically excised, and radiation and chemotherapy can be used for residual tumor. Tumors in this location can be part of upper cervical cord astrocytomas, so that the cervical cord as well as the brainstem should be imaged.

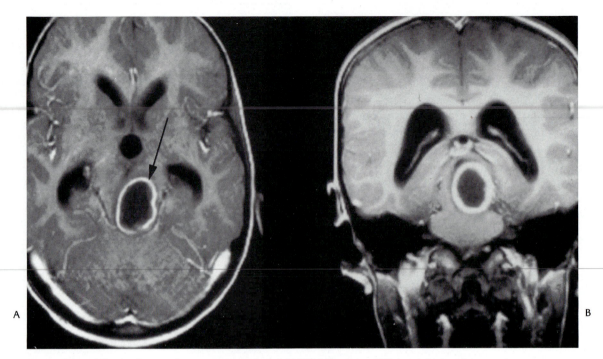

A

B

***Figure 8-8*** **Midbrain, low-grade astrocytoma. A.** Axial T$_1$WI following gadolinium injection shows a ring-enhancing mass (arrow) producing obstructive hydrocephalus. **B.** Coronal T$_1$WI following gadolinium injection shows the same finding.

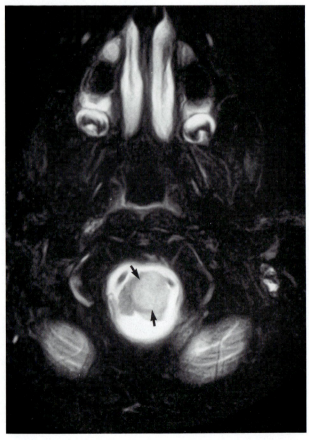

A

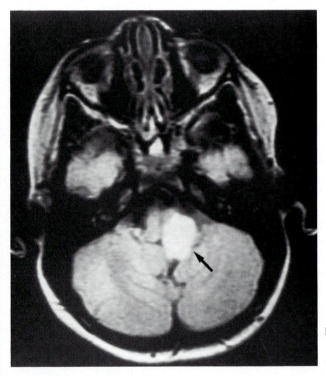

B

***Figure 8-9*** **A. Medullary glioma** is demonstrated as an area of increased signal intensity (arrows) within the medulla oblongata on T$_2$WI. **B.** Axial PDWI on another patient, shows a hyperintense, exophytic medullary mass (arrow).

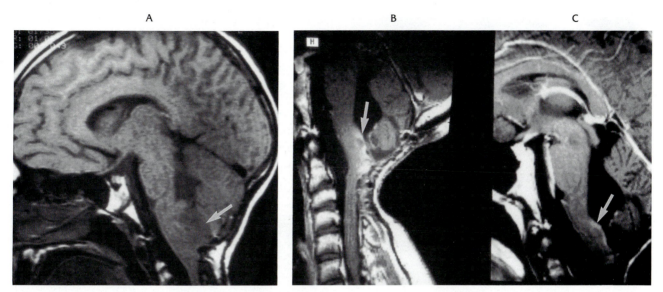

**Figure 8-10** **A.** Sagittal T$_1$WI, 5 years after surgical resection and radiation of a **medullary exophytic brainstem glioma,** shows **recurrent tumor** (arrow). **B.** Sagittal CEMR, 3 years later, shows residual, contrast-enhancing tumor (arrows) following re-resection after the study in **A. C.** Sagittal T$_1$WI 3 years after **B.** Residual contrast enhancing tumor is present (arrow), following multiple re-resections.

The main differential diagnosis of brainstem gliomas includes the occult vascular malformation, other causes of brainstem bleeding, and other causes of brainstem lesions that appear hypodense on CT and hyperintense on T$_2$-weighted MR images. Such hyperintense lesions on T$_2$-weighted MR include multiple sclerosis, acute disseminated encephalomyelitis (Fig. 8-11), dysmyelinating disease, and central pontine myelinolysis (Smith 1990). The occult vascular malformation may be of increased density on CT (Fig. 8-12), shows some contrast

enhancement, and on MR shows mixed signal intensity on both T$_1$WI and T$_2$WI (Savoiardo 1978; Gomori 1986). The presence of subacute blood products, including methemoglobin and hemosiderin, is suggestive (Figs. 8-13, 8-14). Arteriovenous malformations may appear to be quite similar. Acute disseminated encephalomyelitis arising after vaccination or a viral infection affects not only the brainstem but the white matter of the supratentorial space and cerebellum (Dunn 1986; Atlas 1986). The multiplicity of lesions

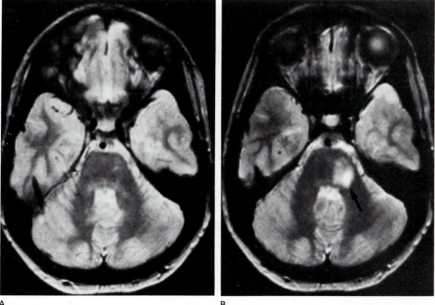

**Figure 8-11** **Acute multiple sclerosis** involving the pons. **A.** Axial PDWI shows no abnormality in the **pons. B.** Repeat axial PDWI 29 days after the first examination shows high-signal-intensity demyelination (arrow) within the left side of the pons.

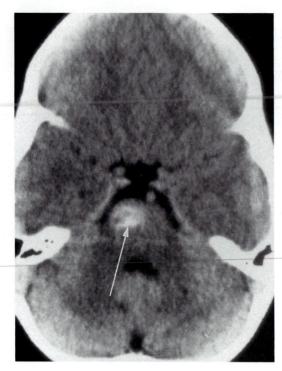

**Figure 8-12**  **Occult vascular malformation** is seen as a zone of increased density due to calcification (arrow).

after prior radiation therapy of a posterior fossa medulloblastoma or of Hodgkin's disease of the cervical region. The presentation in patients with cerebellar astrocytomas usually takes the form of signs of increased intracranial pressure (headache, nausea, vomiting), with the symptoms lasting weeks to years before diagnosis (Geissinger 1971). Cerebellar signs may or may not be evident at the time of diagnosis. Cerebellar astrocytomas tend to be large at diagnosis. Approxi-

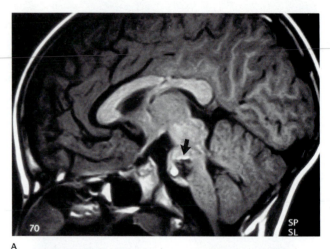

A

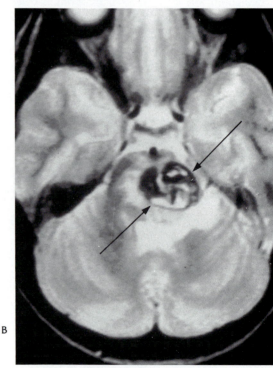

B

**Figure 8-13**  **Occult vascular malformations of the brainstem.** **A.** Sagittal $T_1$WI shows mixed signal intensity, both high and low signal (arrow) within the belly of the pons due to occult vascular malformation. **B.** Occult vascular malformation in pons. Axial $T_2$WI shows hypointense blood products (arrows) surrounded by hyperintense vasogenic edema.

and the relationship to the inciting event help in making the differential diagnosis. Dysmyelinating disease is characterized by its clinical onset, symmetry, and supratentorial components. Central pontine myelinolysis is unusual in infants and children and more common in adults and is associated with episodes of hyponatremia, such as those in ethanol abuse (Koch 1989).

## Cerebellar Astrocytoma

Cerebellar astrocytomas are one of the most common posterior fossa tumors of childhood, often listed as second to primitive neuroectodermal tumors (medulloblastoma) (Zimmerman 1992). Histologically, two types occur most frequently; juvenile pilocytic astrocytomas (75 to 85 percent) and more diffuse fibrillary astrocytomas (15 to 20 percent) (Russell 1989; Lee 1989; Steinberg 1985). A small percentage of cerebellar astrocytomas are malignant, either anaplastic astrocytomas or glioblastomas, and a still smaller percentage are oligodendrogliomas. Pilocytic astrocytomas are characterized by long-term survival of 90 percent or better, whereas fibrillary astrocytomas have a much less favorable outcome (Winston 1977; Auer 1981). Anaplastic astrocytomas and glioblastomas are usually fatal and in our experience often arise as a second primary tumor

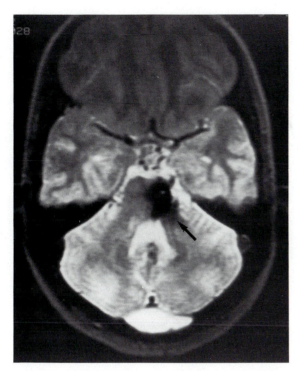

*Figure 8-14* **Occult vascular malformation** in the **pons.** Axial T₂WI shows hypointense hemosiderin (arrow) in the left side of the pons at the site of an old occult vascular malformation that had hemorrhaged 8 years before.

mately half of these tumors are solid masses (Fig. 8-15). In cystic tumors, the cyst walls are often made up of compressed nonneoplastic cerebellar tissue, with the tumor being a mural nodule (Fig. 8-16) (Gol 1959). However, some of these tumors are actually solid tumors that have undergone cystlike central necrosis, so that tumor surrounds the necrotic center. Tumors arise both in the vermis and in the cerebellar hemispheres (Lee 1989).

In most instances hydrocephalus is present at the time of diagnosis. On CT and MR, the lateral and third ventricles are markedly dilated and the fourth ventricle is displaced anteriorly by a vermian mass or contralaterally by a cerebellar hemispheric mass (Fig. 8-17). On CT, the tumor mass is lower in density than is the uninvolved cerebellar tissue (Fig. 8-15A) (Zimmerman 1978*a*). The solid portion of the tumor is usually slightly more dense than the cystic portion (Fig. 8-16). Fluid within the cyst is proteinaceous and usually is slightly denser than cerebrospinal fluid (CSF) (Zimmerman 1978*a*). Calcification is uncommon, between 13 and 20 percent (Gusnard 1990; Zimmerman 1978*a*). Contrast enhancement is common with both CT (Fig. 8-15B) and MR (Fig. 8-19B) (Gusnard 1990). Both the cystic and solid components appear hypointense on

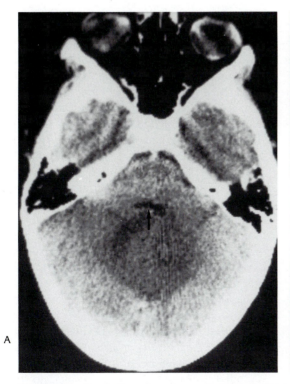
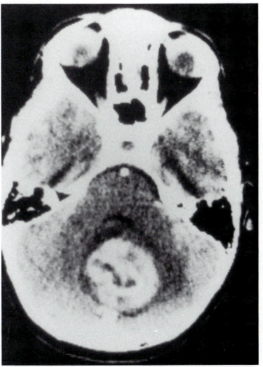

A                                                                    B

*Figure 8-15* **Cerebellar astrocytoma. A.** Axial NCCT injection shows a hypodense mass in the vermis, displacing the fourth ventricle (arrow) forward. **B.** Axial CECT shows enhancement of a cerebellar astrocytoma.

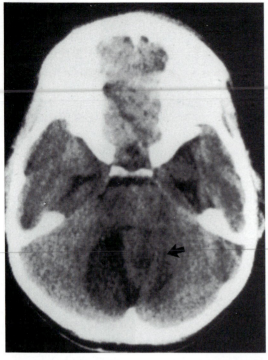

**Figure 8-16   Cystic cerebellar astrocytoma.** Axial NCCT shows a cystic mass in the cerebellar vermis, containing a denser mural nodule (arrow).

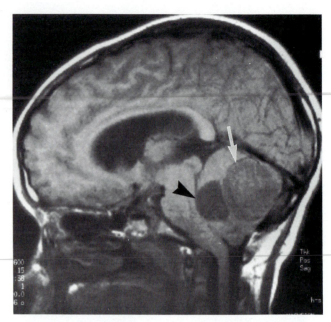

**Figure 8-18   Cerebellar astrocytoma with cysts.** Sagittal T₁WI shows hydrocephalus with dilatation of the lateral ventricles. The aqueduct of Sylvius is deformed by posterior fossa mass effect arising in the vermis, displacing and compressing the fourth ventricle forward. The mass consists of two components. A lower-signal-intensity fluid-filled space (arrowhead) is a cyst on the anterior margin of the solid (arrow) more intense tumor mass.

T₁WI (Figs. 8-18 and 8-19A) (Zimmerman 1992). Both components appear hyperintense on proton density weighted images (PDWI) and T₂WI (Figs. 8-17 and 8-20). Hemorrhage is uncommon in the solid portion of the tumor on MR, but the presence of hemosiderin within the cyst cavity wall, which is seen on long TR

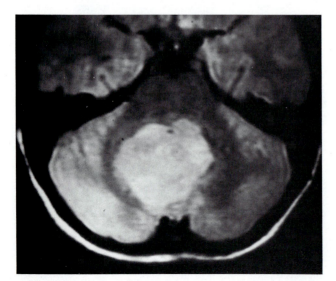

**Figure 8-17   Solid vermian astrocytoma.** Axial PDWI shows a high-signal-intensity vermian mass.

MR as a rim of hypointensity (Fig. 8-20), is not uncommon. This arises from repeated episodes of bleeding into the cystic cavity. Such episodes of bleeding contribute to the high protein content that frequently makes the cystic cavity higher in signal intensity on PDWI than is the solid tumor. While pilocytic astrocytomas show marked enhancement after MR contrast injection (Fig. 8-19), fibrillary astrocytomas may show none. Subarachnoid dissemination of primary cerebellar astrocytomas is uncommon but can be found late in the disease process.

In general, the long-term survival of patients with a cerebellar astrocytoma stems from the relatively benign nature of these tumors. Even patients with a tumor that is subtotally resected often have a survival measured in decades. This is true for pilocytic astrocytomas but not for the more aggressive fibrillary, anaplastic, and malignant ones. Successful treatment depends on surgical resection. If tumor is evident on follow-up examination after an initial surgery and resection is feasible, that is the subsequent therapeutic course. Radiation therapy has proved to be of little value in the management of benign cerebellar astrocytomas. Radiation therapy and chemotherapy have been utilized in treating malignant cerebellar astrocytomas, with results no better than those seen with brainstem gliomas. The differential diagnosis of a cerebellar astrocytoma in childhood in-

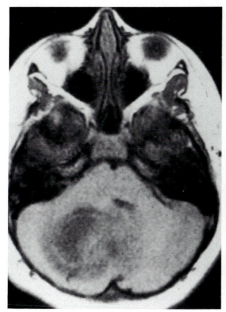
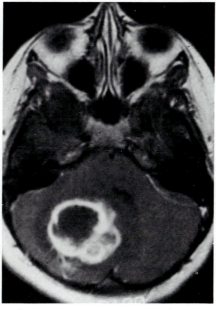

**Figure 8-19** **Cystic cerebellar astrocytoma.** **A.** Axial $T_1WI$ shows a hypointense mass in the right cerebellar hemisphere, displacing the fourth ventricle forward and to the left. **B.** Axial CEMR shows enhancement of the tumor in the wall of the cystic cerebellar astrocytoma.

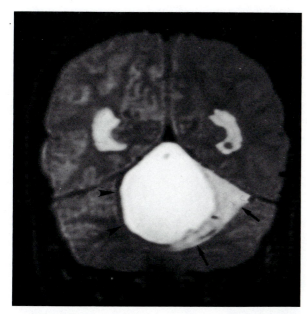

**Figure 8-20** **Cystic cerebellar astrocytoma.** Coronal $T_2WI$ shows a high-signal-intensity cyst cavity with a margin of low-signal-intensity hemosiderin (arrowheads) and a left lateral mass of astrocytoma (arrows) that is less intense than the cystic fluid.

cludes the occult vascular malformation, dysmyelinating disease, Lhermitte-Duclos disease (dysplastic gangliocytoma), and other dysplastic diseases of cerebellar tissue. Occult vascular malformations of the cerebellar hemisphere and vermis as well as arteriovenous malformations (AVMs) are diagnosed by the presence of

mixed blood products and, in the case of AVMs, by feeding arteries, the vascular nidus, and the draining veins. Dysmyelinating diseases such as Alexander's disease can affect the cerebellum and may be differentiated only on the basis of biopsy. Infectious diseases of the cerebellum such as abscesses can cause diagnostic problems. In the preantibiotic era, cerebellar abscesses were not uncommon, usually secondary to mastoiditis. Even in the antibiotic era, cerebellar abscesses occasionally present and require diagnostic consideration.

In general, the solid component that constitutes the wall of a cystic cerebellar astrocytoma is relatively hypodense, whereas the solid component that makes up the enhancing wall of a cerebellar abscess is often isodense to slightly hyperdense (Fig. 8-21) before the injection of iodinated contrast material (Zimmerman 1987b). On MR cerebellar abscesses are often slightly hyperintense on $T_1WI$, whereas cerebellar astrocytomas are usually hypointense (Gusnard 1990; Zimmerman 1987b; Zimmerman 1992). Both abscesses and cerebellar astrocytomas may produce surrounding vasogenic edema in the cerebellar white matter. Tuberculomas are more common in underdeveloped countries and can mimic cerebellar astrocytomas. Parasitic cysts within the fourth ventricle, such as those found with cysticercosis, can produce a mass with a parenchymal reactive change. Today in the United States, with AIDS as a problem, toxoplasmosis can also mimic a cerebellar astrocytoma. It is fortunate that opportunistic infections are relatively uncommon in children with AIDS (States 1996).

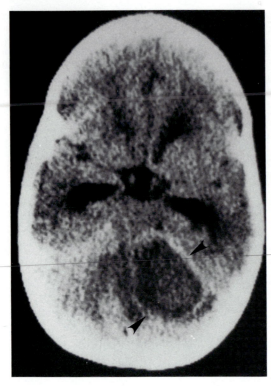

*Figure 8-21* **Cerebellar abscess.** Axial NCCT shows the high-density rim (arrowheads) of a left cerebellar abscess wall.

## Primitive Neuroectodermal Tumors (Medulloblastoma)

Depending on the series, medulloblastoma or cerebellar astrocytoma is the most common primary neoplasm of the pediatric posterior fossa (Zimmerman 1992).

Primitive neuroectodermal tumors of both the supratentorial and infratentorial spaces are the most common primary malignant CNS tumors in the pediatric population (Arseni 1982). Three of four patients with medulloblastoma present within the first decade (Farwell 1977; Chou 1983). These are rapidly growing tumors characterized by a short duration of symptoms, often on the order of weeks to months (Hoffman 1983). The signs are those of a posterior fossa mass, most often associated with obstructive hydrocephalus. Compression or occlusion of the fourth ventricle is responsible for the hydrocephalus. Histologically, these tumors are highly cellular, consisting of cells with scant cytoplasm and large nuclei, and frequently undergo mitosis (Russell 1989). These tumors tend to have a rich vascular supply. Tumors that occur in patients under 3 years of age, those that tend to disseminate early, those that are so large or difficult in location that they are not candidates for gross total resection, and those that show features of histological differentiation along more mature cell lines have a significantly worse prognosis (Rorke 1983; Packer 1985-1986).

On CT and MR, the common findings are a posterior fossa mass, arising in the vermis or cerebellar hemispheres, that compresses and obstructs the fourth ventricle, producing enlargement of the third and lateral ventricles (hydrocephalus) (Figs. 8-22, 8-23) (Gusnard 1990; Zimmerman 1978*b*). On CT, the mass is usually isodense to hyperdense before contrast injection (Fig. 8-23A) (Zimmerman 1978*b*). The mass is most often solid, relatively homogenous, and diffusely enhancing (Fig. 8-23B) (Ramondi 1979). Occasionally small cystic or necrotic areas and even larger ones may be present. Calcification is uncommon, on the order of 10 to 15

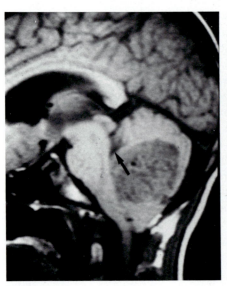

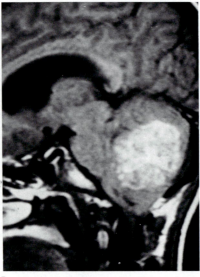

*Figure 8-22* **Primitive neuroectodermal tumor (medulloblastoma type). A.** Sagittal T₁WI, NCMR, shows a slightly hypointense mass within the vermis, compressing the brainstem and fourth ventricle (arrow) and producing hydrocephalus. **B.** Sagittal CEMR shows enhancement of the tumor.

A                                    B

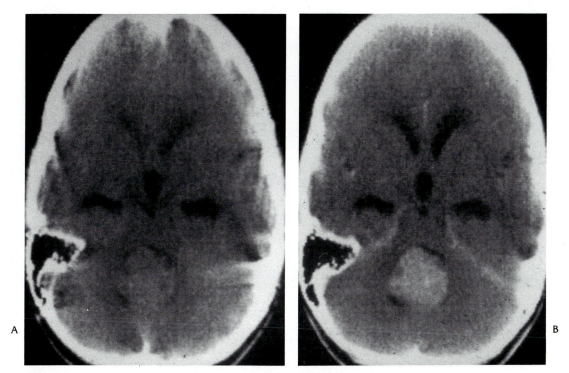

***Figure 8-23*** **Primitive neuroectodermal tumor (medulloblastoma type). A.** Axial NCCT shows an isodense to slightly hyperdense mass in the vermis, filling the fourth ventricle. There is early hydrocephalus with dilatation of the temporal horns and third ventricle. **B.** Axial CECT shows homogeneous enhancement of the mass.

percent (Gusnard 1990; Ramondi 1979). On MR, the mass is hypointense on $T_1WI$ (Fig. 8-22A), often slightly hyperintense on proton density weighted images (PDWI), and most often hypointense to isointense on $T_2WI$ (Fig. 8-24A) (Gusnard 1990); (Zimmerman 1992). This is different from a cerebellar astrocytoma,

which is high in signal intensity on $T_2WI$ (Fig. 8-19). The etiology of the hypointensity to isointensity on $T_2WI$ is most likely the highly cellular nature of the tumor and its relatively low interstitial water content. After contrast injection, enhancement occurs on both CT and MR (Figs. 8-22B and 8-24B,C,F).

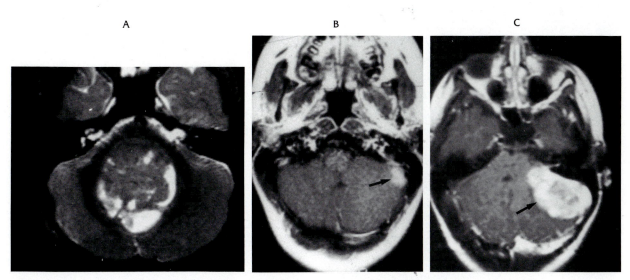

***Figure 8-24*** **Primitive neuroectodermal tumor (medulloblastoma type). A.** Axial $T_2WI$ shows the tumor to be relatively hypointense, having a few high-signal-intensity areas of necrosis both within the tumor and at its margins. **B,C.** CEMR in patient with 6 weeks between studies, showing rapid growth of the tumor (arrow), without treatment. *(Continued on next page.)*

D    E    F

**Figure 8-24 (Continued)**   **D,E,F.** Same patient. **D.** Axial FLAIR shows hydrocephalus with dilatation of the temporal horns and high signal intensity at the site of edema anterior and medial to the right cerebellar hemispheric mass (arrows). Note that the mass is isointense to gray matter. There is edema in the frontal lobes around the inferior aspects of the frontal horns, from reabsorption of CSF. **E.** Axial FLAIR image at the level of the lateral ventricles shows the increased signal intensity surrounding the ventricles from reabsorption of CSF from the obstructive hydrocephalus. **F.** CEMR, axial, shows enhancement of the solid portion of the tumor (arrows).

Fluid attenuated inversion recovery (FLAIR) shows increased signal intensity where there is increased water in tissue, such as at the margins of the lateral ventricles when they are obstructed and there is CSF reabsorption. With primitive neuroectodermal tumor of the cerebellum, on FLAIR imaging, the tumor is isointense to gray matter (Fig. 8-24D) and consequently may be difficult to identify other than by mass effect. Astrocytomas and other glial tumors of the cerebellum show usually high signal intensity on FLAIR images. Subarachnoid dissemination of tumor has been reported at the time of diagnosis (Heideman 1989). This may occur both intracranially (Fig. 8-25) and intraspinally.

Treatment of medulloblastoma is performed with gross total resection (Ramondi 1979) with radiation therapy to the craniospinal axis (Heideman 1989). Adjunctive chemotherapy has been shown to improve survival (Pendergrass 1987). Before gross total resection gadolineum-enhanced MRI of the entire spinal canal is carried out to rule in or out subarachnoid drop metastases. The tumor may be found adherent to the pial surface of the cord, the arachnoid lining the thecal sac, or the nerve roots (Fig. 8-26B) (Kramer 1991). Nonenhanced MR has been unsatisfactory in the evaluation of subarachnoid dissemination.

## Ependymomas

Over two-thirds of ependymomas are infratentorial in location, occurring predominantly in children usually less

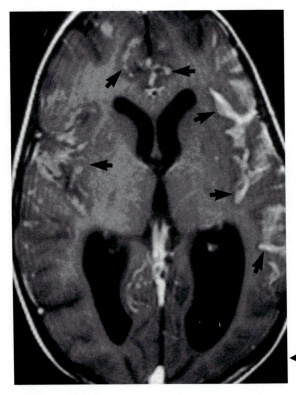

**Figure 8-25   Subarachnoid dissemination of medulloblastoma.** CEMR shows extensive contrast enhancing tumor (arrows) within the subarachnoid space.

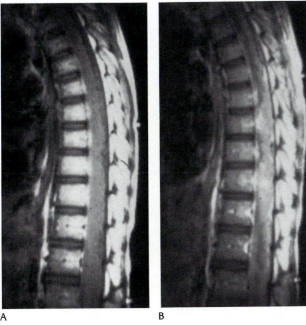

A    B

***Figure 8-26*** **Spinal subarachnoid dissemination of a primitive neuroectodermal tumor (medulloblastoma type). A.** Axial T₁WI before contrast injection shows loss of subarachnoid space in the thoracic spinal canal. **B.** Sagittal CEMR shows an enhanced tumor coating the surface of the thoracic cord.

than 5 years of age, with a later but smaller peak in the third decade in adults (Kun 1988; Swartz 1982). Supratentorial and infratentorial ependymomas constitute under 10 percent of all primary CNS tumors of childhood. In the posterior fossa, ependymomas arise from the ependymal lining of the fourth ventricle or along the course of the tela choroidea, which extends through the lateral recesses of the fourth ventricle into the cerebellopontine angle cisterns (Russell 1989). In the supratentorial space, ependymomas arise both intraventricularly and from ependymal rests in the white matter (Russell 1989).

Ependymomas are classified as benign or malignant (Rorke 1987). Ependymoblastoma has been recategorized as one form of primitive neuroectodermal tumor (Rorke 1985). The tumor tends to expand within the fourth ventricle (Fig. 8-27A), extending in a plasticlike fashion through the lateral recesses (Fig. 8-27B,C and 8-28) and through the foramen of Magendie into the adjacent cisterns. The tumor tends to wrap around the blood vessels (Fig. 8-27B) and cranial nerves, making total surgical resection difficult. Hypervascularity, evidence of previous hemorrhage, and calcification are common features of ependymomas (Russell 1989). In general, histological features, benign versus more malignant, have not been major factors in survival (Liu 1976). Survival has been equally dismal in patients with both the benign and malignant forms. Despite treatment, both types have tended to recur locally and to disseminate with time.

Ependymomas are most often isointense on plain CT and frequently, but not always, show contrast enhancement (Fig. 8-29) (Swartz 1982; Tortori-Donati 1995). Calcification in the form of small round flecks occurs in approximately 50 percent of these patients (Fig. 8-30), making this one of the most common pos-

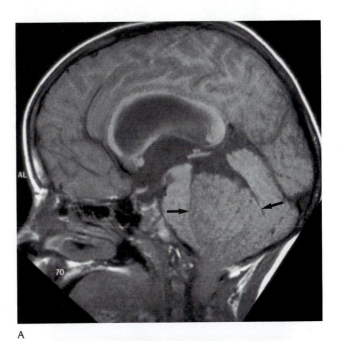

A

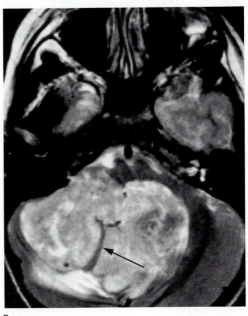

B

***Figure 8-27*** **Ependymoma. A.** Sagittal T₁WI shows an intra-fourth ventricular mass (arrows). The mass extends inferiorly into the upper cervical canal. Hydrocephalus is present with dilatation of the lateral and third ventricles, cerebral aqueduct, and proximal fourth ventricle. The mass is isointense. **B.** Axial T₂WI shows a mass of mixed signal intensity, extending from the fourth ventricle through a markedly dilated lateral recess of the lateral ventricle into the cerebellopontine angle. There is a large vessel, seen as a hypointense flow void (arrow). *(Continued on next page.)*

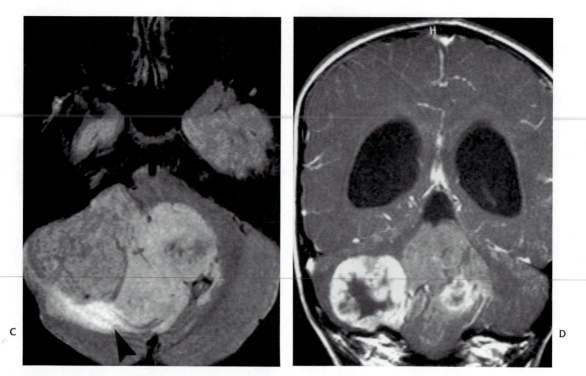

**Figure 8-27 (Continued)  C.** Axial FLAIR image shows the mass to be slightly more intense than the surrounding normal brain. There is edema (arrowhead) in the cerebellum along the posterior margin, which is even brighter in signal intensity. **D.** Coronal CEMR shows irregular enhancement of a portion of the cerebellopontine angle tumor, enhancing more than the central, where there is a more variable degree of enhancement.

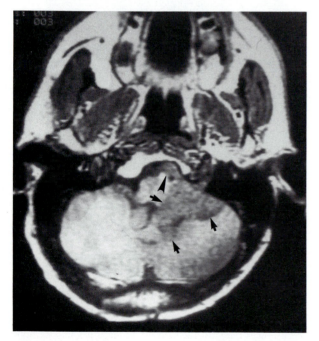

**Figure 8-28    Ependymoma.** Axial T$_1$WI shows a hypointense mass (arrows) in the lateral recess of the fourth ventricle extending anterior to the medulla (arrowhead).

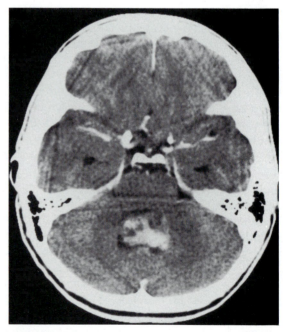

**Figure 8-29    Ependymoma.** Axial CECT shows an intra-fourth-ventricular enhanced tumor.

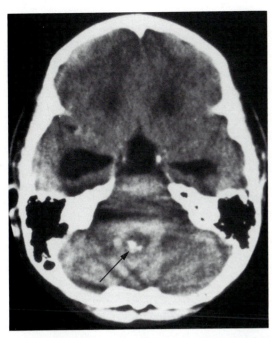

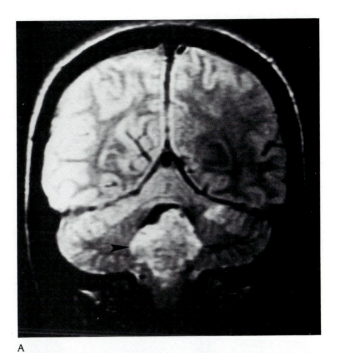

A

**Figure 8-30  Ependymoma.** Axial NCCT shows focal calcification (arrow) in an ill-defined mass in the region of the fourth ventricle. Note that there is marked dilatation of the third ventricle and temporal horns, consistent with hydrocephalus.

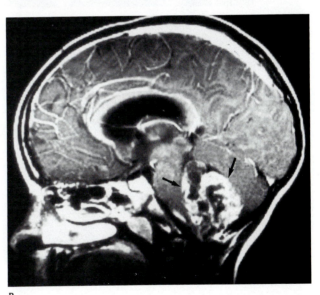

B

**Figure 8-31  A. Ependymoma.** Coronal PDWI shows a hyperintensity mass (arrowheads) filling the fourth ventricle. **B.** Sagittal CEMR shows a irregular enhancing mass (arrows) within the fourth ventricle.

terior fossa tumors to show calcium deposits (Swartz 1982; Tortori-Donati 1995). The incidence of calcification is similar in the supratentorial ependymoma. On MR, the tumor is usually low in signal intensity on $T_1WI$ (Figs. 8-27 and 8-28) and high in signal intensity on $T_2WI$ but often has mixed interspersed signals because of prior hemorrhage, calcification, or tumor blood vessels (Fig. 8-31A) (Gusnard 1990; Zimmerman 1992; Spoto 1992). On CEMR $T_1WI$ following IV gadolinium injection, irregular enhancement is usually seen (Figs. 8-27D, 8-31B). Even with contrast-enhanced MR, the tumor may not enhance in a small percentage of patients. Not infrequently, small seedings of the tumor to the ventricular ependyma, subarachnoid space, or spinal canal do not show contrast enhancement until the tumor reaches a certain degree of enlargement. Thus, recognition of the dissemination of an ependymoma may be difficult in the early stages. Ependymomas are one type of tumor in which water-soluble myelography may remain an important adjunct in staging tumor dissemination.

In general, most patients with posterior fossa ependymomas are young and develop signs and symptoms of increased intracranial pressure due to hydrocephalus from obstruction of the CSF outlets, with the onset of symptoms occurring over a variable period of time (Coulon 1977). Invasion of the cerebellum may lead to cerebellar signs, while cranial nerve palsies may be due to tumor encasing the nerves (Heideman 1989).

The treatment of a posterior fossa ependymoma consists of gross total resection and radiation therapy either by local portals or, if there is a question of dissemination, to the craniospinal axis by craniospinal irradiation. Adjunctive chemotherapy has been used without great success (Heideman 1989). With recurrent ependymoma, (Fig. 8-32) chemotherapy is a mainstay but does not appear to alter the ultimate course. Both benign and malignant ependymomas tend to evolve over several years, with local recurrence followed by dissemination.

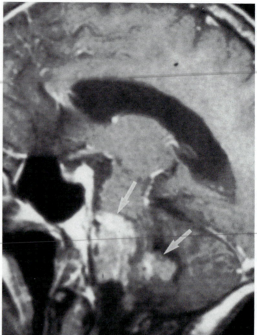

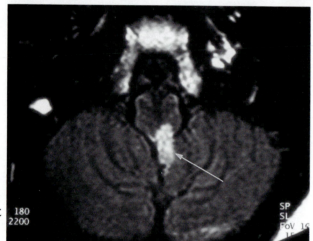

*Figure 8-32* **Recurrent ependymoma. A.** Sagittal T₁WI without contrast. **B.** Sagittal T₁WI with gadolinium. Both show a large cerebellopontine angle and intra-fourth ventricular mass that contrast enhances (arrows). **C.** Residual recurrent ependymoma at the site of prior resection is seen as a zone of increased signal intensity (arrow) on axial FLAIR images.

# Choroid Plexus Papilloma and Carcinoma

Tumors of the choroid plexus represent less than 1 percent of all intracranial tumors, but when they occur, they are found in childhood (Zimmerman 1979c). Most occur within the first decade of life, primarily within the first 2 years (Laurence 1979). The lateral and third ventricles are affected more frequently in those under age 2, while the fourth ventricle is more often affected in adolescents (Laurence 1979). Choroid plexus carcinomas are even less common and are found in infancy (Zimmerman 1979b). Invasion of adjacent neural tissue and loss of the papillary architecture of the tumor are two signs of malignancy. Both choroid plexus papilloma and carcinoma may seed the subarachnoid space and ventricles. Seeding is more common and occurs earlier with carcinoma.

Papillomas appear as reddish cauliflowerlike masses that expand the ventricle within which they grow (Russell 1989). The production of CSF by the tumor can produce a generalized hydrocephalus when CSF production exceeds the reabsorptive capacity of the arachnoid villi (Milhorat 1976). Hydrocephalus can also result from obstruction of the outlets of the fourth ventricle by tumor or occur when a subarachnoid hemorrhage produces adhesions and scarring that prevent CSF flow.

The CT appearance of a choroid plexus papilloma is that of a radiographically dense, often calcified frond-like mass arising at the site of the choroid within the

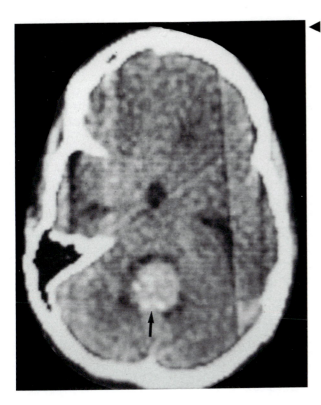

*Figure 8-33* **Choroid plexus carcinoma.** Axial CECT shows increased density within an ill-defined, irregular mass (arrowheads) in the vicinity of the fourth ventricle. There is marked hydrocephalus with dilatation of the lateral ventricles, the third ventricle, and the temporal horns of the lateral ventricles.

fourth ventricle and sometimes extending through the lateral recess into the cerebellopontine angle (Zimmerman 1979c; Coates 1989). Some tumors arise purely within the cerebellopontine angle. The fourth ventricle is expanded, the aqueduct, third ventricle, and lateral ventricles are dilated. After contrast injection, the tumor enhances markedly, usually homogeneously. Vertebral angiography shows dilatation of the posterior inferior cerebellar arteries and their choroidal branches. Dense tumor stain begins in the arterial phase and lasts into the venous phase. Choroid plexus carcinomas show a contrast-enhancing mass that extends into the cerebellum, the brainstem, or the walls of the fourth ventricle (Fig. 8-33). On MR, a choroid plexus papilloma appears as an isointense to hypointense frondlike mass (Fig. 8-34A) on $T_1WI$. On PDWI and $T_2WI$, the tumor tends to be variably hyper- to hypointense to CSF

*Figure 8-34* **Choroid plexus papillomas. A.** Sagittal $T_1WI$ without contrast shows an intra-fourth ventricular mass (arrows). **B.** Coronal $T_2WI$ shows a mass of mixed signal intensity (arrows) expanding the fourth ventricle. **C.** Axial CEMR shows an intra-fourth ventricular mass (arrows) to enhance homogeneously.

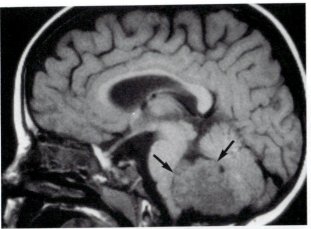

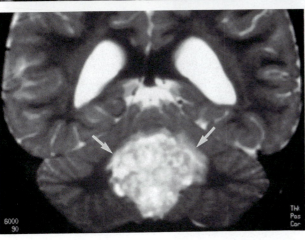

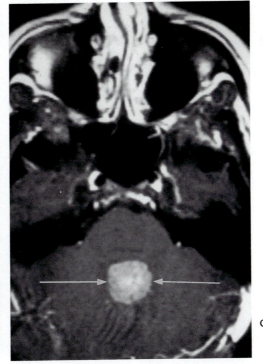

(Fig. 8-34B) (Tien 1991). This most likely reflects both calcification and rich blood flow within the tumor mass. After MR contrast injection, the tumor enhances intensely (Fig. 8-34C). Contrast enhancement is an ideal method of demonstrating cerebellar and brain-stem invasion as well as spread of a carcinoma to distal sites.

Treatment consists of gross total resection of the papilloma or carcinoma (Heideman 1989). A papilloma is often totally resectable, whereas a carcinoma, because of invasion, is not. A postoperative papilloma patient is reexamined by CT or MR to determine whether residual disease is present. Residual disease, if symptomatic, may require reoperation at a future date. Choroid plexus carcinomas are rarely cured by means of surgical resection. Postoperatively, radiation therapy and chemotherapy are utilized. The treatment of choroid plexus carcinomas is complicated by the often young age of the patients, immature myelination, and dangers entailed when radiation is given to an immature brain. Long-term survival of patients with choroid plexus papillomas is excellent, whereas even short-term survival of patients with choroid plexus carcinomas is limited (Heideman 1989).

## Other Posterior Fossa Tumors of Childhood

Congenital inclusion masses such as lipomas, dermoids, and teratomas may be found in the posterior fossa (Zimmerman 1979b). Dermoids may be associ-

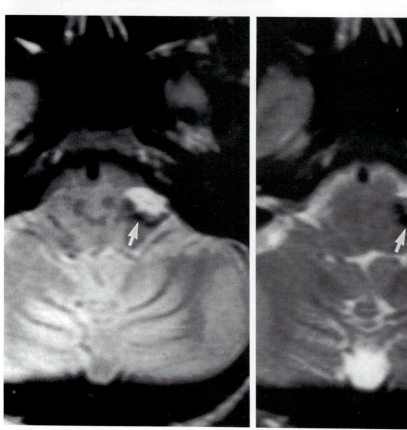

**Figure 8-35 Lipomas, cerebellopontine angle. A.** Axial CECT shows a hypodense, right-sided, cerebellopontine angle mass (arrow). Note that the contrast-enhanced vessel passes through it as does the cranial nerve, going to the internal auditory canal. **B,C.** PDWI and T$_2$WI of a left cerebellopontine angle lipoma. Note the chemical shift artifact (arrow) along the posterior aspect of the lipoma.

ated with a sinus track that leads through the calvarium, in the midline, from an orifice in the skin. As a result, infection of an intracranial dermoid with abscess formation is possible. Lipomas in the vicinity of the tectum of the midbrain are an incidental finding (Zimmerman 1979*b*). Lipomas involving the pars acoustica are less frequent but, with stretching of the seventh and eighth nerves, may become symptomatic (Fig. 8-35).

Acoustic neurinomas are found in childhood, almost exclusively in the circumstance of a patient with neurofibromatosis type 2 (Zimmerman 1990*c*; Aoki 1989; Braffman 1994). In these circumstances, the acoustic neurinomas will eventually be bilateral. Their synchrony, the rate at which they grow, and therefore the ease with which the first entity and then the second is recognized, is variable. CT with contrast enhancement and bone windows is less effective, whereas MR with contrast is the best diagnostic method for demonstrating findings consistent with a bilateral acoustic neurinoma (Fig. 8-36). In addition, neurinomas of other cranial nerves, meningiomas, and spinal cord ependymomas may be demonstrated in these patients (Zimmerman 1990*c*; Aoki, 1989).

In childhood, tumors that involve the bony wall of the posterior cranial fossa are most often metastatic, either neuroblastomas (Fig. 8-37) (Zimmerman 1980*a*) or Ewing's sarcomas. Rare primary bone tumors, such as angiosarcomas and osteogenic sarcomas, may present as posterior fossa cranial masses. Tumors of the bony vault are best evaluated on CT with or without contrast, utilizing soft tissue and bone windows. MR is complementary and adds the ability to evaluate blood flow in the dural venous sinuses. Compromise of the dural venous sinuses by calvarial vault tumor masses can produce venous hypertension, increased intracranial pressure, and papilledema (Zimmerman 1980*a*). Eosinophilic granuloma is an inflammatory osseous vault mass lesion that can produce a tumorlike mass effect. This is usually recognized because of beveled edges at the site of involvement of the cranial vault and intense homogeneous enhancement. Rhabdomyosarcomas of the ear produce destruction of the temporal bone and invasion of the posterior cranial fossa (Zimmerman 1978*c*).

## SUPRATENTORIAL TUMORS

The classic concept that most pediatric brain tumors are infratentorial in location was changed first by CT and then by MR. MR, with its ability to detect small low-grade astrocytomas and gangliogliomas because of their increased water content, has made it possible to detect tumors earlier and altered the ratio of supratentorial to infratentorial tumors. Today, more than 50 percent of pediatric brain tumors are found in the supratentorial space (Zimmerman 1990*b*).

Once a mass has been identified, the differential diagnosis depends primarily on its anatomic localization.

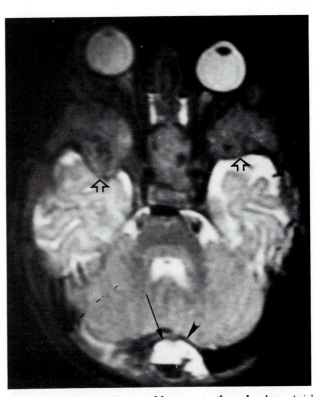

***Figure 8-37*  Metastatic neuroblastoma to the calvarium.** Axial T$_2$WI shows a mixed-signal-intensity mass (arrow) in the vicinity of the torcular herophili (arrowhead), consistent with hemorrhagic neuroblastoma. The torcula and left transverse sinus are compressed by the mass. The walls of both orbits (open arrows) are markedly expanded by the tumor.

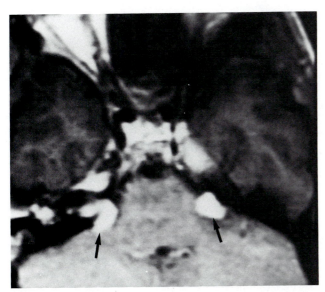

***Figure 8-36*  Neurofibromatosis type 2 with bilateral acoustic neurinomas.** Axial CEMR shows bilateral enhanced (arrows) acoustic neurinomas.

In the pediatric supratentorial space, tumors have been categorized as those that are intrasellar and/or suprasellar, those that arise within the parenchyma of the cerebral hemisphere or basal ganglia, those that are intraventricular, those that arise in the region of the pineal gland, and those that arise superficially from the meninges, pia, or cortex.

## Intrasellar and Suprasellar Tumors

Neoplasms in and around the sella are more common in adults than in children because of the increasing frequency of pituitary adenomas, metastases, and meningiomas with age. Neoplasms and other masses with a predilection for the pediatric population include craniopharyngioma and visual pathway glioma-hypothalamic astrocytoma. Less frequently neurinoma, arachnoid cyst, germinoma, epidermoid, Rathke's cleft cyst, hamartoma, teratoma, histiocytosis, and basilar meningitis produce an intrasellar, suprasellar, or parasellar mass (Zimmerman 1990a,b).

### CRANIOPHARYNGIOMA

Two-thirds of all craniopharyngiomas present before the age of 20. Overall, craniopharyngiomas constitute 6 to 9 percent of all primary CNS tumors (Farwell 1977; Cohen 1983). Craniopharyngiomas arise from epithelial cell rests along the involuted pathway of the hypophysis—Rathke's duct (Russell 1989). These tumors, while smooth, may be solid, cystic, or mixed. The content of the cysts varies from a cholesterol-rich fluid to a gelatinous mass (Russell 1989). Calcification is common within the solid portion. Most craniopharyngiomas are suprasellar and attach to the hypothalamus; a smaller proportion project into the sella turcica from the hypothalamus; and a very small proportion are purely intrasellar in location (Carmel 1982).

The visual field abnormalities are due to compression of the optic chiasm and tract, and the endocrinological disturbances (hypogonadism) are due to involvement of the hypothalamus and infundibular stalk (Thomsett 1980). The growth of the mass is slow, and the symptoms are insidious in their onset.

Plain skull radiographs may show suprasellar calcification, expansion of the sella, and/or erosion of the dorsum sellae. Such findings in a child are highly suggestive of a craniopharyngioma. On CT, the mass is usually less dense than the adjacent brain but of greater density than CSF (Fig. 8-38) (Rao 1977). Calcification occurs frequently in the wall or solid portion (Fig. 8-39). After contrast injection, there is enhancement of the cyst wall and solid portion (Fig. 8-38) (Rao 1977). The cystic component does not enhance. A tumor may be lobulated and may even extend through adjacent CSF spaces such as under the frontal lobe, up against the temporal lobe, down along the clivus, or even into the cerebello-

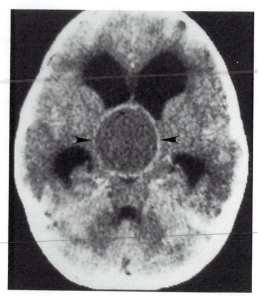

**Figure 8-38  Craniopharyngioma.** Axial CE CT shows a cystic mass with a contrast-enhanced thin wall (arrowheads) and a hypodense cavity that is denser than CSF. There is hydrocephalus with dilatation of the frontal and temporal horns in the lateral ventricle.

pontine angle cistern. Coronal CT sections often complement the axial study. Infrequently, the craniopharyngioma may be hyperdense on NC CT and may be solid. On MR with $T_1WI$, the cystic contents are of variable signal intensity, most often hypointense but occasionally hyperintense (Fig. 8-40) (Young 1987). On PDWI and $T_2WI$, the cystic contents may be slightly to markedly hyperintense (Fig. 8-41) (Pusey 1987). On CEMR, the solid portion and the wall enhance (Figs. 8-42, 8-43) (Zimmerman 1990a). Sagittal and coronal MR studies with thin sections give an anatomic depiction of the re-

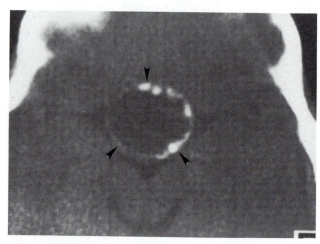

**Figure 8-39  Craniopharyngioma.** Axial NCCT shows the partially calcified wall (arrowheads) of a cystic suprasellar mass, consistent with craniopharyngioma.

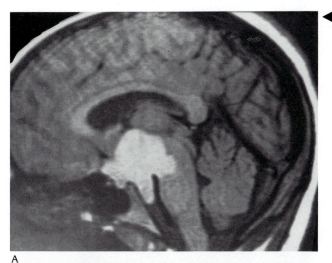

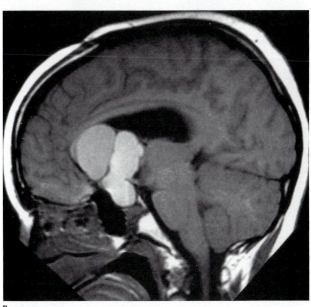

◀*Figure 8-40*  **Craniopharyngioma. A.** Sagittal T₁WI shows an intrasellar, suprasellar, and retrosellar high-signal-intensity mass compressing the midbrain and hypothalamus. **B.** Sagittal T₁WI shows recurrent craniopharyngioma involving the sella and suprasellar space. Note that there are two compartments, one is more hyperintense than the other.

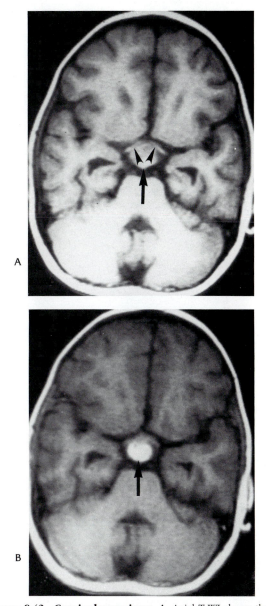

*Figure 8-42*  **Craniopharyngioma. A.** Axial T₁WI shows the optic chiasm pushed forward (arrowheads) by an isointense retrochiasmal mass (arrow). **B.** Axial CEMR shows enhancement of the mass (arrow).

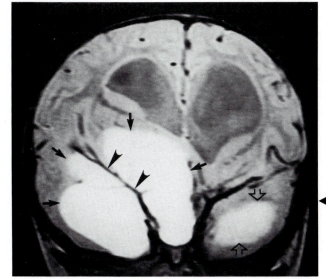

◀*Figure 8-41*  **Craniopharyngioma.** Coronal PDWI shows a mass of high-signal-intensity (arrows) encasing the distal internal carotid and middle cerebral arteries (arrowheads) on the right, involving the sella and the suprasellar and parasellar regions and producing hydrocephalus with marked dilatation of both frontal horns of the lateral ventricles. Tumor (open arrows) is present in the left temporal horn of the lateral ventricle.

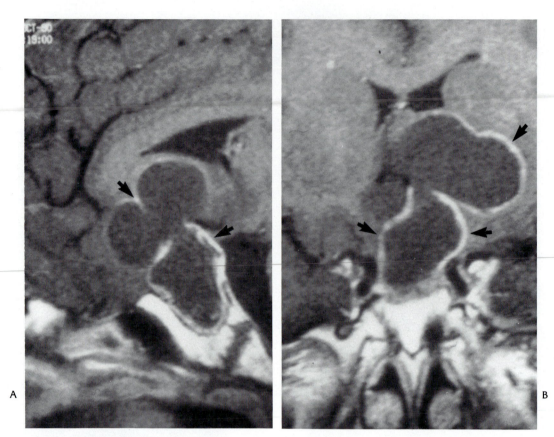

*Figure 8-43*   **Craniopharyngioma. A,B.** Sagittal and coronal CEMR with marginal, ringlike enhancement of the craniopharyngioma wall (arrows).

lationship between the craniopharyngioma and the optic chiasm, optic tracks, and pituitary gland. Differentiation from other suprasellar masses is usually not difficult, except in rare hypothalamic astrocytomas that contain significant calcification or are located inferiorly with exophytic cyst formation. Differentiation is also difficult when one is attempting to distinguish a purely intrasellar craniopharyngioma from an intrasellar Rathke's cleft cyst.

## RATHKE'S CLEFT CYST

Epithelial rests from remnants of Rathke's cleft may persist and form cysts between the anterior and intermediate pituitary lobes. Goblet cells line Rathke's cleft and secrete a mucinous or serous fluid (Fairburn 1964). Often these cysts are found incidentally, but occasionally they are associated with pituitary dysfunction.

The CT appearance of a Rathke's cleft cyst is that of a low-density mass, usually intrasellar, in or near the pars intermedia. It is not calcified and does not enhance. Surrounding normal pituitary tissue does enhance. The MR findings in a Rathke's cleft cyst usually consist of increased signal intensity on $T_1WI$ and $T_2WI$ (Fig. 8-44) (Zimmerman 1990a; Kucharczyk 1987). This is thought

to be related to the high protein and/or starch contents of the mucoid material. They may be hypointense on $T_1WI$. The main differential diagnosis is between Rathke's cleft cyst and craniopharyngioma (Ross 1992).

## VISUAL PATHWAY AND HYPOTHALAMIC ASTROCYTOMA

Visual pathway gliomas (VPGs) include gliomas found within the optic nerves, chiasm, and optic tracts. Together these tumors constitute 5 percent of all primary CNS tumors of childhood (Oxenhandler 1978). They tend to present in the first decade of life. It has been reported that 6 to 45 percent of patients with VPGs have neurofibromatosis type 1 (NF 1) (Hope 1981). The exact incidence and interrelationship between VPG and neurofibromatosis are uncertain, since a VPG may present years before the clinical stigmata of NF 1 are present (Packer 1988).

Histologically, these tumors are either pilocytic astrocytomas or fibrillary astrocytomas (Braffman 1990). In our experience, more are pilocytic, and these tend to be the ones that involve more of the extent of the visual pathway. Thus far, despite the use of CT and MR,

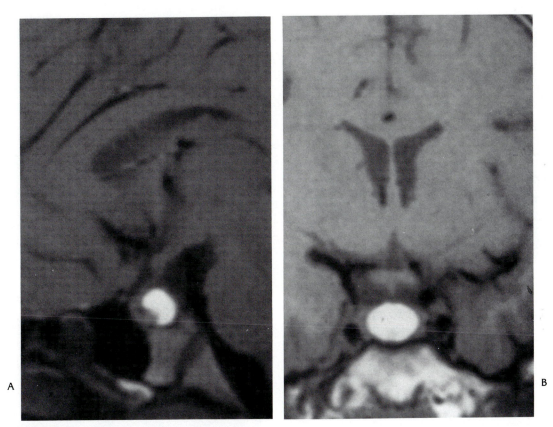

*Figure 8-44* **Cyst of Rathke's pouch. A.** Sagittal $T_1WI$ shows a hyperintense intrasellar mass. **B.** Coronal $T_1WI$ of the same hyperintense mass.

we have not demonstrated that the tumors grow by further extension along the visual pathway; rather, they expand areas that are involved as the tumors slowly grow. Tumor growth is slow, with survival often exceeding decades (Packer 1983*b*).

The signs and symptoms of VPGs relate to the location of the tumor and the age at presentation (Heideman 1989). Developmental difficulties, strabismus and/or nystagmus, and signs of hydrocephalus are the modes of presentation in infants and young children. In older children, proptosis and reduced visual acuity as well as growth disturbances, along with signs of hydrocephalus, are the forms of presentation (Packer 1983*b*).

When only the optic nerve is involved, a differential diagnosis is necessary. In older children, adolescents, and young adults, the differential diagnosis includes perioptic meningioma. Differentiation with MR may be difficult because both optic nerve gliomas and perioptic meningiomas can produce peripheral signal-intensity changes and contrast enhancement around the optic nerve. Calcification is more common in meningiomas, which tend to extend out onto the dural surface surrounding the intracranial portion of the optic nerve canal. When both optic nerves, the optic nerve and chiasm, or the chiasm

and optic tracts are involved, the tumor differential is limited to the VPG. The nontumor portion of the differential diagnosis at that point also includes inflammatory conditions that expand the visual pathway, such as demyelinating disease, and diseases that encase the surface of the visual pathway, such as sarcoid, meningitis, arachnoiditis, and an occasional rare vascular malformation (Armington 1990). In a patient with NF 1, other stigmata of this condition must be looked for, including high-signal-intensity lesions in the globus pallidus, thalamus, brainstem, and cerebellum (Braffman 1990). Brainstem gliomas, cerebellar astrocytomas, and other glial neoplasms also may be present. Neurinomas of the cranial nerves, spinal neurofibromas, and bony dysplasia involving the walls of the orbit, the internal auditory canals, or the spinal canal may be present.

On CT, a VPG appears as an expansile mass involving the optic nerve, chiasm, and tract and/or a mass that infiltrates and expands the hypothalamus (Fig. 8-45) (Zimmerman 1990*a*). They are isodense to hypodense before contrast and usually show enhancement (Fig. 8-45) (Fletcher 1986). The optic nerve may be fusiformly dilated with peripheral enhancement (Fig. 8-46). On MR these tumors are hypointense on $T_1WI$

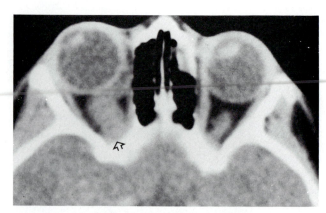

**Figure 8-46  Unilateral optic glioma.** Axial CECT shows marked enhancement of the enlarged right optic nerve (open arrow).

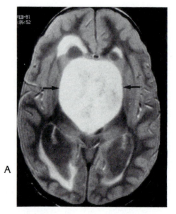

**Figure 8-45  Visual pathway glioma** with hypothalamic involvement. Axial CECT shows a large suprasellar mass contrast-enhancing with posterolateral arachnoid cysts (arrows). Previous surgical changes are present in the left temporal region.

(Fig. 8-47) and hyperintense on PDW and T$_2$WI (Fig. 8-48) (Zimmerman 1987a). Enhancement characteristics are quite variable on CEMR: Some tumors do not enhance, some show peripheral enhancement, and others enhance throughout (Fig. 8-49A), (Zimmerman 1990a). The increased signal intensity of the tumor on PDWI and T$_2$WI identifies the tumor extension posterior to the chiasm along the optic tracts to the genicu-

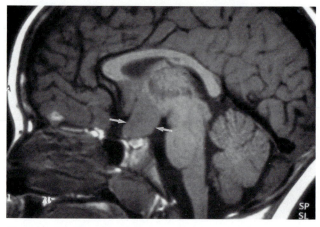

**Figure 8-47  Hypothalamic astroctyoma.** Sagittal T$_1$WI without contrast shows the optic chiasm and adjacent hypothalamus to be expanded (arrows).

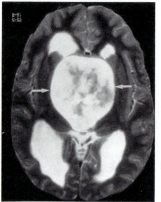

**Figure 8-48  Hypothalamic astrocytoma. A.** Axial PDWI and (**B**). T$_2$WI show a large, high-signal-intensity hypothalamic mass (arrows). Obstructive hydrocephalus is present with reabsorption of CSF seen on the PDWI image as increased signal intensity outlining the margins of the lateral ventricles.

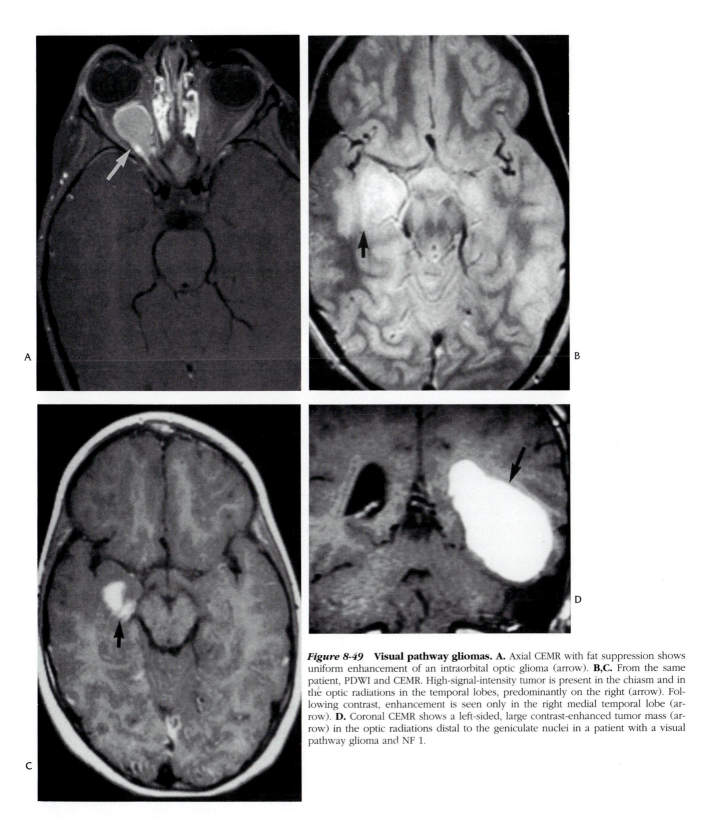

***Figure 8-49*** **Visual pathway gliomas. A.** Axial CEMR with fat suppression shows uniform enhancement of an intraorbital optic glioma (arrow). **B,C.** From the same patient, PDWI and CEMR. High-signal-intensity tumor is present in the chiasm and in the optic radiations in the temporal lobes, predominantly on the right (arrow). Following contrast, enhancement is seen only in the right medial temporal lobe (arrow). **D.** Coronal CEMR shows a left-sided, large contrast-enhanced tumor mass (arrow) in the optic radiations distal to the geniculate nuclei in a patient with a visual pathway glioma and NF 1.

late nuclei into the optic radiations (Fig. 8-49). En-hancement with gadolinium is quite variable within the path of the tumor (Fig. 8-49C,D).

The role of CT and MR is in making the diagnosis of a VPG. In a patient with NF 1 and a VPG, follow-up

may be done in order to ascertain whether the tumor is growing. At the time of growth, with obstruction of the foramen of Monro and the production of hydro-cephalus, shunting and further treatment may be re-quired. Biopsy is often carried out during the early

**Figure 8-50  Suprasellar germinoma. A.** Axial NCCT shows suprasellar mass of increased density (arrows). **B.** Axial CECT shows uniform enhancement of the suprasellar mass.

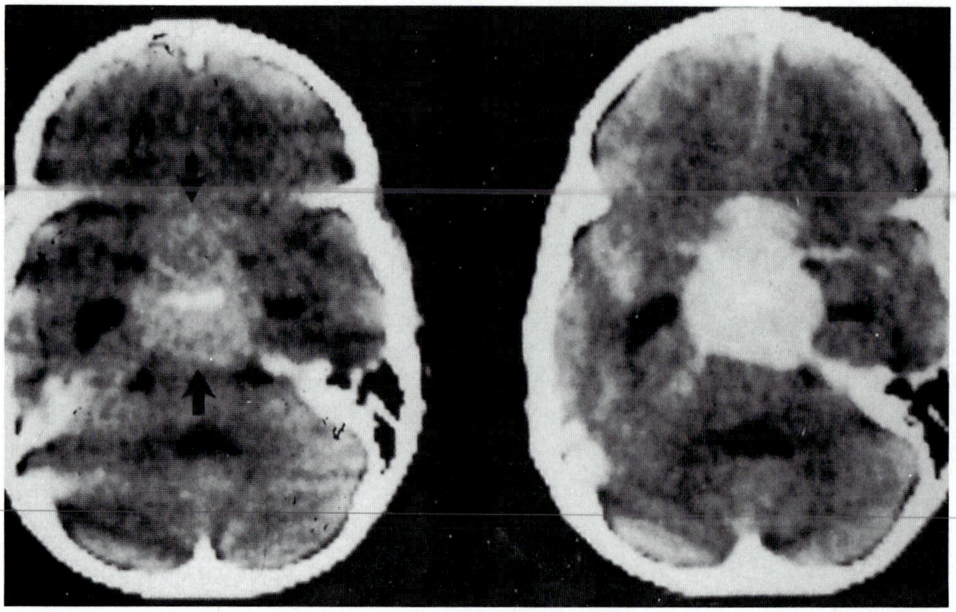

course to establish the histology. If the mass is progressive and the patient is a young child, chemotherapy may be utilized (Rosenstock 1985). In older children with tumor progression, radiation therapy has been the treatment of choice (Danoff 1980). Among children with only optic nerve involvement and no evidence of neurofibromatosis, some of these tumors are resected for cosmetic reasons (Tenny 1982).

## GERMINOMAS

The most frequent type of germ cell tumor originating in the suprasellar area is the germinoma (Jenkin 1978). In the suprasellar area, the male predominance seen in the pineal gland is reversed, so that more often the patient is female. The tumor typically presents as a disturbance of growth or hypothalamic-sexual development. On CT, the mass is isointense to slightly hyperdense before contrast and enhances (Fig. 8-50) (Zimmerman

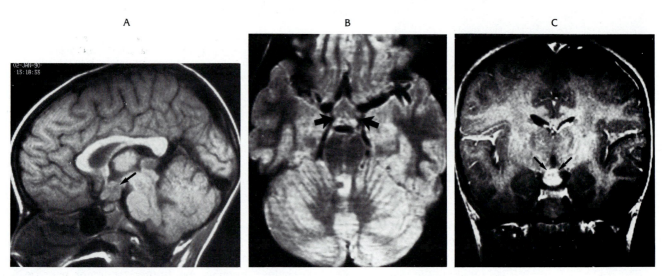

**Figure 8-51  Suprasellar germinoma,** MRI. **A.** Sagittal $T_1WI$ shows an isointense suprasellar mass (arrow) involving the hypothalamus and chiasm. **B.** Axial PDWI (long TR, short TE) shows the mass (arrows) to be isointense. **C.** Coronal CEMR shows the mass (arrows) to be enhanced.

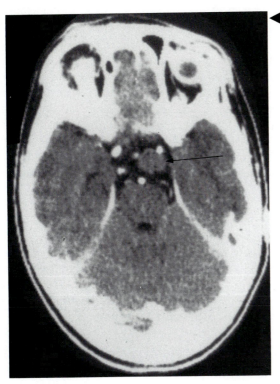

◄ ***Figure 8-52*** **Hypothalamic hamartoma.** Axial CECT shows no enhancement of an isodense suprasellar mass (arrow).

1986; Muller-Forell 1988). The change in signal intensity is thought to be related to the highly cellular nature of the tumor. Treatment consists of biopsy for tissue and then radiation therapy with or without adjuvant chemotherapy (Rustin 1986). The tumor is highly radiosensitive, and in Japan, where there is a high incidence of germinomas, patients have been treated without biopsy and have received radiation doses up to 3000 rad to see whether the tumor responds (Onoyama 1979). If it disappears, it is thought to have been a germinoma. Similarly, patients have also been treated with chemotherapy to see if it responds (Patel 1992).

## HAMARTOMAS OF THE TUBER CINEREUM

These are well-defined masses composed of mature ganglionic tissue attached to the tuber cinereum or the mammillary bodies (Russell 1989). They occur in both men and woman and are associated with precocious puberty (Wolman 1963). Seizures, described as gelastic in nature, consisting of episodes of laughing, may also be seen. Because the tissue is made up of mature cerebral gray matter, the CT appearance is that of a mass isodense to cortex that does not enhance (Fig. 8-52) (Diebler 1983). On MR the mass is isointense to gray matter on $T_1$WI and typically isointense on PDW and $T_2$WI (Fig. 8-53A). Occasionally it is slightly hyperin-

1980*b*; Ganti 1986). On MR the mass is usually isointense to slightly hypointense on $T_1$WI (Fig. 8-51A) and enhances markedly after gadolinium injection (Fig. 8-51B). On PDWI the mass may be isointense or slightly hyperintense, whereas on $T_2$WI it is often hypointense or isointense (Fig. 8-51C) (Zimmerman 1990; Kilgore

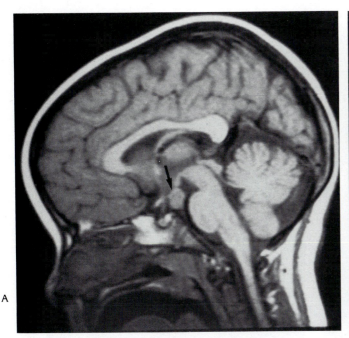

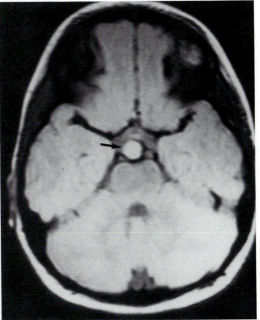

A    B

***Figure 8-53*** **Hypothalamic hamartoma. A.** Sagittal $T_1$WI shows an isointense mass (arrow) at the site of the mamillary body. **B.** Axial PDWI shows a slightly intense hypothalamic mass (arrow) projecting into the chiasmatic cistern.

tense on PDW and T$_2$WI (Fig. 8-53B). After MR contrast injection, there is no enhancement (Boyko 1991). When the diagnosis is in doubt, a biopsy can be performed.

## OTHER SUPRASELLAR TUMORS OF CHILDHOOD

A broad array of conditions, both neoplastic and nonneoplastic, produce masses in the suprasellar region during childhood. These include benign conditions such as arachnoid cysts, inflammatory conditions such as sarcoid and eosinophilic granuloma, and neoplastic conditions such as subarachnoid dissemination of a malignant tumor arising from the brain or orbit (retinoblastoma) (Zimmerman 1990*a*).

# Parenchymal Tumors of the Cerebral Hemispheres and Basal Ganglia

Supratentorial astrocytic tumors represent one-third of pediatric brain tumors when VPGs are included (Heideman 1989). More than half occur in the cerebral hemispheres or basal ganglia outside the VPG. Males are affected more frequently; the age peak occurs between 2 and 4 years with a VPG and occurs in adolescence usually with more hemispheric tumors (Heideman 1989). These tumors are classified as fibrillary, pilocytic, or anaplastic, or as glioblastoma multiforme (Russell 1989). Subcategories are recognized, such as the oligodendroglioma and gliomatosis cerebri, and there are less common types. In general, pilocytic astrocytomas are more frequently diencephalic and have

histological features analogous to those of cerebellar astrocytomas. Fibrillary astrocytomas are densely cellular, tend not to be cystic, and infiltrate (Russell 1989). Within the cerebral hemispheres, fibrillary astrocytomas are more common; this tumor has been implicated in malignant degeneration. So-called malignant or high-grade astrocytomas are labeled as anaplastic and as glioblastoma multiforme. They are highly cellular, undifferentiated tumors with frequent mitosis, areas of necrosis, and hemorrhage. They are widely invasive, grow rapidly, and spread into the subarachnoid pathways over time (Russell 1989).

The clinical presentation of a patient with a cerebral hemispheric astrocytoma is that of increased intracranial pressure (50 to 75 percent) or seizures (25 to 50 percent) (Heideman 1989). The incidence of seizures as a form of presentation is higher with low-grade tumors than it is with high-grade tumors. The location of a tumor is an important factor in determining the type of symptoms with which it presents.

## PILOCYTIC AND FIBRILLARY ASTROCYTOMAS

On CT, low-grade astrocytomas are variable in appearance (Naidich 1984). A fibrillary astrocytoma is found within the white matter of the cerebral hemisphere as a low-density infiltrating lesion on CT (Fig. 8-54A) (Zimmerman 1990*b*). These tumors usually do not enhance after contrast administration. Pilocytic astrocytomas are more often cystic or present as a mural tumor nodule on the margin of a cyst, are of decreased density without contrast, and enhance after contrast in-

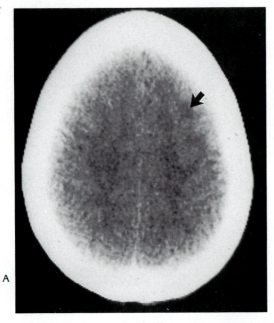 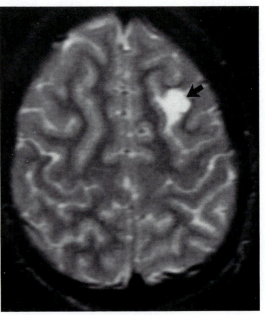

***Figure 8-54*** **Low-grade fibrillary astrocytoma. A.** Axial NCCT shows a faint hypodensity (arrow) in the left frontal lobe. **B.** Axial T$_2$WI shows a hyperintensity lesion in the left frontal lobe (arrow).

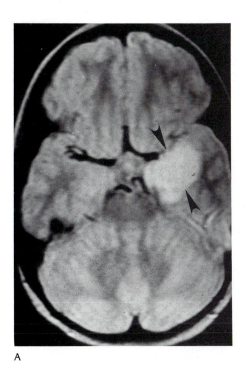

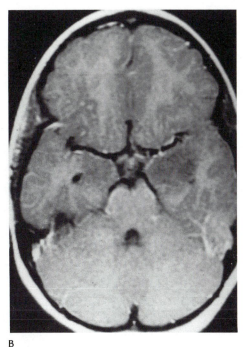

A

B

*Figure 8-55* **Fibrillary astrocytoma** in the left temporal lobe. **A.** Axial PDWI shows a high-signal-intensity mass (arrowheads) in the medial aspect of the left temporal lobe. **B.** Axial T₁WI after MR contrast shows no evidence of enhancement.

jection (Fig. 8-55) (Zimmerman 1990*b*). The solid portion of the tumor tends to be slightly higher in density than is the fluid-filled cystic portion. Calcification can be present but is not as frequent or as marked as it is in oligodendroglioma or ependymoma. On MR, the appearance of both pilocytic and fibrillary astrocytoma is that of a hypointense mass on T₁WI and a hyperintense mass on PDW and T₂WI (Figs. 8-54B and 8-55A). After MR contrast injection there is more frequent enhancement with a pilocytic astrocytoma (Fig. 8-56C)

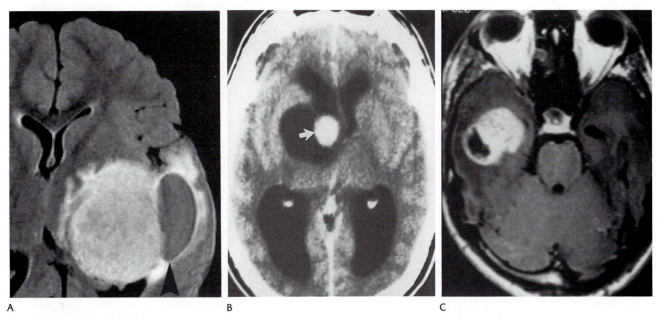

A                                          B                                          C

*Figure 8-56* **Cystic pilocytic astrocytomas. A.** Axial FLAIR image shows a left thalamic, basal ganglionic mass of increased signal intensity that is displacing the midline to the right. A cyst (arrowhead) is present laterally, and is slightly greater in signal intensity than the CSF in the ventricle. **B.** Axial CECT shows a mural enhancing tumor nodule (arrow). The mural tumor nodule lies in the wall of a nonenhancing cyst. The mass produces hydrocephalus with dilatation of both lateral ventricles by compression of the foramen of Monro. **C.** Low-grade pilocytic astrocytoma in the right temporal lobe. Axial T₁WI after MR contrast injection shows a partially cystic contrast-enhancing mass in the right temporal lobe.

than with a fibrillary astrocytoma (Fig. 8-55B), but both may enhance (Zimmerman 1989*b*). Tumor dissemination is not usually present at diagnosis but may be found in a small percentage of cases years after treatment. This is more often a complication of fibrillary astrocytomas (Zimmerman 1990*b*).

## PLEOMORPHIC XANTHOASTROCYTOMA

Pleomorphic xanthoastrocytomas are tumors of the cortex and leptomeninges that arise peripherally in adolescents and children. Seizures and headaches are the usual presenting symptoms. Tumors vary from solid to cystic and may or may not produce vasogenic edema. They are peripherally located and usually enhance with contrast on CT or MR (Fig. 8-57) (Lipper 1993).

## ANAPLASTIC ASTROCYTOMA AND GLIOBLASTOMA

With the more aggressive astrocytoma and **glioblastoma multiforme** there are generally rapidly proliferating, poorly formed tumor blood vessels that result in a disturbance of the blood-brain barrier (BBB) that leads to the formation of surrounding vasogenic edema and permits contrast enhancement of the core of the viable tumor (Zimmerman 1990*b*). These tumors tend to be more widely invasive, producing significant mass effect, and are frequently necrotic. On CT, the tumor masses are low in density, enhance after contrast injec-

tion, have irregular margins, and are surrounded by vasogenic edema (Zimmerman 1989). On T$_1$WI, the lesions are usually hypointense unless a subacute hemorrhage is present in the form of methemoglobin (high

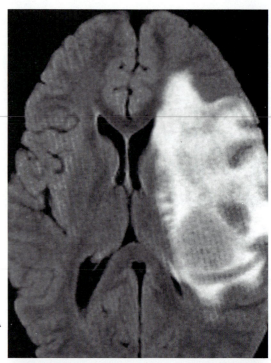

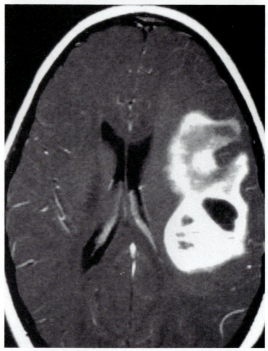

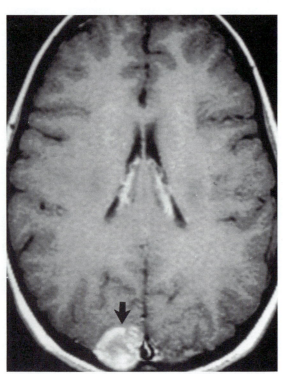

***Figure 8-57 Pleomorphic xanthoastrocytoma.*** Axial CEMR shows a contrast-enhanced peripheral cortical mass (arrow) scalloping the bone.

***Figure 8-58 Glioblastoma multiforme. A.*** Axial FLAIR image at presentation shows extensive vasogenic edema and tumor, which are not individually separable, in the left hemisphere, producing mass effect. **B.** Axial CEMR at presentation, shows contrast enhancement of the solid portion of the tumor. *(Continued on next page.)*

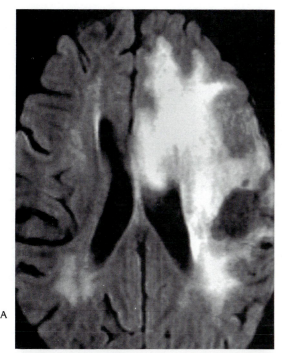

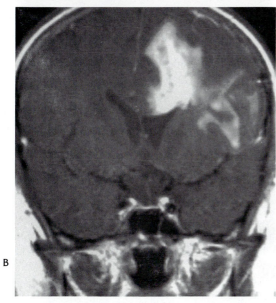

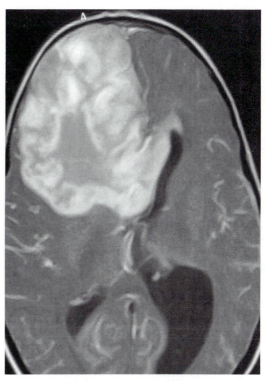

***Figure 8-59*** **Glioblastoma multiforme.** Radiation induced, after treatment for retinoblastoma. Axial CEMR shows a large right frontal lobe mass with peripheral contrast enhancement, crossing the corpus callosum.

***Figure 8-58 (Continued)*** **C,D.** Follow-up study, 1 year later at time of progression, following treatment. **C.** Axial FLAIR image shows the tumor had extended deeper into the midline in the corpus callosum, compressing the anterior portion of the body of the lateral ventricle. There is abnormal signal in the right hemisphere, most likely due to microscopic tumor infiltrating through the corpus callosum. **D.** Coronal CEMR, shows tumor, that has now extended into the right side of the corpus callosum, depressing the body of the lateral ventricle.

in signal intensity). On PDW, FLAIR, and $T_2$WI these tumors are hyperintense (Fig. 8-58A,C). After MR contrast injection, the solid portions of the tumor contrast-enhance (Figs. 8-58B,D and 8-59). Vasogenic edema surrounding the tumor may have the same signal intensity that the tumor has on PDW and $T_2$WI. Hy-

pointense flow voids within tumor blood vessels and may be due to increased tumor vascularity.

In benign pilocytic and fibrillary astrocytomas, survival is measured in years to decades, whereas in anaplastic astrocytoma and glioblastoma multiforme it is measured in months to years (Heideman 1989). Treatment begins with surgical excision of as much of the tumor as is possible, with the realization that in an invasive anaplastic astrocytoma and glioblastoma multiforme, gross total resection is usually impossible (Heideman 1989). Small, noninvasive low-grade tumors can be totally resected provided that they lie in a favorable site such as the anterior temporal lobe. At present, the major form of therapy is radiation therapy but this has not been effective in providing long-term survival in patients with the more aggressive tumors (Sheline 1977). Chemotherapy has been used in children under 3 years of age and as an adjuvant in older children (Pendergrass 1987).

## GANGLIOGLIOMA

This is a common (4.5 percent) pediatric low-grade tumor of the supratentorial white matter and the adjacent gray matter (Zimmerman 1979*a*). The tumors are composed of a mixture of ganglion cells and glial elements (Russell 1989). Eighty percent of gangliogliomas are found in children and young adults. The most frequent

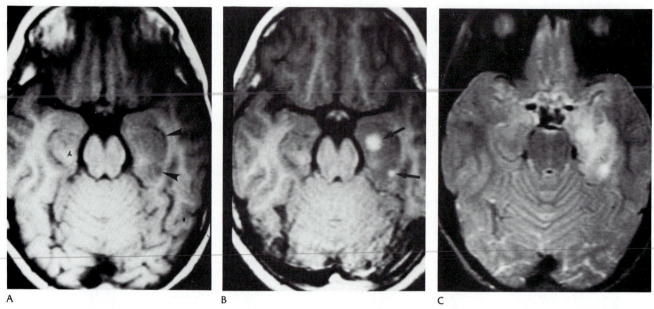

A            B            C

**Figure 8-60  Ganglioglioma. A.** Axial T₁WI shows hypointense expansion of the hippocampal gyrus (arrowheads). **B.** Axial CEMR shows two areas of enhancement (arrows). **C.** Axial T₂WI shows a high-signal-intensity mass involving the medial aspect of the left temporal lobe.

site is the temporal lobe, but no area of the CNS is spared. These tumors are of considerable variability in appearance (Zimmerman 1979*a*). They are usually not hemorrhagic and have a variable contrast-enhancement pattern. Calcification and/or cystic changes may be found. The tumors are usually not necrotic. On CT, they are usually hypodense and may or may not contrast-enhance (Zimmerman 1979*a*; Tampieri 1991;

Castillo 1990). On MR, they are hypointense on T₁WI and hyperintense on PDW, FLAIR, and T₂WI (Figs. 8-60 and 8-61) (Thomsett 1980). Contrast enhancement after MR contrast injection is variable (Fig. 8-60B) (Zimmerman 1991). They should be suspected in a patient who presents with the symptoms of a seizure in whom a cortical or subcortical tumor is found. The differential diagnosis is that of other astrocytic tumors.

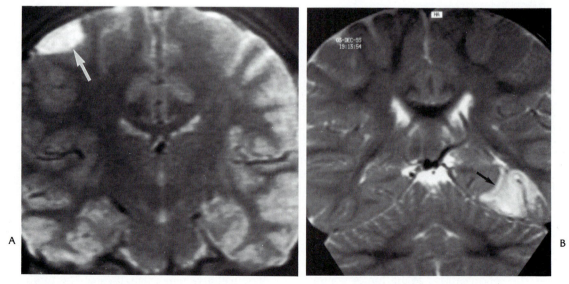

A            B

**Figure 8-61  Ganglioglioma. A.** Coronal PDWI shows a peripheral cortical mass of increased signal intensity (arrow). **B.** Coronal T₂WI shows a peripheral cortical mass (arrow) in the inferior posterior temporal lobe on the left.

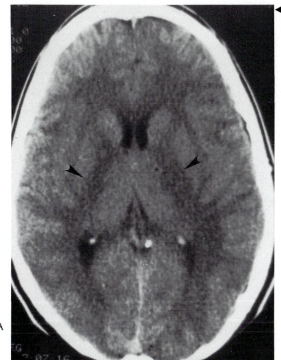

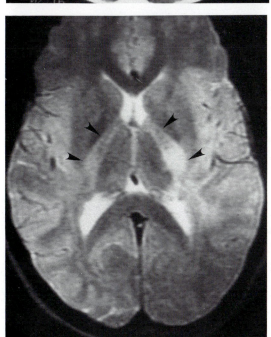

*Figure 8-62* **Gliomatosis cerebri. A.** Axial CECT shows slight fullness in the white matter of both internal capsules (arrowheads). There is no evidence of contrast enhancement and no mass effect **B.** Axial T₂WI shows high signal intensity involving both internal capsules (arrowheads).

and to some extent in the white matter of the fronto-parietal lobes. Usually both hemispheres are involved. These tumors tend not to be hemorrhagic, tend not to enhance, and rarely show calcification (Zimmerman 1990b). On CT, the finding is that of expansion of the white matter, usually not different in density from the white matter (Fig. 8-62A). On MR with T₁WI, the tumor may not be recognizable, as it blends in with the white matter. On PDW and T₂WI, the signal intensity of the white matter appears to be high and is abnormal (Figs. 8-62, 8-49B, and 8-63) (Spagnoli 1987). The characteristic expansion of the white matter by the tumor mass usually helps differentiate it from demyelinating diseases.

### EPENDYMOMAS

One-third of all ependymomas occur in the supratentorial space (Heideman 1989). Within this space they arise from ependymal rests in the white matter or within or adjacent to the ependymal lining of the ventricular system (Russell 1989). They tend to occur early

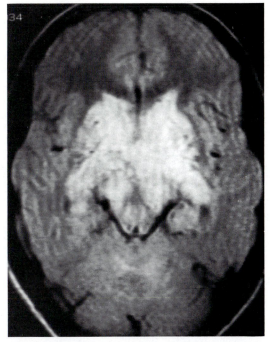

*Figure 8-63* **Gliomatosis cerebri.** Axial PDWI shows high-signal-intensity mass involving the basal ganglia, thalami, upper brainstem, and medial temporal lobes bilaterally.

### GLIOMATOSIS CEREBRI

This is a rare form of a diffusely infiltrating low-grade tumor that often involves major portions of the cerebral hemispheres and most commonly presents in the first or second decade of life. Typically, there is involvement of the internal capsules and adjacent white matter pathways with inferior extension into the brainstem. The tumor also is found in the corpus callosum

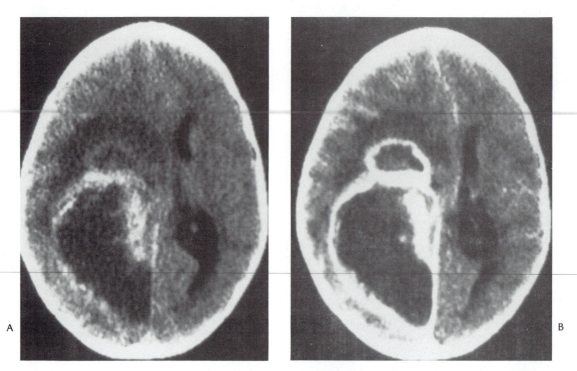

*Figure 8-64* **Ependymoma. A.** Axial NCCT shows a large right parietal occipital mass that is centrally necrotic and contains multiple small calcifications within its walls. **B.** Axial CECT shows enhancement of the necrotic tumor wall.

in life although they are found throughout childhood (Kun 1988; Swartz 1982). They tend to be well demarcated and partially encapsulated and are frequently hemorrhagic and cystic. They vary in grade from those that are "benign" to those that are malignant. Their clinical presentation in the supratentorial space relates to their location and size and the age of the patient. If ependymomas obstruct the CSF pathways, they can produce hydrocephalus, whereas if they occur within the white matter, they present predominantly by mass effect and increased intracranial pressure. More peripheral ependymomas may produce seizures. On CT, calcification is common (50 percent), with the tumor tissue usually being hypodense on plain CT (Fig. 8-64A) (Swartz 1982; Armington 1985). Enhancement occurs frequently, and the tumor is often centrally necrotic (Fig. 8-64B). On $T_1WI$ the signal intensity is low, whereas on PDWI and $T_2WI$ signal intensity is quite variable (Fig. 8-65A) (Zimmerman 1990*b*). Rarely, the supratentorial ependymoma may occur intraventricularly (Fig. 8-65B,C). Contrast enhancement is frequent on $T_1$ images after gadolinium (Fig. 8-65C) (Spoto 1990). Tumor dissemination is usually not present at

the time of diagnosis but occurs with some frequency after local recurrence (Packer 1985). Treatment consists of surgical resection when possible. Radiation therapy is used, but the overall results suggest that it is not very effective. Chemotherapy has been used, but again, the results have not been promising.

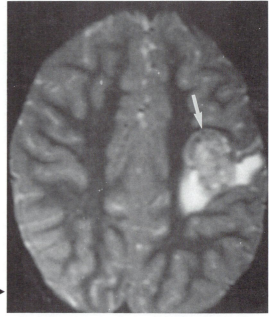

*Figure 8-65* **Ependymomas. A.** Axial $T_2WI$ shows a mass (arrow) that is isointense to gray matter and is partially surrounded by vasogenic edema. *(Continued on next page.)*

A

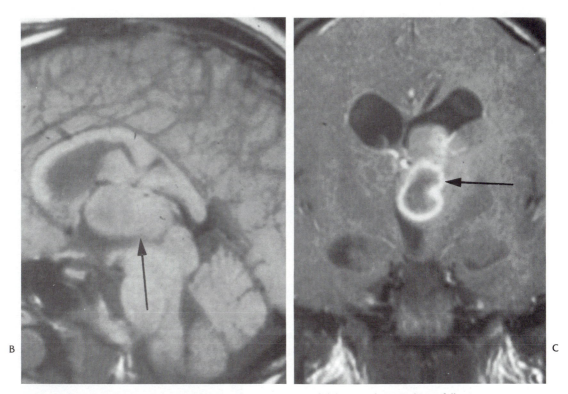

***Figure 8-65 (Continued)*** **B.** Sagittal T₁WI without contrast and (**C**) coronal CEMR (T₁WI following gadolinium injection) shows a mass (arrow) arising in the wall of the third and lateral ventricle, from the left side, with marginal contrast enhancement.

## PRIMITIVE NEUROECTODERMAL TUMORS OF THE CEREBRAL HEMISPHERE

Remnants of the germinal matrix can give rise to tumors in the white matter near the margins of the lateral ventricle. In the past these have been called cerebral neuroblastomas; today they are labeled as one of the varieties of primitive neuroectodermal tumors (PNET). They fall among the 5 to 10 percent of supratentorial tumors of childhood that are PNETs. They have a marked tendency to grow rapidly, reaching the ependymal or pial surface of the brain to disseminate through the CSF pathways. On CT they are iso- to hyperdense and frequently have some calcification. Necrosis is not uncommon, and contrast enhancement of the solid portion of the tumor is the rule. Surrounding vasogenic edema can be seen both on CT and on MRI. Signal intensity is hypointense on T₁WI, hyperintense on PDWI, and often isointense to gray matter on both FLAIR and T₂WI (Fig. 8-66A,B). Contrast enhancement is the rule (Fig. 8-66C). Hemorrhage occurs in approximately 10 percent (Fig. 8-66).

## Intraventricular Tumors

In addition to ependymomas, the two major intraventricular tumors seen in childhood are choroid plexus papillomas and choroid plexus carcinomas (Zimmerman 1990*b;* Jelinek, 1990). In other children, intraventricular meningiomas may be found in association with neurofibromatosis (Fletcher 1986; Braffman 1994). Glial tumors arising within the brain parenchyma can extend into the ventricle, appearing as primary intraventricular masses.

## CHOROID PLEXUS TUMORS

Tumors of the choroid plexus account for up to 10 to 20 percent of brain tumors occurring during the first year of life but represent only 3 percent of all pediatric brain tumors (Zimmerman 1979*c;* Laurence 1979). Choroid plexus papillomas occurring during the first year of life are found within the lateral ventricle (Laurence 1979). Most of these papillomas are benign, and some are capable of CSF production (Milhorat 1976). Only 10 to 20 percent of choroid plexus tumors are carcinomas (Carpenter 1982). Choroid plexus carcinomas have a tendency to invade the margin of the ventricle and involve the subependymal white matter, producing vasogenic edema. They also have a tendency to disseminate within the ventricular system and the subarachnoid spaces (Carpenter 1982).

Choroid plexus papillomas are often calcified or hyperdense on plain CT (Fig. 8-67) and enhance homogeneously after contrast administration (Fig. 8-68) (Zimmerman 1979*c*). Hydrocephalus is a frequent find-

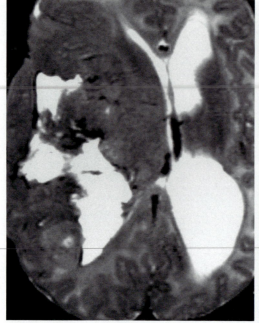
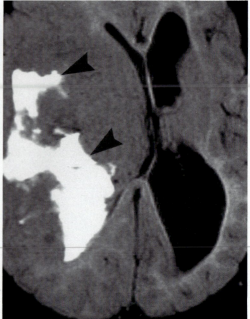

**Figure 8-66 Supratentorial primitive neuroectodermal tumor (neuro-blastoma). A.** Axial T₂WI shows a mass involving the right hemisphere that is isointense to cortex. Mass effect produces contralateral hydrocephalus. Within the mass are areas that are of increased signal intensity, most of which are outlined by marginal hypointensities. This is the site of old hemorrhage. Note multiple linear hypointense flow voids within the tumor. These are enlarged vessels. **B.** Axial FLAIR image shows the tumor mass to be isointense to gray matter. The high signal intensity, seen in the tumor mass in the right hemisphere, is blood (arrowheads) in the form of methemoglobin. **C.** CEMR shows enhancement of tumor surrounding the site of hemorrhage. Note some of the enhancement is linear (arrows), occurring within vessels.

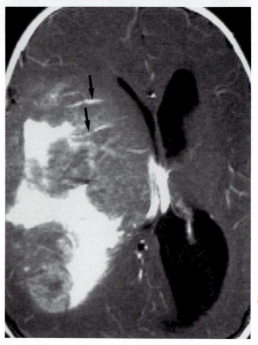

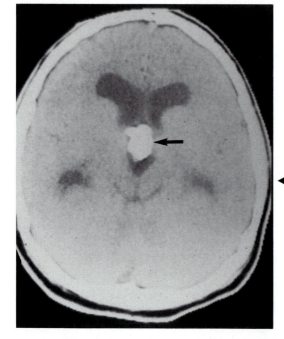

**◄ Figure 8-67 Choroid plexus papilloma** in the third ventricle. Axial NCCT shows a calcified mass (arrow) in the anterior third ventricle; hydrocephalus is present.

ing that possibly is caused by overproduction of CSF (Milhorat 1976) or episodes of subarachnoid hemorrhage with resultant hydrocephalus (Zimmerman 1990*b*). On MR, they are hypointense to isointense on T₁WI and of hypointensity on PDW and T₂WI (Fig. 8-

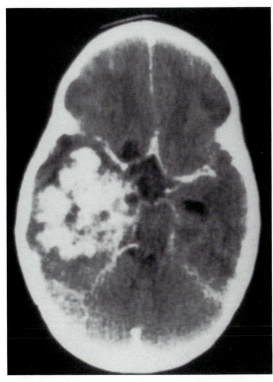

*Figure 8-68* **Choroid plexus papilloma.** Axial CECT shows an enhanced frondlike mass in the anterior aspect of the right temporal lobe.

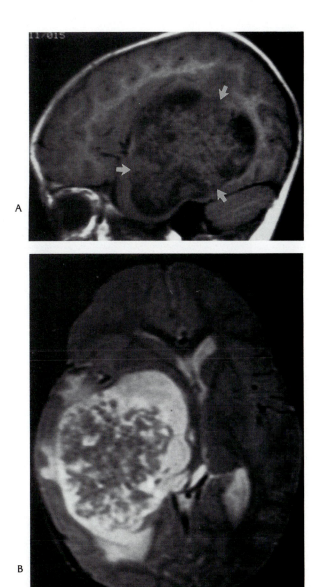

*Figure 8-69* **Choroid plexus papillomas. A,B.** Lateral ventricle. **A.** Sagittal $T_1$WI shows that the right temporal horn is expanded and is filled with a papillary appearing isointense mass (arrows). **B.** Axial $T_2$WI shows marked dilatation of the temporal horn, which is filled with a hypointense frondlike or papillarylike mass.

69A,B) (Zimmerman 1990*b*). They enhance intensely after contrast injection (Fig. 8-69C,D).

### SUBEPENDYMAL GIANT CELL ASTROCYTOMA

Subependymal giant cell astrocytomas complicate tuberous sclerosis in 2 to 10 percent of patients. They most commonly are found between the ages of 8 and 18, arising from subependymal nodules near the foramen of Monro. They contrast-enhance on CT and MR (Fig. 8-70). On MR, this does not differentiate the potential giant cell astrocytoma from the other subependymal nodules. On CT, contrast enhancement is seen in giant cell astrocytomas (Fig. 8-70A) and not usually seen in the routine subependymal nodule. Growth of the tumor mass does differentiate a giant cell astrocytoma from the other subependymal nodules. These masses eventually produce obstructive hydrocephalus at the foramen of Monro.

### INTRAVENTRICULAR MENINGIOMAS

In childhood, these meningiomas are most often found in association with neurofibromatosis (Braffman 1990). An intraventricular meningioma appears as a mass of increased density (Fig. 8-71), with or without calcification, that enhances on CT and is usually located within the atrium of the lateral ventricle. Hydrocephalus is due to compression of the third ventricle or trapping of the atria of the lateral ventricle, producing the signs and symptoms of increased intracranial pressure. Compression of the visual pathway and the optic radiations produces a homonymous hemianopsia. On MR, a meningioma is isointense on $T_1$WI, may be slightly hy-

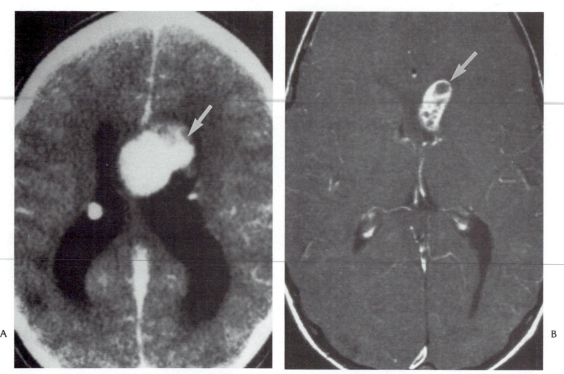

**Figure 8-70    Giant cell astrocytomas. A.** Axial CECT shows an enhancing mass (arrow) producing obstructive hydrocephalus, arising near the left foramen of Monro. **B.** Axial CEMR shows a contrast-enhancing left-sided mass (arrow). This has not reached the size that would produce obstructive hydrocephalus.

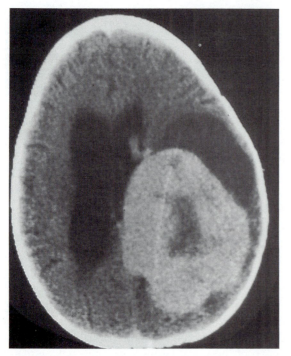

**Figure 8-71    Intraventricular meningioma.** Axial NCCT shows a high-density mass in an atrium of the left lateral ventricle capped by CSF trapped in the obstructed and markedly expanded temporal horn.

perintense on PDWI, and is usually isointense to hypointense on $T_2WI$ (Spagnoli 1986). These entities enhance intensely after MR contrast injection.

## Pineal Tumors

Tumors of the pineal region are a heterogeneous group representing 0.5 to 2 percent of all childhood CNS tumors (Zimmerman 1980b). Tumors of the pineal parenchyma, pineoblastomas (a primitive neuroectodermal tumor), and pineocytomas represent one major group. Germ cell tumors, including germinomas, embryonal cell carcinomas, teratomas (benign and malignant), and choriocarcinomas represent the other major group (Zimmerman 1980b). Germ cell tumors are found more frequently in men and tend to occur in the second decade of life, whereas pineal parenchymal tumors occur more frequently in the first decade of life and are more equally distributed between the sexes (Packer 1984). The third category includes tumors that arise from the supporting structures of the pineal gland and are of an astrocytic nature. Tumors of adjacent structures can arise and simulate tumors of the pineal region. From the adjacent meninges, meningiomas can involve the pineal region, while enlargement of the vein of Galen as a result of an arteriovenous malformation can simulate a pineal tumor. The most common difficulty encountered with CT in which the cuts are done in the axial plane occurs when a tumor in the tectum of the midbrain projects superiorly into the pineal region, mimicking a pineal neoplasm. This differentiation can be made on sagittal and coronal MR images.

The signs and symptoms of tumors in the pineal area are often nonspecific and nonlocalizing (Packer 1984). They arise primarily from obstruction of the outlet of the third ventricle, with the production of hydrocephalus. Compression of the collicular plate may produce vertical gaze paresis (Parinaud's syndrome).

Pineocytomas and pineoblastomas appear on CT as tumors of slightly increased density often with calcification, and contrast-enhancement (Fig. 8-72) (Zimmerman 1980b; Zimmerman 1996). They infiltrate the surrounding structures, and hydrocephalus is found frequently. On MR, these tumors are usually low in signal intensity on $T_1WI$ (Fig. 8-73A) and frequently have mixed signal intensity on PDW and $T_2WI$ (Zimmerman 1990b) (Fig. 8-74A). On PDWI they may be slightly increased in signal intensity, but they are usually lower in signal intensity on $T_2WI$. This is thought to reflect the highly cellular nature of these tumors. They enhance intensely with MR contrast (Fig. 8-73B and 8-74B) (Zimmerman 1991; Muller-Forell 1988). The best method of evaluating these tumors is with thin $T_1WI$ sagittal and coronal sections before and after MR contrast injection. Subarachnoid dissemination should be looked for, since it is not uncommon and in fact may be the presenting manifestation of a pineoblastoma or germinoma (Fig. 8-74B). There is an increased incidence of pineoblastoma in association with congenital bilateral retinoblastoma (Bader 1982). Given the history of bilateral retinoblastoma, any early calcification in the pineal gland (before age 6) should be looked at on CT as the initial manifestation of a pineoblastoma (Zimmerman 1982). This combination of retinoblastoma and pineoblastoma has been labeled *trilateral retinoblastoma* (Fig. 8-73) (Bader 1982; Bagley 1996).

On CT, germ cell tumors are usually of increased density (Fig. 8-75A), contrast-enhance (Fig. 8-75B) and may have calcifications (Zimmerman 1980b). In a germinoma the calcifications are usually found in the invaded pineal gland but may occur throughout the tumor matrix after treatment. In an embryonal cell carcinoma, calcifications are seen frequently through-

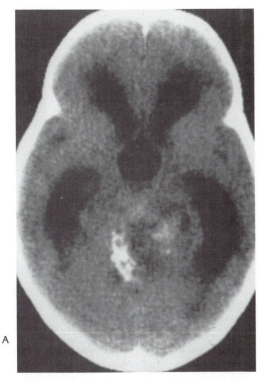
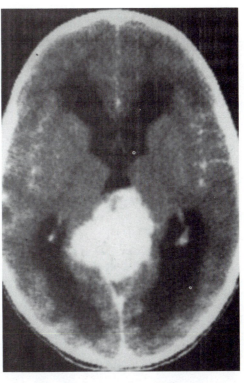

*Figure 8-72* **Primitive neuroectodermal tumor (pineoblastoma type). A.** Axial NCCT shows a poorly marginated, isodense, partially calcified pineal gland mass. There is hydrocephalus with dilatation of the third and lateral ventricles. **B.** Axial CECT shows that the mass enhances.

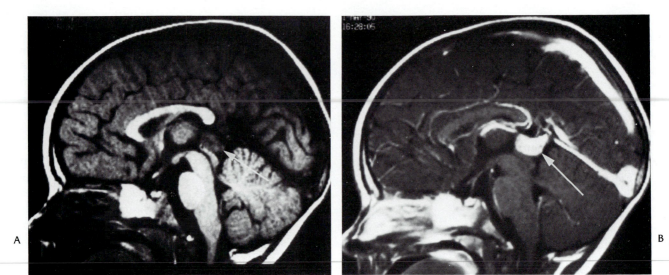

**Figure 8-73** **Primitive neuroectodermal tumor (pineoblastoma type)** associated with bilateral congenital retinoblastoma **(trilateral retinoblastoma)**. **A.** Sagittal T₁WI, NCMR shows a large pineal gland, consistent with a small tumor mass (arrow). **B.** Sagittal CEMR shows an enhanced pineal mass (arrow).

out the tumor matrix. Benign or malignant teratomas frequently have calcification or ossification, such as in teeth. Embryonal carcinomas tend to undergo necrosis. All malignant germ cell tumors are invasive and have a potential for CSF dissemination (Packer 1984). Germinomas like the pineoblastoma have a isointense to cor-

tex appearance on T₂WI (Fig. 8-76A) and enhance with gadolinium (Fig. 8-76B). Teratomas, pineal tumors, frequently have a mixture of fat, calcium, bone and soft tissue on CT (Fig. 8-77) or MRI.

Surgical resection is recommended; when surgery is not feasible, biopsy is performed so that treatment can

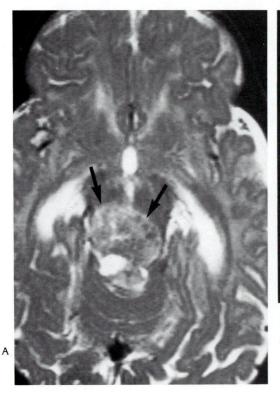

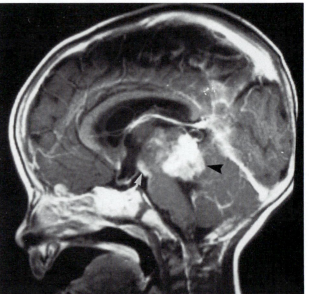

**Figure 8-74** **Primitive neuroectodermal tumor (pineoblastoma type).** **A.** Axial T₂WI shows an isointense pineal mass (arrows). The temporal horns are dilated. The patient is postshunting for obstructive hydrocephalus. **B.** Sagittal CEMR the pineal tumor to be enhanced (arrowhead) and there to be tumor disseminated to the interpeduncular cistern (arrow).

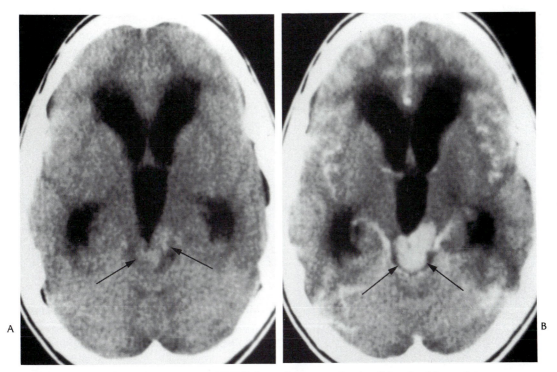

***Figure 8-75*** **Pineal germinoma. A.** Axial NCCT shows the mass at the site of the pineal (arrows) to be isodense and producing obstructive hydrocephalus with dilatation of the third and lateral ventricles. **B.** On CECT, the mass enhances (arrows).

be appropriate to the type of lesion (Packer 1984). Radiotherapy is curative in germinomas (Onoyama 1979). Chemotherapy may also be curative in some germinomas (Rustin 1986). The response to therapy of pineoblastomas, pineocytomas, and embryonal cell carci-

nomas has generally been disappointing (Packer 1984). Cysts of the pineal gland are common, appearing on CT as low-density, sometimes partially calcified ringlike lesions. Contrast enhancement occurs in the adjacent veins and the residual portion of the pineal gland. On

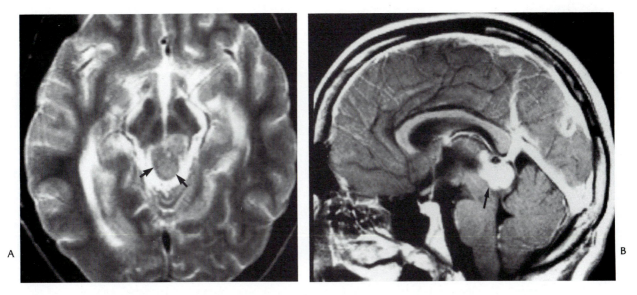

***Figure 8-76*** **Pineal germinoma. A.** Axial T$_2$WI shows pineal mass (arrows) to be isointense to cortical gray matter. **B.** Sagittal CEMR shows the pineal mass to be enhanced (arrow).

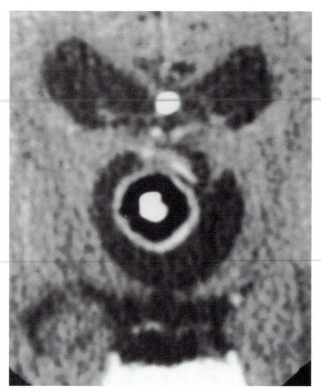

***Figure 8-77*** **Pineal teratoma.** Coronal CT shows a mass containing fat and ossification and calcification at the posterior third ventricle. The mass is producing some ventricular enlargement.

MR, pineal cysts are hypointense on $T_1$WI (Fig. 8-78) and hyperintense on PDWI; they are isointense to CSF on $T_2$WI. Pineal cysts may get larger than the normal upper limits of the pineal gland (1 cm in diameter) but do not appear to produce hydrocephalus or compression of the collicular plate and cerebral aqueduct.

Pineal cysts are thought to arise as a degeneration of the pineal gland and contain slightly proteinaceous fluid.

## Superficial Tumors of the Meninges, Pia, or Cortex

There is a small but real incidence of meningiomas in childhood. Their appearance is usually not different from that in adults (Spagnoli 1986); even in the young, the tumor can be large. There is an increased incidence in childhood of meningiomas that are more aggressive ("malignant"), and some of these tumors burrow within the brain parenchyma. Identification of large meningiomas is not a problem, since they can be recognized by their mass effect. Small meningiomas may not be seen on CT or MR unless contrast is given. Meningiomas have an increased incidence in patients with either type of neurofibromatosis and should be looked for in that clinical setting (Braffman 1990). Other tumors that arise from the calvarium or dura in children include chondrosarcomas, metastases due to neuroblastoma and Ewing's sarcoma, metastatic rhabdomyosarcomas, and rhabdomyosarcomas invading extracranial to intracranial through the bone or along the neural foramina and the nerves they contain. Superficial cortical astrocytomas are uncommon but can be found in childhood. An uncommon mass that is probably related to the phacomatoses is referred to as *meningoencephaloangiomatosis* (MEAN) (Duhaime 1985). Subarachnoid tumor dissemination should also be considered, as should meningitis and sarcoid, when there is enhancement of the pial surface of the brain.

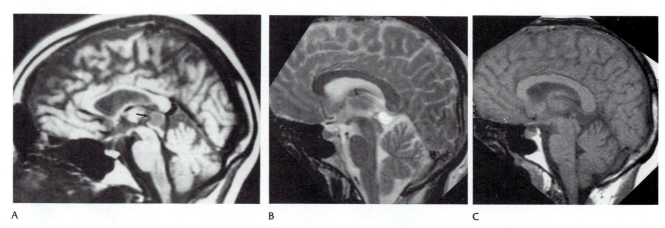

A                                B                                C

***Figure 8-78*** **Pineal cyst. A.** Sagittal $T_1$WI shows cystic expansion of the pineal gland (arrow) without hydrocephalus or compression of the aqueduct or tectum of the midbrain. **B.** On $T_2$WI, isointensity to CSF is noted. **C.** CEMR shows no contrast enhancement.

# References

ALBRIGHT AL, PRICE RA, GUTHKELCH AN: Brain stem gliomas of children: A clinicopathologic study. *Cancer* 52: 2313–2319, 1983.

AOKI S, BARKOVICH AJ, NISHIMURA K, et al: Neurofibromatosis types 1 and 2: cranial MR findings. *Radiology* 172: 527–534, 1989.

ARMINGTON WG, OSBORN AG, CUBBERLEY DA, et al: Supratentorial ependymoma: CT appearance. *Radiology* 157:367–372, 1985.

ARMINGTON WG, ZIMMERMAN RA, BILANIUK LT: Imaging of the retroorbital visual pathway, in Som PM, Bergeron RT (eds), *Head and Neck Imaging*, St. Louis, CV Mosby, 1990, pp 829–873.

ARSENI C, CIURZA AV: Statistical survey of 276 cases of medulloblastomas (1935–1978). *Acta Neurochir (Wien)* 57:159–162, 1982.

ATLAS SW, GROSSMAN RI, GOLDBERG HI, et al: MR diagnosis of acute disseminated encephalomyelitis. *J Comput Assist Tomogr* 10(5):798–801, 1986.

AUER R, RICE JG, HINTON G, et al: Cerebellar astrocytoma with benign histology and malignant clinical course. *J Neurosurg* 54:128–132, 1981.

BADER JL, MEADOWS AT, ZIMMERMAN LE, et al: Bilateral retinoblastoma with ectopic intracranial retinoblastoma: Trilateral retinoblastoma. *Cancer Genet Cytogenet* 5:203–213, 1982.

BAGLEY LJ, HURST RW, ZIMMERMAN RA, et al: Imaging in the trilateral retinoblastoma syndrome. *Neuroradiology* 38:166–170, 1996.

BILANIUK L, ZIMMERMAN R, LITTMAN P, et al: Computed tomography of brain stem gliomas in children. *Neuroradiology* 134:89–95, 1980.

BOYKO OB, CURNES JT, OAKES WH, et al: Hamartomas of in tuber cinereum: CT, MR, and pathologic findings. *AJNR* 12:309–314, 1991.

BRAFFMAN BH, BILANIUK LT, ZIMMERMAN RA: MR of central nervous system neoplasia of the phakomatoses. *Semin Roentgenol* 25(2):198–217, 1990.

BRAFFMAN B, NAIDICH TP: The Phakomatoses: Part I: Neurofibromatosis and tuberous sclerosis. *Neuroimag Clin North Am* 4(2):299, 1994.

BUETOW PC, SMIRNIOTOPOULOS JG, DONE S: Congenital brain tumors: A review of 45 cases. *AJNR* 11:793–799, 1990.

CARMEL PW, ANTUNES JL, CHANG CH: Craniopharyngiomas in children. *Neurosurgery* 11:382–389, 1982.

CARPENTER DB, MICHELSON WG, HAYS AP: Carcinoma of the choroid plexus. *J Neurosurg* 56:722–727, 1982.

CASTILLO M, DAVIS PC, TAKEI Y, et al: Intracranial ganglioglioma: MR, CT, and clinical findings in 18 patients. *AHNR* 11:109–114, 1990.

CHOU M, LENA G, HASSOUN J: Prognosis and long term followup in patients with medulloblastoma. *Clin Neurosurg* 30:246–277, 1983.

COATES TL, HINSHAW DB Jr, PECKMAN N, et al: Pediatric choroid plexus neoplasms: MR, CT and pathologic correlation. *Radiology* 173:81–88, 1989.

COHEN ME, DUFFNER PK: Craniopharyngiomas, in *Brain Tumors in Children*, New York, Raven Press, 1983, pp 193–210.

COULON RA, TILL K: Intracranial ependymomas in children: A review of 43 cases. *Childs Brain* 3:154–168, 1977.

DANOFF BF, KRAMER S, THOMPSON N: The radiotherapeutic management of optic gliomas of children. *Int J Radiat Oncol Biol Phys* 6:45–50, 1980.

DIEBLER C, PONSOT G: Hamartomas of the tuber cinereum. *Neuroradiology* 25:93–101, 1983.

DUHAIME AC, SCHUT L, RORKE LB, et al: The MEAN disease, *Concepts Pediatr Neurosurg* 5:154–164, 1985.

DUNN V, BALE JF, ZIMMERMAN RA, et al: MRI in children with postinfectious disseminated encephalomyelitis. *Magn Reson Imaging* 4:25–32, 1986.

EDWARDS MSB, WARA WM, CIRCILLO SG, et al: Focal brainstem astrocytomas causing symptoms of involvement of the facial nucleus: long-term survival in six pediatric cases. *J Neurosurg* 80:20–25, 1994.

FAIRBURN B, LARKIN IM: A cyst of Rathke's cleft. *J Neurosurg* 21:223–225, 1964.

FARWELL JR, DOHRMANN GJ, FLANNERY JT: Central nervous system tumors in children. *Cancer* 40:3123–3132, 1977.

FLETCHER WA, IMES RK, HOYT WF: Chiasmal gliomas: Appearance and long-term changes demonstrated by computerized tomography. *J Neurosurg* 65:154–159, 1986.

GANTI SR, HILAL SK, STEIN BM, et al: CT of pineal region tumors. *Am J Roentgenol* 146:451–458, 1986.

GEISSINGER J, BUCY P: Astrocytomas of the cerebellum in children: Long term study: *Arch Neurol* 29:125–135, 1971.

GOL A, MCKISSACK W: The cerebellar astrocytomas: A report on 98 verified cases. *J Neurosurg* 16:287–296, 1959.

GOMORI JM, GROSSMAN RI, GOLDBERG HI, et al: Occult cerebral vascular malformations: High field MR imaging. *Radiology* 158:707–713, 1986.

GUSNARD DA: Cerebellar neoplasms in children. *Semin Roentgenol* 25(3):263–278, 1990.

HEIDEMAN RL, PACKER RJ, ALBRIGHT LA, et al: Tumors of the central nervous system, in Pizzo RA, Poplack DG (eds), *Principles and Practice of Pediatric Oncology*, Philadelphia, Lippincott, 1989, pp 505–553.

HOFFMAN HJ, HENDRICK EB, HUMPHREYS RP: Management of medulloblastoma. *Clin Neurosurg* 30:226–245, 1983.

HOPE DG, MULVIHILL JJ: Malignancy in neurofibromatosis, in Riccardi VM, Mulvihill JJ (eds), *Neurofibromatosis*. Advances in Neurology, vol 29, New York, Raven Press, 1981, pp 33–35.

JELINEK J, SMIRNIOTOPOULOS JG, PARISH JE, et al: Lateral ventricular neoplasms of the brain: differential diagnosis based on clinical, CT and MR findings. *AJNR* 11:567–574, 1990.

JENKIN RDT, SIMPSON WJK, KEEN CW: Pineal and suprasellar germinomas. *J Neurosurg* 48:99–107, 1978.

KILGORE DP, STROTHER CM, STARSHAK RJ, et al: Pineal germinoma: MR imaging. *Radiology* 158:435–438, 1986.

KOCH KJ, SMITH RR: Gd-DTPA enhancement in MR imaging of central pontine myelinolysis. *AJNR* 10(suppl):558, 1989.

KRAMER ED, RAFTO S, PACKER RJ, et al: Comparison of myelography with computed tomography follow-up vs. gadolinium magnetic resonance imaging for subarachnoid metastatic disease in children. *Neurology* 41:46–50, 1991.

KUCHARCZYK W, PECK WW, KELLY WM, et al: Rathke cleft cysts: CT, MR imaging, and pathological features. *Radiology* 165:491–495, 1987.

KUN LE, KOVNER EH, SANFORD RA: Ependymomas in children. *Pediatr Neurosci* 14:57–63, 1988.

LAURENCE KM: The biology of choroid plexus papilloma in infancy and childhood. *Acta Neurochir (Wien)* 50:79–90, 1979.

LEE Y, VAN TASSEL P, BRUNER JM, et al: Juvenile pilocytic astrocytomas: CT and MR characteristics. *AJNR* 10:363–370, 1989.

LIPPER MH, EBERHARD DA, PHILLIPS CD, et al: Pleomorphic xanthoastrocytoma, a distinctive astroglial tumor: Neuroradiologic and pathologic features. *AJNR* 14:1397–1404, 1993.

LIU HM, BOGGS J, KIDD J: Ependymomas of childhood: I. Histological survey and clinicopathological correlation. *Childs Brain* 2:92–110, 1976.

MANTRAVADI R, PHATAK R, BELLUR S, et al: Brain stem gliomas. An autopsy study of 25 cases. *Cancer* 49:1294–1296, 1982.

MILHORAT TH, HAMMOCK MK, DAVIS DA, et al: Choroid plexus papilloma: Proof of cerebrospinal fluid overproduction. *Childs Brain* 2:273–289, 1976.

MULLER-FORELL W, SCHROTH G, EGAN PJ: MR imaging in tumors of the pineal region. *Neuroradiology* 30:224–231, 1988.

NAIDICH TP, ZIMMERMAN RA: Primary brain tumors in children. *Semin Roentgenol* 19:100–114, 1984.

ONOYAMA Y, ONO K, NAKAJIMA T, et al: Radiation therapy of pineal tumors. *Radiology* 130:757–760, 1979.

OXENHANDLER DC, SAYERS MP: The dilemma of childhood optic gliomas. *J Neurosurg* 48:34–41, 1978.

PACKER R, ALLEN J, NIELSON S, et al: Brainstem glioma: Clinical manifestations of meningeal gliomatosis. *Ann Neurol* 14:177–182, 1983a.

PACKER RJ, SAVINO PJ, BILANIUK L, et al: Chiasmatic gliomas of childhood: A reappraisal of natural history and effectiveness of cranial irradiation. *Childs Brain* 10:393–403, 1983b.

PACKER RJ, SUTTON LN, ROSENSTOCK JG, et al: Pineal region tumors of childhood. *Pediatrics* 74:97–103, 1984.

PACKER RJ, SIEGEL KR, SUTTON LN, et al: Leptomeningeal dissemination of primary central nervous system tumors of childhood. *Ann Neurol* 18:217–227, 1985.

PACKER RJ, SUTTON LN, D'ANGIO G, et al: Management of children with primitive neuroectodermal tumors of the posterior fossa/medulloblastoma. *Pediatr Neurosci* 12:272–282, 1985–1986.

PACKER RJ, LITTMAN PA, SPOSTO RM, et al: Results of a pilot study of hyperfractionated radiation therapy for children with brain stem gliomas. *Int J Radiat Oncol Biol Phys* 13:1647–1651, 1987.

PACKER RJ, BILANIUK LT, COHEN BH, et al: Intracranial visual pathway: gliomas in children with neurofibromatosis. *Neurofibromatosis* 1:212–222, 1988.

PATEL SR, BUCKNER JC, SMITHSON WA, et al: Cisplatin-based chemotherapy in primary central nervous system germ cell tumors. *J Neurooncol* 12:47–52, 1992.

PENDERGRASS TW, MILSTEIN JM, GEYER RJ, et al: Eight drugs in one-day chemotherapy for brain tumors: Experience in 107 children and rationale for preradiation chemotherapy. *J Clin Oncol* 5:1221–1231, 1987.

PUSEY E, KORTMAN KE, FLANNIGAN BD, et al: MR of craniopharyngiomas: Tumor delineating and characterization. *AJNR* 8:439–444, 1987.

RAMONDI A, TOMITA T: Medulloblastoma in childhood: Comparative results of partial and total resection. *Childs Brain* 5:310–328, 1979.

RAO KCVG, FITZ CR, HARWOOD-NACH DC: Craniopharyngiomas in children: Neuroradiological evaluation. *Rev Interam Radiol* 2:149–157, 1977.

ROBERTSON PL, MURASZKO KM, BRUNBERG JA, et al: Pediatric midbrain tumors: a benign subgroup of brainstem gliomas. *Pediatr Neurosurg* 22:65–73, 1995.

RORKE LB: The cerebellar medulloblastoma and its relationship to primitive neuroectodermal tumors. *J Neuropathol Exp Neurol* 42:1–15, 1983.

RORKE LB, GILES FH, DAVIS RL, et al: Revision of the World Health Organization classification of brain tumors for childhood brain tumors. *Cancer* 56:1869–1886, 1985.

RORKE LB: Relationship of morphology of ependymoma in children to prognosis. *Prog Exp Tumor Res* 30:170–174, 1987.

ROSENSTOCK JG, PACKER RJ, BILANIUK LT, et al: Chiasmatic optic glioma treated with chemotherapy: A preliminary report. *J Neurosurg* 63:862–866, 1985.

ROSS DA, NORMAN D, WILSON CB: Radiologic characteristic and results of surgical management of Rathke's cysts in 43 patients. *Neurosurgery* 39(2):173–178, 1992.

RUSSELL DS, RUBINSTEIN LJ: *Pathology of Tumours of the Nervous System,* Baltimore, Williams & Wilkins, 1989.

RUSTIN GJ, NEWLAND ES, BAGSHAWE KD, et al: Successful management of metastatic and primary germ cell tumors of the brain. *Cancer* 57:2108–2113, 1986.

SAVOIARDO M, PASSERINI A: CT, angiography and RN scans in intracranial cavernous hemangiomas. *Neuroradiology* 16:256–260, 1978.

SEGALL HD, BATNITZKY'S S, ZEE C, et al: Computed tomography in the diagnosis of intracranial neoplasms in children. *Cancer* 56:1748–1755, 1985.

SHELINE GE: Radiation therapy of brain tumors. *Cancer* 39:873–881, 1977.

SMITH RR: Brain stem tumors. *Semin Roentgenol* 25(3): 249–262, 1990.

SMITH RR, ZIMMERMAN RA, PACKER RJ, et al: Pediatric brainstem glioma: Post-radiation MR follow-up. *Neuroradiology* 32:265–271, 1990.

SPAGNOLI MV, GOLDBERG HI, GROSSMAN RI, et al: High-field MRI of intracranial meningiomas. *Radiology* 161: 369–375, 1986.

SPAGNOLI MV, GROSSMAN RI, PACKER RJ, et al: Magnetic resonance imaging determination of gliomatosis cerebri. *Neuroradiology* 29:15–18, 1987.

SPOTO GP, PRESS GA, HESSELINK JR, et al: Intracranial ependymoma and subependymoma: MR manifestations. *AJNR* 11:83–91, 1990.

STATES LJ, RUTSTEIN R, ZIMMERMAN, RA: Imaging of pediatric central nervous system HIV infection. *Int J Neuroradiol* 3:42–56, 1997.

STEINBERG GK, SHUER LM, CONLEY FK, et al: Evolution and outcome in malignant astroglial neoplasms of the cerebellum. *J Neurosurg* 62:9–17, 1985.

SWARTZ JD, ZIMMERMAN RA, BILANIUK LT: Computed tomography of intracranial ependymomas. *Radiology* 143: 97–101, 1982.

TAMPIERI D, MAMDJIAN R, MELANSON D, et al: Intracerebral gangliogliomas in patients with partial complex seizures: CT and MR imaging findings. *AJNR* 12:749–755, 1991.

TENNY RT, LAWS ER, YOUNGE BR, et al: The neurosurgical management of optic glioma. *J Neurosurg* 57:452–458, 1982.

THOMSETT MJ, CONTE FA, KAPLAN SL, et al: Endocrine and neurologic outcome in children with craniopharyngioma: Review of effect of treatment in 42 patients. *J Pediatr* 97:728–738, 1980.

TIEN RD: Intraventricular mass lesions of the brain: CT and MR findings. *Am J Roentgenol* 157:1283–1290, 1991.

TORTORI-DONATI P, FONDELLI MP, CAMA A, et al: Ependymomas of the posterior cranial fossa: CT and MRI findings. *Neuroradiology* 37:238–243, 1995.

WINSTON K, GILLES FH, LEVITON A, et al: Cerebellar gliomas in children. *JNCI* 58:833–838, 1977.

WOLMAN L, BALMFORTH CG: Precocious puberty due to a hypothalamic hamartoma in a patient surviving to late middle age. *J Neurol Neurosurg Psychiatry* 26:275, 1963.

YOUNG J, MILLER R: Incidence of malignant tumors in U.S. children. *J Pediatr* 86:254–258, 1975.

YOUNG SC, ZIMMERMAN RA, NOWELL MA, et al: Giant cystic craniopharyngiomas. *Neuroradiology* 29:468–473, 1987.

ZIMMERMAN RA, BILANIUK LT, BRUNO L, et al: Computed tomography of cerebellar astrocytoma. *AJR* 130:170–174, 1978a.

ZIMMERMAN RA, BILANIUK LT, PAHLAJANI H: Spectrum of medulloblastomas demonstrated by computed tomography. *Radiology* 126:137–141, 1978b.

ZIMMERMAN RA, BILANIUK LT, LITTMAN P, et al: Computed tomography of pediatric craniofacial sarcoma. *CT: J Comput Tomogr* 2:113–121, 1978c.

ZIMMERMAN RA, BILANIUK LT: Computed tomography of intracerebral gangliogiomas. *CT: J Comput Tomogr* 3:24–30, 1979a.

ZIMMERMAN RA, BILANIUK LT: Cranial CT of epidermoid and congenital fatty tumors of maldevelopmental origin. *CT: J Comput Tomogr* 3:40–50, 1979b.

ZIMMERMAN RA, BILANIUK LT: Computed tomography of choroid plexus lesions. *CT: J Comput Tomogr* 3(2):93–103, 1979c.

ZIMMERMAN RA, BILANIUK LT: Computed tomography of primary and secondary craniocerebral neuroblastoma. *AJNR* 1:431–434, 1980a.

ZIMMERMAN RA, BILANIUK LT, Wood JH, et al: Computed tomography of pineal, para pineal and histologically related tumors. *Radiology* 137:669–677, 1980b.

ZIMMERMAN RA, BILANIUK LT: Age related incidence of pineal calcification detected by CT. *Radiology* 142:659–662, 1982.

ZIMMERMAN RA, BILANIUK LT, HACKNEY DB: Applications of magnetic resonance imaging in diseases of the pediatric central nervous system. *Magnet Reson Imaging* 4:11–24, 1986.

ZIMMERMAN RA, BILANIUK LT, SCHUT L, et al: Medical imaging of pediatric brain tumors. *Prog Exp Tumor Res* 30:61–80, 1987*a*.

ZIMMERMAN RA, BILANIUK LT, SZE G: Intracranial infection, in Brant-Zawadski M, Norman D (eds), *Magnetic Resonance Imaging of the Central Nervous System,* New York, Raven Press, 1987*b*, pp 235–257.

ZIMMERMAN RA, BILANIUK LT: CT and MR: Diagnosis and evolution of head injury, stroke, and brain tumors. *Neuropsychology* 3:191–230, 1989*a*.

ZIMMERMAN RA: Imaging of intrasellar, suprasellar, and parasellar tumors. *Semin Roentgenol* 25(2):174–197, 1990*a*.

ZIMMERMAN RA: Pediatric supratentorial tumors. *Semin Roentgenol* 25(3):225–248, 1990*b*.

ZIMMERMAN A: The phakomatoses, In Ishibashi Y, Hori Y (eds), *Tuberous, Sclerosis and Neurofibromatosis: Epidemiology, Pathophysiology, Biology and Management,* Amsterdam, Elsevier, 1990*c*, pp 249–280.

ZIMMERMAN RA, GUSNARD DA, BILANIUK LT: Gadolinium DTPA enhanced MR evaluation of pediatric brain tumors. *Am J Pediatr Hematol Oncol,* 1991.

ZIMMERMAN RA, BILANIUK LT, REBSAMEN S: Magnetic resonance imaging of pediatric posterior fossa tumors. *Pediatr Neurosurg* 18:58–64, 1992.

ZIMMERMAN RA: Pineal region masses: imaging, in Wilkins RH, Rengachary SS (eds): *Neurosurgery,* New York, McGraw-Hill, 1996, pp 1003–1018.

# 9 INTRACRANIAL METASTATIC DISEASE

*Carl E. Johnson*

*Gordon Sze*

## CONTENTS

Metastasis to the central nervous system is a relatively common occurrence in patients with systemic cancer. Approximately 15 percent of patients with a systemic malignancy can be expected to develop neurological signs or symptoms during the course of illness (Posner 1978). Among these patients, intracranial metastatic disease is one of the most common causes of the neurological disorder. Headache is the most frequent presenting symptom, occurring in about 50 percent of patients (Posner 1979). Motor signs are more common than are mental and personality changes. Extrapyramidal signs are uncommon even with metastases to the basal ganglia (Lesse 1954). In approximately 15 percent of patients, a seizure is the presenting event (Posner 1979). Seizures are more common in children younger than 15 years, constituting an initial symptom in about 50 percent (Graus 1983).

Intracranial metastases have been found in 11 to 35 percent of patients with systemic malignancies in various autopsy series (Posner 1978; Abrams 1950; Lesse 1954; Earle 1954). The incidence of intracranial metastases may be considerably higher, however, when specific tumor types are considered. For example, melanoma and lung carcinoma commonly metastasize to the brain, while brain metastases are an infrequent occurrence in patients with ovarian carcinoma. Consequently, a patient with malignant melanoma who presents with neurological symptoms is likely to have brain metastases, while the opposite is true for a patient with ovarian carcinoma (Posner 1978).

The site and type of intracranial metastasis also vary in accordance with the primary tumor type. For instance, lung carcinoma most often metastasizes to the brain parenchyma, while lymphoma and leukemia most frequently involve the leptomeninges. Intracranial prostate metastases are commonly dural in location, with parenchymal metastases being rare (Posner 1978; Lynes 1986; Castaldo 1983).

Although series differ in regard to the most frequently encountered metastatic lesions, in adults common primary tumors that metastasize to the brain are, in decreasing order of frequency, lung, breast, melanoma, genitourinary tract, and gastrointestinal tract. Lymphoma or leukemia often metastasize to the leptomeninges, whereas direct or perineural tumor extension occurs in head and neck neoplasms (Posner 1978; Potts 1980; Lesse 1954; Vieth 1965). In children, solid tumors that metastasize intracranially include sarcomas (especially osteogenic), germ cell tumors, Wilms' tumors, and uncommonly, neuroblastoma (Table 9-1) (Graus 1983). Pulmonary metastases usually precede brain metastases in children (Graus 1983; Chee 1987). The rarity of pulmonary metastases in patients with neuroblastoma probably explains the infrequent occurrence of brain metastases in this disease.

## Table 9-1 Common Parenchymal Brain Metastases

| ADULTS | CHILDREN |
| --- | --- |
| Lung | Sarcomas |
| Breast | Germ cell tumors |
| Melanoma | Wilms' tumor |
| Genitourinary tract | Neuroblastoma |
| Gastrointestinal tract | |

## Table 9-2   Sources of Intracranial Metastases

Hematogenous spread to the brain or meninges
Cerebrospinal fluid dissemination
Intracranial extension of skull base or calvarial metastases
Perineural or direct extension of head and neck neoplasms

Metastatic lesions arise through a number of routes. The most common is hematogenous spread of a tumor to the brain and meninges through the arterial circulation. Dissemination of malignant cells in the cerebrospinal fluid, secondary invasion of the meninges and brain by metastatic disease involving the calvarium and skull base, and direct or perineural intracranial extension of head and neck neoplasms are alternative routes (Table 9-2). Contrast-enhanced MR (CEMR) is the most sensitive imaging method and procedure of choice for the detection of intracranial metastases, though computed tomography maintains an important role.

## PARENCHYMAL METASTASES

Metastases to the brain may occur anywhere within the parenchyma, though they are most frequently located at the corticomedullary junction in the anatomic water shed area of the main cerebral arteries, in keeping with arterial tumor microemboli (Delattre 1988). Multiple metastases are more common though single lesions occur almost as often, particularly with some primary tumors (Posner 1978; Delattre 1988; Bindal 1993). Certain tumors tend to have a single metastasis, while others have a propensity to present with multiple lesions. Renal cell carcinoma metastases and metastases arising from tumors of the pelvis and abdomen are much more likely to be single lesions, while those of lung carcinoma and melanoma are usually multiple. Breast carcinoma metastases are about evenly divided between single and multiple lesions.

In general, metastases are evenly distributed between the supratentorial and infratentorial compartments when the respective proportion of the brain in each of these structures is considered (Posner 1978; Pechova'-Peterova' 1986). However, single metastasis of renal cell carcinoma and of pelvic or abdominal tumors are very often infratentorial (Posner 1978; Delattre 1988). The reasons for this phenomenon are unknown. Batson's vertebral venous plexus is not a probable source of tumor spread, since there is not an increased incidence of spine or skull base lesions in patients with pelvic and abdominal tumors. These tumors may have an affinity for different parts of the brain and meninges because of unique biological and surface properties (Delattre 1988; Brunson 1978). Another reason for this phenomenon may be related to the "fertile-soil" hypothesis; that is, circulating tumor cells arrest in a variety of regions, but metastases occur only in certain locations (Delattre 1988; Cairncross 1983). In addition to lesions in the brain parenchyma, metastases may arise within the pineal gland, the pituitary gland, and the ventricles (Fig. 9-1) (Schreiber 1982; Morrison 1984; Kart 1986; Jelinek 1990).

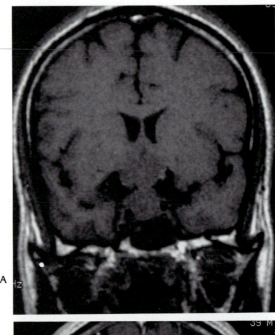

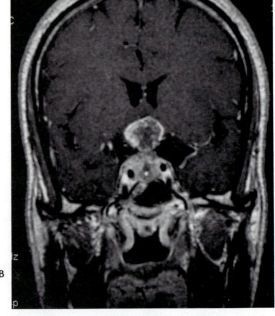

***Figure 9-1*** **Breast carcinoma metastasis to the pituitary gland.** **A.** Coronal precontrast and **B.** CEMR through the sella show an enhancing intrasellar mass with suprasellar extension. The optic chiasm is compressed.

Metastases may be hypodense, isodense, or hyperdense relative to the adjacent brain on non-contrast-enhanced CT (NCCT). Low-density lesions are often encountered with metastases arising from lung, breast, or kidney. (Potts 1980; Deck 1976; Tarver 1984). There is usually associated surrounding white matter edema, which is also of decreased density. The tumor margin may be difficult if not impossible to separate from surrounding edema.

Hyperdense lesions are frequently seen on NCCT in lesions arising from the gastrointestinal tract or small round cell tumors, or with hemorrhagic metastases such as melanoma or choriocarcinoma (Fig. 9-2) (Potts 1980; Deck 1976; Ruelle 1987). Calcification rarely causes increased attenuation since, with the exception of osteogenic sarcoma metastases, calcification is uncommon in untreated metastases (Fig. 9-3) (Table 9-3) (Anand 1982; Hwang 1993). Although secondary lymphoma usually metastasizes to the leptomeninges, parenchymal

## Table 9-3    Calcified Metastases

Osteogenic sarcoma
Mucinous adenocarcinoma
Treated metastases (radiotherapy or chemotherapy)

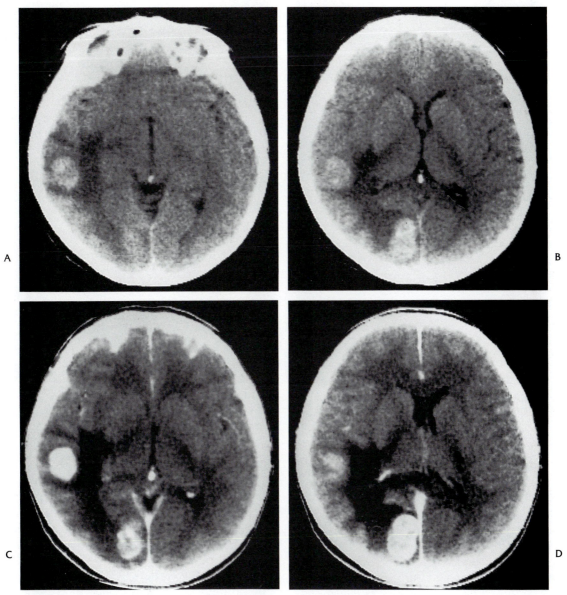

***Figure 9-2*** **Colon carcinoma metastases. A, B.** NCCT shows two hyperdense masses in the right posterior temporal and occipital lobes with surrounding edema. **C, D.** The lesions enhance homogeneously following contrast administration.

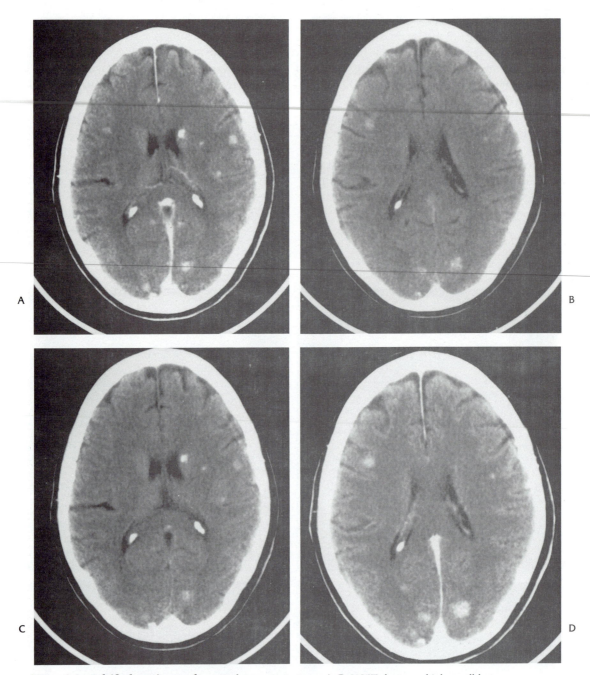

***Figure 9-3*** **Calcified mucinous adenocarcinoma metastases A, B.** NCCT shows multiple small hyperdense lesions. Calcification was found on biopsy. **C, D.** After contrast administration, the lesions enhance. Additional enhancing lesions are seen which were inapparent on the NCCT.

lesions occur that are often isodense to mildly hyperdense (Yang 1985; Bennett 1983; Brant-Zawadzki 1978; Holtas 1984). Similarly, leukemic parenchymal metastases (chloromas), though rare, are usually hyperdense (Barnett 1986). The higher attenuation of lymphoma, leukemia, and other metastases in which neither calcification nor hemorrhage is found on pathological examination may be caused by a more compact cellular density and high nuclear to cytoplasmic ratio.

Different lesions from a single primary source may have both increased and decreased attenuation from hemorrhage in some but not all the lesions. This is frequently the case with melanoma. Variable densities may also be found in metastases from renal cell and lung carcinomas.

Finally, metastases may be isodense on NCCT. In these instances, their presence must be inferred from associated mass effect and edema. Lesions without a

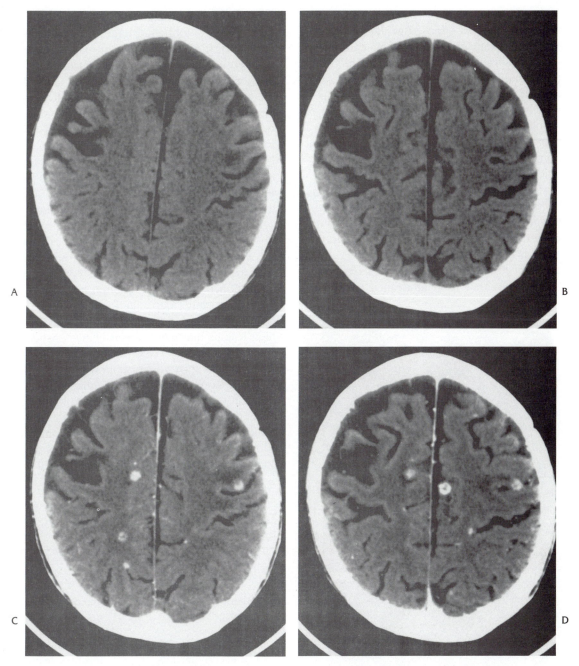

***Figure 9-4*** **Metastatic lung carcinoma. A, B.** NCCT images do not show any apparent lesions. A small area of low-density edema is seen in left posterior frontal subcortical white matter, which could be interpreted as ischemic change. **C, D.** Multiple lesions are seen following contrast injection.

significant amount of surrounding edema can be extremely difficult to visualize without the use of contrast material (Fig. 9-4). In addition, multiple bilateral lesions may exert equal "balanced" pressure, obscuring any apparent focal mass effect. Consequently, it is necessary to obtain a CECT study when searching for metastases, both to better define the borders of the neoplasm from surrounding edema and to detect lesions that are inapparent on NCCT.

Most metastases enhance after a standard dose of intravenous contrast (approximately 40 g of iodine), though in a number of cases additional lesions may be identified with delayed scans obtained about 1 to 1.5 hours after a high-dose contrast infusion (80 to 85 g of iodine) (Hayman 1980; Shalen 1981). Contrast enhancement occurs secondary to breakdown of the blood-brain barrier.

After contrast infusion, a metastasis may show diffuse,

nodular, or ringlike enhancement. The ringlike enhancement is frequently thick, as opposed to the thin rim of enhancement more often seen surrounding an abscess. However, it is not always possible to differentiate a ring-enhancing metastasis from an abscess or a resolving hematoma on CT. Occasionally, delayed scans show permeation of contrast throughout the lesion in the case of a tumor but not in an abscess or hematoma. Regions of metastases that fail to enhance are related to central necrosis. Contrast may accumulate within a necrotic cystic cavity and produce a fluid-fluid level. Some metastases may have true nonnecrotic cystic components (Fig. 9-5). These components typically are more sharply marginated than are regions of necrosis. Hemorrhagic fluid levels have been described in cystic renal cell carcinoma and other metastases (Kaiser 1983).

Contrast-enhanced MR is the procedure of choice for the detection and evaluation of intracranial metastases

(Haughton 1986; Healey 1987; Russell 1987; Sze 1990*b*, Davis 1991). Nonhemorrhagic metastatic lesions typically appear as masses that are subtly hypointense to isointense compared with white matter on $T_1$-weighted images ($T_1$WI). On proton density and $T_2$-weighted images ($T_2$WI), metastases are usually hyperintense. Hemorrhagic metastases have variable signal intensity on both $T_1$- and $T_2$-weighted sequences owing to the metabolic products of hemoglobin that are present. Melanoma metastases may also have a variable appearance related both to hemorrhage and melanin content in the tumor. Metastatic mucin-secreting adenocarcinomas or highly cellular tumors with a high nuclear to cytoplasmic ratio may be hypointense on $T_2$-weighted images (Egelhoff 1992). Surrounding edema may also be seen as subtle white matter hypointensity on $T_1$WI with increased signal intensity on $T_2$WI (Table 9-4).

On noncontrast MR, it is often not possible to distinguish metastatic deposits from regions of ischemic change, edema, and demyelination or from other benign lesions that have similar characteristics (Sze 1988; Graif 1985; Bydder 1984). Metastases typically enhance following contrast administration (Felix 1985; Claussen 1985). Lesions which do not enhance are unlikely to be metastases (Elster 1992). Like CT, lesions may show solid, ring, or nodular enhancement.

Surgical resection of a solitary brain metastasis with adjuvant radiotherapy may improve length of survival and functional independence (MacGee 1971; Sundare-

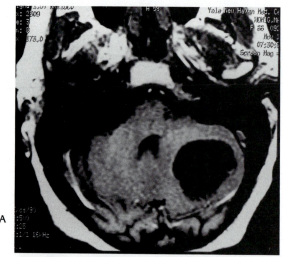

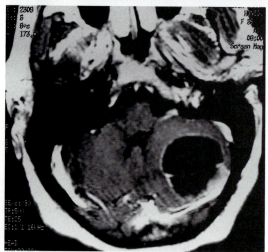

***Figure 9-5*** **Renal cell carcinoma metastasis A.** Axial precontrast and **B.** Postcontrast $T_1$-weighted images show a solitary cystic left cerebellar renal cell carcinoma metastasis. (*Reprinted from Hussman 1996.*)

### Table 9-4    Imaging Findings of Parenchymal Metastases

| CT | MRI |
|---|---|
| Hypodense (most common) or isodense mass | Isointense to mildly hypointense mass on $T_1$WI |
| Hyperdense mass—hemorrhagic metastases, or in GI tract or mucin producing adenocarcinomas, small round cell tumors including lymphoma and leukemia, and calcified metastases (rare) | Hyperintense mass on $T_2$WI or FLAIR—may be relatively hypointense to surrounding edema |
| | Hyperintense lesions on $T_1$WI—hemorrhagic metastases or melanoma |
| | Hypo-intense mass on $T_2$WI—mucinous adenocarcinoma or hemorrhagic metastases |
| Nodular, diffuse, or ring-like enhancement, surrounding low-density edema (common) | Nodular, diffuse ring-like enhancement |
| | Edema—hypointense on $T_1$WI and hyperintense on $T_2$WI or FLAIR images (common) |

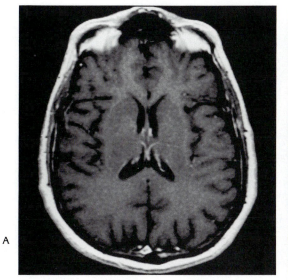

A

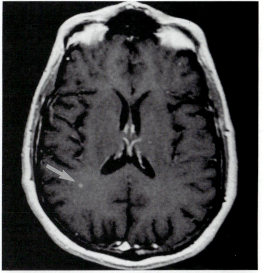

B

C

san 1985; Magilligan 1986; Mandell 1986; Patchell 1986, 1990; Smalley 1992). It is desirable to perform CEMR before undertaking surgical resection of a presumed solitary lesion to ensure that there are not small lesions that are not apparent on CT. Care must be taken in interpreting punctate foci of enhancement in the basal ganglia or white matter in elderly patients as metastases, since these foci may represent subacute enhancing lacunar infarcts (Sze 1990*b*). If there is doubt about whether a punctate region of enhancement is a metastasis or a subacute lacunar infarct, a follow-up scan can help differentiate the two.

Delayed images do not show a consistent advantage over those obtained immediately after contrast infusion, though in some cases metastases are better seen on delayed CEMR scans (Sze 1990*a,b*; Haustein 1992; Yuh 1995). Although the usual dose of contrast is 0.1 mmol/kg, a higher dose (0.2 to 0.3 mmol/kg) may improve tumor visualization (Niendorf 1987; Yuh 1994; Yuh 1995). Also contrast-enhanced magnetization transfer MR imaging in which an off-resonance pulse selectively saturates protons bound to macromolecules may better demonstrate lesions (Finelli 1994; Mehta 1995). Magnetization transfer MR imaging may also show white matter abnormalities not detected on other sequences, which may provide better delineation of radiation portals (Boorstein 1994). It has been advocated that routine use of high-dose contrast is cost-effective by showing additional lesions in patients thought to have solitary metastases on standard dose studies, thereby eliminating surgery in some patients (Mayr 1994). However, most patients have multiple lesions on a single-dose study. Finding more lesions with high-dose MR imaging does not change therapy in these patients. Also, it is not clear that patients with one or

*Figure 9-6* **Punctate enhancing lesion in a patient with melanoma. A.** Single-dose and **B.** triple-dose CEMR. A punctate-enhancing lesion is seen only on the triple-dose study. **C.** Six-month follow-up CEMR with triple-dose gadolinium shows this lesion less apparently, suggesting this is more likely a small vascular structure than a metastasis.

more additional punctate enhancing lesions would not benefit from surgery or that a solitary punctate enhancing lesion should be resected, since studies showing the effectiveness of surgical resection of metastases did not consider high-dose versus standard-dose MR (Black 1994). Also, in some cases, high-dose MR may lead to greater uncertainty in diagnosis. Small nonneoplastic lesions such as telangiectasias or other vascular structures may be apparent only on high-dose studies (Fig. 9-6) (Kamamura 1995). This may inappropriately preclude resection of a true solitary metastasis or suggest a small metastasis when one is not actually present.

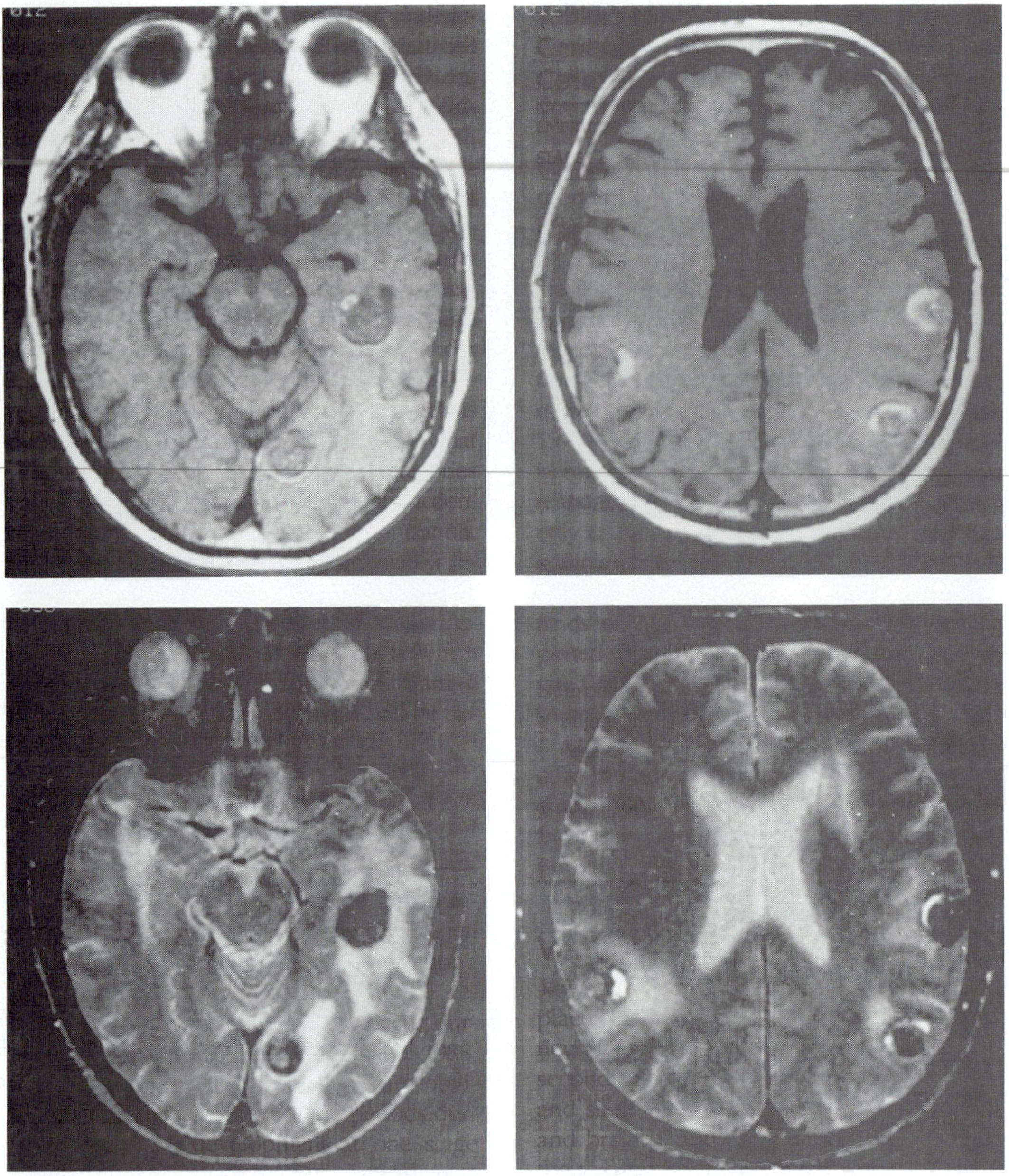

***Figure 9-7*** **Melanoma metastases. A.** and **B.** T$_1$WI (SE 600/20) show multiple heterogeneous metastases with regions of decreased and increased signal intensity. **C** and **D.** On comparable T$_2$WI (SE 2000/80), the lesions become predominantly markedly hypointense. Small regions of hyperintensity are seen, especially at the peripheral aspect of the lesions. The appearance is consistent with multiple hemorrhagic metastases with hemorrhage of variable age. Hyperintense white matter edema is seen surrounding the metastases.

Some additional consideration can be given to hemorrhagic metastases and melanoma. A number of metastatic lesions have a tendency to *hemorrhage*. These lesions include metastases from melanoma, renal cell carcinoma, choriocarcinoma, and thyroid carcinoma (Fig. 9-7) (Weisberg 1985*b*; Mandybur 1977). Although metastases from bronchogenic carcinoma do not have a high propensity to hemorrhage, hemorrhagic lesions are seen because lung carcinoma metastases are so frequently encountered (Table 9-5).

Hemorrhagic metastases may present clinically with the sudden onset of a neurological deficit caused by acute hemorrhage (Gildersleeve 1977; Mandybur 1977; Weir 1978; Little 1979; Bitoh 1984; van den Doel 1985; Weisberg 1985b). CT typically shows a hyperdense lesion secondary to hemorrhage. After contrast injection, there may be nodular, ringlike, or diffuse enhancement. CT features that aid in distinguishing hemorrhagic metastatic lesions from simple hemorrhage include: (1) hemorrhage in association with a mass of lower density,

## Table 9-5    Hemorrhagic Metastases

Melanoma
Renal cell carcinoma
Choriocarcinoma
Thyroid carcinoma
Bronchogenic carcinoma

(2) atypical location of a hemorrhage, (3) ring enhancement around a lesion at a time when interval enhancement would not be expected, and (4) a multiplicity of hemorrhagic lesions (Gildersleeve 1977).

MR is uniquely suited for the evaluation of hemorrhagic metastases. Simple intracerebral hemorrhage normally follows a complex but orderly progression of evolutionary changes in signal intensity on MR that are related to the metabolism of hemoglobin, clot retraction, changes in protein concentration, red cell lysis, and the accumulation of water in a hematoma (Bradley 1985; Gomori 1985, 1987; Di Chiro 1986; Zimmerman 1988; Hayman 1989a,b).

A number of MR features of hemorrhagic metastases distinguish these metastases from simple hematomas (Atlas 1987a). On spin-echo MR imaging, tumors may have a prolonged phase of decreased signal intensity on $T_2$WI (Fig. 9-6). This is secondary to the persistent presence of deoxyhemoglobin, perhaps related to continued oozing of blood from the lesion or rapid reabsorption of hemoglobin metabolites before methemoglobin can form (Atlas 1987a; Destian 1988). Unlike nonneoplastic bleeds, hemorrhagic tumors can demonstrate persistent hypointensity for weeks or even months. In addition, because of multiple episodes of bleeding, a heterogeneous appearance of a tumor hemorrhage is also common, with the simultaneous occurrence of multiple hemoglobin breakdown products from hemorrhages of different ages in the same lesion (Fig. 9-7). The complete hemosiderin rim that is characteristic of chronic nonneoplastic hematomas may be seen with metastatic lesions but is often diminished. Areas of abnormal soft-tissue signal are sometimes seen corresponding to nonhemorrhagic tumor tissue (Fig. 9-8). CEMR may be expected to show regions of nodular or ringlike enhancement, as are found on CECT.

Malignant melanoma metastases may also show variable MR signal intensity not only because of the propensity of a melanoma to hemorrhage but also because of the inherent paramagnetic effects of melanin (Woodruff 1987; Atlas 1987b; Atlas 1990). On NCCT melanoma has a variable appearance that depends on the presence or absence of hemorrhage, with decreased, mixed, or increased density (Enzmann 1978; Ginaldi 1981; Holtas 1981). Contrast enhancement is usually homogeneous, though ringlike enhancement does occur (Weisberg 1985a). Although the signal char-

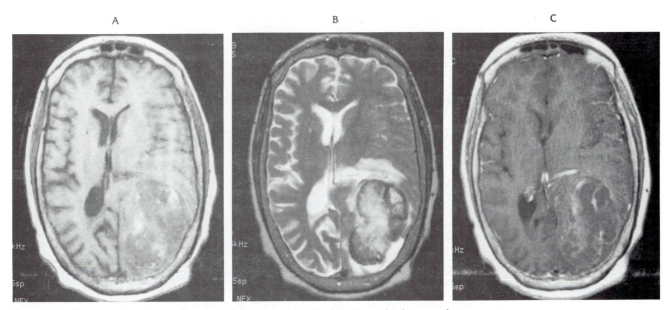

**A**            **B**            **C**

*Figure 9-8*  **Choriocarcinoma metastases. Axial A.** $T_1$-weighted and **B.** $T_2$-weighted images show a large left occipital mass of heterogeneous increased and decreased signal on both pulse sequences consistent with hemorrhage of variable age. Areas of hypointense signal on the $T_1$-weighted image are seen with corresponding hyperintensity on the $T_2$-weighted image, which are consistent with nonhemorrhagic soft tissue mass. **C.** Mild ringlike peripheral and ill-defined or linear central enhancement is seen.

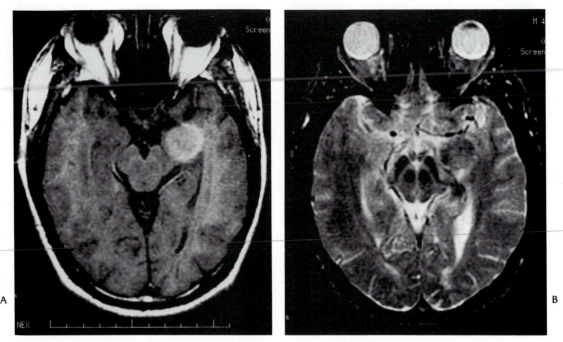

***Figure 9-9*** **Metastatic melanotic melanoma. A.** Axial noncontrast $T_1$-weighted and **B.** axial $T_2$-weighted images show a hyperintense and hypointense left temporal mass, respectively. Recent hemorrhage could have this appearance though the signal intensity of this lesion did not change on follow-up. The signal characteristics are related to the paramagnetic effects of melanin. *(Reprinted from Hussman 1996.)*

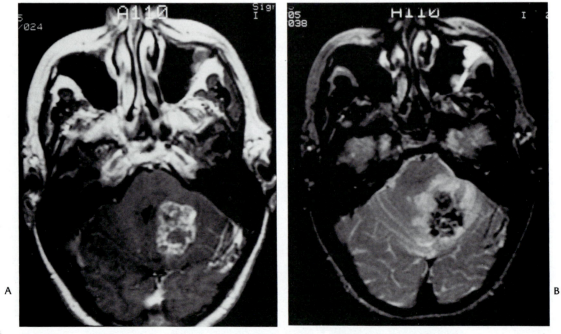

***Figure 9-10*** **Metastatic colon adenocarcinoma. A.** Axial postcontrast $T_1$-weighted image shows a heterogenously enhancing left cerebellar mass. **B.** The lesion is hypointense on the axial $T_2$-weighted image. No hemorrhage was found pathologically. *(Reprinted from Hussman 1996.)*

acteristics of melanoma on NCMR are also predominantly related to the presence or absence of hemorrhage, various melanoma subtypes may be able to be differentiated on the basis of signal intensity patterns (Atlas 1987*b*). Nonhemorrhagic melanotic melanoma is hyperintense on $T_1WI$ and mildly hypointense or isointense on $T_2WI$ (Fig. 9-9). Nonhemorrhagic amelanotic melanoma is mildly hypointense or isointense on $T_1WI$ and mildly hyperintense or isointense on $T_2WI$. The signal intensity of hemorrhagic melanoma depends on the age of the hemorrhage. As with CT, homogeneous enhancement is usually seen after contrast administration.

Another tumor that may have an unusual MR appearance is gastrointestinal carcinoma. Gastrointestinal adenocarcinoma metastatic to the brain may be hypointense and/or isointense on $T_1WI$ and hypointense on $T_2WI$ (Fig. 9-10). These are mucinous adenocarcinomas without blood or increased iron deposition histologically. The low signal intensity on $T_2WI$ has been proposed to be related to the proteinaceous mucin content within the lesion (Egelhoff 1992), though others have found no histological correlation to mucin content. Instead, the hypointensity of GI metastases was believed to represent the relatively shorter $T_2$ relaxation time of the primary tumor compared to the $T_2$ relaxation time of white matter (Camer 1994).

## LEPTOMENINGEAL CARCINOMATOSIS

Leptomeningeal metastases, or arachnoid-subarachnoid metastases, have been estimated to account for 8 to 10 percent of intracranial metastatic disease (Posner 1978; Lee 1984), though isolated leptomeningeal tumor is rare (Gonzalez-Vitale 1976). A patient with leptomeningeal carcinomatosis often has neurological symptoms more widespread than can be accounted for by the presence of a single lesion (Posner 1979). Furthermore, signs demonstrable on neurological examination are often more numerous than the patient's symptomatology would indicate (Wasserstrom 1982). This results from the widespread distribution of tumor cells throughout the CSF. Focal symptoms occur as a result of cell proliferation at multiple locations.

Tumor most often spreads to the leptomeninges through thin-walled meningeal vessels, with subsequent dissemination into the subarachnoid space (Wasserstrom 1982; Fischer-Williams 1955). There is diffuse or widespread multifocal tumor infiltration of the leptomeninges. Direct leptomeningeal invasion of tumor from adjacent structures can occur, as in a superficially placed parenchymal tumor, but is less common owing to a fibrotic meningeal reaction that walls off tumor, preventing its dissemination within the subarachnoid space.

Primary CNS tumors associated with leptomeningeal tumor spread include medulloblastoma, ependymoma, pineoblastoma, and retinoblastoma (Fig. 9-11) (Nadich 1984; Rippe 1990; Mackay 1984). Spread occurs through dissemination of cells in the subarachnoid

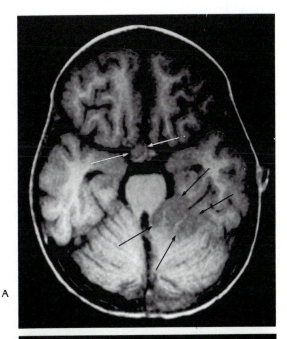

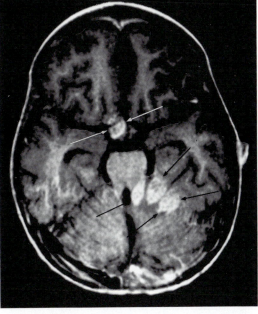

***Figure 9-11***  **Medulloblastoma with subarachnoid seeding. A.** NCMR shows a mass in the suprasellar cistern (white arrows). Subtle subarachnoid deposits are also seen along the left tentorial edge (black arrows). **B.** The contrast-enhanced $T_1$-weighted image shows enhancement of these subarachnoid metastases (arrows).

## Table 9-6   Leptomeningeal or Subarachnoid Metastases

| SYSTEMIC TUMORS | CNS PRIMARY |
| --- | --- |
| Lymphoma | Glioblastoma (adults) |
| Leukemia | Medulloblastoma |
| Melanoma | Ependymoma |
| Breast | Pineal tumors |
| Lung | Retinoblastoma |
| Neuroblastoma (children) | |

space. Glioblastomas may infrequently disseminate in the subarachnoid space. Among systemic malignancies, leptomeningeal carcinomatosis most commonly arises from lymphoma, leukemia, and melanoma, followed by breast and lung carcinoma (Table 9-6) (Lee 1984). In a patient with lymphoma, leptomeningeal tumor spread usually is from non-Hodgkin's lymphoma; intracranial Hodgkin's disease is rare (Sapozink 1983).

With leptomeningeal metastases CT may demonstrate obliteration of the subarachnoid space, basal cisterns, and sulci. After contrast infusion there may be sulcal-cisternal enhancement (Lee 1984; Ito 1986), especially in the basal cisterns, in the sylvian fissures, and along the high-convexity cortical sulci. Tentorial enhancement can also occur. The enhancement can be diffuse or localized. Since the tentorium normally enhances, enhancement should be considered significant only if it occurs over a widened area or is irregular in configuration. Within the ventricles, there may be ependymal or subependymal enhancement in a diffuse or a nodular pattern. This appearance is particularly characteristic of lymphoma (Dubois 1978). Leptomeningeal enhancement is not specific for meningeal carcinomatosis, and infectious and inflammatory processes or ischemic change may mimic meningeal metastases. Enhancement due to periventricular tumor spread must be differentiated clinically from ventriculitis.

Communicating hydrocephalus with or without leptomeningeal enhancement is the second most common abnormality found on CT after sulcal-cisternal enhancement (Lee 1984). Leptomeningeal disease impairs the reabsorption of CSF, resulting in mild to moderate symmetrical dilatation of the ventricular system with the subsequent development of increased intracranial pressure. Leptomeningeal metastases should be strongly considered in any patient with a systemic neoplasm who has communicating hydrocephalus on CT and MRI. Lumbar puncture may be required in making the diagnosis; repeated CSF examinations may be necessary.

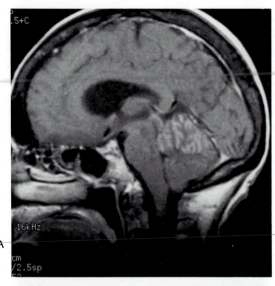

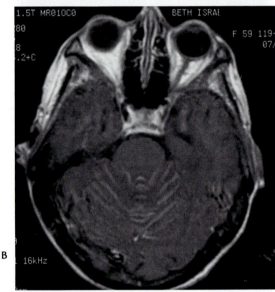

*Figure 9-12* **Leptomeningeal metastases from breast carcinoma. A.** Sagittal and **B.** axial contrast-enhanced MR images show cerebellar vermian sulci and folia enhancement secondary to leptomeningeal tumor.

CEMR is the most useful imaging test for the detection of leptomeningeal metastases (Sze 1989; Rippe 1990; Frank 1988). NCMR is relatively insensitive for showing leptomeningeal tumor (Krol 1988; Davis 1987). On MR, as on CT, meningeal enhancement is often seen within the basal cisterns, sylvian fissures, sulci, and along the tentorium (Fig. 9-12). Normal meningeal enhancement on MR is characteristically thin and discontinuous, primarily of the dura. Normal arachnoid and pia do not enhance (Sze 1993). Meningeal enhancement in carcinomatosis tends to show a nodular pattern, whereas a diffuse linear pattern is commonly present with inflammatory conditions (Phillips 1990). Less frequently, leptomeningeal metas-

## Table 9-7   Leptomeningeal Tumor— Imaging Findings

Sulcal, cisternal or ventricular enhancement
Hydrocephalus
Effacement of sulci and basilar cisterns
Diffuse or asymmetric (dural) enhancement on MRI
Cranial nerve enhancement

## Table 9-8   Meningeal Enhancement— Differential Considerations

Leptomeningeal tumor
Meningitis
Sarcoidosis
Vasculitis
Prior craniotomy
Shunt placement
Extra-axial fluid collections
Prior intrathecal chemotherapy or radiotherapy
Hydrocephalus

tases present as lobulated and isolated lesions (Lee 1989), including cranial nerve enhancement (Fig. 9-13). Enhancing subependymal metastases may also be found. Diffuse meningeal enhancement applied to the inner table of the skull, although not apparent on CECT, is frequently seen (Table 9-7) (Sze 1989). However, the presence of contrast enhancement does not necessarily indicate the presence of tumor, because meningeal enhancement related to other causes, such as meningitis, sarcoidosis, vasculitis, prior craniotomy, shunt placement, extra-axial fluid collections, prior intrathecal chemotherapy or radiotherapy, and hydrocephalus (Schumacher 1994), may appear identical with meningeal tumor spread (Table 9-8). Conversely, the absence of contrast enhancement does not exclude the possibility of leptomeningeal metastases. In some cases of recurrent medulloblastoma, subependymal metastases that do not enhance may be shown on $T_2WI$ but not on CEMR (Rollins 1990). Positive cytology is necessary to confirm the diagnosis.

A rare form of metastatic disease which does not in fact involve the leptomeninges, but which may also be considered here, is carcinomatous encephalitis. In this entity there are diffuse miliary punctate tumor nodules in a perivascular distribution. $T_2$-weighted images show multiple punctate hyperintensities in the basal ganglia and cortical gray matter which may not enhance (Nemzek 1993, Olsen 1987).

## CALVARIAL, SKULL BASE, AND DURAL METASTASES

Metastases to the skull or dura may occur from a variety of tumors. In adults, metastases from carcinoma of the lung, breast, and prostate are common. In the pe-

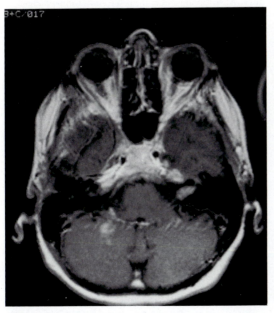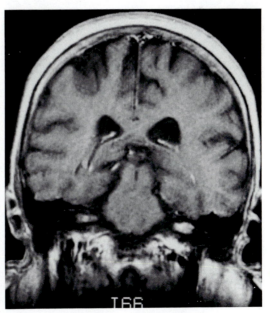

*Figure 9-13* **Leptomeningeal metastases from lung carcinoma. A, B.** Axial and coronal contrast-enhanced $T_1$-weighted images show enhancement of the cranial nerves within the internal auditory canals secondary to leptomeningeal tumor.

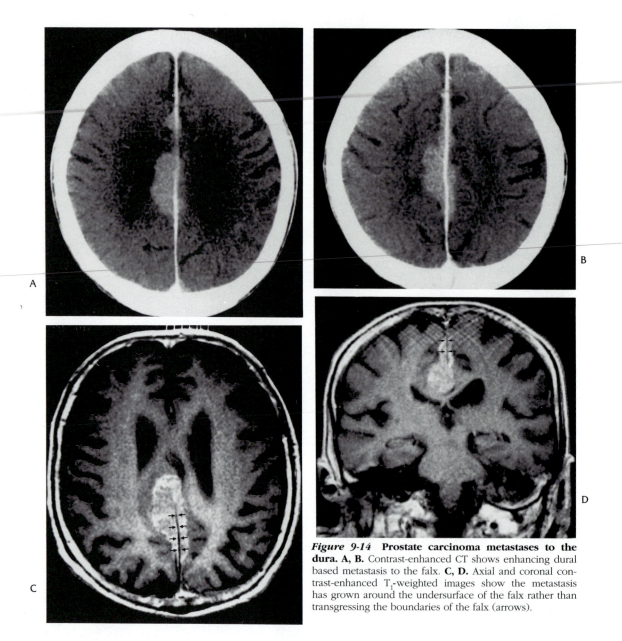

**Figure 9-14** **Prostate carcinoma metastases to the dura. A, B.** Contrast-enhanced CT shows enhancing dural based metastasis to the falx. **C, D.** Axial and coronal contrast-enhanced $T_1$-weighted images show the metastasis has grown around the undersurface of the falx rather than transgressing the boundaries of the falx (arrows).

diatric age group, neuroblastomas or sarcomas are more often seen (Posner 1978; Healy 1981).

Unless they are very aggressive, metastatic tumors generally do not transgress dural boundaries. Consequently, calvarial and epidural metastases do not usually involve the brain parenchyma (Posner 1978). Similarly, metastases generally do not cross the falx to invade the contralateral hemisphere.

Dural-based metastases, as can be found in prostate carcinoma, are easily recognized on CECT or MR (Fig. 9-14). Differentiation from meningioma may be difficult. Metastatic disease to the dura must be differentiated from the normal enhancement of the falx and tentorium seen on both CT and MR. Normal linear enhancement of sections of the dura, more pro-

nounced in the parasagittal regions near the pacchionian granulations, is present on MR (Sze 1989; West 1990). Dural or parenchymal carcinomatosis is a rare entity, in which there is diffuse infiltration of the dura by neoplastic cells. An enhancing thickened dural membrane is seen covering the brain (Tyrell 1987). Subdural hematomas occur in conjunction with dural carcinomatosis (Fig. 9-15).

In adults, metastases to the calvarium are usually lytic. However, prostate carcinoma can produce either a mixed lytic and blastic or a purely osteoblastic response. In the pediatric age group, rhabdomyosarcoma, neuroblastoma, lymphoma, and Langerhans' giant cell granulomatosis may produce bone destruction with intracranial extension of mass (Scotti 1982). In

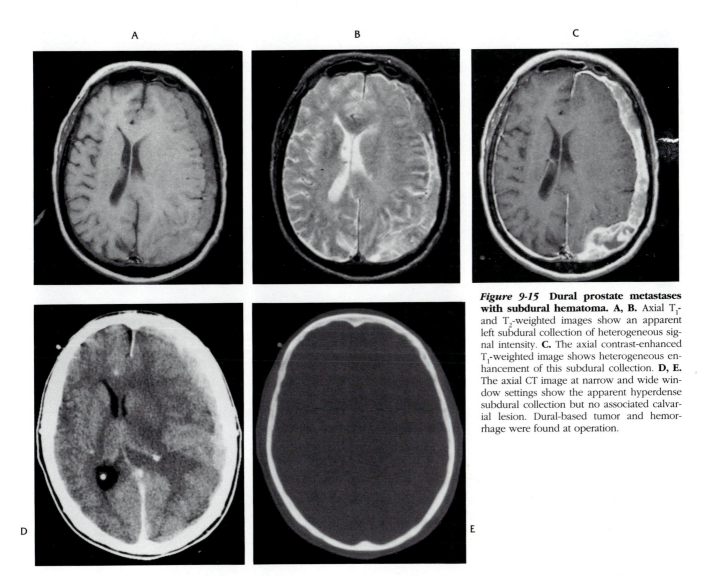

*Figure 9-15* **Dural prostate metastases with subdural hematoma. A, B.** Axial $T_1$- and $T_2$-weighted images show an apparent left subdural collection of heterogeneous signal intensity. **C.** The axial contrast-enhanced $T_1$-weighted image shows heterogeneous enhancement of this subdural collection. **D, E.** The axial CT image at narrow and wide window settings show the apparent hyperdense subdural collection but no associated calvarial lesion. Dural-based tumor and hemorrhage were found at operation.

neuroblastoma there may be a mixed osteolytic and blastic response. CT readily shows lytic calvarial and skull base lesions. Intracranial extension of the mass is also well shown. Sclerotic metastases to the calvarium can be somewhat more subtle.

On NCMR, recognition of skull metastases may require recognition of asymmetry of the normal diploic space marrow signal (West 1990). The normal diploic space may have several appearances, including (1) uniform high signal intensity on $T_1$WI owing to fatty marrow, (2) patchy nonuniform areas of hypointensity within hyperintense fatty marrow, or (3) predominantly low signal intensity (West 1990). The distribution of the diploic marrow signal, however, is usually uniform from side to side. Metastatic lesions may be seen on NCMR as regions of hypointense tumor replacing the normal hyperintense marrow signal in an asymmetrical fashion (West 1990; Daffner 1986). This is most easily recognized in regions of high fat concentration, such as the skull base. If the calvarial diploic space is of predominantly low-signal intensity, metastases can be difficult to recognize on NCMR.

After contrast injection, the normal calvarial diploic space in adults does not show significant enhancement except in occasional diploic venous channels or at the site of previous surgical intervention, such as the region of a previous burr hole placement. Metastatic calvarial lesions, however, enhance after contrast administration, allowing detection (Fig. 9-16). CEMR is more sensitive than is NCMR in detecting calvarial metastases (West 1990), though careful comparison of both images is required for the evaluation of the calvarium and skull base to ensure that lesions are not masked by enhancing to isointensity with normal adjacent fatty marrow. Fat-suppressed images would be useful in this respect, though they are not routinely obtained. Intracranial extension of mass is easily recognized on MR (Fig. 9-17). In general, CEMR is more sensitive than is NCMR in showing intracranial extension.

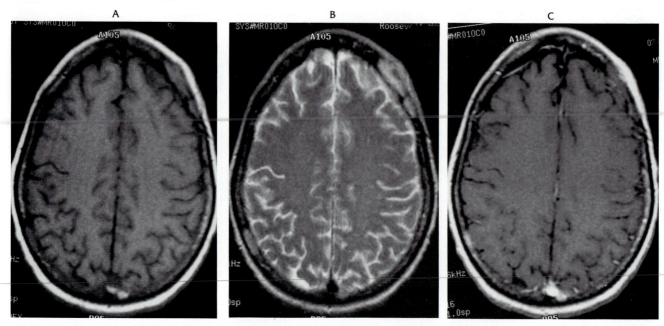

**Figure 9-16   Calvarial metastases from lung carcinoma. A.** Axial $T_1$- and **B.** $T_2$-weighted images show left frontal and right parietal calvarial metastases. **C.** The axial contrast-enhanced $T_1$-weighted image shows enhancement of the lesions, particularly the right parietal lesion.

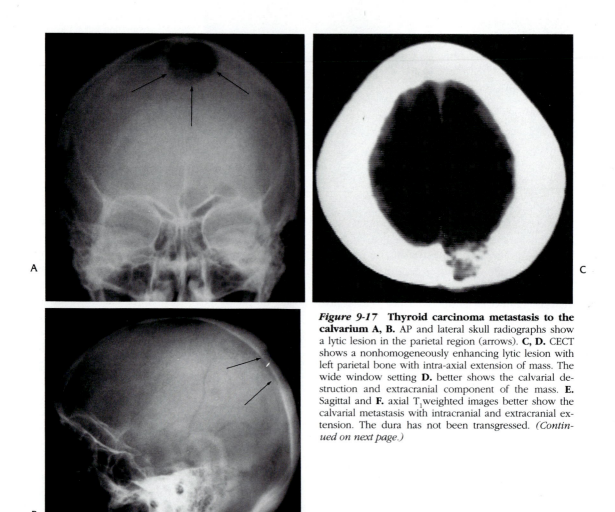

**Figure 9-17   Thyroid carcinoma metastasis to the calvarium A, B.** AP and lateral skull radiographs show a lytic lesion in the parietal region (arrows). **C, D.** CECT shows a nonhomogeneously enhancing lytic lesion with left parietal bone with intra-axial extension of mass. The wide window setting **D.** better shows the calvarial destruction and extracranial component of the mass. **E.** Sagittal and **F.** axial $T_1$weighted images better show the calvarial metastasis with intracranial and extracranial extension. The dura has not been transgressed. *(Continued on next page.)*

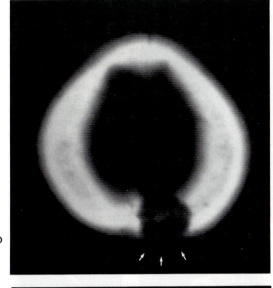

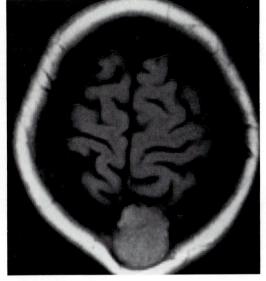

Figure 9-17   (continued)

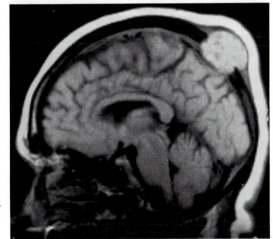

## DIRECT OR PERINEURAL EXTENSION OF EXTRACRANIAL TUMORS

Malignancies of the head and neck may erode through the skull base with direct intracranial extension or may extend along neural pathways to gain intracranial access (Lee 1985; Laine 1990). Tumor extends in a retrograde fashion along the perineural or endoneural spaces, entering the intracranial compartment through the basal foramina (Ballantyne 1963; Laine 1990). Multiple tumors of the head and neck, including squamous cell carcinoma, basal cell carcinoma, melanoma, adenoid cystic carcinoma, lymphoma, and neurofibroma, may enter the intracranial cavity in this manner (Laine 1990; Dodd 1970; Woodruff 1986). Among these tumors, adenoid cystic carcinoma, though less common than head and neck carcinoma arising from the skin and mucous membranes, has a predilection for perineural extension (Spiro 1974; Lee 1985; Laine 1990). Entrance along the mandibular division of the trigeminal nerve through the foramen ovale is a relatively common pathway for intracranial tumor extension. Intracranial metastases arising from a perineural tumor extension are often noncontiguous with "skip" metastases, producing the appearance of a distinct intracranial extra-axial mass (Lee 1985; Laine 1990; Curtin 1985). Consequently, a mass with the appearance of meningioma in a patient with a head and neck neoplasm should be considered a metastasis until proved otherwise (Lee 1985).

The extracranial mass and intracranial extension of head and neck neoplasms can be demonstrated on CT. These lesions typically demonstrate homogeneous contrast enhancement. Associated findings of perineural tumor extension include widening of the basal foramina and muscle denervation atrophy. MR has several advantages, including superior contrast resolution, absence of beam-hardening artifact related to scanning through the skull base, and ease of obtaining multiple planes. MR findings of perineural tumor extension include isointense thickening of the involved nerve and enlargement of the basal foramen, lateral bulging of

Wiley RG (ed): *Neurologic Complications of Cancer.* New York, Marcel Dekker, 1995, pp 219–232.

KAISER MC, RODESCH G, CAPESIUS P: Blood-fluid levels in multilobulated cystic brain metastases of a hypernephroma: A case report. *Neuroradiology* 25:339–341, 1983.

KALKMAN PH, ALLAN S, BIRCHALL IWJ: A MRI of limbic encephalitis. *J Can Assoc Radiol* 44:121–124, 1993.

KAMAMURA Y, JOHNSON C, GOLDBERG SN, et al: Clinical utility of triple dose contrast for the MR screening of brain metastases. *Poster session Society of Magnetic Resonance 3rd Society Meeting and Exhibition.* Nice, France, May 19–25, 1995.

KART BH, REDDY SC, RAO GR, et al: Choroid plexus metastasis: CT appearance. *J Comput Assist Tomogr* 10:537, 1986.

KODAMA T, NUMAREDRI Y, GELLA FE, et al: Magnetic resonance imaging of limbic encephalitis. *Neuroradiol* 33:520–523, 1991.

KROL G, SZE G, MALKIN M, et al: MR of cranial and spinal meningeal carcinomatosis: Comparison with CT and myelography. *AJNR* 9:709–714, 1988; *AJR* 151:583–588, 1988.

LACOMIS D, KHOSHBIN S, SCHICK RM: MR imaging of paraneoplastic limbic encephalitis. *J Comp Asst Tomogr* 14:115–117, 1990.

LAINE FJ, BRAUN IF, JENSEN ME, et al: Perineural tumor extension through the foramen ovale: Evaluation with MR imaging. *Radiology* 174:65–71, 1990.

LEE YY, CASTILLO M, NAUERT C: Intracranial perineural metastases of adenoid cystic carcinoma of the head and neck. *J Comput Assist Tomogr* 9:219–223, 1985.

LEE YY, GLASS JP, GEOFFRAY A, et al: Cranial computed tomographic abnormalities in leptomeningeal metastasis. *AJNR* 5:559–563, 1984; *AJR* 143:1035–1039, 1984.

LEE YY, TIEN RD, BRUNS JM, et al: Lobulated intracranial leptomeningeal metastasis: CT and MR characteristics. *AJNR* 10:1171–1179, 1989.

LESSE S, NETSKY MG: Metastasis of neoplasms to the central nervous system and meninges. *Arch Neurol Psych* 77:133–153, 1954.

LITTLE JR, DIAL B, BELANGER G, et al: Brain hemorrhage from intracranial tumor. *Stroke* 10:283–288, 1979.

LYNES WL, BOSTWICK DG, FREIHA FS, et al: Parenchymal brain metastases from adenocarcinoma of prostate. *Urology* 28:280–287, 1986.

MACGEE EE: Surgical treatment of cerebral metastases from lung cancer. The effect on quality and duration of survival. *J Neurosurg* 35:416–420, 1971.

MACKAY CJ, ABRAMSON DH, ELLSWORTH RM: Metastatic patterns of retinoblastoma. *Arch Ophthalmol* 102:391–396, 1984.

MAGILLIGAN DJ Jr, DUVERNOY C, MALIK G, et al: Surgical approach to lung cancer with solitary cerebral metastasis: Twenty-five years, experience. *Ann Thorac Surg* 42:360–364, 1986.

MANDELL L, HILARIS B, SULLIVAN M, et al: The treatment of single-brain metastases from nonoat cell-lung carcinoma: Surgery and radiation versus radiation therapy alone. *Cancer* 58:641–649, 1986.

MANDYBUR TI: Intracranial hemorrhage caused by metastatic tumors. *Neurology* 27:650–655, 1977.

MAYR NA, YUH WTC, MUHONEN MG, et al: Cost-effectiveness of high-dose MR contrast studies in the evaluation of brain metastases. *AJNR* 15:1053–1061, 1994.

MEHTA RC, PIKE GB, HAROS SP, et al: Central nervous system tumor infection, and infarction: Detection with gadolinium enhanced magnetization transfer MR imaging. *Radiology* 195:41–46, 1995.

MORRISON D, SOBEL DF, KELLY WM, et al: Intraventricular mass lesions. *Radiology* 153:435–442, 1984.

NADICH TP, ZIMMERMAN RA: Primary brain tumors in children. *Semin Roentgenol* 19:100–114, 1984.

NEINDORF HP, LANIADO M, SEMMLER W, et al: Dose administration of gadolinium-DTPA in MR imaging of intracranial tumors. *AJNR* 8:803–815, 1987.

NEMZEK W, POIRER V, SALAMAT MS, et al: Carcinomatous encephalitis (Miliary metastases): Lack of contrast enhancement. *AJNR* 14:540–542, 1993.

OLSEN WL, WINKLER ML, ROSS DA: Carcinomatous encephalitis: CT and MR findings. *AJNR* 8:553–554, 1987.

PATCHELL RA, CIRRINCIONE C, THALER HT, et al: Single brain metastases: Surgery plus radiation or radiation alone. *Neurology* 36:447–453, 1986.

PATCHELL RA, TIBBS PA, WALSH JW, et al: Randomized trial of surgery in the treatment of single metastases to the brain. *N Engl J Med* 332:494–500, 1990.

PECHOVA'-PETEROVA' V, KALVACH P: CT findings in cerebral metastases. *Neuroradiology* 28:254–258, 1986.

PHILLIPS ME, RYALS TJ, KAMBHU S, et al: Neoplastic vs. inflammatory meningeal enhancement with Gd-DTPA. *J Comput Assist Tomogr* 14(4):536–541, 1990.

POSNER JB: Neurologic complications of systemic cancer. *Med Clin North Am* 63:783–800, 1979.

POSNER JB, CHERNIK NL: Intracranial metastases from systemic cancer. *Adv Neurol* 19:579–591, 1978.

POTTS DG, ABBOTT GF, VON SNEIDERN JV: National Cancer Institute study: Evaluation of computed tomography in the diagnosis of intracranial neoplasms: III. Metastatic tumors *Radiology* 136:657–664, 1980.

RIPPE DJ, BOYKO OB, FRIEDMAN HS, et al: Gd-DTPA-enhanced MR imaging of leptomeningeal spread of primary intracranial CNS tumor in children. *AJNR* 11:329–332, 1990.

ROLLINS N, MENDELSOHN D, MULNE A, et al: Recurrent medulloblastoma: Frequency of tumor enhancement on Gd-DTPA-MR imaging. *AJNR* 155:153–158, 1990.

RUELLE A, BAMBINI C, MACCHIA G, et al: Brain metastasis from colon cancer: Case report showing a clinical and CT unusual appearance. *J Neurosurg Sci* 31:31–36, 1987.

RUSSELL EJ, GEREMIA GK, JOHNSON CE, et al: Multiple cerebral metastases: Detectability with Gd-DTPA-enhanced MR imaging. *Radiology* 165:609–617, 1987.

SAPOZINK MD, KAPLAN HS: Intracranial Hodgkin's disease: A report of 12 cases and review of the literature. *Cancer* 52:1301–1307, 1983.

SCHREIBER D, BERNSTEIN K, SCHNEIDER J: Metastases of the central nervous system: A prospective study, 3rd communication: Metastases in the pituitary gland, pineal gland, and choroid plexus. *Zentralbi Allg Pathol* 126:64–73, 1982.

SCHUMACHER DJ, TIEN RD, FRIEDMAN H: Gadolinium enhancement of the leptomeninges caused by hydrocephalus: A potential mimic of leptomeningeal metastasis. *AJNR* 15:639–641, 1994.

SCOTTI G, HARWOOD-NASH DC: Computed tomography of rhabomyosarcomas of the skull base in children. *J Comput Assist Tomogr* 6:33–39, 1982.

SHALEN PR, HYMAN LA, WALLACE S, et al: Protocol for delayed contrast enhancement in computed tomography of cerebral neoplasia. *Radiology* 139:397–402, 1981.

SMALLEY SR, LAWS ER Jr, O'FALLON JR, et al: Resection for solitary brain metastases. Role of adjuvant radiation and prognostic variables in 229 patients. *Neurosurg* 77:531–540, 1992.

SPIRO RH, HUVOS AG, STRONG EW: Adenoid cystic carcinoma of salivary origin: A clinicopathologic study of 242 cases. *Am J Surg* 128:512–520, 1974.

SUNDARESAN N, GALICICH JH: Surgical treatment of brain metastases: Clinical and computerized tomography evaluation of the results of treatment. *Cancer* 55:1382–1388, 1985.

SZE G: Magnetic resonance imaging of the brain in oncology, in Breit A (ed): *Magnetic Resonance in Oncology.* Berlin, Springer-Verlag, 1990a.

SZE G: Diseases of the intracranial meninges: MR imaging features. *AJR* 160:727–733, 1993.

SZE G, MILANO E, JOHNSON C, et al: Detection of brain metastases: Comparison of contrast-enhanced MR with unenhanced MR and enhanced CT. *AJNR* 11:785–791, 1990b.

SZE G, SHIN J, KROL G, et al: Intraparenchymal brain metastases: MR imaging vs contrast-enhanced CT. *Radiology* 168:187–194, 1988.

SZE G, SOLETSKY S, BRONEN R, et al: MR imaging of the cranial meninges with emphasis on contrast enhancement and meningeal carcinomatosis. *AJNR* 10:965–975, 1989; *AJR* 153:1039–1049, 1989.

TARVER RD, RICHMOND BD, KLATTE BC: Cerebral metastases from lung carcinoma: Neurologic and CT correlation. *Radiology* 153:689–692, 1984.

TYRELL RL, BUNDSCHUH CV, MODIC MT: Dural carcinomatosis: MR demonstration. *JCAT* II:329–332, 1987.

VAN DEN DOEL EM, VAN MERRIENBOER FJ, TULLEKEN CA: Cerebral hemorrhage from unsuspected choriocarcinoma. *Clin Neurol Neurosurg* 87:287–290, 1985.

VIETH RG, ODOM GL: Intracranial metastases and their neurosurgical treatment. *J Neurosurg* 23:375–383, 1965.

WASSERSTROM WR, GLASS JP, POSNER JB: Diagnosis and treatment of leptomeningeal metastases from solid tumors: Experience with 90 patients. *Cancer* 49:759–772, 1982.

WEIR B, MACDONALD N, MIELKE B: Intracranial vascular complications of choriocarcinoma. *Neurosurgery* 2:138–142, 1978.

WEISBERG LA: Computerized tomographic findings in intracranial metastatic malignant melanoma. *Comput Radiol* 9:365–372, 1985a.

WEISBERG LA: Hemorrhagic metastatic intracranial neoplasms: Clinical computed tomographic correlations. *J Comput Assist Tomogr* 9:105–114, 1985b.

WEST M, RUSSELL EJ, BREIT R, et al: Calvarial and skull base metastasis: Comparison of nonenhanced and Gd-DTPA enhanced MR images. *Radiology* 175:85–91, 1990.

WOODRUFF WW Jr, DJANG WT, MCLENDON RE, et al: Intracerebral malignant melanoma. High-field strength MR imaging. *Radiology* 165:209–213, 1987.

WOODRUFF WW Jr, YEATES AE, MCLENDON RE: Perineural tumor extension to the cavernous sinus from superficial facial carcinoma: CT manifestations. *Radiology* 161:395–399, 1986.

YANG PJ, KNAKE JE, GABRIELSEN TO, et al: Primary and secondary histiocytic lymphoma of the brain: CT features. *Radiology* 154:683–686, 1985.

YUH WTC, FISHER DJ, RUNGE VM et al: Phase III multicenter trial of high-dose gadoteridol in MR evaluation of brain metastases. *AJNR* 15:1037–1051, 1994.

YUH WTC, TALI T, NGUYEN HD, et al: The effect of contrast dose, imaging time and lesion size in the MR detection of intracranial metastasis. *AJNR* 16:373–380, 1995.

ZIMMERMAN RD, HEIER LA, SNOW RB, et al: Acute intracranial hemorrhage: Intensity changes on sequential MR scans at 0.5T. *AJNR* 9:47–57, 1988.

# CRANIOCEREBRAL TRAUMA

*Robert A. Zimmerman*

## CONTENTS

Head injuries are responsible for 200 to 300 hospital admissions per 100,000 population per year in the United States (Bakay 1980). Most admissions are brief, with the patient discharged within 48 hours, and most of the patients are men. Serious head trauma occurs in only 3 percent of nonvehicular and 15 percent of vehicular injuries (Caveness 1979). However, craniocerebral trauma still constitutes the major cause of accidental death in the United States and represents more than 50 percent of deaths between ages 15 and 24 (Caveness 1979). Nine deaths per 100,000 population per year result from head injuries in the United Kingdom (Jennett 1981); this constitutes 1 percent of all deaths,

25 percent of traumatic deaths, and 50 percent of deaths due to road accidents.

Thus, in the United States and other economically developed countries, head injury represents not only a serious cause of loss of life but also a significant source of financial burden, resulting in a prolonged loss of earnings and a financial loss in terms of the health care resources expended in treating and caring for these patients. In the pediatric population, head trauma, either alone or in combination with other injuries, represents 95,000 emergency room visits in the United States per year (Kraus 1986). The incidence of trauma (50% of which are head injuries) in the first year of life is approximately 86 per 1000 children (McCormick 1981). Trauma in infants and young children may be accidental or nonaccidental (child abuse) (Rivera 1988). Severe accidental head trauma is relatively uncommon in children before 2 years of age (Bruce 1989). Nonaccidental injury accounts for 80% or more of deaths from head trauma in this under 2 year age population. That is even though accidental injury is 10 to 15 times more common than nonaccidental injury. It is furthermore estimated, that in the United States, that there are 3000 deaths per year from nonaccidental head injury and that at least 10% of children with mental retardation and cerebral palsy are presumed to have been damaged by child abuse (Radkowski 1983).

When a patient has a head injury, there is an urgent need to understand the nature, extent, and rapidity of its progression (Zimmerman 1978*a*). If this can be accomplished, it may be possible to correct certain problems and institute measures that protect the brain from greater or irreversible damage.

The evaluation and treatment of the trauma patient starts at the scene of the injury. The emergency medical personnel ensure a patent airway, that the patient breathes, that blood pressure is maintained, and that hemorrhage is stopped. Assessment of the patient's consciousness is made, the spine is immobilized so that no further spinal cord injury occurs, and transport to the emergency care facility occurs. Assessment of the patient's status utilizes the Glasgow Coma Score (GCS), which is based on a scale that evaluates the degree of coma. A mild head injury is a GCS of 13 to 15, a moderate one is a GCS of 9 to 12, and a severe one is GCS of 8 or less. In general, patients with a GCS of less than 13 are observed and have an imaging study to evaluate the brain and to help determine the care necessary. Further clinical deterioration requires further reevaluation by imaging and an aggressive approach to control hemorrhage and mass effect or brain swelling.

A variety of factors contribute to the way in which a head injury occurs, and other factors act to mitigate this process (Zimmerman 1984). It is the interplay between the factors that produce the traumatic event and those that protect a person from it that produces the end result. Physical factors include the thickness of the scalp and hair, the density of ossification, and the dimensions and thickness of the calvarium. The position of the head at the time of injury, the protection afforded by objects surrounding the head, and the direction and nature of the force that produces the injury are variables that affect the traumatic outcome.

Newborns, infants, and young children with open sutures and a thin calvarium have an advantage in that a greater impact can be absorbed by a more flexible skull (Zimmerman 1981). Also, the lack of myelination in younger persons contributes to greater plasticity of the cerebral hemispheres. Calvarial flexibility and cerebral plasticity, however, permit more severe distortion between the skull and the dura relative to the cerebral hemispheres and their superficial vessels. When they are severe, such forces produce posterior fossa subdural hematomas, tentorial dura venous sinus tears, and other lesions rarely seen in older children and adults (Zimmerman 1981). Posttraumatic swelling appears to be a more rapid and more diffuse problem in a young child (Zimmerman 1978b); a similar degree of swelling is rarely seen in an adult. The patterns of brain injury change as a child ages; the sutures fuse, the calvarium thickens, myelination progresses, and cerebrovascular responsiveness matures (Zimmerman 1978b). Cerebral injury patterns in adults are different from those in children.

Not only are there differences in head injuries between infants and adults (Alberico 1987), there is also a difference in the nature of the cervical spinal injuries that occur as a component of the overall traumatic episode. Weakness of the neck muscles, a proportionately larger head mass relative to that of the body, open ossification centers, and ligamentous elasticity are all present in an infant and permit greater motion between the occiput, C1, and C2 (Melzak 1969). This elasticity results in a variety of subluxations, dislocations, and fractures that are found less frequently in older children and adults. With further maturation, adult proportions between the head and the body are reached, the epiphyses fuse, muscular development takes place, ligamentous elasticity decreases, and cervical spine injuries become analogous to those in adults (Ogden 1982). There is also a significant difference in the incidence of cervical spine injury in young children (1 in 230) as opposed to adults (1 in 20) (Henrys 1977). Thus, it is important for physicians who perform posttraumatic brain and spine imaging studies to recognize the limitations of these studies caused by differences in biomechanical factors in an infant or a young child.

## IMAGING TECHNIQUES

The equipment necessary for evaluation of trauma patients must be available 24 hours a day, 7 days a week. The access to the equipment must be rapid. Plain skull radiographs, CT, arteriography, and MR can be used to assess skull and brain injury (Gentry 1994). With a cervical spine injury, plain spine radiographs, CT, myelography, and MR are utilized. The choice of technique depends on several factors, including availability, speed of performance, diagnostic information desired, information derived, limitations of the technology, clinical circumstances, and cost (Zimmerman 1984). For example, the demonstration of an operable intracranial hematoma with a technology that takes more time (MR) rather than with one that is faster but less elegant (CT) delays the removal of the hematoma, perhaps resulting in increased disability or the death of the patient. An imaging procedure that is more rapid but insensitive, such as a skull radiograph, when one is attempting to determine whether there has been parenchymal brain damage only delays the diagnosis and the treatment of the patient (Zimmerman 1983).

In the emergency room, after the institution of support and monitoring and after the patient has been stabilized, the immediate radiographic question is stability of the spine to ensure that cord injury does not occur as a result of movement. This requires a good-quality lateral radiograph of the cervical spine that shows the relationship between the skull, C1, and the cervical vertebrae through C7. Such alignment on a lateral radiograph does not assure that ligamentous injury has not occurred or demonstrate with clarity the presence of fractures and epiphyseal separations that require a more complete cervical spine radiographic examination or CT study. However, at this point the patient usually can be moved with a physician and nurse in attendance so that a CT study can be performed. The CT examination is done to evaluate the brain and/or spine.

## Computed Tomography

CT is the first and most important step in evaluating for head and contiguous spine injuries (Bernardi 1993). CT does not show every calvarial fracture, but shows a sufficient number of depressed ones and reveals basilar skull fractures that plain radiographs do not demonstrate. CT is also the method of choice for demonstrating fractures of the facial bones, including the paranasal sinuses and orbits. CT's main role, however, is to separate patients into three categories: those with normal intracranial structures (brain and subarachnoid space), those with focal intraaxial or extraaxial hematomas, and those with a more diffuse pattern of brain injury (Schunk 1996). In general, in those with normal brain and subarachnoid spaces, observation is all that is required, unless there is superimposed but, as yet unrecognized, hypoxic-ischemic, metabolic, or electrolyte disturbance that may lead to brain swelling and further deterioration (Marion 1991). Patients with intra axial or extra axial hematomas may require surgical evaluation or further medical management. Patients with more diffuse brain injury, such as brain swelling and diffuse axonal injury (DAI) may require medical management to control intracranial pressure. CT is rapid and can be repeated as often as is necessary, provided that the patient can be transported to the scanner room.

Current CT scanners have data acquisition times of less than 1 to 3 seconds per slice (Gibbey 1992). Because of interscan delay, tube cooling, and reconstruction, the total examination time for a brain study is between 5 and 10 minutes. A more detailed examination that requires thin sections for the evaluation of facial injury or cervical spine trauma requires a longer period of time. Patient motion during data acquisition degrades or destroys the image quality of a scan done while the motion occurred. When the motion stops, the scans will again be of good quality. With CT, it is easy to rescan sections that were made useless by motion. This should be done routinely by the technician unless the patient's clinical condition is deteriorating.

Spiral or helical CT scanning is the acquisition of data by continuously rotating x-ray tube and detectors while the patient is continuously moving on a table at a set rate of speed (Zimmerman 1992). A volume of density information is acquired and reconstructed into axial slices at a predetermined slice thickness. For instance, brain can be examined with a series of 5-mm-thick slices from the foramen magnum to the vertex, the imaging time being the matter of only a minute or less. The cervical spine from the occiput to C7 can be examined with 2-mm-thick slices, again in a relatively short time span. Images acquired in this fashion can often be done without motion of the patient, so that when thin enough, sagittal and coronal reformatting

can be done, such as with the cervical spine, to detect fractures or subluxations. Even three-dimensional reconstructions of the vertebral bodies or skull base can be made when the sections are thin enough. Monitoring and support equipment function in the CT scanner room and do not pose a management problem. Anesthesiologists accompanying the patient are shielded from the scatter radiation by wearing lead aprons. The CT scan that is generated is photographed onto x-ray film to make a hard copy, or displayed on monitors from which it is interpreted.

In a typical head injury, windows and window levels are (1) optimized for the brain (brain window) (Fig. 10-1); (2) used to assess the presence or absence of blood adjacent to the inner table of the skull, as is seen in a subdural or epidural hematoma (intermediate windows) (Fig. 10-2); and (3) used to determine the presence or absence of a bony fracture (bone windows) (Fig. 10-3). In the spine, usually one set of windows is used for the spinal cord and one for the bony anatomy. Rapidity and resolution of spiral CT in evaluating cervical spine injuries and head injured patients has made this a convenient and useful procedure (Figs. 10-4 to 10-6). If a spinal subdural or epidural hematoma is sus-

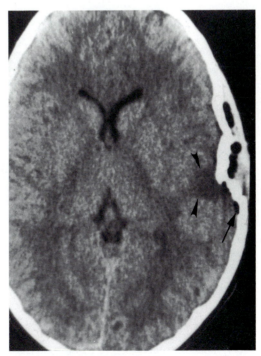

***Figure 10-1*** **Depressed fracture** within an underlying contusion in a 10-year-old male hit on the left side of the head. Axial CT shows gas within the subgaleal region, intracranial air (arrow) in the subdural space, and a depressed fracture. There is an underlying area of hypodensity (arrowheads) consistent with nonhemorrhagic contusion.

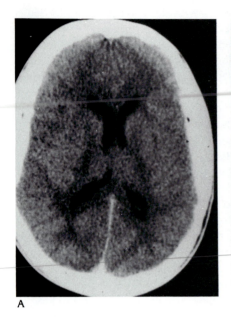
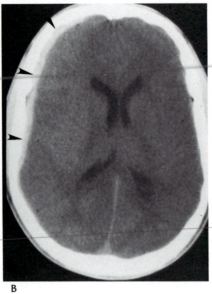

A

B

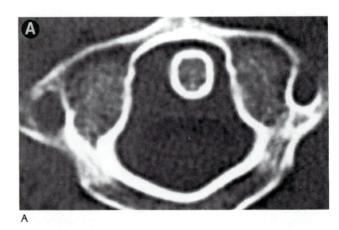

*Figure 10-2* **Acute subdural hematoma** in a 17-year-old man rendered comatose in a motor vehicle accident. **A.** Axial CT with brain windows shows no definite extracerebral collection of blood. **B.** Same section displayed with intermediate windows demonstrates a small, peripheral acute subdural hematoma (arrowheads) encompassing the anterior two-thirds of the right cerebral hemisphere.

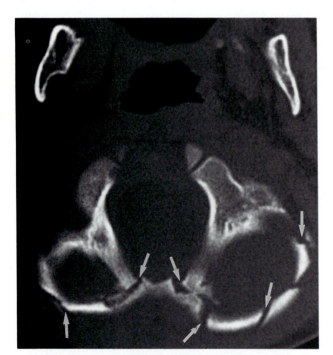

A

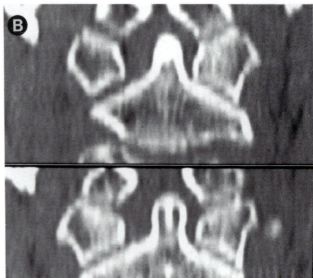

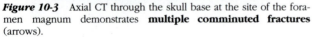

*Figure 10-3* Axial CT through the skull base at the site of the foramen magnum demonstrates **multiple comminuted fractures** (arrows).

*Figure 10-4* **Rotatory Subluxation of C1 on C2.** Spiral CT with ▶ reconstruction. **A.** Axial spiral CT section through C1 shows the relationship between the lateral masses of C1 and the odontoid process to be offset. **B.** Coronal reconstruction of the spiral CT slices depicts the relationships between the lateral masses of C1 and the particular surface of the C2 vertebral body. The slight offset of C1 relative to C2 is shown.

B

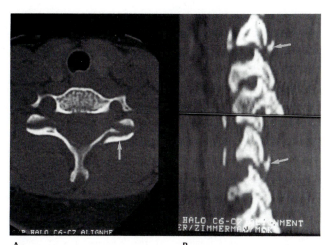

*Figure 10-5*  **A.** Axial CT slice shows a **fracture of the articular facet** joint at C6 on the left (arrow). **B.** Contiguous reconstructed sagittal sections from axial spiral data shows the fractured articular facet (arrow).

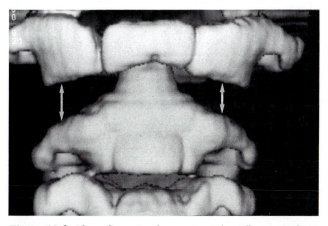

*Figure 10-6*  Three-dimensional reconstructed axially acquired spiral CT sections demonstrate **distraction of the C1 vertebral body** from the C2 vertebral body (arrows).

pected, intermediate windows can be useful. If intermediate windows are not used in the head, small but significant life-threatening extracerebral hematomas may be missed. The studies can always be rephotographed, but it is important to have the critical information early so that an appropriate management decision can be made prospectively.

## Magnetic Resonance Imaging

Magnetic resonance imaging of traumatic brain injury is valuable for several reasons. First, it is multiplanar and can separate cortex from extra-axial blood collections

in the subdural and epidural spaces that lie at the vertex and at the skull base, which are missed on axial CT imaging. MR scanning can show nonhemorrhagic parenchymal lesions, such as those associated with diffuse axonal injury which are not visible on CT. MR is also extremely useful in demonstrating small areas of hemorrhage, by their susceptibility effects, that is the loss of signal at the site of the blood products that throws the spins of the protons out of phase, and such sites of small hemorrhage are usually not visible on CT sections. Where magnetic resonance imaging fails is primarily in the demonstration of subarachnoid hemorrhage, which is generally shown much better with CT, especially within the first 48 hours after injury, and in the demonstration of calvarial fractures, where the contrast between hypointense cortical bone on MR and the fracture line is quite difficult (Orrison 1994). MRI is utilized in our institution, following CT, when CT does not resolve the nature of the brain injury, and it is used to demonstrate whether there is or is not injury to the cervical cord and to the soft tissue and disk structures of the cervical spine.

Data acquisition periods for a $T_1$-weighted set of images are on the order of several minutes, whereas those for a set of proton and $T_2$-weighted multiecho images require 8 or more minutes (Zimmerman 1989). Long acquisition times can cause problems in regard to motion. Image quality is degraded by motion, and the scans may be uninterpretable.

$T_2$-weighted imaging has become faster, with acquisition times dropping to the order of 3 to 5 minutes with techniques that fall under the category of fast or turbo spin echo. Even faster $T_2$-weighted images can be obtained by techniques that utilize a single-shot half-Fourier turbo spin echo, capable of producing an image every second, as a single acquisition, so that when motion occurs, it is only that slice during which the motion occurs that is ruined. These techniques have the rapidity of CT, but relative to fast spin echo and conventional spin-echo imaging, lack some of the sharpness, and are not as sensitive to the presence of blood products in the form of a susceptibility effect (loss of signal) that occurs with deoxyhemoglobin and intracellular methemoglobin and hemosiderin at the site of prior hemorrhage. Even faster is echo planar imaging (EPI), which requires higher millitesla gradients and more sophisticated software. These techniques give images on the order of 50 milliseconds per section and can examine the entire brain in acquisition times of between 2 and 8 seconds. However, there are trade-offs: image resolution is not as good as turbo spin-echo images, and there are artifacts due to susceptibility that are magnified on EPI, adjacent to sites where there is bone- or air-containing structures, such as the paranasal sinuses and mastoid air cells. However, susceptibility produced by hemorrhages are extremely well shown by such EPI techniques.

Motion can also be controlled by means of sedation, but sedation eliminates the ability to evaluate a patient's neurological signs. However, many seriously injured comatose patients are intubated and paralyzed; these patients can be examined in the acute situation when support, the monitoring equipment, and the intubation devices utilized are compatible with the requirements of the MR scanner (Zimmerman 1989). Nonferromagnetic equipment must be used because it cannot be pulled into the magnetic field of the MR magnet. Ultra-low-field MR systems and some permanent magnets are exceptions. The fields generated by these units are so low that it may be possible to use ferromagnetic equipment. However, plastic intubation devices and subarachnoid bolts are a standard part of the neuroanesthesiologist's and neurosurgeon's armamentarium today. Electronic monitoring equipment becomes a matter of concern in the MR room if it generates a radiofrequency (RF) signal that interferes with the signals of the scanner. An extraneous RF source degrades the image quality. The magnetic field can interfere with the readout or the functioning of monitoring devices. For instance, strong magnetic fields deflect the output of the electron gun on an ECG monitor, making the readout uninterpretable. At present, nonferromagnetic respirators, shielded cables for ECGs, pulse oximeters that work in the magnetic field, and a variety of other monitoring and support devices allow MR examination of emergency head injury patients. With experience, the setup times have decreased, and studies have been done in as little as 30 minutes.

Two other MR techniques in investigations of head injuries are worth noting here. MR scanners can generate MR angiographic (MRA) images of blood vessels with fast flow by utilizing the three-dimensional (3D) time of flight (3D TOF) techniques with gradient-echo $T_1$-weighted images ($T_1$WI) processed by means of a maximum-intensity projection (Masaryk 1989). At present the entire brain can be examined. MRA can show the integrity of the circle of Willis and its branches.

Three-dimensional time of flight MRAs incorporate the high-signal-intensity flow-related enhancement to make the MRA image. Unfortunately, the mapped image also incorporates high-signal-intensity blood products in the form of methemoglobin into the MRA. Thus, if a traumatic aneurysm or dissection is being looked for, the 3D TOF MRA may not be adequate. An alternative MRA method is phase contrast (PC) angiography. With this method, only blood that is moving produces the image of the blood vessel. Thus, high-signal-intensity methemoglobin is not incorporated into the MRA image. PC MRA have problems in that the acquisition times are long and the volumes that can be acquired are relatively limited. The potential of this technique is realized in the demonstration of traumatic vascular injury resulting in obstruction of a major vessel or the production of a pseudoaneurysm. Magnetic resonance spectroscopy (MRS) is another technique that has research applications in the evaluation of head injury patients (Schnall 1987) (Sutton 1995). Acquisition times for spectroscopic data are long. Proton spectra can be acquired for a region of interest measuring 2 by 2 by 2 cm in 10 minutes, following a 5-minute period of shimming. A proton spectrum can show whether lactates are elevated in the brain (Detre 1990) secondary to a hypoxic-ischemic insult. A longer data acquisition time displays the relative concentration of phosphorous metabolites in the brain (Sutton 1990). The relationship between inorganic phosphorous and phosphocreatine gives a relative measure of brain pH.

## Cerebral Angiography

Prior to the availability of CT, cerebral angiography was routinely used to assess the presence or absence of intracranial mass lesions. Today it is reserved for the demonstration of vascular injury in the form of dissections, ruptures, pseudoaneurysms, and fistulas (Davis 1983). Invasive cerebral angiography is time-consuming, requiring several hours, and necessitates control of patient motion during the injection of dye and filming. Support and monitoring equipment are not a problem.

## Myelography

Prior to the availability of CT and spinal MR, myelography was widely used to demonstrate posttraumatic cord compression. Myelographic procedures are invasive, requiring puncture of the subarachnoid space and the introduction of radiographic contrast media. These studies take an hour or more and necessitate patient compliance or motion control. Support and monitoring equipment are not a problem.

## SKULL FRACTURE

A calvarial or even a vertebral fracture provides evidence of bone injury from trauma. However, a fracture does not mean that the brain or spinal cord has been injured. In general, in cases of trauma, what has happened to the brain and/or spinal cord tissue is the most important factor. Osseous injury is significant not only as a sign of injury but often as a pathway for the spread of infection when the fracture is associated with disruption of the overlying soft tissues. A finding of cranial nerve palsy in association with trauma indicates the necessity of identifying a fracture through the foramen or canal in which that nerve passes. The two most effective ways of demonstrating calvarial injury are

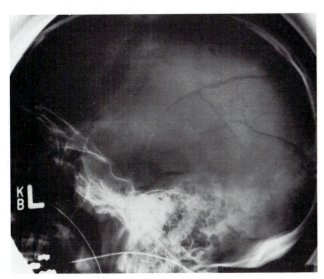

*Figure 10-7* Multiple **calvarial fractures.** Lateral skull radiograph shows multiple irregular lucent fracture lines within the temporoparietal region.

skull radiographs (Fig. 10-7) and CT (Fig. 10-3). Both studies show bone as high density and the fracture within it as a lucency.

MR does not usually show fractures, because the protons of cortical bone are nonmobile; as a result, the cortical bone appears as a linear hypointensity or blackness that is not discernible from air or cerebrospinal fluid (CSF). When the cortical bone lies in apposition to a tissue with higher signal intensity, such

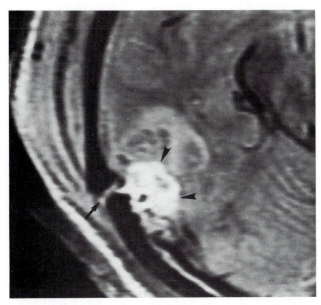

*Figure 10-8* **Calvarial fracture** underlying hemorrhagic contusion. Axial proton density image shows a disruption of the hypointense line of cortical bone (arrow). A high-signal-intensity cortical hemorrhagic contusion (arrowheads) underlies the fracture site.

as far within the scalp, the bone may be visualized in contrast as a structure with low signal intensity. The intradiploic marrow may be seen in older patients because of its fatty nature. On $T_2$-weighted images ($T_2$WI) when the CSF is made high in signal intensity, it outlines the inner table, with the skull appearing as a hypointense line. In some instances fractures can be recognized on MR if the observer knows how to look for them. Zimmerman and coworkers (Zimmerman 1987) evaluated seven patients with temporal bone fractures and found that six of eight fractures were visible with MR. Fractures were recognized by (1) interposition between the fracture fragments of higher-signal-intensity posttraumatic tissue (CSF, hemorrhage, or brain) (Fig. 10-8), (2) disruption of the hypointense black line of cortical bone, (3) displacement of the hypointense line of cortical bone, and (4) orbital fat displaced through a fractured defect.

With an increase in the severity of brain injury, there is an increase in the incidence of fractures. Eighty-one percent of 151 fatal injuries examined at autopsy had associated skull fractures (Adams 1975). The converse—that 19 percent of those fatal injuries did not include a skull fracture—is also of interest. The yield of fractures varies from a high of 15 percent to a low of 2.7 percent in general urban hospital emergency rooms (St. John 1968; Balasubramaniam 1981; Strong 1978). Significant fractures—those associated with the presence of intracranial air or a foreign body, those in which the fracture passes through an air-containing space such as the paranasal sinus and mastoid air cells, a fracture that is associated with laceration of the overlying scalp, and a depressed fracture over the motor strip or major dural venous sinus—are rare. Among 570 children with 49 fractures, only 2 fractures were significant (Roberts 1972). In this series the overall incidence of fractures was 8.25 percent, whereas the incidence of significant fractures was only 0.35 percent.

However, skull fractures are found in approximately 50 percent of children with intracranial injury that results from child abuse (Merten 1984, Tsai 1980). Fifty percent of children with intracranial injury as a result of abuse, however, do not have fractures. Fractures of the long bones are more frequent than those of the skull in victims of child abuse (Merton 1983). Even though overall linear skull fracture is most frequent, depressed, diastatic, and comminuted fractures are more frequent in victims of child abuse than in accidental injury patients (Merton 1984). Often the history is not consistent with the skull findings. A fall from a stroller onto a rug or a fall from a couch onto the floor 2 feet away does not produce a depressed fracture and a brain injury.

Since most patients seen in the emergency room with head injuries do not have fractures, it is easy to guess right in predicting their absence. Among 7970 patients, the physician was correct in predicting the absence of a skull fracture in 96.6 to 99 percent (Balasubramaniam 1981; Royal College of Radiologists 1980). It is more difficult to predict a positive examination. Among 2102 patients, the correct positive diagnosis of fracture was made by means of clinical examination in only 17.4 percent (Balasubramaniam 1981). It should be noted that among patients in whom the physician correctly predicted a fracture, the incidence of brain injury was higher (24 percent) (Balasubramaniam 1981). When the physician predicted a skull fracture but it was absent, brain injury was less frequent (7.5 percent) (Balasubramaniam 1981). High-yield criteria (Bell 1971) exist for obtaining a trauma emergency skull radiograph; adherence to these criteria decreases the number of skull radiographs performed in the emergency room. However, the current practice in emergency medicine in the United States is to obtain a CT scan for most of these indications. Today the skull radiograph is complementary to CT in demonstrating depressed fractures, in localizing foreign bodies, and as another method for assessing and following craniofacial fractures (Zimmerman 1986a). Skull radiographs may be useful in an emergency situation by demonstrating a calvarial fracture in a comatose patient when a history is lacking and CT is negative. This situation is relatively uncommon.

When a patient has minimal evidence of head injury, it must be decided whether a skull radiograph should be done if a CT scan is not performed. A very small percentage of these patients may have acute subdural or epidural hematomas, and some of them would be observed more closely if a skull fracture were demonstrated. Even with the use of the high-yield criteria for the ordering of skull radiographs, it has been noted that a proportion of patients who might benefit from the information derived from the skull radiographs would not be examined. It has been pointed out that 50 percent of patients with compound depressed fractures do not suffer loss of consciousness and that 40 percent of patients with intracranial hematomas do not have an initial loss of consciousness (Jennett 1981). Thus, there is a small ill-defined population of patients who fall through the high-yield criteria. Some of these patients represent a potential catastrophe. Finally, if a fracture is present, there is a possibility of an associated intracranial hematoma. If there is scalp laceration and a fracture, there is a possibility of infection (Jennett 1980). Ultimately, if skull radiographs are performed, they should be adequate in their projections and well penetrated, and the person interpreting the study should be trained in the recognition of these abnormalities.

## Linear Skull Fractures

These fractures appear more lucent than do vascular grooves and closed cranial sutures (Fig. 10-9). Linear fractures are wider in the midportion and narrower at either end (Zimmerman 1986a). Typically, they are less than 3 mm in overall width. A young child with a thin calvarium or an adult with a thin temporal squama may present problems, since the fracture line in these areas may be more difficult to identify. Linear fractures are most common in the temporoparietal, frontal, and occipital regions. These fractures tend to extend from the calvarium toward the cranial base. The fractures should be able to be identified on more than one projection, but it is not uncommon to have difficulty identifying a fracture on all views.

Currently, many fractures are visualized only on the scout image for the CT and/or on the CT scan itself

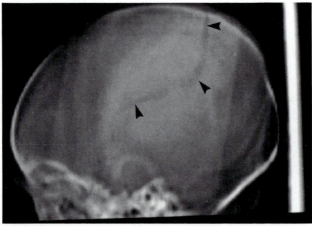

A

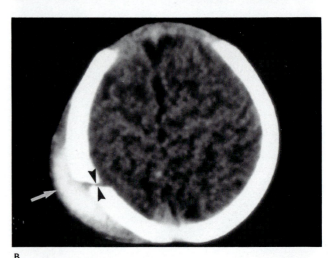

B

***Figure 10-9*** **A.** Sagittal scout for CT shows a large **parietal skull fracture** (arrowheads). **B.** Axial non-contrast-enhanced CT shows a scalp hematoma (arrows) with an underlying parietal fracture (arrowheads). There is slight depression of the posterior fracture fragment.

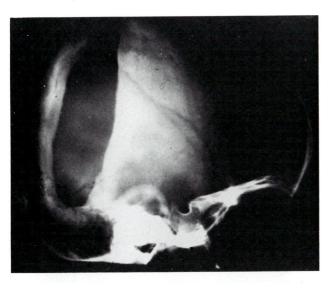

***Figure 10-10*** **Leptomeningeal cyst.** Lateral skull radiograph shows a widened fracture line with beveled edges that has increased in size over the course of the year. The etiology was a leptomeningeal cyst.

(Fig. 10-9). Soft tissue scalp swelling often demarcates the site to be examined for the underlying fracture (Fig. 10-6B). As a fracture heals, the line becomes less distinct and the fracture becomes more difficult to distinguish from normal structures such as vascular grooves and sutures (Zimmerman 1986*a*). A linear fracture in a young patient such as an infant heals in less than 3 to 6 months, whereas in an adult this often takes 2 to 3 years (Zimmerman 1986*a*). If a fracture line does not heal but continues to enlarge (Fig. 10-10), the presence of a leptomeningeal cyst or brain hernia should be considered (Taveras 1953). Both conditions occur as a result of a compound fracture that rends the dura mater so that either brain tissue or arachnoid is interposed between the dura and the fracture fragments. As a result, brain pulsations are transmitted to the CSF at the fracture edges, preventing healing and eventually leading to widening of the defect (Fig. 10-11) (Taveras 1953). Leptomeningeal cysts

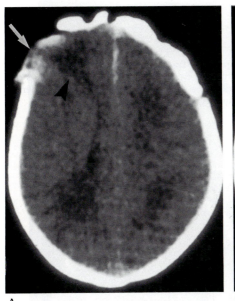

A

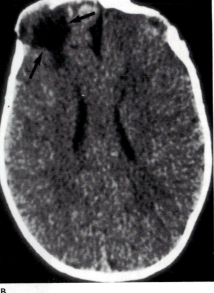

B

***Figure 10-11*** **A.** Axial CT following **raccoon bite** of right frontal bone and brain. A defect is present in the cranium (arrow). There is hypodensity in the underlying brain tissue (arrowhead). A small amount of hemorrhage is present along the falx cerebri. **B.** Follow-up CT examination a year later shows a **leptomeningeal cyst** (arrows) bulging through the defect in the calvarium. **C.** Three-dimensional reconstructed sagittal image from 2-mm axially acquired scans shows large right-sided defect due to the leptomeningeal cyst (arrowhead). **D.** AP 3D view shows that there is not only the right-sided leptomeningeal cyst, but a second defect (arrow) in the left frontal region due to a previously unrecognized site of trauma.

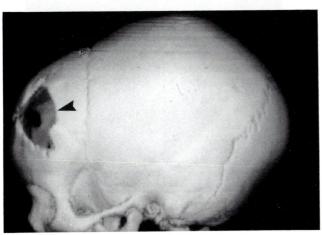

C

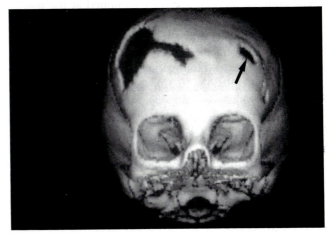

D

of a posttraumatic infection (Zimmerman 1986*a*). They indicate a need for a diagnostic workup to determine the source of infection and the nature of the infecting organism so that appropriate treatment can be instituted.

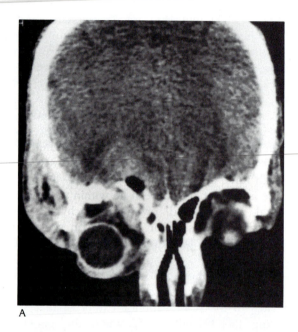

A

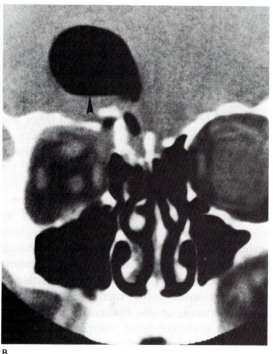

B

***Figure 10-20*** Development of **posttraumatic pneumatocele. A.** Coronal CT shows fracture of the roof of the orbit with contusion of the frontal lobe, intracranial pneumocephalus, and an intraorbital subperiosteal hematoma. **B.** Coronal CT 6 weeks later shows air extending through the fracture site into an intraparenchymal cavity at the site of the contused brain. An air-filled level (arrowhead) is present within the cavity.

## SEQUENTIAL CHANGES OF BLOOD PRODUCTS ON CT AND MR

To understand the interpretation of CT and MR images relative to posttraumatic bleeding, it is necessary to understand the evolution of such hematomas as they are depicted with medical imaging. On CT, a hematoma has high density as a result of the relative density of the globin molecule in stopping the x-ray beam (Dolinskas 1977). Clot retraction occurs over the hours following hematoma formation, and serum is extruded. The hematoma becomes higher in density after clot retraction. Clots typically measure 60 to 100 HU. As the globin molecule breaks down, the density of the clot is progressively lost. Clot density decreases from the periphery and progresses centrally. A 2.5-cm clot becomes isodense in 25 days (Dolinskas 1977). The clot is not gone, but it is no longer visible on CT. With enough time, the clot is completely reabsorbed by macrophages that digest the blood products. A small or larger cavity will typically be the residuum of an old hematoma.

Blood within the vascular system is in the oxyhemoglobin state. When it is extruded into a clot, deoxygenation changes it to deoxyhemoglobin (Gomori 1986). With MR, on $T_1WI$ the deoxyhemoglobin is hypointense to isointense (Fig. 10-21), whereas on $T_2WI$ it is markedly hypointense (a susceptibility effect) (Fig. 10-22) (Gomori 1985*b*). *Susceptibility* refers to the inherent magnetic fields within the different tissues that constitute the brain. Intact red blood cells containing deoxyhemoglobin have a susceptibility different from that of the surrounding extracellular fluid. A proton that is exposed to the varying local fields, one due to intracellular deoxyhemoglobin, or one due to surrounding extracellular fluid has its spin thrown out of phase so that it does not give back a signal. This susceptibility effect appears as an area of blackness on the MR study. Deoxyhemoglobin is subsequently oxidized to methemoglobin. Evidence of this is seen about 3 days after the formation of the hematoma. It appears as a high signal intensity on $T_1WI$ (Fig. 10-23), first at the periphery of the hematoma. Unpaired electrons in methemoglobin produce a paramagnetic $T_1$ shortening effect (Schnall 1987). At this point the red blood cell membrane is still intact, containing intracellular methemoglobin within it. Because the inherent fields within the cell differ from the field surrounding it, the susceptibility effect is found on $T_2WI$. Thus, the hematoma appears black on $T_2WI$. Subsequently, the red blood cell membrane dies as a result of failure of nutrient supply. With the rupture of the red blood cell membranes, a solution of methemoglobin is formed which is bright on both $T_1WI$ and $T_2WI$ (Zimmerman 1986*b*).

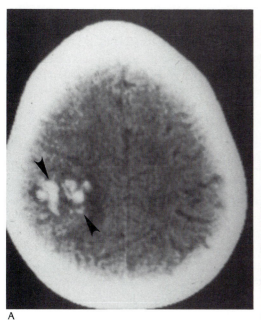
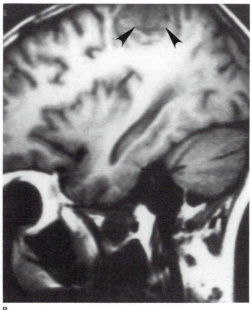

A                                              B

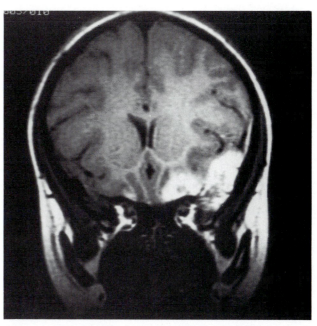

*Figure 10-21* **Acute intra-cerebral hematoma. A.** Axial CT shows a high-density parietal hematoma (arrowheads). **B.** Sagittal T₁-WI shows a slightly hypointense hematoma (arrowheads) composed of deoxyhemoglobin.

Intracellular methemoglobin is found first around 3 days after the formation of a hematoma. The formation of intracellular methemoglobin progresses from the periphery of the hematoma centrally (Zimmerman 1985). Extracellular methemoglobin is found about the end of the first week. Deoxyhemoglobin within the center of the hematoma may persist for weeks. Macrophages are

mobilized and move in to digest the hematoma. As a result of the ingestion of the blood products, hemosiderin is found within the lysosomes of the macrophage (Gomori 1985a). Hemosiderin within the lysosome again creates a susceptibility effect that makes the area of hemosiderin black on T₂WI (Fig. 10-24). It is found within the brain tissue at sites of trau-

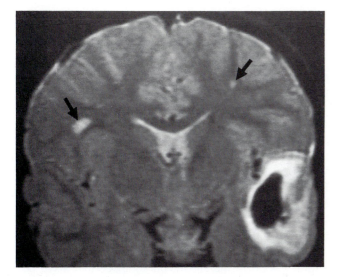

*Figure 10-22* A 5-year-old male involved in a motor vehicle accident, suffering from **intracerebral hematoma** and **diffuse axonal injury.** Coronal T₂-WI shows a left temporal lobe hematoma that is markedly hypointense, surrounded by high-signal-intensity edema. The hypointense hematoma consists of deoxyhemoglobin, methemoglobin, or both. A T₁-WI is needed to determine whether it is deoxyhemoglobin or methemoglobin. Two areas of high signal intensity (arrows) are present in the frontal white matter and are consistent with areas of diffuse axonal injury.

*Figure 10-23* **Contrecoup hemorrhagic contusions** in the methemoglobin state. Coronal T₁-WI shows a predominately left-sided subfrontal and anterior temporal high-signal-intensity peripheral cortical hemorrhagic contusion. A small contusion is present in the right inferior frontal lobe.

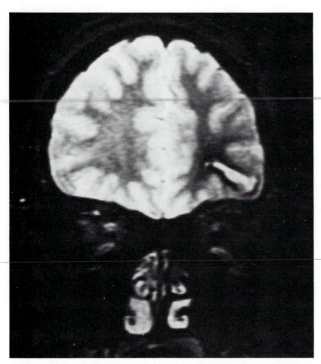

**Figure 10-24** **Old hematoma cavity** lined by hemosiderin and filled with high-signal-intensity fluid. Coronal T$_2$-WI shows a left inferior frontal hematoma cavity that is old, with the hematoma having been reabsorbed. The cavity is lined by hemosiderin which is markedly hypointense. Hemosiderin and ferritin extend into the surrounding white matter, producing hypointensity. The cavity is filled with high-signal-intensity fluid.

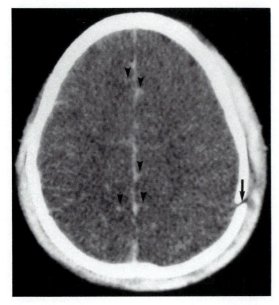

**Figure 10-25** **Traumatic subarachnoid hemorrhage** axial, NCCT shows increased density along the falx cerebri, extending into adjacent sulci (arrowheads). A fracture of the left parietal bone (arrow) is present. There is bilateral scalp swelling with hematomas.

matic bleeding, perhaps for the rest of the patient's life. Extracellular methemoglobin has been found months to years after an injury but is eventually reabsorbed. MR can demonstrate subacute and old bleeding when CT is no longer able to show such blood products (Zimmerman 1989).

## SUBARACHNOID HEMORRHAGE

Subarachnoid hemorrhage occurs as a result of injury to surface vessels, veins, and arteries on the pia or the arachnoidal meninges and as a result of cerebral laceration associated with contusion (Zimmerman 1986a). Rupture of an intracerebral hematoma into the ventricular system with dissemination of blood through the intraventricular fluid to the fourth ventricle, exiting through the foramina of Magendie and Luschka, is another source of subarachnoid hemorrhage (Zimmerman 1986a). Hemorrhage within the subarachnoid space may be focal or diffuse, with the diffuse form being more common in rupture of an aneurysm than it is in head injury. In our experience, after injury subarachnoid blood has often been focal, overlying the area of contusion or found in the interhemispheric fissure along the falx cerebri (Dolinskas 1978).

CT is the procedure of choice in identifying the radiographic findings of a subarachnoid hemorrhage because blood that occupies the full thickness of a CT slice shows the increased density as a distinct area of brightness (Fig. 10-25). When the blood lies parallel to the plane of the slice, it occupies only a part of the volume. Thus, there is volume averaging of the blood with brain, a process that tends to obscure the presence of a subarachnoid hemorrhage. The normal falx may be slightly dense and may be even calcified or ossified, and so it may be mistaken for a parafalcine subarachnoid hemorrhage (Osborn 1980). The increased density of the falx and its calcification and ossification are normal findings in older adolescents and adults. When a subarachnoid hemorrhage is present along the falx, it typically disappears over the ensuing week (Dolinskas 1978). In our experience with children, the incidence of subarachnoid hemorrhage as seen on CT increases with the increasing severity of a head injury.

When the patient is examined long after the initial trauma, blood in the subarachnoid space may have decreased in density to isodense so that the subarachnoid spaces appear obliterated (but are not), or it may have decreased to a point where the sulci and cisterns appear to be of CSF density. Thus, subarachnoid hemorrhage is difficult to appreciate when the CT study is done more than several days after trauma. A complication of sub-

and fluid-attenuated inversion recovery images (FLAIR) (Noguchi 1995, 1997) on occasion can show subarachnoid hemorrhage as areas of increased signal intensity within the subarachnoid space (Fig. 10-26), more so than with other MR pulse sequences. Blood that is clotted and has undergone clot retraction may be seen subacutely as an area of high-signal-intensity methemoglobin on $T_1WI$ (Bradley 1984).

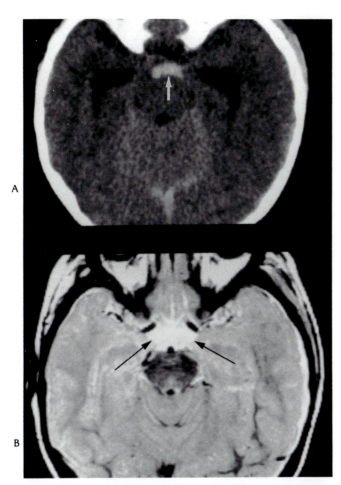

*Figure 10-26* **A.** Axial NCCT shows **subarachnoid hemorrhage** in the interpeduncular cistern (arrow) as well as on the surface of the cerebellum. The temporal horns are dilated as a result of hydrocephalus related to the subarachnoid hemorrhage. **B.** Axial MR-PDWI shows increased signal intensity in the suprasellar cistern (arrows) due to subarachnoid blood.

arachnoid hemorrhage—fibroblastic proliferation within the subarachnoid space and the arachnoid villi—may lead to the production of communicating hydrocephalus. Intraventricular blood can produce ependymitis, which can obstruct the aqueduct of Sylvius or the outlets of the fourth ventricle, leading to obstructive hydrocephalus.

Subarachnoid hemorrhage is poorly demonstrated or not shown at all on MR (Atlas 1993). Oxyhemoglobin is not paramagnetic and does not produce a change in signal intensity. Blood in the subarachnoid space may remain in the oxyhemoglobin state for a longer period than it does in the brain parenchyma. This is thought to occur because of higher oxygen tension in CSF (Kemp 1986). Flowing blood that is not clotted is usually not seen. Proton density weighted images (PDWI)

## CONTUSIONS

A contusion is a bruise of the surface of the brain. The apex of the gyrus is damaged from its outer surface inward to its junction with the white matter and beyond. The degree of involvement of subcortical white matter is variable. The mechanism of contusion has been classically subdivided into two types: coup and contrecoup (Gurdjian 1976). A coup contusion occurs when an object impacts on the stationary head so that the overlying calvarium moves inward, physically distorting the contiguous brain tissue (Figs. 10-1, 10-27, 10-28). As a result, petechial hemorrhages and torn capillaries, along with evidence of mechanical damage to adjacent neurons, are found. Contrecoup contusions are produced at a site remote from the point of initial impact. For this to occur, the brain has to be set in motion relative to the calvarium. Thus, the site of the contusion occurs at a point remote from the site of the initial impact. With a blow to one temporal region, a contrecoup contusion of the opposite temporal lobe may occur (Fig. 10-29C). With a fall on the occiput, contrecoup contusions are often found in the anterior temporal lobes and inferior frontal lobes (Fig. 10-29D and E). It is possible to have a mixture of coup and contrecoup lesions in the same patient. Coup contusions occur most frequently in the frontal and temporal regions, and contrecoup lesions occur most often in the inferior frontal, anterior temporal, and lateral temporal lobes.

Contusions are examined by means of two diagnostic radiological methods: CT and MR. With CT, contusions may produce a high-density (hemorrhagic) or low-density (nonhemorrhagic or hemorrhagic with partial voluming of hemorrhagic elements with necrotic or edematous brain) areas of mass effect (Figs. 10-1, 10-30). Depressed fractures, which frequently accompany a coup contusion, are usually well seen on CT, especially when bone windows are done. The problem with CT is in recognizing small superficial contusions when a thin stripe of high-density cortical blood lies next to high-density bone. Beam-hardening artifacts

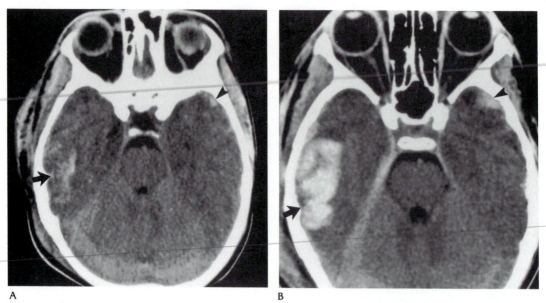

A                                          B

***Figure 10-27*** **A.** CT immediately following trauma shows a **coup contusion** within the inferior right temporal lobe as a high density (arrow). Contrecoup contusion to the left anterior temporal lobe (arrowhead) is also seen. **B.** Follow-up CT scan a day later shows delayed bleeding into both sites of contusion. There is now an intracerebral hematoma present on the right (arrow). There is enlargement of the contrecoup contusion of the left temporal lobe (arrowhead).

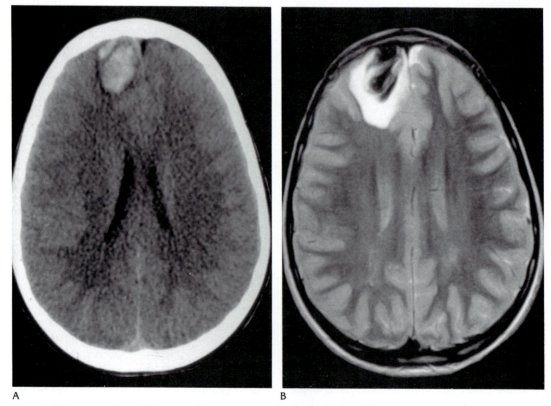

A                                          B

***Figure 10-28*** **A.** Axial CT following trauma shows a frontal **intracerebral hemorrhage** arising from a coup contusion. This has now reached the hematoma stage. **B.** Axial MRI: T$_2$-WI, shows the hematoma to be hypointense and surrounded by hyperintense edema.

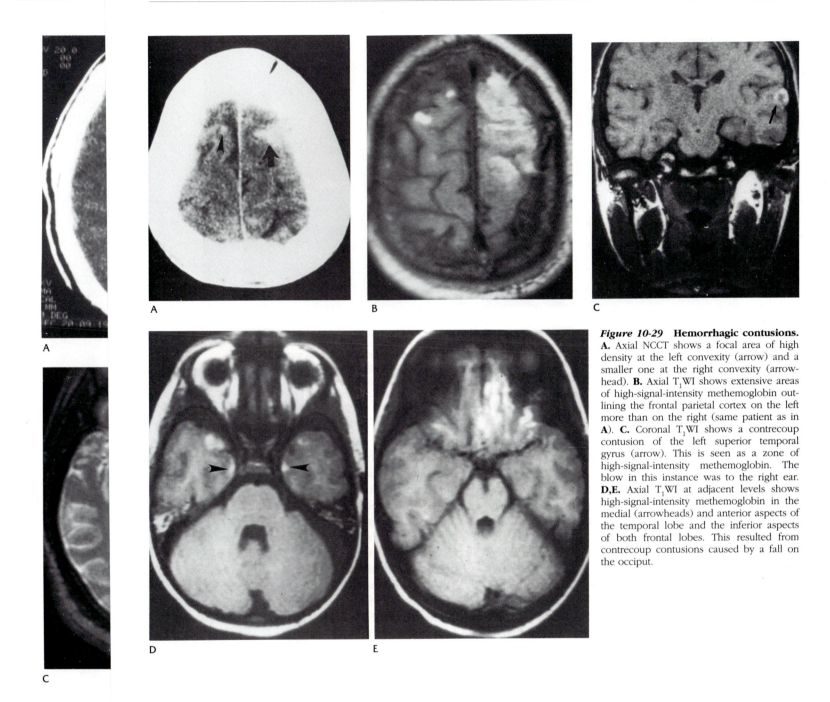

A

C

***Figure 10-29*  Hemorrhagic contusions. A.** Axial NCCT shows a focal area of high density at the left convexity (arrow) and a smaller one at the right convexity (arrowhead). **B.** Axial T$_1$WI shows extensive areas of high-signal-intensity methemoglobin outlining the frontal parietal cortex on the left more than on the right (same patient as in **A**). **C.** Coronal T$_1$WI shows a contrecoup contusion of the left superior temporal gyrus (arrow). This is seen as a zone of high-signal-intensity methemoglobin. The blow in this instance was to the right ear. **D,E.** Axial T$_1$WI at adjacent levels shows high-signal-intensity methemoglobin in the medial (arrowheads) and anterior aspects of the temporal lobe and the inferior aspects of both frontal lobes. This resulted from contrecoup contusions caused by a fall on the occiput.

pointensity outli
tusion (Fig. 10-31

A fourth stage
place in which tl
tic cavities are fc
ing 6 to 12 moi
may be sloughec
regular surface c
sphere results. C
within the brain
of the overlying
size of the cortic

may obscure blood on the surface of the brain adjacent to bone. Contusions of the parietal vertex and inferior temporal lobe may be partially volumed with contiguous bone on the axial slice, resulting in an overall bony density that obscures the presence of the contusion (Fig. 10-29). Unless coronal images are obtained, such contusions are frequently missed. Wider windows than are customary for examination of brain tissue are also effective in separating blood from adjacent bone and should be utilized when there is a possibility of superficial hemorrhagic contusions.

The single most frequent traumatic hemorrhagic parenchymal lesion seen on CT is a hemorrhagic contusion (Zimmerman 1978a). In a series of 286 head injuries, hemorrhagic contusions were present in 21.3 percent and multiple in 29 percent (Koo 1977). Thirty-nine percent of these patients with contusions had other significant focal mass effects, such as subdural hematomas.

MR is an ideal way of examining the brain for the presence or absence of hemorrhagic contusions (Zimmerman 1986b). Acutely, hemorrhagic contusions con-

tracerebral hematomas is lower than that of hemorrhagic contusions. It has been reported to be relatively low (5 percent) (Koo 1977), but when it is present, there is an associated high incidence of other traumatic lesions, such as subdural hematomas and/or epidural hematomas (56 percent) (Zimmerman 1978a). Traumatic intracerebral hematomas appear to occur more frequently in adults than they do in children. Intraventricular extension was found in a CT series of traumatic cases in one-third of the intracerebral hematomas studied (Zimmerman 1978a).

Most intracerebral hematomas are visible on CT and MR immediately after trauma (Figs 10–32, 10–33, and 10–34). They are hyperdense, measuring from 50 to 100 HU (Dolinskas 1977), and may be found to have a surrounding rim of hypodensity caused by extravasated serum from a retracting clot. Subsequently, during the week after the formation of the hematoma, edema develops around the hematoma, extending through the white matter pathways and increasing the mass effect. Although most intracerebral hematomas are demonstrated on the initial day of injury, a small percentage develop in a delayed fashion, appearing 1 to 7 days after the injury (Dolinskas 1977). These hematomas occur most often at the site of contusion or the site of parenchymal ischemia. They are found most often in the frontotemporal and temporal regions. A factor in the formation of delayed intracerebral hematoma may be the removal by surgery of an intracranial mass such as a subdural hematoma. It has been hypothesized that in these instances the removed hematoma produced a tamponade effect on a torn vessel and the removal of the tamponading mass allowed the vessel to rebleed. Vascular necrosis may also result from tissue lactate acidosis or ischemia of a blood vessel wall as a result of spasm. A delayed intracerebral hematoma is an important and treatable cause of secondary deterioration after head injury (Zimmerman 1986a).

In the weeks after hematoma formation, the hematoma decreases in size and density because of chemical breakdown of the globin molecule (Dolinskas 1977). At some point the density of the hematoma on CT will approximate that of the adjacent brain. Usually the decrease in mass effect does not correspond to the decrease in density (Dolinskas 1977). Thus, while the hematoma may not be apparent as a density difference, the mass effect persists. New vessel formation occurs in the tissue surrounding the hematoma; new vessels lack a tight endothelial juncture and as a result, when a contrast agent is injected, there is enhance-

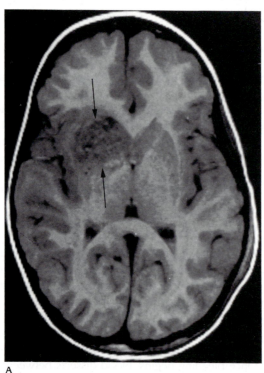 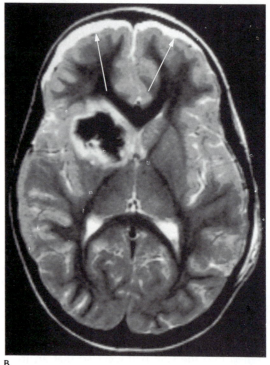

A                                          B

*Figure 10-32*  **Acute intracerebral hematoma: A.** MRI: Axial $T_1$-WI shows hypointense mass effect in the right basal ganglia (arrows). The finding is consistent with deoxyhemoglobin. **B.** Axial $T_2$-WI at the same slice location as shown in **A,** shows the hematoma to be hypointense, surrounded by a small amount of edema. The finding is consistent with deoxyhemoglobin within an intracerebral hematoma. Note the bilateral frontal subdural hygromas (arrows). These are of CSF signal intensity.

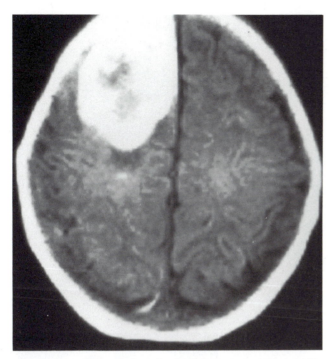

*Figure 10-33* **Subacute intracerebral hematoma.** MRI: Axial $T_1$-WI shows a large right frontal intracerebral hematoma of high-signal-intensity methemoglobin.

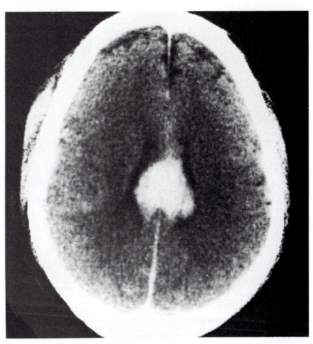

*Figure 10-34* **Shearing injury** with corpus callosal hemorrhage. Axial NCCT shows a high-density hemorrhage within the posterior portion of the corpus callosum.

ment of a rim of tissue surrounding the hematoma (Zimmerman 1986*a*). With CT, when a previous study is not available or the history is not helpful, this may be useful in identifying a subacute hematoma that is isodense. On MR, an intracerebral hematoma has the same signal intensity characteristics that are described in the section on hemorrhagic contusion. An acute intracerebral hematoma in the deoxyhemoglobin state is hypointense on $T_2$WI (Fig. 10-32), whereas a subacute hematoma composed of methemoglobin is hyperintense on $T_1$WI (Fig. 10-33).

Thus, when the clot is no longer visible on CT, it is highly visible on MR. Exactly how long the clot will remain visible on MR is uncertain, but we have followed a patient for over 4 years, during which time we have seen residual high-signal-intensity methemoglobin on $T_1$WI. Macrophages that carry off blood breakdown products produce hemosiderin, giving the rim of the hematoma cavity a hypointense signal intensity on $T_2$WI. Follow-up MR studies show that the hematoma cavity decreases in size with time, just as follow-up CT studies show a subsequent CSF density residuum. Frequently, with both techniques there is a demonstration of overlying cortical sulcal enlargement and adjacent ventricular dilatation, changes that correlate with parenchymal brain damage from injury.

## Diffuse Axonal Injury (DAI) or Shearing Injury

When one cerebral hemisphere is put in motion relative to the other, shearing stresses are produced along the courses of the white matter axons that connect the two hemispheres (Meaney 1995). As a result of these stresses, disruption of axons occurs, along with the rupture of the small accompanying blood vessels (Zimmerman 1978*c*). This type of injury occurs most often among drivers and passengers in high-speed motor vehicle accidents. Often the patient is rendered comatose at the time of the accident, undergoes emergency imaging evaluation, and is hospitalized for a prolonged period, not infrequently in a persistent vegetative state that may last months or years and often necessitates institutionalization (Zimmerman 1978*c*). A CT examination may be unremarkable, may show some degree of cerebral swelling, or may show small focal hemorrhages (Fig. 10-35) or even more extensive injury (Zimmerman 1978*c*). Characteristically, the lesions in DAI occur in four sites: (1) corpus callosum (Fig. 10-35C), (2) corticomedullary junctures (Fig. 10-36), (3) upper brainstem (Fig. 10-35B), and (4) basal ganglia (Strich 1961). Axonal tears occur not only where the hemor-

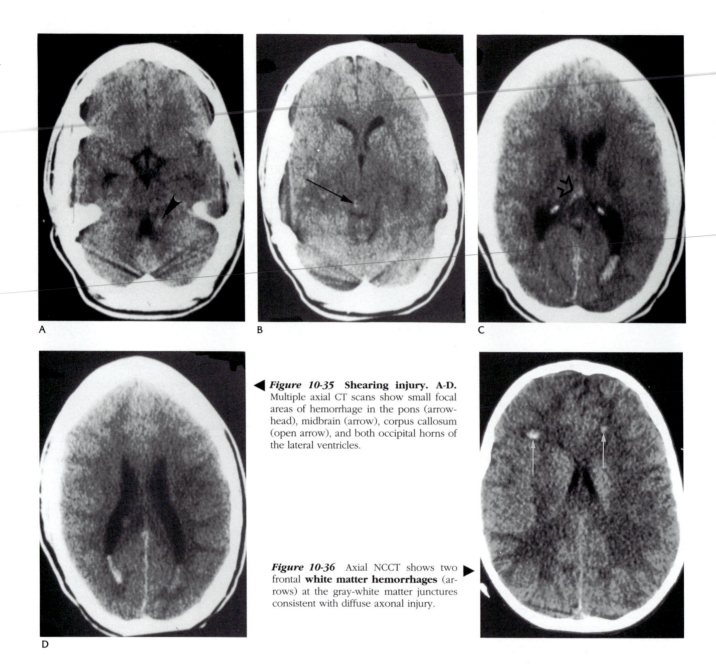

A

B

C

◀ *Figure 10-35* **Shearing injury. A-D.** Multiple axial CT scans show small focal areas of hemorrhage in the pons (arrowhead), midbrain (arrow), corpus callosum (open arrow), and both occipital horns of the lateral ventricles.

*Figure 10-36* Axial NCCT shows two ▶ frontal **white matter hemorrhages** (arrows) at the gray-white matter junctures consistent with diffuse axonal injury.

D

rhages are found but throughout the white matter as well (Gentry 1988). CT can show only the hemorrhagic component and the brain swelling that may accompany it. The presence of a small amount of intraventricular blood in the occipital horn of one or both ventricles should arouse suspicion that there has been a tear of the corpus callosum with transependymal extension of the bleeding (Abraszko 1995). Often it is not possible to see small hemorrhages in the corpus callosum on CT.

MR has proved to be superior to CT in demonstrating findings consistent with DAI. The sites of disrupted axonal bundles that are unaccompanied by hemorrhage are shown by MR as zones of high-signal-intensity edema on $T_2WI$ (Figs. 10-37, 10-38A) (Zimmerman 1986b; Gentry 1988). Depending on their chemical

state, hemorrhages are shown at the classic locations in the corpus callosum, corticomedullary junctures, dorsal midbrain, and basal ganglia (Zimmerman 1988) (Fig. 10-39). Gradient echo susceptibility scanning in the form of a 2D FLASH gradient echo sequence is a useful adjunct to MRI in traumatic brain injury. This shows the hemorrhagic foci, such as in DAI as multiple areas of signal loss at the site of bleeding (Fig. 10-40). The course of brain injury after DAI is one of secondary Wallerian degeneration of torn axons (Zimmerman 1978c). As a result, brain atrophy occurs over months to years, with enlargement of the sulci and ventricles (Fig. 10-38B). The white matter may be seen to undergo a loss of volume with scattered areas of high signal intensity on $T_2WI$ at sites of Wallerian degeneration. MR is particularly successful in examining a

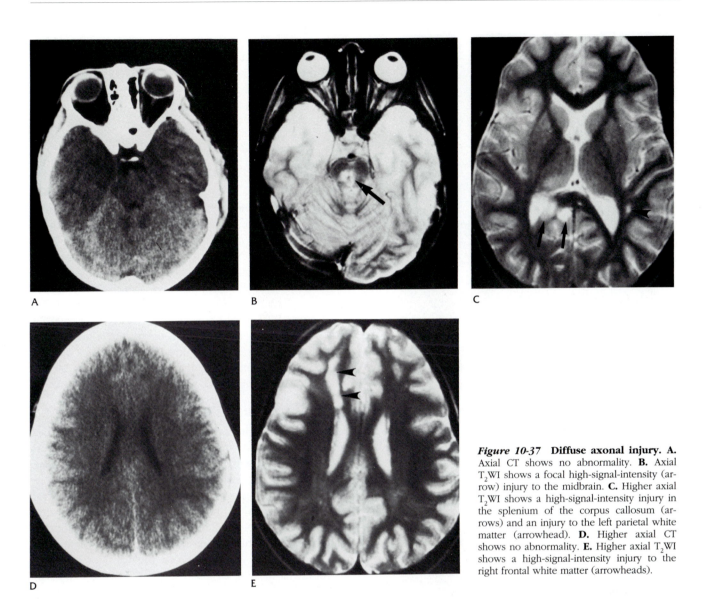

*Figure 10-37* **Diffuse axonal injury. A.** Axial CT shows no abnormality. **B.** Axial T₂WI shows a focal high-signal-intensity (arrow) injury to the midbrain. **C.** Higher axial T₂WI shows a high-signal-intensity injury in the splenium of the corpus callosum (arrows) and an injury to the left parietal white matter (arrowhead). **D.** Higher axial CT shows no abnormality. **E.** Higher axial T₂WI shows a high-signal-intensity injury to the right frontal white matter (arrowheads).

*Figure 10-38* **Acute shearing injury** and subsequent follow-up. **A.** T₂WI at the time of an acute injury shows multiple basal ganglionic and corpus callosal areas of high-signal-intensity injury. **B.** Follow-up MR scan many months later shows the absence of the foci of high signal intensity but dilatation of the ventricles and sulci as a result of atrophy. One focal area of low signal intensity is present at the site of an old hemorrhage (arrow).

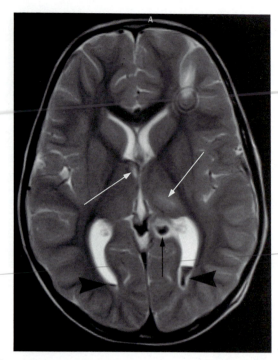

**Figure 10-39** Axial T$_2$-WI in a patient with **diffuse axonal injury** shows edema in both thalami (white arrows). A hypointense site of hemorrhage (black arrow) is present in the left splenium of the corpus callosum. Hypointense blood products are present in a dependent portion in both lateral ventricles (arrowheads). Note the blood fluid levels. Artifact is present in the left frontal lobe from a subarachnoid pressure bolt.

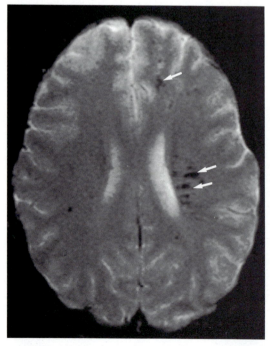

**Figure 10-40** Axial gradient echo susceptibility scan done with 2D FLASH technique shows multiple deep white matter sites of hemorrhage in the left hemisphere (arrows). Fewer areas are found on the right. The findings are consistent with **diffuse axonal injury.**

mystery patient who has been rendered comatose by a prior DAI. The atrophy, tears in the corpus callosum, and the presence of old blood products in the form of hemosiderin at characteristic sites help in making a diagnosis of a prior DAI (Fig. 10-38B).

## Subdural Hematoma

The subdural space is a potential space that lies between the dura and the arachnoid. With trauma, tearing, and separation of the arachnoid from the dura, there may be associated bleeding and hematoma formation. Hematomas within the subdural space are classified as either acute or chronic. Posttraumatic subdural collections may be filled with CSF when there is a tear in the arachnoid so that CSF dissects between the arachnoid and dura. A CSF-filled collection of this type is called a *subdural hygroma*. In general, acute and chronic subdural hematomas and subdural hygromas differ in their history, their significance, and often their pattern of resolution (Zimmerman 1986*a*).

### ACUTE SUBDURAL HEMATOMAS

Acute subdural hematomas follow acute trauma, becoming manifest within hours after injury. They are often associated with an underlying brain injury. The damage to the cerebral substance results not only from the mass effect produced by the clot in the subdural space but also from the brain injury and swelling that accompany it. Despite modern methods of treatment, acute subdural hematomas associated with parenchymal brain injury, most often in the form of an intracerebral hematoma or contusion, contiue to carry significant morbidity and mortality (Fobben 1989). On CT, an acute subdural hematoma is seen as a peripheral collection of blood-density clot lying between the inner table and the cerebral hemisphere (Figs. 10-2, 10-41, 10-42). Subdural hematomas tend to extend around the hemisphere from front to back and frequently extend around the occipital pole or frontal pole into the interhemispheric fissure, under the temporal lobe to the floor of the middle cranial fossa, or under the occipital lobe onto the tentorium (Fig. 10-43) (Zimmerman 1986*a*). The full extent of the clot and the space that it occupies intracranially reduce the amount of space available for the brain within the cranial vault. In addition, there is a further decrease in intracranial volume as a result of the associated brain injury (Figs. 10-41, 10-42) and swelling, which also raise the intracranial pressure, leading to herniation or impaired cerebral perfusion. Surgery is utilized to decrease the size of an acute subdural hematoma. However, the degree of mass effect postoperatively may be larger than it is preoperatively because parenchymal injury has be-

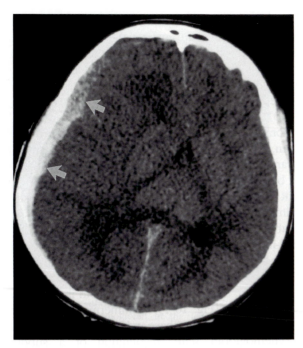

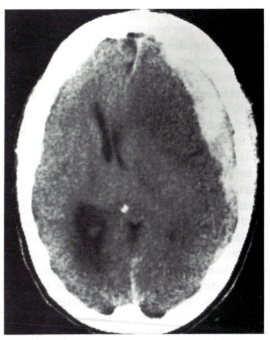

*Figure 10-41*  **Acute subdural** is shown on axial NCCT as a high-density hematoma (arrows) on the right, producing marked mass effect.

*Figure 10-42*  **Acute subdural hematoma.** Axial NCCT shows a peripheral high-density extracerebral collection within the subdural space that compresses and displaces the left cerebral hemisphere. There is a subfallaceal midline shift. The falx is bent to the right. The pineal gland, which is calcified, is shifted. There is hypodensity in the underlying left cerebral hemisphere, notably below the region of the subdural hematoma.

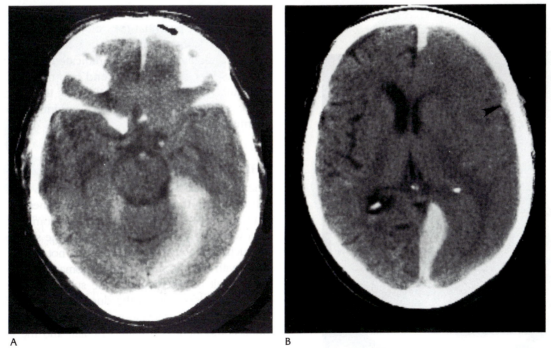

A                                                                      B

*Figure 10-43*  **Acute subdural hematoma. A.** Axial NCCT at the level of the tentorium shows high-density blood conforming to the medial aspect of the tentorium, representing an infratemporal and infraoccipital extension of a subdural hematoma. **B.** A higher section shows a subdural hematoma in the interhemispheric fissure between the left occipital lobe and the falx as well as in the interhemispheric fissure between the left frontal lobe and the falx. There is a smear of subdural hematoma adjacent to the inner table of the skull (arrowhead).

## CONCLUSION

CT remains the first diagnostic step in the definitive evaluation of an emergency patient with craniocerebral trauma. It is used in determining whether surgical evacuation of a hematoma or medical management is indicated. However, it can no longer be said that CT is the most accurate noninvasive imaging modality for showing the morphological manifestations of brain injury. MR in many instances is more accurate though more difficult to obtain. The advent of MR angiography and spectroscopy will add important aspects to our understanding of brain injury.

# References

ABRASZKO RA, ZURYNSKI YA, DORSCH NW: The significance of traumatic intraventricular hemorrhage in severe head injury. *Br J Neurosurg* 9(6):769–773, 1995.

ADAMS JH: The neuropathology of head injury, in Vinken PJV, Bruyn GW (eds), *Handbook of Clinical Neurology,* vol 23, New York, American Elsevier, 1975, pp 35–65.

ALBERICO AM, WARD JD, CHOI SC, et al: Outcome after severe head injury. Relationship to mass lesions, diffuse injury, and ICP course in pediatric and adult patients. *J Neurosurg* 67:648–656, 1987.

ATLAS SW: MR imaging is highly sensitive for acute subarachnoid hemorrhage . . . not! *Radiology* 186:319–332, 1993.

BAKAY L, GLASAUER FE: *Head Injury,* Boston, Little, Brown, 1980.

BALASUBRAMANIAM S, KADAPIA T, CAMPBELL JS, et al: Efficacy of skull radiography. *Am J Surg* 142:366, 1981.

BELL R, LOOP JW: The utility and futility of radiographic skull examinations in trauma. *N Engl J Med* 284:236, 1971.

BERNARDI B, ZIMMERMAN RA, BILANIUK LT: Neuroradiologic evaluation of pediatric craniocerebral trauma. *Topics Magn Reson Imag* 5(3):161–173, 1993.

BILLMIRE ME, MYERS PA: Serious head injury in infants: Accident or abuse? *Pediatrics* 75:340–342, 1985.

BIRD CR, MCMAHAN JR, GILLES FH, et al: Strangulation in child abuse: CT diagnosis. *Radiology* 163:373–375, 1987.

BRADLEY WG, SCHMIDT PG: Effect of methemoglobin formation on the MR appearance of subarachnoid hemorrhage. *Radiology* 156:99–103, 1984.

BRUCE DA, ALAVI A, BILANIUK L, et al: Diffuse cerebral swelling following head injuries in children: The syndrome of "malignant brain edema." *J Neurosurg* 54:170–178, 1981.

BRUCE DA, ZIMMERMAN RA: Shaken impact syndrome. *Pediatr Ann* 18:482–494, 1989.

CAFFEY J: Multiple fractures in the long bones of infants suffering from chronic subdural hematoma. *AJR* 56:163–173, 1946.

CAFFEY J: The whiplash shaken infant syndrome: Manual shaking by the extremities with whiplash-induced intracranial and intraocular bleedings, linked with residual permanent brain damage and mental retardation. *Pediatrics* 54:396–403, 1974.

CAVENESS WF: Incidence of cranio-cerebral trauma in 1976 with trend from 1970 to 1975, in Thompson RA, Green JRG (eds), *Advances in Neurology,* vol 22, New York, Raven Press, 1979, pp 1–3.

DAVIS JM, ZIMMERMAN RA: Injury of the carotid and vertebral arteries. *Neuroradiology* 25:55–69, 1983.

DETRE JA, WANG Z, BOGDAN AR, et al: Regional variation in brain lactate in Leigh syndrome by localized $^1$H magnetic resonance spectroscopy. *Ann Neurol* 29:218–221, 1991.

DOLINSKAS C, BILANIUK LT, ZIMMERMAN RA, et al: Computed tomography of intracerebral hematomas: I. Transmission CT observations of hematoma resolution. *AJR* 129:681–688, 1977.

DOLINSKAS C, ZIMMERMAN RA, BILANIUK LT: A sign of subarachnoid bleeding on cranial computed tomograms of pediatric head trauma patients. *Radiology* 126:409, 1978.

DOLINSKAS CA, ZIMMERMAN RA, BILANIUK LT, et al: Computed tomography of post-traumatic extracerebral hematomas: Comparison to pathophysiology and responses to therapy. *J Trauma* 19:163, 1979.

DUHAIME AC, GENNARELLI TA, THIBAULT LE, et al: The shaken baby syndrome. A clinical, pathological, and biochemical study. *J Neurosurg* 66:409–415, 1987.

FOBBEN ES, GROSSMAN RI, ATLAS SW, et al: MR characteristics of subdural hematomas and hygromas at 1.5 T. *AJNR* 10:687–693, 1989.

GENTRY LR, GODERSKY JC, THOMPSON B: MR imaging of head trauma: Review of the distribution and radiopathologic features of traumatic lesions. *AJNR* 9:101, 1988.

GENTRY LR: Imaging of closed head injury. *Radiology* 191: 1–17, 1994.

GIBBY WA, ZIMMERMAN RA: X-Ray Computed Tomography, in Mazziotta and Gilman (eds), *Clinical Brain Imaging: Principles and Applications*, Philadelphia, Davis, 1992.

GOMORI JM, GROSSMAN RI, BILANIUK LT, et al: High-field MR imaging of superficial siderosis of the central nervous system. *J Comput Assist Tomogr* 9(5):972–975, 1985*a*.

GOMORI M, GROSSMAN RI, GOLDBERG HI, et al: High field magnetic resonance imaging of intracranial hematomas. *Radiology* 157:87–93, 1985*b*.

GOMORI JM, GROSSMAN RI: Mechanisms responsible for the MR appearance and evolution of intracranial hemorrhage. *Radiology* 161(P):364, 1986.

GURDJIAN ES: Cerebral contusions: Reevaluation of the mechanism of their development. *J Trauma* 16:35, 1976.

HARWOOD-NASH DC: Fractures of the petrous and tympanic parts of the temporal bone in children: A tomographic study of 35 cases. *AJR* 110:598, 1970.

HARWOOD-NASH DC: Abuse to the pediatric central nervous system. *AJNR* 13:569–575, 1992.

HENRYS P, LYNE ED, LIFTON C, et al: Clinical review of cervical spine injuries in children. *Clin Orthop* 129:172, 1977.

ITO J, MARMAROU A, BARZO P, et al: Characterization of edema by diffusion-weighted imaging in experimental traumatic brain injury. *J Neurosurg* 84:97–103, 1996.

JENNETT B: Skull x-rays after recent head injury. *Clin Radiol* 31:463, 1980.

JENNETT B, TEASDALE G: *Management of Injuries,* Philadelphia, Davis, 1981.

KANTER RK: Retinal hemorrhage after cardiopulmonary resuscitation or child abuse. *J Pediatr* 108:430–432, 1986.

KEMP SS, GROSSMAN RI: The importance of oxygenation in the appearance of acute subarachnoid hemorrhage on high field magnetic resonance imaging (abst). XIII Symposium Neuroradiologicum, Stockholm, June 1986.

KOO AH, LA ROQUE RI: Evaluation of head trauma by computed tomography. *Radiology* 123:345, 1977.

KRAUS J, FIFE D, COX P, et al: Incidence, severity and external cause of pediatric brain injury. *Am J Dis Child* 140: 687–693, 1986.

LANTZ EJ, FORBES GS, BROWN MI, et al: Radiology of cerebrospinal fluid rhinorrhea. *AJR* 135:1023, 1980.

LINDENBERG R: Pathology of craniocerebral injuries, in Newton TH, Potts DS (eds), *Radiology of the Skull and Brain: Anatomy and Pathology,* vol 3, St. Louis, CV Mosby, 1977.

MANELFE C, CELLERIER P, SOBEL D, et al: Cerebrospinal fluid rhinorrhea: Evaluation with metrizamide cisternography. *AJR* 138:471, 1982.

MARION DW, DARBY J, YONAS H: Acute regional cerebral blood flow changes caused by severe head injuries. *J Neurosurg* 74:407–414, 1991.

MASARYK TJ, MODIC MT, RUGGIERI PM, et al: Three-dimensional (volume) gradient-echo imaging of the carotid bifurcation: Preliminary clinical experience. *Radiology* 171: 801, 1989.

MCCORMICK MC, SHAPIRO S, STARFIELD BH: Injury and its correlates among one year old children. *Am J Dis Child* 135:159–163, 1981.

MEANEY DF, SMITH DH, SHREIBER DI, et al: Biomechanical analysis of experimental diffuse axonal injury. *J Neurotrauma* 12:689–694, 1995.

MELZAK J: Paraplegia among children. *Lancet* ii:45, 1969.

MERTEN DF, OSBORNE DRS, RADKOWSKI MA, et al: Craniocerebral trauma in the child abuse syndrome: Radiological observations. *Pediatr Radiol* 14:272–277, 1984.

MERTEN DF, RADKOWSKI MA, LEONIDAS JC: The abused child: A radiological reappraisal. *Radiology* 146:377–381, 1983.

NAIDICH TP, MORAN CJ, PUDLOWSKI RM, et al: CT diagnosis of the isodense subdural hematoma, in Thompson RA, Green JR (eds), *Advances in Neurology,* vol 22, New York, Raven Press, 1979.

NAIDICH TP, MORAN CJ: Precise anatomic localization of atraumatic sphenoethmoidal cerebrospinal fluid rhinorrhea by metrizamide CT cisternography. *J Neurosurg* 53:222, 1980.

NOGUCHI K, OGAWA T., IMGAMI A, et al. Acute subarachnoid hemorrhage: MR imaging with fluid-attenuated inversion recovery pulse sequences. *Radiology* 196:773–777, 1995.

NOGUCHI K, OGAWA T, SETO H, et al. Subacute and chronic subarachnoid hemorrhage: Diagnosis with fluid-attenuated inversion-recovery MR imaging *Radiology* 203:257–262, 1997.

OGDEN JA: *Skeletal Injury in the Child,* Philadelphia, Lea & Febiger, 1982.

ORRISON WW, GENTRY LR, STIMAC GK, et al: Blinded comparison of cranial CT and MR in closed head injury evaluation. *AJNR* 15:351, 1994.

OSBORN AG, DAINES JH, WING SD, et al: Intracranial air on computerized tomography. *J Neurosurg* 48:355, 1978.

OSBORN AG, ANDERSON RE, WING SD: The false falx sign. *Radiology* 134:421, 1980.

RADKOWSKI MA, MERTEN DR, LEONIDAS JC: The abused child: Criteria for the radiological diagnosis. *Radiographics* 3:262–297, 1983.

RIVERA FP, KAMITSUKA MD, QUAN L: Injuries to children younger than one year of age. *Pediatrics* 81:93–97, 1988.

ROBERTS F, SHOPFNER CE: Plain skull roentgenograms in children with head trauma. *AJR* 114:230, 1972.

ROBINSON AE, MEARES BM, GOREE JA: Traumatic sphenoid sinus effusion: An analysis of 50 cases. *Am J Radium Ther Nucl Med* 101:795, 1967.

ROYAL COLLEGE OF RADIOLOGISTS: A study of the utilization of skull radiography in nine accidents and emergency units in the UK. *Lancet* i:1234, 1980.

SATO Y, YUH WTC, SMITH WL, et al: Head injury in child abuse: Evaluation with MR imaging. *Radiology* 173:653–657, 1989.

SCHNALL MD, BOLINGER I, RENSHAW PF, et al: Multinuclear MR imaging: Technique for combined anatomic and physiologic studies. *Radiology* 162:863, 1987.

SCHUNK JE, RODGERSON JD, WOODWARD GA: The utility of head computed tomographic scanning in pediatric patients with normal neurologic examination in the emergency department. *Pediatr Emerg Care* 12(3):160–165, 1996.

ST. JOHN EG: The role of the emergency skull roentgenogram in head trauma. *AJR* 76:315, 1968.

STRICH SJ: Shearing of nerve fibers as a cause of brain damage due to head injury: A pathological study of twenty cases. *Lancet* ii:443, 1961.

STRONG I, MACMILLAN R, JENNETT B: Head injuries in accident and emergency departments at Scottish hospitals. *Injury* 10:154, 1978.

SUTTON LN, WANG Z, DUHAIME AC, et al: Tissue lactate in pediatric head trauma: A clinical study using 1HNMR spectroscopy. *Pediatr Neurosurg* 22: 81–87, 1995.

TASI FY, ZEE CS, APTHORP JS, DIXON GH: Computed tomography in child abuse head trauma. *J Comput Tomogr* 4:277–286, 1980.

TAVERAS JM, RANSOHOFF J: Leptomeningeal cysts of the brain following trauma, with erosion of the skull. *J Neurosurg* 10:223, 1953.

YOSHIHARU T, HANAFEE WN: Cerebrospinal fluid rhinorrhea: The significance of an air-fluid level in the sphenoid sinus. *Radiology* 135:101, 1980.

ZIMMERMAN RA, BILANIUK LT, DOLINSKAS C, et al: Computed tomography of acute intracerebral hemorrhagic contusion. *J Comput Tomogr* 1:271–280, 1977.

ZIMMERMAN RA, BILANIUK LT, GENNARELLI T, et al: Cranial computed tomography in diagnosis and management of acute head trauma. *AJR* 131:27, 1978a.

ZIMMERMAN RA, BILANIUK LT, BRUCE D, et al: Computed tomography of pediatric head trauma: Acute general cerebral swelling. *Radiology* 126:403, 1978b.

ZIMMERMAN RA, BILANIUK LT, GENNARELLI T: Computed tomography of shearing injuries of the cerebral white matter. *Radiology* 127:393–396, 1978c.

ZIMMERMAN RA, BILANIUK LT, BRUCE D, et al: Computed tomography of pediatric head trauma: Acute general cerebral swelling. *Radiology* 126:403–408, 1978.

ZIMMERMAN RA, BILANIUK LT, BRUCE D, et al: Computed tomography of craniocerebral injury in the abused child. *Radiology* 10:687, 1979.

ZIMMERMAN RA, BILANIUK LT, BRUCE D, et al: Computed tomography of craniocerebral injury in the abused child. *Radiology* 130:687–690, 1979.

ZIMMERMAN RA, BILANIUK LT: Computed tomography in pediatric head trauma. *J Neuroradiol* 8:257, 1981.

ZIMMERMAN RA, BILANIUK LT: Computed tomographic staging of traumatic epidural bleeding. *Radiology* 144:809, 1982.

ZIMMERMAN RA: The effectiveness of skull plain films in the evaluation of traumatic coma. *J Neuroradiol* 10:145, 1983.

ZIMMERMAN RA, BILANIUK LT: Head trauma, in RN Rosenberg (ed), *The Clinical Neurosciences,* Edinburgh, Churchill Livingstone, 1984, p 483.

ZIMMERMAN RA, BILANIUK LT, GROSSMAN RI, et al: Resistive NMR of intracranial hematomas. *Neuroradiology* 27:16–20, 1985.

ZIMMERMAN RA: Evaluation of head injury: Supratentorial, in Taveras J, Ferrucci E (eds), Philadelphia, Lippincott, 1986a.

ZIMMERMAN RA, BILANIUK LT, HACKNEY DB, et al: Head injury: Early results of comparing CT and high-field MR. *AJNR* 7:757–764, 1986b.

ZIMMERMAN RA, BILANIUK LT, HACKNEY DB, et al: Magnetic resonance imaging in temporal bone fracture. *Neuroradiology* 29:246–257, 1987.

ZIMMERMAN RA: Magnetic resonance of head injury, in Taveras J, Ferrucci E (eds), *Radiology: Diagnosis-Imaging-Intervention,* Philadelphia, Lippincott, 1988, pp 1–12.

ZIMMERMAN RA, BILANIUK LT: CT and MR: Diagnosis and evolution of head injury, stroke, and brain tumors. *Neuropsychology* 3:191–230, 1989.

ZIMMERMAN RA, GUSNARD DA, BILANIUK LT: Pediatric craniocervical spiral CT. *Neuroradiology* 34:112–116, 1992.

ZIMMERMAN RA, BILANIUK LT: Pediatric head trauma. *Neuroimag Clin North Am* 4(2):349, 1994.

# 11 INFECTIOUS DISEASES

*Gordon Sze*
*S. Howard Lee*

## CONTENTS

## GENERAL CONSIDERATIONS

The brain and spinal cord are well protected from direct spread of infectious disease processes by osseous and membranous coverings, including the pachymeninges (dura) and leptomeninges (pia-arachnoid) and also by the blood-brain and blood-CSF barriers at a microscopic level (Gray 1997). Possible reasons for the peculiar CNS response to microorganisms include certain structural peculiarities of the brain and its coverings, such as the absence of true lymphatics; differences in vascular supply in gray and white matter; the absence of capillaries in the subarachnoid space; direct intercommunication between intra- and extracra-

nial venous systems via diploic and emissary veins; and the presence of a perivascular arachnoid space around the veins as well as the large vessels (Virchow-Robin spaces) and the perivascular glial membrane. Cerebrospinal fluid also is an excellent culture medium for bacterial growth.

An infectious process varies with time and the intrinsic ability of the host to react and with the nature of the infectious agent. Infectious agents are considered *pathogenic* when a normal individual is infected by an adequate inoculum and *opportunistic* when the host is compromised (Scavanilli 1997). An effective treatment often depends on the exact identification of the etiological agents. This chapter discusses the various groups of organisms—bacterial, granulomatous, viral, fungal, and parasitic—that affect the brain. In addition, a final section is devoted to acquired immune deficiency syndrome (AIDS), because many of its manifestations form a characteristic constellation and because it is almost certainly the most common cause of infections of the CNS today.

## BACTERIAL INFECTION

Bacterial agents reach the brain or meninges predominantly by two routes: (1) hematogeneous dissemination from a distant infective focus to the meninges, corticomedullary junction, and choroid plexus, and (2) direct extension by bony erosion from an adjacent focus of suppuration (otitis, mastoiditis, sinusitis) or (3) by transmission along cranial nerves with or without surgery or traumatic craniocerebral wound.

### Subdural Empyema

Subdural infection accounts for about 13 to 20 percent of all cases of intracranial bacterial infection and 5.1 percent of all space-occupying lesions in the subdural space (Weinman 1972; Galbraith 1974; Danziger 1980; Blaquiere 1983). It is frequently associated with epidural abscess (Kaufmann 1975; Zimmerman 1984) and usually presents a fulminating clinical course and an emergent neurosurgical condition. Before the era of CT, subdural empyema was associated with a mortality rate as high as 40 percent; since the advent of CT (Bhardari 1970; Weinman 1972; LaBeau 1973), mortality has dropped significantly (Schroth 1987), but it remains considerable. The high morbidity and mortality are related more to the response of the cerebral vasculature and brain to the inflammatory process than to the mass effect of the extraaxial collection (Sadhu 1980; Zimmerman 1984). Whenever progressive neurological deterioration coexists with a systemic manifestation of infection, this diagnosis should be strongly considered.

The most common cause of subdural empyema is paranasal sinusitis (Kaufmann 1975; Carter 1983). In Zimmerman's (1984) series of 49 patients, frontal sinusitis was the most common cause of empyema; more than 40 percent of these patients had preceding frontal sinusitis. Less frequently, subdural empyema may be secondary to otitic infection, a penetrating wound of the skull, craniectomy, or osteomyelitis of the skull.

The mechanism of subdural infection may be twofold: progressive retrograde thrombophlebitis or (less likely) direct spread after penetration of the dura. The most common location of a subdural empyema is over the convexity of one or both hemispheres (80 percent). The interhemispheric fissure is the next most frequent location (12 percent). In this space, subdural empyema may occur as an extension of the convexity collection (Stephanov 1979). Convexities or combined convexities-interhemispheric empyemas have a predilection for the anterior aspects of the cranial cavity near the frontal lobes, whereas an isolated interhemispheric empyema may occur at the base of the brain or beneath the tentorium (Weinman 1972; Grinelli 1977).

CT findings of acute subdural empyema may be subtle and not apparent initially. Noncontrast CT (NCCT) demonstrates a crescentic or, more frequently, lentiform-shaped area of low density (0 to 16 HU) adjacent to the inner border of the skull or the falx, representing pus (Fig. 11-1). Frequently, mass effect of the underlying brain may be more prominent than the subtle extracerebral collection. The white matter may appear hypodense as a result of edema, cerebritis, or infarction (Enzmann 1984). On contrast-enhanced CT (CECT), a zone of enhancement separates the hypodense extracerebral collection from the brain surface (Fig. 11-2). This curvilinear enhancement is due to granulation tissue formation at the boundary of the

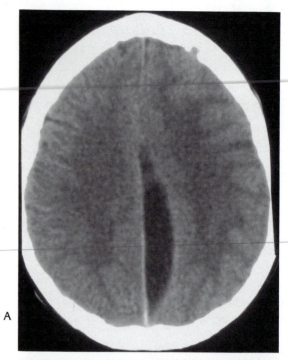

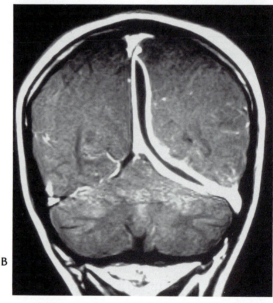

***Figure 11-1*** **Subdural empyema** in a 14-year-old male with sinusitis. **(A)** Axial NCCT shows a large left-sided posterior parafalcine collection of fluid that was slightly higher in density than CSF. **(B)** CEMR: Coronal $T_1$WI shows a subdural collection with contrast enhancing walls extending from the falx down onto the tentorium. Thick, intense dural and marginal contrast enhancement is conspicuous.

empyema on its leptomeningeal surface and perhaps inflammation or ischemia in the subjacent cerebral cortex (Grinelli 1977; Weisberg 1986) (Fig. 11-1). The margins of the enhanced zone may show varying degrees of irregularity and thickness (Stephanov 1979; Sadhu 1980; Zimmerman 1984).

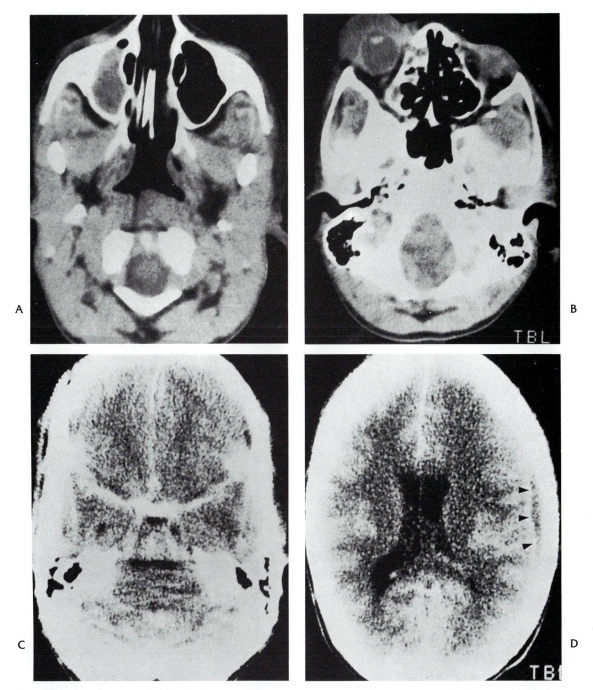

**Figure 11-2** **Subdural empyema** associated with **leptomeningitis** and **cerebritis.** NCCT **(A)•(B):** Right maxillary sinusitis **(A)** extends into the right orbit **(B).** CECT **(C)** shows marked contrast enhancement at the basal cistern representing extensive leptomeningi-tis. CECT **(D):** A thin, crescentic, left hemispheric subdural empyema (arrowheads) with marked contrast enhancement of the underlying gyri and of the interhemispheric fissure (leptomeningitis, cerebritis, and/or venous thrombosis). (*Continued on next page*)

Currently, MR has become the modality of choice in the evaluation of suspected subdural empyema (Weingarten 1989). MR offers several advantages over CT. First, it is considerably more sensitive in the detection of extracerebral fluid collections. Although fluid collec-tions may be obscured on CT because of the adjacent skull, on MR even small crescentic empyemas are read-ily visible since the bony inner table appears as a signal void. This is more evident in paratentorial and subtem-poral locations on coronal MR images. Second, MR can

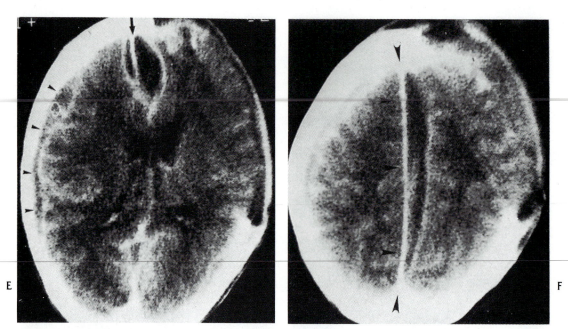

**Figure 11-2 (continued)**   CECT (**E**) following surgical evacuation of the left subdural empyema demonstrates occurrence of the right subdural empyema (arrowheads) with underlying cerebritis. Frontal interhemispheric subdural empyema can be seen on both sides of the falx cerebri (arrow). **F.** On CECT, convexity level shows a large interhemispheric subdural empyema delineated by a thick falx cerebri on the medial side (arrowheads) and an early membrane formation on the lateral side. Note also gyral contrast enhancement on both hemispheres.

often differentiate subdural from epidural empyemas (Fig. 11-3). The dura itself can be detected in an epidural empyema as a hypointense medial rim separating the fluid collection from the underlying subarachnoid space and brain parenchyma. Third, MR can provide better characterization of the contents of extraaxial fluid (Brant-Zawadzki 1985). Very purulent collections have decreased $T_1$ and $T_2$ relaxation times and are hyperintense on $T_1$ and $T_2$WI compared with pure CSF using routine parameters. Whereas both chronic hematoma and empyema appear as hypodense collections on CT, MR is able to differentiate the two easily (Weingarten 1989). Subacute to chronic hematomas have a markedly increased signal on both $T_1$ and $T_2$WI as a result of hemoglobin degradation, unlike pure empyemas, which exhibit signal characteristics similar to those of a proteinaceous fluid. Fourth, MR is superior in the detection of concomitant parenchymal alterations and venous thrombosis (Figs. 11-3 and 11-4). Edema is underlying parenchyma and secondary infarcts resulting from vasculitis or thrombosis are easily seen.

Sulcal alterations such as effacement and reversible cortical hyperintensities on $T_2$WI are also more readily assessed with MR than with CT (Fig.11-3). These cortical hyperintensities were thought to represent cortical hyperemia or edema resulting from ischemia induced by inflammatory vasospasm (Weingarten 1989; Sze 1988b).

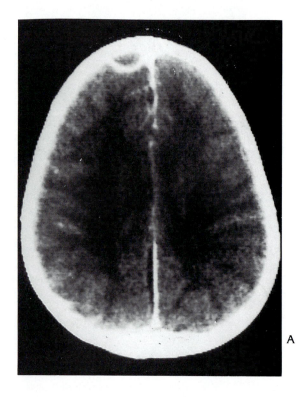

On contrast enhanced MR (CEMR), enhancement can be seen on both the inner and outer surfaces of a subdural empyema, unlike in CT (Sze 1989) (Fig. 11-1). Since the inner table of the skull is not visualized, con-

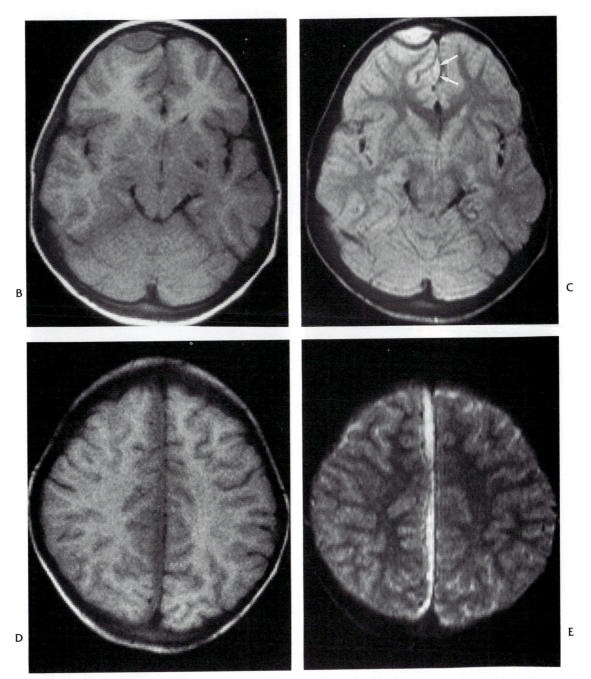

◄ *Figure 11-3* **Subdural and epidural empyemas** in a 9-year-old boy with postsinusitis. **A.** CECT shows extraaxial collections in posterior interhemispheric fissure and anterior to right frontal lobe. Note thickening of falx and marginal enhancement of right frontal collection. **B–E.** MR images the same day. Axial $T_1WI$ (500/30) and $T_2WI$ (2150/60, 120) scans show collections seen on CT. Note superior delineation of anterior interhemispheric subdural collection (arrows), hyperintensity of collections relative to CSF, and presence of hypointense rim of dural margin between right frontal epidural collection and underlying cortex.

trast enhancement of the inflamed dura stands out. Often the outer aspect of the subdural fluid collection enhances more significantly and evenly than does the inner aspect adjacent to the brain parenchyma.

## Epidural Empyema

Extension of infection from the paranasal sinuses or mastoids is the most frequent route of infection of the skull and epidural space (Sharif 1982). The infectious process is localized outside the dural membrane and beneath the inner table of the skull. The frontal region is most frequently affected, probably because of its close relationship to the frontal sinuses and the ease

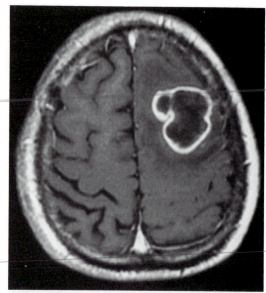

C

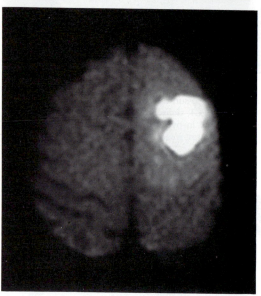

D

**Figure 11-12 (continued)**

products, such as deoxyhemoglobin, or other aspects of clot formation. Alternatively, it has been suggested that the presence of free radicals produced by actively phagocytosing macrophages is responsible for the marked hypointensity of some abscess capsules (Haimes 1989). As on CT, after the administration of contrast, the abscess capsule can be seen to enhance on MR (Grossman 1984). Other features of the enhancing wall, such as thinness and evenness, are known from CT.

Surrounding the abscess capsule, prominent edema is seen in 80 to 90 percent of patients (Paxton 1974; Nielsen 1977; Haimes 1989). The volume of the surrounding edematous white matter is often greater than that of the abscess and is therefore responsible for much of the mass effect (Figs. 11-13 and 11-14). On $T_1WI$ the edematous regions appear to be of slightly low intensity; on $T_2WI$ they become high-intensity. Fingers of vasogenic edema often follow white matter tracts.

The majority of abscesses are supratentorial. Two special circumstances—cerebellar abscesses and intrasellar abscesses—deserve mention. Cerebellar abscesses constitute 2 to 18 percent of all brain abscesses (Fig. 11-14). They are less likely to be encapsulated but have a better prognosis than do supratentorial abscesses if they are recognized early and treated surgically prior to the onset of irreversible brainstem damage (Morgan 1975). Pituitary or intrasellar abscesses should be suspected if a rapidly expanding mass in the sella is seen in a patient with a history of recurrent episodes of meningitis and rhinorrhea. CECT can demonstrate focal contrast enhancement or ring en-

The abscess rim displays changes in signal intensity very different from those of the necrotic core (Figs. 11-13, 11-14). Against the hypointense center, it often appears as isointense to normal brain parenchyma or, occasionally, hyperintense on $T_1WI$. The hyperintensity may be related to hemorrhage. Although hemorrhage is usually not associated with abscess formation on CT, MR is able to detect very small amounts of blood. On $T_2WI$, the rim may appear isointense or become hypointense. The etiology of the hypointense rim surrounding many abscesses has been the subject of speculation (Haimes 1989, Cox 1992, Ostrow 1994). It may be due to the presence of hemoglobin breakdown

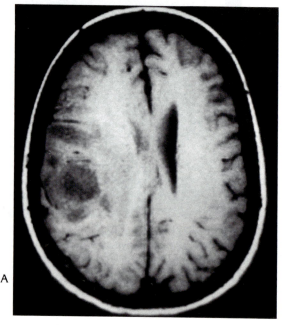

A

**Figure 11-13** (Continued on next page)

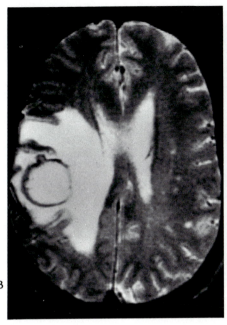

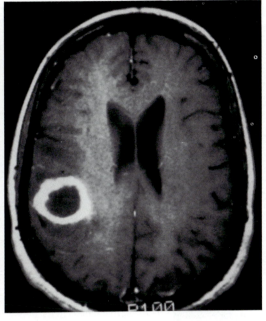

**Figure 11-13 (continued) H. influenzae abscess,** NC and CEMRI. A 36-year-old woman with tetralogy of Fallot and left-sided weakness. **A, B.** T₁WI CEMR shows the enhancing capsule surrounding the necrotic central core. (*Courtesy A. Haimes and R.D. Zimmerman, New York, NY.*)

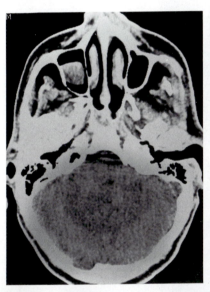

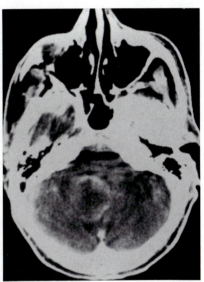

*Figure 11-14* **Cerebellar abscess** in a 42-year-old woman with a history of breast carcinoma. **A.** NCCT demonstrates mass effect in the right cerebellum, with mild shift of the fourth ventricle toward the left. **B.** CECT shows enhancement of the periphery of the lesion, with low density centrally. **C, D.** MRI sagittal (**C**) and axial (**D**) T₁WI disclose mass effect and an ill-defined low-intensity region in the right cerebellum, extending to the vermis. Compression of the brainstem is well documented on the sagittal scan. Again noted is shift of the fourth ventricle toward the left. (*Continued on next page*)

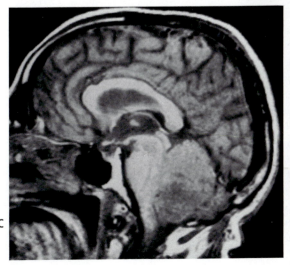

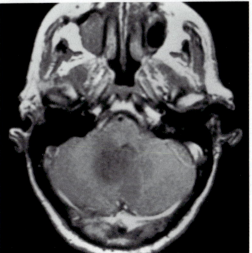

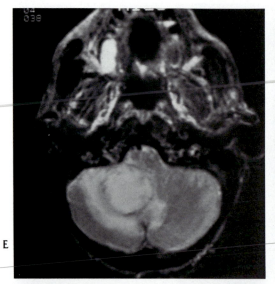

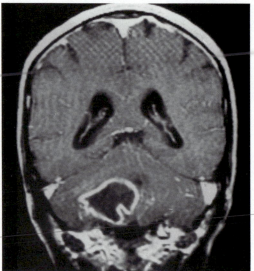

E

H

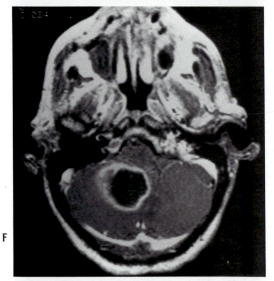

F

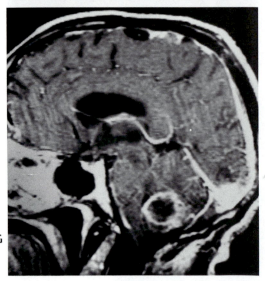

G

*Figure 11-14 (continued)*   **E.** Axial T$_2$WI (2000/70) shows that the lesion has become of high intensity centrally, with an isointense to mildly hypointense fairly even rim. Surrounding high intensity caused by edema is also noted. **F–H.** T$_1$WI (600/12) axial, sagittal, and coronal MR scans demonstrate enhancement of the rim of the lesion, with hyperintensity centrally. At surgery this proved to be a cerebellar abscess caused by mixed gram-negative bacilli.

hancement within the sella (Fig. 11-15). MR discloses a pituitary mass with enhancement (Fig. 11-15). Differentiation from tumor may be difficult. In some cases, hemoglobin breakdown products may produce hyperintensity on T$_1$WI.

In patients with abscesses, clinical improvement with medical therapy has been correlated with a decrease in both the degree of contrast enhancement of the ring and the amount of surrounding edema (Robertheram 1979; Kamin 1981). Delayed postsurgical contrast enhancement may be due to vascular granulation tissue present about the circumference of the previous abscess and may not represent persistence of the abscess capsule. Steroids may reduce the inflammatory edema associated with brain abscesses (Wallenfang 1981) but can also suppress the contrast enhancement of the capsule completely. Also, withdrawal of steroids may result in a rebound increase in the degree of enhancement (Robertheram 1979).

Complications of abscess formation include raised intracranial pressure with the potential risk of cerebral herniation and rupture of the abscess into the ventricle. It is thus extremely important to determine the severity of the associated edema and to determine the size of an abscess accurately. The multiplanar capability of MR is particularly useful. In addition, demonstration of an abscess associated with contrast enhancement of an adjacent ventricular wall indicates rupture of an abscess into the ventricle with secondary ependymitis. The prognosis in this situation is usually poor.

offer
tates
into t
cereb
spon:
cular
The 1
main
subpi:
of the
tory re
In
(Clave
to be 1
equate
sity in
choroi
late co
binatio
leptom
hemorr
interhe:
eral and
and ext
spaces
swelling
matous
less sev
podensi
normal
gyral co
zones n
congesti
blood-br
Chang
mild dise
more sev
tensity ca
interhem:
date (Sze
CSF in ot
is necessa
addition,
in signal
of the su
with areas
of Sylvius,
Verificat
obtained I
and 11-18
seen and
1989). Enl
surroundin
located, fo
lobe (Figs.

## Mycotic Aneurysms and Septic Thrombophlebitis

Aneurysms of inflammatory origin may be bacterial, syphilitic, or mycotic. Although the term mycotic is used in the general sense of microorganisms, a bacterial etiology is the most common. These aneurysms originate mainly as a septic emboli from the lung or infected endocarditis; less commonly, they form as a complication of cardiac surgery, meningitis, cavernous sinus thrombophlebitis, or osteomyelitis. The most frequent location is the peripheral branches of the middle cerebral artery, followed by the anterior cerebral artery, the internal carotid artery, and the basilar artery, where abscesses are often multiple. Progressive weakening of the elastica and the media of the aneurysm wall may result in enlargement and rupture, with hemorrhage into the adjacent cortex or the subarachnoid or subdural spaces, or may cause multiple coalescent infarcts (Gray 1997).

CT and MR clearly demonstrate the complications of septic emboli as well as "mycotic" aneurysms at the peripheral branches near the cortex. On CECT, a small enhancing focus may be noted in the parenchyma. An enhancing vessel leading to the focus is strongly suggestive of an aneurysm but is not always seen because of its small size. On MR, a small area of signal void is visualized associated with adjacent parenchyma alteration (Fig. 11-16). Angiography may confirm the presence of the aneurysm itself. Complications of mycotic aneurysms include meningitis, cerebral abscess, and cerebral infarction in addition to hemorrhage.

Septic intracranial thrombophlebitis most frequently follows infection of paranasal sinuses, middle ear, mastoid, face or oropharynx. The infection spreads centrally along the emissary veins. Septic thrombophlebitis may also occur in association with epidural abscess, subdural empyema or meningitis. Rarely the infection is metastatic from lungs or other distant infective sites.

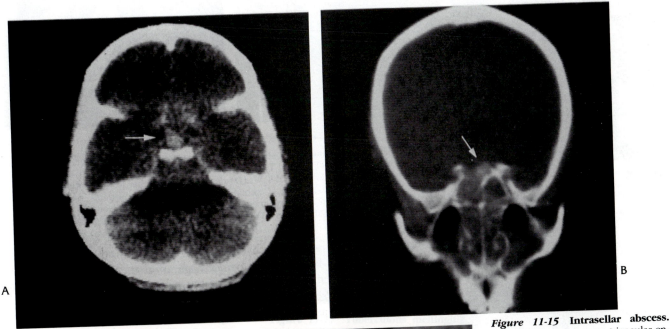

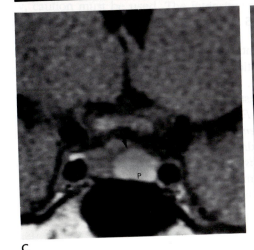

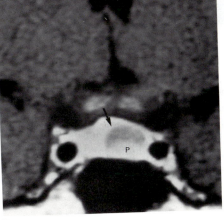

***Figure 11-15* Intrasellar abscess. (A)** CECT demonstrates a triangular enhancement in the sella (arrow). **(B)** Coronal view discloses pansinusitis with opacification and fluid levels. Opacified sphenoid sinus with infected mucocele communicates with the intrasellar abscess (arrow) by way of the destroyed floor of the sella. Complete resolution of intrasellar abscess occurred following surgery and vigorous antibiotic therapy. Intrasellar abscess NCMR **(C)** and CEMR **(D)** in another patient show hypointense signal within the sella (arrow) **(C)** and hypointense signal (arrow) on CEMR in contrast to intense enhancement of the entire pituitary gland **(D)**

known sarcoidosis have CNS involvement (Silverstein 1965). Rarely, CNS involvement may be the only manifestation of this disease (Cahill 1981; Griggs 1973). Sarcoid may present at any age but is most common in the third and fourth decades and usually occurs in women. Two major patterns of intracranial involvement are (1) meningeal or ependymal and (2) parenchymal findings (Hollander 1998). Granulomatous leptomeningitis may occur diffusely or as a circumscribed process at the skull base involving the optic chiasm, the pituitary gland, the floor of the third ventricle, and the hypothalamus. Communicating hydrocephalus is a common result. The second pattern of CNS sarcoid, which is less commonly seen, consists of noncaseating granulomas scattered diffusely in the brain parenchyma or occurring as a single large mass which mimics a brain neoplasm (Saltzman 1958; Silverstein 1965; Robert 1948; Griggs 1973).

On CT, patients with neurosarcoidosis may have normal scans, as was seen in 60 percent of cases in a review of 32 patients (Ketonen 1986). Leptomeningeal sarcoid can appear similar to bacterial meningitis, with enhancement of the meninges along the inner table of the skull (Fig. 11-28). It can also present initially as hydrocephalus (Morehouse 1981). Hydrocephalus may occur as a result of an obstructing mass lesion (Bahgr 1978; Kendall 1978; Kumpe 1979). Differentiation from other causes of communicating hydrocephalus may be difficult unless the patient has proven pulmonary sarcoidosis. Parenchymal sarcoid is seen as a hyperdense area on NCCT, with further homogeneous enhancement on CECT (Fig. 11-28). Another common abnormality that involves the parenchyma is the occurrence of hypodense white matter lesions attributed to small vessel involvement. Finally, linear or nodular meningeal contrast enhancement extending deep into the parenchyma is highly suggestive of a meningeal infiltrative process with secondary parenchymal extension through the Virchow-Robin spaces, another path of spread in neurosarcoidosis (Mirfakharee 1986).

On MR, sarcoid involvement of the leptomeninges is difficult to detect without contrast, although large deposits may be seen as masses compressing the underlying brain parenchyma (Fig. 11-29). Dural-based neurosarcoidosis of CSF spaces, for example, in the suprasellar cistern, may also be detected, as it is with other types of meningitis (Sze 1989). On CEMR, marked enhancement of the sarcoid granulation tissue occurs. Enhancement can be seen throughout the meninges or may be very localized, especially in the suprasellar cistern. Compared with bacterial meningitis, meningeal sarcoid often, although not always, appears more focal and nodular. Contrast MR is not specific, but is the most accurate modality for documenting disease. As with CT, linear or nodular enhancement extending into the parenchyma can represent infiltration of disease into the sulci and Virchow-Robin spaces. Again, white matter involvement resulting from small vessel disease may occur and is seen as areas of high signal intensity on $T_2WI$ (Fig. 11-27).

On MR, sarcoid granulomas are generally isointense or hypointense relative to cerebral cortex on $T_1WI$ and hyperintense on $T_2WI$ (Hayes 1987) (Fig. 11-30). They enhance homogeneously with contrast. When there is no evidence of peripheral sarcoidosis, differentiation from neoplasm or multiple sclerosis may be difficult unless a biopsy is performed (Smith 1989). Of note, sarcoid granulomatous masses within the parenchyma rarely demonstrate significant surrounding edema. In addition, they decrease in size dramatically after treatment with steroids (Lexa 1994) (Fig. 11-30).

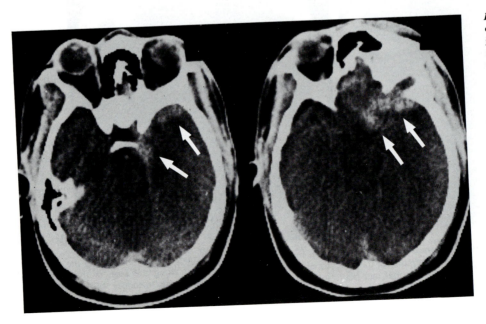

*Figure 11-28* **A, B. Meningeal sarcoid granulomas**. On CECT, extensive granulomas present as nonhomogeneous densities in the temporal fossa along the sphenoid bone (arrows) and in the parasellar region (arrows).

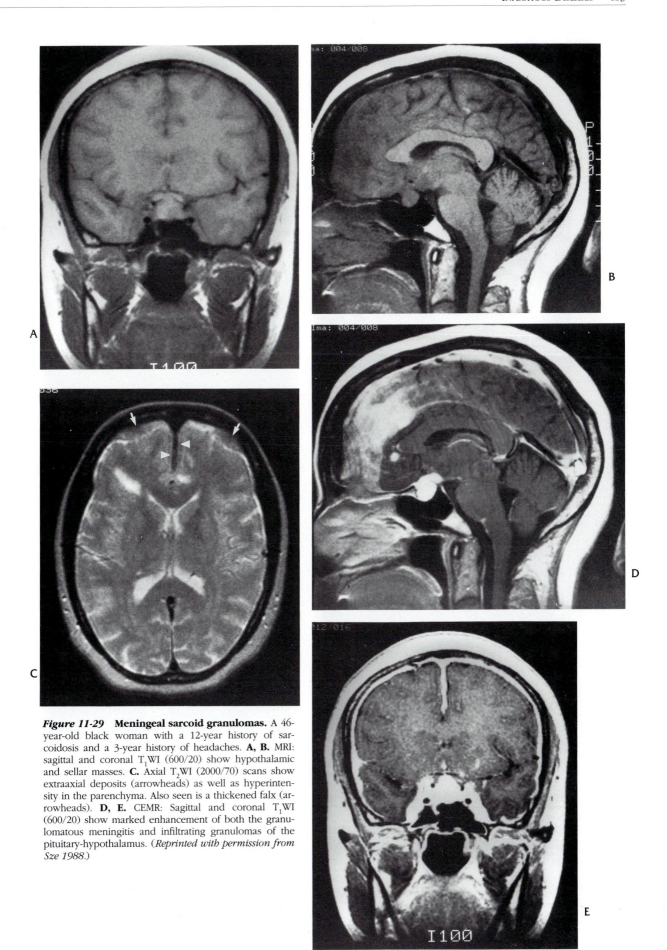

*Figure 11-29* **Meningeal sarcoid granulomas.** A 46-year-old black woman with a 12-year history of sarcoidosis and a 3-year history of headaches. **A, B.** MRI: sagittal and coronal $T_1$WI (600/20) show hypothalamic and sellar masses. **C.** Axial $T_2$WI (2000/70) scans show extraaxial deposits (arrowheads) as well as hyperintensity in the parenchyma. Also seen is a thickened falx (arrowheads). **D, E.** CEMR: Sagittal and coronal $T_1$WI (600/20) show marked enhancement of both the granulomatous meningitis and infiltrating granulomas of the pituitary-hypothalamus. (*Reprinted with permission from Sze 1988.*)

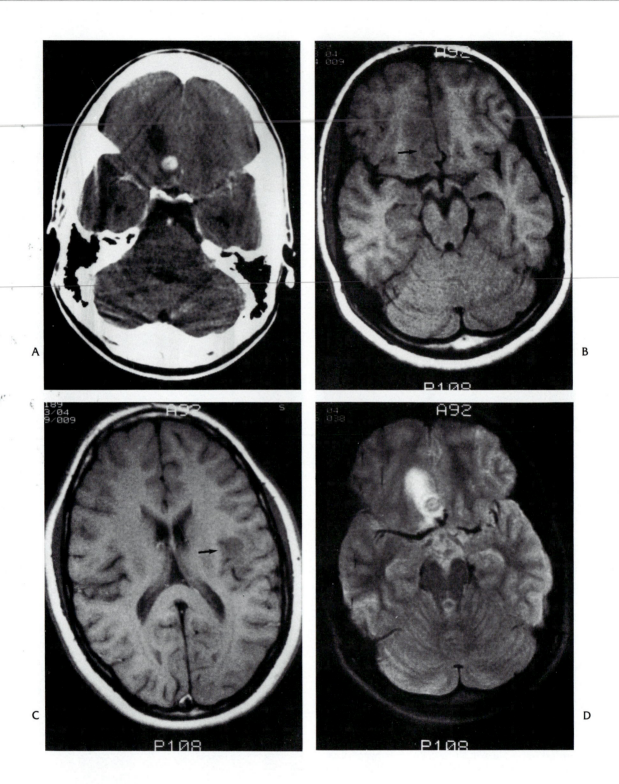

# FUNGAL INFECTION

Fungal infections generally affect the CNS as opportunistic granulomatous disease which may be acute and fulminant or chronic and indolent. Fungi may exist either in hyphal or yeast form. Many fungi are dimorphic. At body temperature, most dimorphic organisms are yeasts. *Hyphae* form larger colonies, which limit access to the microvasculature. Therefore, the organisms tend to spread along large vessels in a retrograde fashion, commonly involving the orbits and sinuses. The smaller size of *yeasts* allows hematogenous spread with a predilection for involvement of the meningeal microvasculature leading to parenchymal invasion

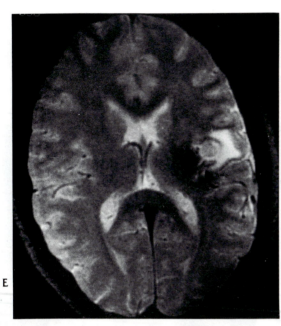

E

**Figure 11-30** **Parenchymal sarcoid granulomas. A.** CECT demonstrates an enhancing sarcoid granuloma in the right basal frontal lobe. It is surrounded by relatively small amounts of edema. **B–E.** MRI: T₁WI (500/20) and T₂WI (2000/70) disclose round, slightly isointense lesions surrounded by a relative paucity of edema in the right frontal lobe and left parietal lobe. After treatment with steroids, lesions resolved totally; follow-up MR scan was negative.

(Harris 1997). Infection may be meningeal, parenchymal (fungal "abscess"), or both. In most instances the primary portal of entry is the lungs, but fungal osteomyelitis or lymphadenitis may also precede brain involvement. The frequency of CNS fungal infection has increased significantly in recent years because of the growing numbers of immunosuppressed patients due to the combination of AIDS and the use of aggressive chemotherapy (Britt 1981; Harris 1997).

Although a variety of opportunistic organisms may involve the CNS, few of these entities have a characteristic pattern that suggests the diagnosis purely on the basis of imaging findings. Most often CT and MR are used to demonstrate and localize the parenchymal or meningeal involvement; confirmation of the specific fungus involved is based on a variety of CSF studies, especially CSF culture. CT and MR features of fungal infection are varied and nonspecific (Enzmann 1980; Mikhael 1985; Riccio 1989). In general, ringlike contrast enhancement on CT and MR probably reflects the host's ability to wall off the organisms.

*Cryptococcus neoformans* infection of the CNS occurs rarely in immunocompetent individuals as a manifestation of disseminated pulmonary cryptococcosis. In AIDS patients, CNS cryptococcosis is the most common fungal infection (Riccio 1989) and the incidence cryptococcal meningitis in patients with AIDS has been es-

timated to be about 10 percent in the United States (Wright 1997). Overall, cryptococcus is the most common fungal infection to involve the CNS. As in *Listeria* infection, meningitis is more prevalent than parenchymal involvement in cryptococcosis. MR and CT findings can be grouped into four patterns (Tien 1991): (1) parenchymal cryptococcoma (toruloma), (2) multiple miliary parenchymal and leptomeningeal nodules, (3) symmetrical perivascular spread in the basal ganglia and midbrain, and (4) a mixed pattern. Types 1 and 2 are different presentations of hematogenous dissemination of the fungi. Intracranial torulomas may exhibit ringlike contrast enhancement (Long 1980; Arrington 1984) or focal homogeneous nodules with or without circumferential edema on CT (Fujita 1981). Tan (1987) and Popovich (1990) reported a variety of CT changes such as hydrocephalus, diffuse cortical atrophy, nonspecific white matter changes, and basal meningeal enhancement. Forty-three to fifty percent of the patients in their series showed normal CT scans.

MR findings demonstrate hypointense lesions on T₁WI and hyperintense lesions on T₂WI. Postcontrast T₁WI can clearly demonstrate the lesions and are essential, especially for miliary nodules in the leptomeninges and parenchyma (Riccio 1989, Harris 1997). Fungal invasion of the perivascular spaces (Virchow-Robin spaces) in the basal ganglia is better seen on MR than on CT (Tien 1991). This presents as symmetrical, bilateral hypointensity or isointensity relative to gray matter on T₁WI and SDWI and as hyperintensity on T₂WI (Fig. 11-31). Also, production of voluminous mucoid material may enlarge the perivascular spaces and form gelatinous pseudocysts (Harris 1997). Very little edema is associated with these lesions; this is most likely due to the intact blood-brain barrier and the extraaxial location. For similar reasons, very little contrast enhancement is generally apparent. These lesions, as well as granulomas of the choroid plexus, are relatively specific for *Cryptococcus* (Andreula 1993).

*Coccidioides imitis* is a dust-borne dimorphic fungus endemic to the southwestern part of the United States, especially the San Joaquin Valley of California, as well as portions of Mexico and central South America (Fraser 1978). It is spread by inhalation of the spore, which is present in soil. Only 0.02 to 0.2 percent of cases progress to the disseminated form involving the brain, meninges, and other systemic organs (Einstein 1974, Harris 1997). Pathologically, CNS coccidiodomycosis is characterized by thickened, congested leptomeninges with multiple granulomas, which are especially prominent in the basal cisterns. Complications include communicating hydrocephalus, vasculitis, ependymitis, and periventricular lesions (focal granulomas without calcification) (McGahan 1981). The most

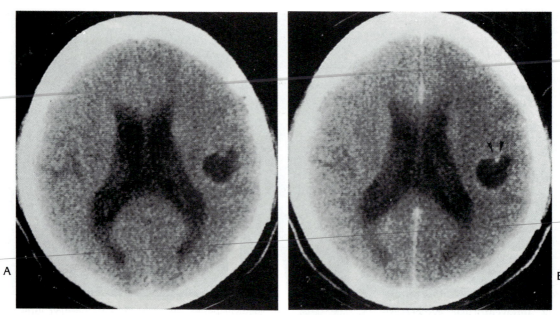

**Figure 11-44  Living intraparenchymal cysticercus. A.** NCCT demonstrates a rounded cystic structure of CSF-equivalent density in the white matter of the parietal lobe. No surrounding edema is present. **B.** CECT shows no contrast enhancement around the cyst, but the scolex (arrowheads) is slightly enhanced, indicating the living cysticercus. Note also the absence of adjacent edema or mass effect. (*Courtesy of S.Y. Kim, Seoul, Korea.*)

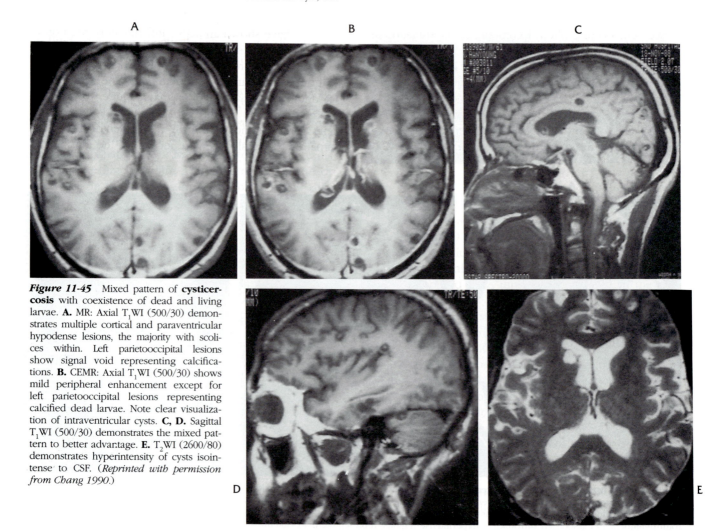

**Figure 11-45** Mixed pattern of **cysticercosis** with coexistence of dead and living larvae. **A.** MR: Axial $T_1WI$ (500/30) demonstrates multiple cortical and paraventricular hypodense lesions, the majority with scolices within. Left parietooccipital lesions show signal void representing calcifications. **B.** CEMR: Axial $T_1WI$ (500/30) shows mild peripheral enhancement except for left parietooccipital lesions representing calcified dead larvae. Note clear visualization of intraventricular cysts. **C, D.** Sagittal $T_1WI$ (500/30) demonstrates the mixed pattern to better advantage. **E.** $T_2WI$ (2600/80) demonstrates hyperintensity of cysts isointense to CSF. (*Reprinted with permission from Chang 1990.*)

or the gray-white matter junction, but they are sometimes seen in the basal ganglia or the deep white matter (Santin 1966). Calcifications may involve both the wall and contents of the cyst. They typically appear round and slightly oval and range from 7 to 16 mm in size (Carbajal 1977). These wholly or partially calcified spheres frequently contain an eccentric small nodular calcification measuring 1 to 2 mm in diameter that represents the scolex of the erupted larva (Janowski 1979). Both dead larvae with calcifications and living larvae

may coexist in cases of reinfestation (Fig. 11-41). Vasculitis may develop in the vicinity of these lesions and lead to cortical arterial occlusion and infarction.

MR is more sensitive than CT in the recognition of parenchymal, intraventricular, and subarachnoid cysts; perifocal edema; and internal changes indicative of cyst death (Suss 1986; Martinez 1989; Suh 1989). CT is far superior in the demonstration of calcification (Teitelbaum 1989). Therefore, if parenchymal cysticercosis is suspected, CT is the preferred initial screening modality.

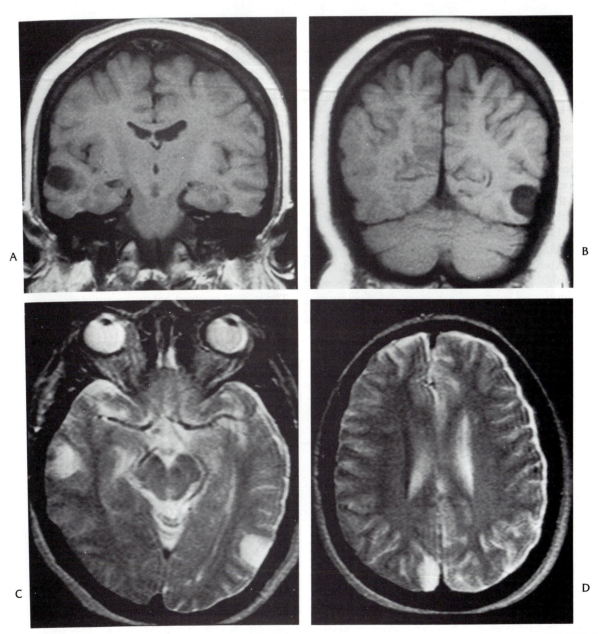

***Figure 11-46*** **Intraparenchymal cysticerci. A, B.** $T_1WI$ (600/20) coronal MR clearly show two cystic lesions. The signal intensity of the lesions is slightly higher than that of CSF in the ventricles. No definite scolices can be determined. **C, D.** $T_2WI$ (2000/70) show hyperintensity of the cystic lesions. *(Continued on next page)*

WHELAN MA, KRICHEFF H, HANDLER M, et al: Acquired immunodeficiency syndrome: Cerebral CT manifestations. *Radiology* 149:477–484, 1983.

WHITEMAN ML, POST MJ, BERGER JR, et al: Progressive multifocal leukoencephalopathy in 47 HIV-seropositive patients: Neuroimaging with clinical and pathologic correlation. *Radiology* 187(1):233–240, 1993.

WHITLEY RJ, NAHMIAS AJ, VISTINE AM, et al: The natural history of herpes simplex virus infection of mother and newborn. *Pediatric* 66:489–494, 1980.

WRIGHT D, SCHNEIDER A, BERGER JR: CNS opportunistic infections. *Neuroimaging Clin N Am* 7(3):513–525, 1997.

ZEE CS, SEGALL HD, MILLER C, et al: Unusual features of intracranial cysticercosis. *Radiology* 137:397–407, 1980.

ZEE CS, SEGALL HD, BOSWELL W, et al: MR imaging of neurocysticercosis. *J Comput Assist Tomogr* 12:927–934, 1988.

ZEGERS DE, BEYL D, NOTERMAN J, et al: Multiple cerebral hematoma and viral encephalitis. *Neuroradiology* 20:47–48, 1980.

ZIMMERMAN RA, PATEL S, BILANIUK LT: Demonstration of purulent bacterial intracranial infections by computed tomography. *AJR* 127:155–165, 1976.

ZIMMERMAN RA, BILANIUK LT, GALLO E: CT of the trapped fourth ventricle. *AJR* 130:503–506, 1978.

ZIMMERMAN RD, RUSSELL EJ, LEEDS NE, et al: CT in the early diagnosis of herpes simplex encephalitis. *AJR* 134:61–66, 1980.

ZIMMERMAN RD, LEEDS NE, DANZIGER A: Subdural empyema CT findings. *Radiology* 150:417–422, 1984.

# 12 INTRACRANIAL ANEURYSMS AND VASCULAR MALFORMATIONS

*Karel G. TerBrugge*
*Krishna C.V.G. Rao*

## CONTENTS

Intracranial aneurysms and vascular malformations commonly present with a history of intracranial hemorrhage. With aneurysms, there often are a variety of clinical findings, such as transient ischemic attacks and signs of cranial nerve involvement. By contrast, with vascular malformations, seizures may be the presenting clinical symptom. CT is the first modality of examination that provides an approach to selecting patients who need further investigation. MRI can be performed to further characterize the lesion, but angiography is often necessary for the definitive examination before treatment planning. CT, MRI, and angiography have been shown to be complementary, with each modality playing a role in the diagnosis and treatment planning of patients with cerebral vascular anomalies.

## INTRACRANIAL ANEURYSMS AND SUBARACHNOID HEMORRHAGE

An *aneurysm* is an abnormal focal enlargement of an artery. Aneurysms can be classified according to their appearance as saccular or fusiform. The etiologic classification of aneurysms includes congenital (genetically induced); developmental (shear stress induced); arteriosclerotic; infectious; traumatic; dissecting; and pseudoaneurysms. The traditional concept is that most aneurysms are congenital and are caused by a defect in the tunica media (Crawford 1959; Crompton 1966). With advancing age, arteriosclerotic changes are thought to cause further weakening of an already defective tunica media, and this may result in enlargement or rupture of the aneurysm (Crompton 1966; Nystrom 1963; DuBoulay 1965; Sarwar 1976a). However, this concept has been questioned in the absence of congenital, developmental, or inherited weakness of the vessel wall (Stehbens, 1989). Aneurysms are most likely degenerative lesions which result from hemodynamic stress. Hypertension and connective tissue disorders may be aggravating factors.

The incidence of intracranial aneurysms in the general population is approximately 3 percent (Chason 1958; Housepian 1958). The aneurysm involves the carotid system in 96 percent of cases. The anterior communicating artery is the single most common site (30 percent), followed by the posterior communicating artery (25 percent) and the middle cerebral artery (20 percent) (Locksley 1966). Approximately 20 percent of patients with an intracranial aneurysm have more than one aneurysm demonstrated at angiography (McKissock 1964; Locksley 1966; Kendall 1976b). Sporadic instances of a familial incidence of aneurysms have been reported (Acosta-Rua 1978; Norgard 1987) and the incidence of multiple aneurysms in such patients may be as high as 40 percent (Jain 1974). The incidence of aneurysms in patients with autosomal dominant polycystic kidney disease varies between 15 and 40 percent (Chapman 1992). Aneurysmal disease in children is rare and differs significantly in its clinical and radiological features. There is a male dominance (3:1), a higher incidence of posterior fossa aneurysms, and a greater number of large and giant size aneurysms. There is also a higher incidence of traumatic and infectious etiologies (Laughlin 1997; Lasjaunias 1997). In adults the great majority of aneurysms presenting with subarachnoid hemorrhage are small in size (diameter less than 1 cm) (DuBoulay 1965; Locksley 1966). Large (diameter between 1 and 2.5 cm) and giant (diameter greater than

1986c). An intracerebral cavernous hemangioma is not a neoplasm and should therefore be identified as a cavernoma or cavernous malformation. An increase in the size of the malformation may occasionally be demonstrated and progressive destruction of the adjacent brain tissue may occur, but there is no evidence of neural tissue proliferation and therefore no evidence of neoplastic disease. It is not unusual to identify different types of vascular malformations in the same patient, which raises questions about etiological linkages and predisposing factors among the vascular disorders (Rigamonti 1991, Putnam 1996, Van Roost 1997).

## Capillary Telangiectasis

These lesions are composed of dilated capillary blood vessels which vary greatly in caliber. These vessels are separated by normal neural tissues. These lesions are a relatively common incidental finding at autopsy and are most often located in the pons but may be seen in the cerebral cortex and subcortical white matter. These lesions by themselves are not symptomatic and are unlikely to be associated with hemorrhage. Capillary telangiectasis are unlikly to show on MCCT but may reveal as a small area of faint enhancement on CECT (Fig. 12-15). The lesion on MRI appears isointense on $T_1WI$, with slight hyperintensity on $T_2WI$, revealing enhancement with gadolinium (Barr 1996, Van Roost 1997). Angiographically, a blush may be demonstrated in the capillary phase within the malformation, but most often the angiogram is negative (Poser 1957, Robertson 1974). Other associated vascular disorders, such as development venous anomalies and cavernomas in the vicinity (Fig. 12-15), may produce combined imaging features characteristic of each vascular entity.

## Cavernous Malformations

Cavernous malformations are composed of large sinusoidal vascular spaces closely clustered together; the vessels are not separated by normal neural tissue. Cavernomas represent about 15 percent of all vascular malformations with an estimated incidence of about 0.1 percent (Jellinger 1988; Robinson 1991; Zabramski 1994). Not all cavernomas are associated with symptoms, but once they become symptomatic 40 to 50 percent present with seizures, 20 percent with focal neurological deficit, and 10 percent with hemorrhage (Simard 1986; Del Curling 1991; Zabramski 1994). The risk of hemorrhage is not well established, but has been estimated between the 0.2 and 2 percent per lesion per year. These numbers may be higher for those patients presenting with brain stem cavernomas (Porter 1997). About 90 percent of the lesions are supratentor-

ial in location and 10 percent within the posterior fossa. Multiple cavernomas are seen in about 15 percent of patients. A familial form of the disorder exists and is inherited as an autosomal dominant trait with variable expression. Multiple lesions can be seen in 60 percent of patients with the familial form (Rigamonti 1988; Duong 1991; Zabramski 1994). Increasingly developmental venous anomalies (DVA, venous angioma) are noted in association with cavernomas (Rigamonti 1988; Zimmerman 1991), but clinical symptoms under such circumstances are believed to be caused by the cavernoma. In cavernomas angiography is invariably normal, although prolonged injection angiography may demonstrate an abnormal capillary blush (Numaguchi 1979). CT findings consist of a hyperdense and often partially calcified lesion which shows fairly homogeneous enhancement of a minimal degree (Fig. 12-16) or no appreciable enhancement, depending on whether the lesions are partially or completely thrombosed. The lesion is not associated with mass effect or surrounding edema except when recent hemorrhage is present (Fig. 12-17) or enlargement has occurred, presumably due to multiple small successive hemorrhages (Fig. 12-18).

The MRI appearance of cavernous malformations has been well described (Savoiardo 1983; Augustin 1985; Lee 1985; Biondi 1988b; Imakita 1989; Rapacki 1990). An MRI classification for cavernomas has been proposed which combines the MRI findings with clinical and pathological characteristics (Zabramski 1994). The type I lesions are characterized by subacute hemorrhage and exhibit a hyperintense core on $T_1$ (methemoglobin), whereas on $T_2$ the initial hyperintense signal changes to hypointensity in time with a faint hypointense rim. The type II lesions demonstrate loculated areas of hemorrhage of varying age and thrombus surrounded by gliosis and hemosiderin. On $T_1$ and $T_2WI$ a reticulated core with high and low signal intensities is seen surrounded by a hypointense ring (Fig. 12-15). Clinically these lesions are active, and thrombosis and hemorrhage are ongoing in a repetitive process. The type III lesions represent chronic mostly inactive lesions with residual hemosiderin in and around the lesion creating hypointensity on $T_1$ and $T_2WI$ (Fig. 12-17). The type IV lesions are poorly visualized on $T_1$ and $T_2$ and are best seen with gradient echo sequences as small punctate hypointense foci (Fig. 12-19). Subacute hemorrhage associated with a microarteriovenous malformation or brain tumor may mimic a type I lesion, and follow-up MRI and angiography is indicated under such circumstances (Willinsky 1993). The type II lesions were thought to be pathognomonic for cavernoma, but thrombosed arteriovenous malformations (AVMs) and hemorrhagic metastases may have a similar appearance (Griffin 1987; Riga-

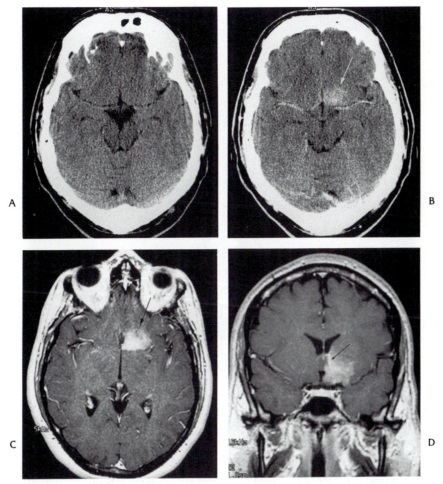

***Figure 12-15*** **Capillary telangiectasia. A.** NCCT shows no abnormality. **B.** CECT shows slight enhancement of poorly defined lesion (arrow). **C.** MRI following gadolinium administration shows on axial and coronal T₁WI **(D)** enhancement of lesion which did show on T₁WI, Flair 1 or T₂WI. Possible associated DVA is noted on coronal imaging **(D)** (arrow). Patient was asymptomatic and imaging did not change over 9 month period.

monti 1987; Sze 1987; Biondi 1988*b*; Rapacki 1990). Type III and IV lesions may be mimicked by radiation-induced telangiectasis (Gaensler 1994). CT and MRI can both be used in the follow-up of patients with known cavernomas, in particular when hemorrhagic events are suspected (Figs. 12-17, 12-18). Although the MRI appearance of cavernomas is not helpful in predicting future bleeds (Willinsky 1996), MRI is the method of choice in the long-term follow-up of patients with cavernomas and the assessment of family members suspected of intracerebral cavernoma malformations (Zabramski 1994).

## Arteriovenous Malformations

In vascular malformation there is an intimate topographic admixture of arteries and veins. It represents the most common form of vascular malformation with an esti-

mated incidence of about 0.3 percent. Brain AVMs are clinically important because they are often symptomatic (Crawford 1986; Brown 1988; Ondra 1990). According to LeBlanc (1979), 55 percent of AVMs present with intracranial hemorrhage, 36 percent with a seizure disorder, and 9 percent with headaches and a progressive neurological deficit. Patients with an unruptured brain AVM have a 3 to 4 percent risk per year of bleeding from the malformation, and each bleeding episode is associated with a 10 percent risk of death. Multiple brain AVMs are uncommon but do occur sporadically or in patients with Rendu-Osler-Weber disease and Wyburn-Mason syndrome (Willinsky 1990; Ericson 1994; Putman 1996). The brain parenchyma adjacent to an AVM shows destructive and atrophic changes (TerBrugge 1977; Russell 1977). Calcifications are often present within the vascular channels as well as in the adjacent brain parenchyma.

The angiographic appearance of an AVM is one of abnormally dilated and tortuous feeding arteries and a

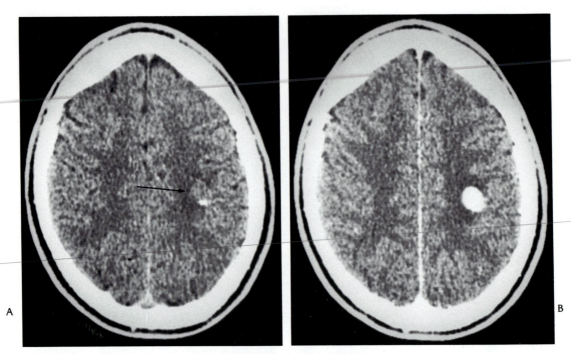

**Figure 12-16** **Cavernous malformation. A.** An isodense lesion (arrow) with a small calcification is shown on NCCT. **B.** CECT reveals homogeneous enhancement of the surgically proven cavernoma.

racemose tangle of increased vascularity which drain into tortuous and elongated veins. Cerebral microarteriovenous malformations (micro AVMs) have been identified as lesions with a nidus less than 1 cm, fed by normal-size arteries with rapid shunting into normal-size veins (Willinsky 1988*b*). Occasionally the malformation becomes partially or completely thrombosed, and angiography may fail to show any evidence of it (angiographically occult) (Wakai 1985).

The CT appearance of an intracranial AVM that is not associated with a recent hemorrhage is fairly characteristic (Pressman 1975*a*; Kendall 1976*a*; TerBrugge 1977; Brunelle 1983; Kumar 1984). The lesion most commonly presents on NCCT as an area of mixed density in which focal areas of hyperdensity are interspersed with areas of decreased density. The margins of the lesions are poorly defined and irregular in outline. After contrast infusion, the lesion shows heterogeneous enhancement (Fig. 12-20). Feeding arteries and draining veins may be recognized on CT. The lesion may be associated with focal atrophy or localized mass effect, but surrounding edema is extremely uncommon.

A significant number of AVMs do not show as an abnormality on NCCT and become apparent only after contrast infusion, which is therefore a mandatory part of the examination. CECT often shows heterogeneous enhancement and poorly defined margins of the lesion (Fig. 12-20). In the presence of a recent hemorrhage the AVM can often be demonstrated on CT following contrast enhancement (Fig. 12-21); however depending

on the size of the AVM versus that of the hematoma, the AVM may be demonstrated only on follow-up examinations (Figs. 12-22 to 12-24).

Areas of increased density may be observed, usually in the range of 40 to 50 HU, on NCCT. Postulated explanations for this baseline increased density imply the presence of local gliosis and hemosiderosis (New 1975), mural thrombus or calcification, or an increased blood pool (Pressman 1975*a*). CECT demonstrates enhancement of the central angiomatous mass and visualizes the adjacent vessels (Figs. 12-20 to 12-22).

A small number of AVMs exhibit a predominantly hyperdense appearance and are heavily calcified. Enhancement may be difficult to detect in these often angiographically occult malformations with high CT number measurements (Kramer 1977; Golden 1978; Sartor 1978; Bell 1978; Teraco 1979; LeBlanc 1981; Chin 1993; Yeates 1983).

Unusual patterns of AVM on CT have been described in which a well-defined area of decreased density is a prominent feature (Fig. 12-21). These cases frequently involve patients who have had previous episodes of hemorrhage associated with the AVM, with subsequent resolving hematoma and "cyst" formation (Daniels 1979; Britt 1980). Occasionally, in rupture of AVMs, extravasation of blood into the preexisting cystic cavities presents as intraparenchymal blood-fluid levels (Richmond 1981).

The MRI appearance of an intracerebral AVM has been extensively described (Lee 1985; Kucharczyk

1985; LeBlanc 1987; Biondi 1988*b*; Smith 1988; Edelman 1989). A low intensity signal (flow void) on both $T_1WI$ and $T_2WI$ is noted to involve the nidus as well as the feeding arteries and veins (Fig. 12-20). Slow flow within parts of the malformation associated with arterial and venous ectasias may result in a mixed signal on $T_1$ and $T_2WI$. Recent hemorrhage may be revealed as a bright signal on both $T_1$ and $T_2WI$. To separate these phenomena special gradient echo imaging techniques can be used with sequential acquisition, gradient refocus, and limited flip angle techniques (Edelman 1989; Huston 1991; Wasserman 1995).

MR angiographic techniques can eloquently depict brain AVMs and for the purpose of diagnosis may replace conventional cerebral angiography (Edelman 1989; Huston 1991). On the other hand, recent advances in superselective angiography have shown pre-, intra-, and postnidal vascular ectasias and pseudo-aneurysms not apparent on MRA or nonselective angiography. These ectasias are believed to be markers for increased risk of hemorrhage and as such need to be identified (Willinsky 1988*a*; Marks 1990, 1992; Garcia-Monaco 1993; Perata 1994; Turjman 1994). In addition to MRI and MRA, superselective angiography is recommended as part of the workup of patients with brain AVM in preparation for treatment.

A characteristic but rare form of AVM has been described in the midbrain, associated with ipsilateral angiomatosis of the retina and the presence of a cuta-

neous nevus in the distribution of the trigeminal nerve; it is called *Wyburn-Mason syndrome* (Wyburn-Mason 1943). CECT and MRI usually demonstrate a vascular malformation of varying size, most commonly in the midbrain (Fig. 12-24). The orbital component of a vascular malformation around the optic nerve, which is always on the same side as the retinal angioma and the intracranial AVM, may not be detected by means of CT unless high-resolution thin sections are obtained or the orbital vascular component is very large and is often better shown with MRI. The extent of the orbital as well as the intracranial vascular anomaly can be confirmed with angiography.

Approximately 50 percent of patients with an AVM present with intracranial hemorrhage (LeBlanc 1979, Willinsky 1988*a*). Bleeding may occur into the subarachnoid space or more often into the ventricular system or the brain parenchyma (Figs. 12-21, 12-22). They rarely bleed into the subdural space (Rengachary 1981). Recent intracerebral hemorrhage may occasionally obscure a small sized AVM on the initial CT, MRI, or angiogram, and follow-up examination subsequent to the absorption of the hematoma may be necessary to demonstrate the underlying cause. MRI is more helpful than CT in the follow-up of such cases and may demonstrate the cause of the hemorrhage to be a neoplasm, a cavernoma, or a small-size AVM. If no cause is apparent on follow-up MRI, then a delayed angiogram is indicated to exclude the possibility of a

C

micro AVM
vascular m
on repeat
cult based
*cryptic vasc*
cause it der
tained by m

A rare co
vascular occ
Lichtor 198

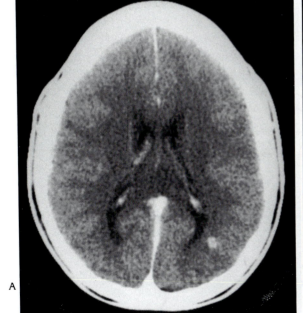
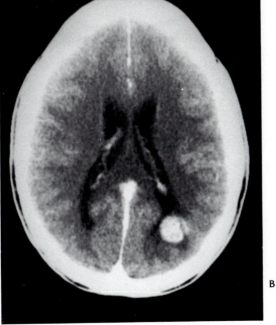

*Figure 12-17*  **Cavernous malformation. A.** The CECT shows a hyperdense lesion adjacent to the occipital horn. **B.** Repeat CECT (3-year interval) showed an increase in the size of this lesion after recent onset of acute headaches. NECT showed similar findings (associated hemorrhage). *(Continued on next page.)*

A

B

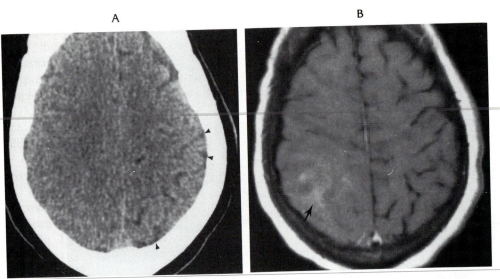

***Figure 13-8*** **Sulcal effacement.** **A.** Right hemispheric sulcal efface-ment is present on the unen-hanced CT image. **B.** MR confirms the sulcal effacement; minimal meningeal enhancement is identi-fied. *(Reprinted with permission from Johnson MH: CT evaluation of the earliest signs of stroke. The Radiologist 1(4):189–199, 1994.)*

the detection rates of early cerebral infarction from 40 to 50 percent at 48 h to 50 percent within 12 h. All scans obtained between 25 and 35 days after the ictus revealed a focal abnormality in this series. Wall (1981) demonstrated subtle mass effects and/or focal areas of hypodensity corresponding to regions of clinical deficit in 79 percent of cases, and 65 percent of the positive scans were obtained by 12 h following the clinical ic-tus (Wall 1981).

## Hyperacute-acute Infarction

Within the first few hours after ictus, the stroke may be referred to as hyperacute. This stage corresponds with the earliest cellular changes of cytotoxic edema and early neutrophilic infiltration. A number of subtle CT

findings, indicative of hyperacute and acute stroke, have been described and correlated with the earliest pathophysiologic changes of acute ischemia (Ng 1970; Sypert 1975; Arimitsu 1977; Wall 1981; Yock 1981; Truwit 1990; Horowitz 1991; Manelfe 1991; Johnson 1994). These signs include loss of gray-white matter differentiation, sulcal effacement, the hyperdense artery sign, loss of the insular ribbon, and obscuration of the lentiform nucleus. Each of these early CT signs of hyperacute to acute cerebral infarction may be ob-served alone or in combination in patients with clinical stroke syndromes. Recognition of these subtle abnor-malities within discrete vascular territories, is key to the diagnosis of hyperacute stroke and has clinical implica-tions for both prognosis and treatment (Johnson 1994).

*Loss of gray-white differentiation,* in the setting of

A

B

C

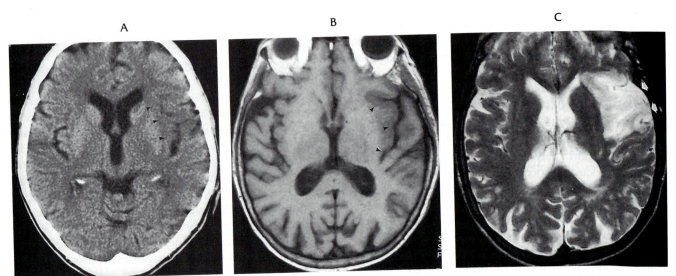

***Figure 13-9*** **Insular ribbon sign of MCA infarction. A.** Noncon-trast CT demonstrates the hypodensity of the right insular cortex without mass effect on the adjacent sylvian cistern (arrowheads). **B.** $T_1$-weighted axial image (TE15/TR600) obtained 2 days later demon-strates hypointense signal in the left insular cortex with mild efface-

ment of the sulci compared with the normal right side. **C.** $T_2$-weighted axial image (TE90/TR4000) demonstrates $T_2$ prolongation in both the insular and opercular cortex, consistent with MCA infarc-tion.

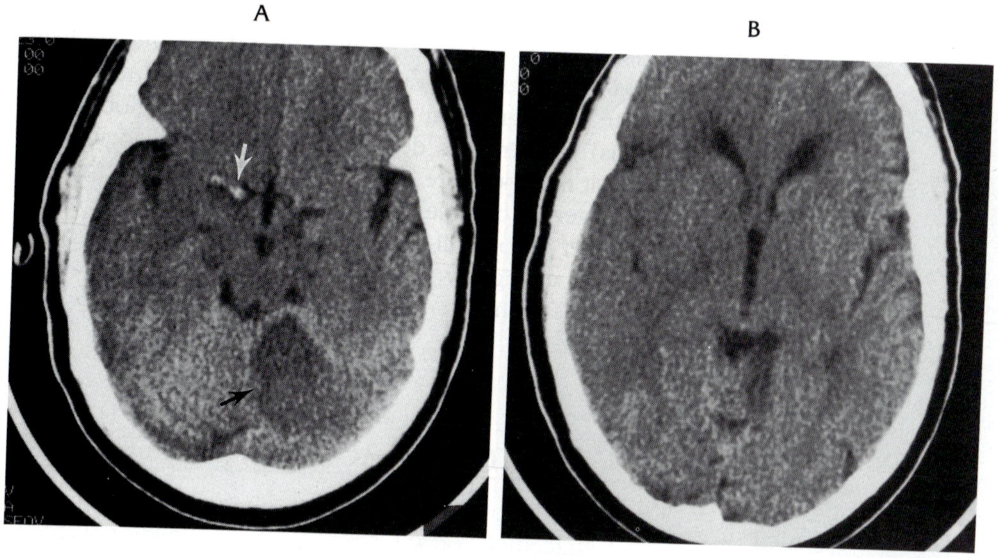

A

B

**Figure 13-10 MCA infarction with hyperdense MCA and branches. A.** Dense clot is identified in the right middle cerebral artery (arrow). Note the cerebellar infarct on the left (arrow). **B.** CT demonstrates loss of gray-white differentiation and sulcal effacement in the MCA territory on the right. *(Reprinted with permission from Johnson MH: CT evaluation of the earliest signs of stroke. The Radiologist 1(4):189–199, 1994.)*

cerebral ischemia, can be attributed to cellular changes resulting from ischemia and secondary edema within a given territory (Ng 1970; Hayman 1981b; Johnson 1994). It can be identified as early as 3 to 6 h following the ictus, particularly when the infarction involves a large vascular territory. The area of hypodensity is initially ill-defined, becoming progressively hypodense, and better defined, during the subsequent 24 to 48 h (Fig. 13-3) (Ng 1970; Sypert 1975; Arimitsu 1977; Wall 1981). Cytotoxic edema, identified within neurons and astrocytic processes within hours of the onset of ischemia, and the subsequent influx of protein-free fluids into the extracellular space, vasogenic edema, *results in early sulcal effacement* (Ng 1970; Wall 1981; Johnson 1994) (Fig. 13-8). This sign may be evident even before significant loss of gray-white differentiation has occurred. The insular ribbon sign, indicating early middle cerebral artery (MCA) infarction, was described by Truwit in 1990 (Truwit 1990) (Fig. 13-9). The insular ribbon refers to the gray and white matter tracts of the most lateral aspect of the insula, the claustrum, extreme capsule, and island of Reil. The insula is supplied by the claustral arteries and other insular branches of the MCA. With impaired insular vascular supply, potential collateral branches are available from the adjacent lentiform nucleus, via the lenticulostriate arteries and the recurrent artery of Heubner. However, when there is occlusion of the MCA distal to the lenticulostriate arteries, the insula is isolated from these potential sources of collateral supply and thus is essentially a border zone (Truwit 1990; Johnson 1994). Focal loss of gray-white differentiation with hypodensity on CT involving the insular ribbon is one of the earliest imaging manifestations of MCA infarction. The hyperdense artery sign can be one of the earliest CT findings of infarction and may precede other imaging signs (Yock 1981; Gacs 1983; Manelfe 1991; Johnson 1994). It is inconstant and, as such, may be overutilized and

its importance overestimated. Although most frequently reported in the MCA, this sign may be seen in the basilar artery, or occasionally, in a branch artery (Figs. 13-10, 13-11). Yock (1981) first reported the association between increased density in the middle cerebral artery, and the presence of intraluminal thrombus (Yock 1981). Gacs (1983) and Pressman (1987) demonstrated that the hyperdense vessel corresponded to vascular occlusion at angiography, owing to embolus or local thrombus (Gacs 1983; Pressman 1987). The hyperdense cerebral artery sign has been reported to occur on 2.5 to 20 percent of CT scans in patients with acute stroke, particularly those with larger infarcts (Yock 1981; Gacs 1983; Pressman 1987; Manelfe 1991). The hyperdense MCA must be of higher density than both the surrounding brain and the

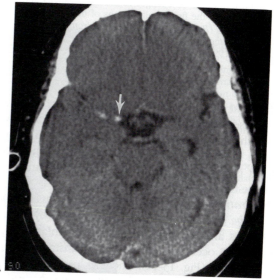

A

**Figure 13-11 Hyperdense MCA, obscuration of the lentiform nucleus. A.** Noncontrast CT demonstrates hyperdensity within the right MCA, indicative of thrombosis. *(Continued on next page)*

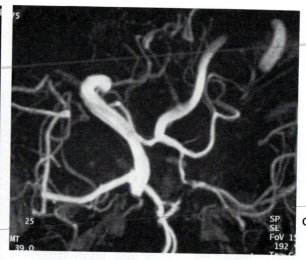

***Figure 13-27 (continued)*** **B.** Axial $T_2$-weighted image confirms the lack of flow void within the cavernous sinus. **C.** Axial MIP time-of-flight MRA image with caudal rotation demonstrates flow within the internal carotid artery on the right with absence of flow on the left. Note the posterior communicating artery filling the middle cerebral artery branches on the left. Anterior cerebral artery branches fill bilaterally, probably owing to right-to-left flow via the anterior communicating artery.

attacks. Hypoperfusion may lead to infarction in the supratentorial border zones. Interestingly, the pattern or distribution of infarction seen on CT or MRI imaging following internal carotid artery occlusion may vary from a large, almost holohemispheric infarction to a small cortical infarct in the periphery of the vascular territory at risk (Johnson 1994) (Figs. 13-25, 13-26, 13-27). The latter scenario may occur when abundant collateral vascular flow exits through the circle of Willis, from external carotid arterial branches as well as from leptomeningeal sources, and is able to maintain rCBF over the major portion of the internal carotid artery territory.

## Hemorrhagic Infarction

The majority of ischemic infarctions are "bland," that is, nonhemorrhagic infarctions (Mohr 1992b). This is particularly true when vascular occlusion persists without the rapid reperfusion that follows clot lysis. When revascularization rapidly follows vascular occlusion, "hemorrhagic transformation" of the infarction may occur. In this situation, the ischemic, initially bland, infarction may develop variable amounts of hemorrhage, often petechial, within 2 h to 2 weeks following vascular occlusion. Hemorrhagic infarction occurs most commonly with strokes caused by emboli from carotid or other sources. It may also occur with atherosclerotic thrombotic infarcts in patients with coagulation disorders or in those on anticoagulant therapy (Hayman 1981b; Mohr 1992b; Hornig 1993). Hypertension may also predispose to hemorrhagic transformation of bland ischemic infarctions (Brott 1986). Minor petechial

hemorrhage in an area of infarction may be clinically silent, although larger areas of hemorrhage are associated with worsening edema, increased intracranial pressure, clinical deterioration, and worsened prognosis. The overall incidence of hemorrhagic infarction has been reported at between 18 and 23 percent (Kase 1992; Lee 1996; Schneider 1996).

Hemorrhagic infarction results when an embolus lodges in a cerebral vessel, rendering the corresponding vascular territory ischemic (Fisher 1951; Torvik 1966). Unlike the vascular obstruction in thrombotic infarction, the embolus lyses, the fragments distally migrate, and perfusion returns to the initially ischemic tissue. There is high-pressure reperfusion of ischemic brain tissue following clot lysis and flow restoration, which often results in the development of hemorrhagic infarction (Fig. 13-28). Angiography may demonstrate evidence of cerebral embolus and/or subsequent fragmentation with reperfusion and distal migration of clot fragments (Fisher 1951; Pessin 1980; Yamaguchi 1987; Bozzao 1991; Bryan 1991; Lee 1996). As a clinical example of reperfusion of infarcted tissue resulting in infarction, consider the case of a carotid endarterectomy performed in the first few weeks following cerebral infarction with subsequent hemorrhagic transformation of the infarcted territory (due to reestablished perfusion pressure within the internal carotid artery circulation). Reperfusion of previously infarcted tissue is, by far, the most common cause of hemorrhagic infarction in both clinical and autopsy series (Torvik 1966; Yamaguchi 1987; Schneider 1996).

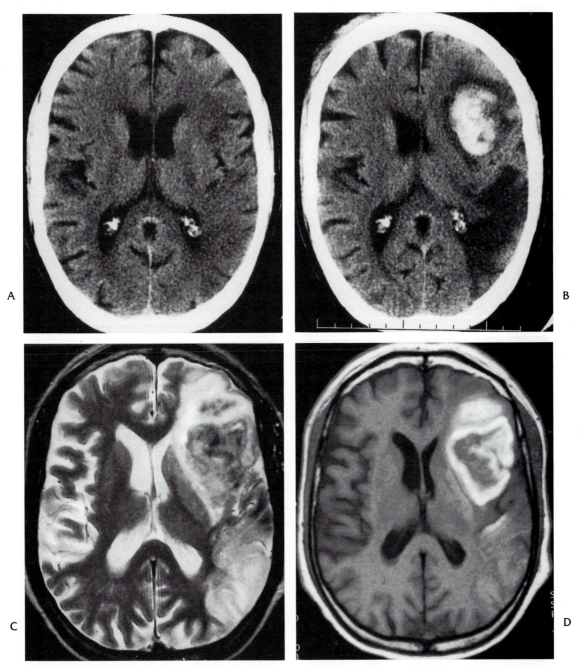

**Figure 13-28 Hemorrhagic infarction. A.** Noncontrast CT demonstrates loss of gray-white matter differentiation in the posterior watershed zone on the left. A second area of hypodensity is identified in the periventricular white matter in the watershed zone on the left anteriorly (arrowheads). **B.** Noncontrast CT obtained 3 days later demonstrates hemorrhage into the anterior watershed region on the left with increasing edema and mass effect with partial effacement of the ipsilateral frontal horn and cortical sulci. The watershed infarct in the posterior border zone is better defined. **C.** Axial T$_2$-weighted image (TE90/TR4000) obtained at 6 days following **B** demonstrates heterogeneous signal in the anterior watershed zone with surrounding edema. **D.** Noncontrast T$_1$-weighted image (TE15/TR600) demonstrates heterogeneously increased signal intensity in the periphery of hematoma with central isointense signal with adjacent mass effect. Notice also the more subtle increased signal intensity in the posterior border zone, which may represent small amounts of petechial hemorrhage within the area of infarction.

Hemorrhagic infarction is characterized pathologically by petechial hemorrhages spread diffusely throughout the infarcted tissue, predominating in the gray matter (Yenari 1997). The cortex at the depth of the sulci is particularly vulnerable to hemorrhagic transformation. Ischemic endothelium may not only leak fluid into the extracellular space, but may also leak blood into the extracellular space, especially when there is severe tissue injury and necrosis. The longer the period of ischemia before reperfusion occurs, the greater the tissue injury, and the greater the risk of hemorrhagic transformation (Jorgensen 1966).

The CT and MRI appearance of hemorrhagic infarction reflects the diffuse, petechial nature of the hemorrhage detected on pathologic examination (Bryan 1991; Zyed 1991). On CT, hemorrhage may be seen at the depths of sulci as a diffuse ribbon of increased density following the gyri or may extend into the subjacent white matter, mimicking a primary parenchymal hematoma (Lee 1996). There is residual hypodensity in the subjacent white matter. The hemorrhage occurs within the original territory of the bland infarct, although when severe, it may extend to involve adjacent parenchyma. Minimal amounts of petechial hemorrhage may be isodense with gray matter on CT, owing to volume averaging, and may be detectable only when images are compared with an earlier CT scan (Schneider 1996). On MRI, the cortical hemorrhage is initially isointense to slightly hypointense on $T_1WI$ and hypointense on $T_2WI$. By the end of the first week following hemorrhagic transformation, the $T_1WI$ frequently demonstrates gyriform cortical hyperintensity, whereas, on $T_2WI$ there is cortical hyperintensity (Zyed 1991). Peripheral contrast enhancement may be identified surrounding the areas of hemorrhage; however, often this enhancement pattern will be superimposed on the enhancement of the initially infarcted tissue.

## Hypertensive Hemorrhage

Severe, chronic hypertension is a significant risk factor for stroke (Wolf 1992; Anderson 1995). CT readily permits identification of parenchymal hematoma or petechial hemorrhage. These are important to identify since this will affect subsequent management of clinical stroke with thrombolytic or anticoagulant therapy. MRI is useful for the detection of blood products in various stages of hemoglobin degradation and reflects the timing of the hemorrhage (Table 13-2). This can be helpful in establishing differential diagnosis of the intracranial process. Hypertensive hematomas tend to occur in the elderly and are most commonly located in the basal ganglia and internal capsule (Fig. 13-29). The lateral putamen is the most common site of origin, although the caudate nucleus, brainstem, and thalamus are all frequent locations (Mohr 1978). Supratentorial white matter hematomas may also occur. On occasion, a small hemorrhagic hypertensive hematoma may present without a "catastrophic" ictus, and may in fact mimic an occlusive (bland) stroke. Larger parenchymal hematomas frequently rupture into the ventricular system resulting in hydrocephalus ventricular obstruction and mass effect on the adjacent normal parenchyma. Enlargement of the ventricles due to obstruction from blood products following hemorrhagic infarction may require ventricular drainage for clinical management and preventing subsequent hydrocephalus. Pathologically, the hypertensive hematoma is thought to arise from rupture of microaneurysms on small penetrating arteries (Charcot 1868). These were described by Charcot and Bouchard (1868) and are referred to Charcot-Bouchard aneurysms (Charcot 1868). These aneurysms involve the penetrating arteries within the basal ganglia and brainstem, thus explaining the propensity of hypertensive hematomas to occur in these locations.

On noncontrast CT, the acute hypertensive parenchymal hematoma appears as a homogeneously dense, well-defined lesion with mass effect, and initially little surrounding edema. On MRI, the hematoma is initially iso- to slightly hypointense to gray matter on $T_1WI$ and markedly hypointense on $T_2WI$ and on gradient-echo sequences (Taber 1996). This appearance is consistent with the presence of deoxyhemoglobin. After 3 to 4

## Table 13-2   Intraparenchymal Hemorrhage and MR Features

| AGE OF HEMORRHAGE | $T_1$-WEIGHTED MR | $T_2$-WEIGHTED MR |
|---|---|---|
| Hyperacute: (<24 h) Oxyhemoglobin begins changing to deoxyhemoglobin within 3h | Isointense | Initially hyperintense, becomes hypointense within 1–2 days |
| Acute: (1–3 days) deoxyhemoglobin | Iso- to hypointense | Hypointense |
| Subacute: (early 1–2 weeks) Intracellular methemoglobin (late 2–4 weeks) extracellular methemoglobin | Hyperintensity begins peripherally, solid hyperintensity at 2–3 weeks | Hypointense until 2 weeks, then peripheral hypointensity progresses to solid hyperintensity at 2–3 weeks |
| Chronic: >1 month | Isointense to mildly hypointense the periphery becomes more hypointense with time | Hypointense periphery progresses to complete hypointensity |

*Modified from Johnson MH: Magnetic resonance imaging of cerebrovascular disease in childhood. In: Faerber EM (ed), Magnetic Resonance Imaging of the Cranial Nerve in Infants and Children. London, MacKeith Press, 1995.*

days, the hematoma is surrounded by hypodensity (edema) on CT and high signal appears surrounding the hematoma on $T_2WI$ images corresponding to the surrounding edema. Hypertensive hematomas can often be distinguished from those originating from tumor or vascular malformation because of their usual homogeneous appearance. In the case of tumoral hemorrhage, a heterogeneous appearance owing to the combined presence of tumor and hematoma is common. With hematoma secondary to arteriovenous malformations, contrast enhancing vessels on CT and/or flow voids on MR may be demonstrated adjacent to the hemorrhage, confirming the diagnosis (Graves 1990; Pessin 1991).

## Hypertensive Encephalopathy

Hypertensive encephalopathy may occur in patients with known hypertension or may occur in a normotensive patient who suffers a sudden elevation in blood pressure (Dinsdale 1992). Generalized parenchymal edema is present, often with associated petechial hemorrhage due to endothelial ischemic injury. Pathophysiologically, the inability of the cerebral vessels to respond appropriately to the elevation in blood pressure due to the impairment of normal cerebrovascular autoregulatory function is thought to represent the mechanism for the cerebral edema (Schwartz 1998). CT and MR demonstrate generalized cerebral edema, with lesser changes in the posterior fossa. There is good correlation between the level of the blood pressure elevation over baseline and the degree of parenchymal edema. A variation of hypertensive encephalopathy is preeclampsia (Mantello 1993). In preeclampsia, a marked elevation of blood pressure in the peripartum period results in a disturbance in autoregulation. There are areas of loss of gray-white matter differentiation on CT. Frequently, fleeting areas of increased $T_2$ signal are identified on MRI, consistent with edema and ischemic or infarcted territories (Fig 13-30). These imaging findings may resolve, in time, without significant sequelae, following delivery and return of blood pressure to more normal levels.

## Amyloid Angiopathy

Amyloid angiopathy is an infrequent cause of nonhypertensive massive spontaneous intracerebral hemorrhage in older persons. Deposition of amyloid in the cerebral parenchymal blood vessels primarily involves the arterioles of the cortex, usually in persons beyond the age of 70 years. The cortical arterioles most frequently involved are those within the parietal cortex.

There is a high association in many of these patients with dementia, and pathological Alzheimer's plaque may be found in association with the vascular deposits

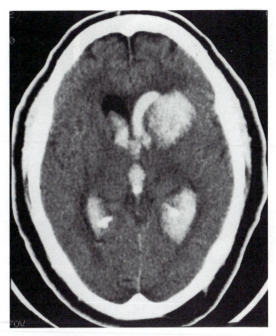

*Figure 13-29* **Hypertensive hemorrhage.** Axial noncontrast CT shows acute hemorrhage involving the left caudate nucleus and anterior limb of the internal capsule with a small amount of surrounding edema. Rupture of the hematoma into the ventricle system is evident, with blood in the lateral, third, and fourth ventricles. There is mass effect generated by both the hematoma and the mildly obstructed ventricles, with resultant effacement of the cortical sulci.

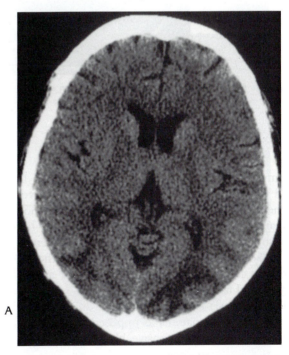

*Figure 13-30* **Hypertensive encephalopathy in eclampsia.** 26-year female with eclampsia presenting with coma and seizures. Axial CT demonstrates bilateral focal areas of hypodensity in the occipital lobes. **(A, B)**. *(Continued on next page)*

techniques, although they are limited by high-signal substances, such as fat or methemoglobin (Medlock 1992). For an overall assessment of both sinuses and cortical veins, a three-dimensional data set is useful. To differentiate slow flow from thrombus, a two-dimensional time of flight data set, oriented perpendicular to the sinus of interest, is most useful. The clarity and accuracy of time of flight techniques are improved by using presaturation of the arterial inflow. Phase contrast angiography is time-intensive, but eliminates the artifactual high signal from fat or methemoglobin. A three-dimensional phase contrast data set with a low (10 ml/s or less) velocity encoding is our preferred sequence. Whichever technique is selected, serial MRI/MRA can be utilized to assess treatment efficacy (Medlock 1992).

## SUMMARY

The identification of stroke on imaging is an important diagnosis. Differentiation from other central nervous system processes such as tumor, infection, and vascular malformation is critical to appropriate patient management. The initial goal of imaging is to assess for the presence or absence of hemorrhage within the territory of suspected infarction. The presence of hemorrhage would preclude the utilization of thrombolytic agents or heparin for management and attempts at reduction of long-term morbidity. Follow-up imaging can be useful in assessing the degree of parenchymal damage that correlates with long-term outcome and functional performance.

# References

ADAMS RD, VICTOR M: Cerebrovascular disease. In: Adams RD, Victor M (eds): *Principles of Neurology*. 2d ed. New York, NY, McGraw-Hill, 1981, pp 529–593.

AMARENCO P, HAUW JJ: Cerebellar infarction in the territory of the superior cerebellar artery: A clinicopathologic study of 33 cases. *Neurology* 40:1383–1390, 1990.

AMARENCO P, HAUW JJ, CAPLAN LR: Cerebellar infarctions. In: Lechtenberg R (ed), *Handbook of Cerebellar Diseases*. New York, NY, Dekker, 1993, pp 251–290.

ANDERSON CS, LINFO J, STEWART-WYNNE EG: A population-based assessment of the impact and burden of caregiving for long-term stroke survivors. *Stroke* 26:843–849, 1995.

ANDERSON DC, COSS DT, JACOBSON RL, et al: Tissue pertechnetate and iodinated contrast material in ischemic stroke. *Stroke* 11:617–622, 1980.

ARIMITSU T, DI CHIRO G, BROOKS RA, SMITH PB: White-gray matter differentiation in computed tomography. *J Comput Assist Tomogr* 1:437, 1977.

ARKAKI G, MIHARA H, SHIZUKA M, et al: CT and arteriographic comparison of patients with transient ischemic attacks: correlation with small infarction of basal ganglia. *Stroke* 14:276, 1983.

Asymptomatic Carotid Artery Stenosis Trial (ACAS): Randomized trial of endarterectomy for recently symptomatic carotid stenosis: Final results of the MRC European Carotid Surgery Trial. *Lancet* 351(9113):1379–1387, 1998.

BECKER H, DESCH H, HACKER H, PENCZ A: CT fogging effect with ischemic cerebral infarcts. *Neuroradiology* 18:185, 1979.

BELL CL, PARTINGTON C, ROBBINS M, et al: Magnetic resonance imaging of central nervous system lesions in patients with lupus erythematosus. *Arthritis Rheum* 34:437–441, 1991.

BERMAN SA, HAYMAN LA, HINCK VC: Correlation of CT cerebral vascular territories with function. I. Anterior cerebral artery. *AJNR* 135:352, 1980.

BERMAN SA, HAYMAN LA, HINCK VC: Correlation of CT cerebrovascular territories with function. 3. Middle cerebral artery. *AJNR* 5(2):161–166, 1984.

BOZZAO L, ANGELONI U, BASTIANELLO S, et al: Early angiographic and CT findings in patients with hemorrhagic infarction in the distribution of the middle cerebral artery, *AJNR* 12:1115–1121, 1991.

BRANDT-ZAWADZKI M, PEREIRA B, WEINSTEIN P, et al: MR imaging of acute experimental ischemia in cats. *AJNR* 7:7, 1986.

BROTT T, THALINGER K, HERTZBERG V: Hypertension as a risk factor for spontaneous intracerebral hemorrhage. *Stroke* 17:1078, 1986.

BRYAN RN, LEVY LM, WHITLOW WD, et al: Diagnosis of acute cerebral infarction: Comparison of CT and MR imaging. *AJNR* 12:611–620, 1991.

CAPLAN LR: Are terms such as completed stroke or RIND of continued usefulness? *Stroke* 14:431, 1983.

CAPLAN LR, PESSIN MS, MOHR JP: Vertebrobasilar occlusive disease, In: Barnett HJM, Mohr JP, Stein BM, Yatsu FM (eds): *Stroke: Pathophysiology, Diagnosis, and Management*. 2d ed. New York, Churchill Livingstone, 1992, pp 443–515.

MARK
    arte
    inte
    126

MASAl
    giog
    tion
    1991

MASDE
    cent
    Arch

MCCAL
    tory,
    Acka
    36–1

MCCOR
    scien
    stone

MEDLO
    with
    reson
    Neuro

MILANI
    territo1
    five ca

MOHR JF
    erative
    (NY) 2

MOHR JF
    disease
    (eds),
    ment. 2
    285–33

MOHR JP,
    Barnett
    Pathopk
    Churchi

MONAJATI
    infarcts:
    3:251, 1

MORAN C
    imaging
    311–321

MOSER F, l
    MR abno
    cooperati

MUELLER D
    in acute c
    tion. AJNI

The Nationa
    Proceedin
    tion and
    4239, Aug

CAPTAIN LR: Top of the basilar syndrome. *Neurology* 30:72–79, 1980.

CARROLL BA: Carotid sonography. *Neuroimaging Clin N Am* 2:3:533–557, 1992.

CHARCOT JD, BOUCHARD C: Nouvelles recherches sur la pathogenie de l'hemorrhagie cerebrale. *Arch Physiol Norm Path* (Paris) 1:110–127, 1868.

CHIEN D, KWONG K, GRESS D, et al: MR diffusion imaging of cerebral infarction in humans. *AJNR* 13:1097, 1992.

CORMIER PJ, LONG ER, RUSSELL EJ: MR imaging of posterior fossa infarctions: Vascular territories and clinical correlates. *Radiographics* 12:1079–1096, 1992.

CRAIN M, YUH W, GREENE G, et al: Cerebral ischemia: evaluation with contrast enhanced MR imaging. *AJNR* 12:631, 1991.

CROSBY DL, TURSKI PA, DAVIS WL: Magnetic resonance angiography and stroke: techniques, applications and limitations. *Neuroimaging Clin N Am* 2:3:509–531, 1992.

DAMASIO H: A computed tomographic guide to the identification of cerebral vascular territories. *Arch Neurol* 40:138, 1983.

DAVIS KR, ACKERMAN RH, KISTLER JP, et al: Computed tomography of cerebral infarction: hemorrhagic, contrast enhancement, and time of appearance. *Comput Tomogr* 1:71–86, 1977.

DAVIS KR, TAVERAS JM, NEW PJF, et al: Cerebral infarction diagnosis by computerized tomography: analysis and evaluation of findings. *AJNR* 124:643, 1975.

DEMAEREL P, CASAER P, CASTEELS-VAN DAELE M, et al: Moyamoya disease: MRI and MR angiography. *Neuroradiology* 33(suppl): 50–52, 1991.

DINSDALE HB: Hypertensive encephalopathy. In: Barnett HJM, Mohr JP, Stein BM, Yasu FM (eds). *Stroke: Pathophysiology, Diagnosis, and Management*. 2d ed. Churchill Livingstone, New York, 1992, pp 787–792.

DUDLEY AW Jr, LUNZER S, HAYMAN A: Localization of radioisotope (chlormerodrin He-203) in experimental cerebral infarction. *Stroke* 1:143–148, 1970.

ELLIS GG, VERITY MA: Central nervous system involvement in systemic lupus erythematosus: a review of neuropathologic changes in 57 cases 1955–1977. *Semin Arthritis Rheum* 8:212–221, 1979.

ELSTER A, MOODY D: Early cerebral infarction: Gadopentetate dimeglumine enhancement. *Radiology* 177:627, 1990.

ESSIG M, VON KUMMER R, EGLEHOF T, et al: Vascular MR contrast enhancement in cerebrovascular disease. *AJNR* 16:223, 1995.

Executive Committee for the Asymptomatic Carotid Atherosclerosis Study: Endarterectomy for symptomatic carotid artery stenosis. *JAMA* 273(18):1421–1428, 1985.

FEATHERSTONE HJ: Clinical features of stroke migraine; a review. *Headache* 26:128, 1988.

FISHER CM: Observation of brain embolism with special reference to the mechanism of hemorrhagic infarction. *J Neuropathol Exp Neurol* 10:92–94, 1951.

FISHMAN RA: Brain edema. *N Engl J Med* 293:706–711, 1977.

GACS G, FOX AJ, BARNETT HJM, et al: CT visualization of intracranial arterial thromboembolism. *Stroke* 14:756, 1983.

GADO MH, PHELPS ME, COLEMAN RE: An extravascular component of contrast enhancement in cranial computed tomography. *Radiology* 117:595–597, 1975.

GAMACHE FW: Comparison of global and focal cerebral ischemia. In: Wood JH (ed), *Cerebral Blood Flow*. McGraw-Hill, New York, 1987, p 518.

GAMMAL T, ADAMS R, NICHOLS F, et al: MR and CT investigation of cerebral vascular disease in sickle cell patient. *AJNR* 7:1043, 1986.

GARCIA JH, KAMIJYO Y: Cerebral infarction: evolution of histopathological changes after occlusion of a middle cerebral artery in primates. *J Neuropathol Exp Neurol* 33:409, 1974.

GARCIA JH, LOSSINSKY A, CONGER KA, et al: Neuronal ischemic injury: light microscopy, ultrastructure and biochemistry. *Acta Neuropath* 43:85, 1978.

GOLDBERG AL, ROSENBAUM AE, WANG H, et al: Computed tomography of dural sinus thrombosis. *J Comput Asst Tomgr* 10:16–20, 1989.

GOLDBERG HI: Angiography of extracranial and intracranial occlusive cerebrovascular disease. *Neuroimaging Clin N Am* 2:3:487–507, 1992.

GRAVES VB, DUFF TA: Intracranial arteriovenous malformations: Current imaging and treatment. *Invest Radiol* 25:952–960, 1990.

GREENAN TJ, GROSSMAN RI, GOLDBERG HI: Cerebral vasculitis MR imaging and angiographic correlation. *Radiology* 182:65–72, 1992.

HALEY EC, BRASHEAR HR, BARTH JT, et al: Deep cerebral venous thrombosis. *Arch Neurol* 46:337–340, 1989.

HAYMAN A, LEVITON A, NEFZGER D, et al: Transient focal cerebral ischemia: epidemiological and clinical aspects. *Stroke* 5:277, 1974.

HAYMAN LA, BERMAN SA, HINCK VC: Correlation of CT cerebral vascular territories with function. II. Posterior cerebral artery. *AJNR* 137:13, 1981a.

HAYMAN LA, EVANS RA, BASTION FO, et al: Delayed high dose contrast CT: identifying patients at risk of massive hemorrhagic infarction. *AJNR* 2:139–147, 1981b.

HAYMAN LA, SAKAI F, MEYER JS, et al: Iodine enhanced CT patterns after cerebral arterial embolization in baboons. *AJNR* 1:233–238, 1980.

HEIER L: White matter disease in the elderly: Vascular etiologies. *Neuroimaging Clin N Am* 2:441, 1992.

connatal form (Wang 1995). The basal ganglia may be hypointense on $T_2$-weighted images, possibly due to iron deposition (Silverstein 1990). On occasion, scattered small areas of normal signal intensity may be seen in the cerebral WM on MRI, which may correspond to the "tigroid" myelination pattern seen on histology (Shimomura 1988).

## Alexander's Disease

Alexander's disease is a rare, sporadic leukodystrophy of unknown etiology. Most biopsy proven cases are isolated, without evidence of genetic inheritance (Pridmore 1993).

Three age-dependent clinical subgroups have been suggested. The infantile form presents early with spastic quadraparesis, psychomotor retardation, and seizures. Macrocephaly and/or hydrocephalus is present. The juvenile form presents from 7 to 14 years of age with bulbar signs, spastic quadraparesis, and ataxia. Mental status is normal. An adult variant is said to mimic multiple sclerosis (Pridmore 1993).

On gross pathological examination, the enlarged brain has a thickened, indurated cortex. The WM is discolored and is soft or jellylike. Microscopically, there is diffuse demyelination and rarefaction of the WM. A distinctive feature is the presence of numerous Rosenthal fibers. These are elongated, irregularly shaped hyaline eosinophilic bodies in astrocytic cell processes (Allen 1992). Both alpha B-crystallin and a related small heat shock protein (HSP27) are found within the characteristic Rosenthal fibers. This suggests that they may be stress protein inclusions formed as a chronic stress response to an unknown stimulus (Head 1993). Smaller numbers of Rosenthal fibers are found in other conditions associated with neoplastic and inflammatory astrocytosis (Allen 1992).

The clinical diagnosis of Alexander's disease may be difficult because of the variable age of onset and the nonspecific symptoms. The definitive diagnosis is made by brain biopsy (Pridmore 1993).

Neuroimaging may suggest the diagnosis. The most common finding is symmetrical deep WM disease. The frontal lobes are usually affected first and most severely. With time, the WM disease extends to most of the cerebral hemispheres including the internal capsules. The cerebellar WM may also be involved. The affected WM is low density on CT. On MRI, the abnormal WM is low signal intensity on $T_1$WI and high signal intensity on $T_2$WI. There is no mass effect (Fig. 14-28A). On CT, the subependymal borders of the lateral ventricles, fornices, and proximal forceps minor appear normal or increased in density. Also, the subependymal borders of the lateral ventricles, the fornices, the proximal forceps minor, the basal ganglia, and the restiform bodies may demonstrate pathological enhance-

ment (Fig. 14-28B). If seen, the enhancement decreases as the disease progresses. Atrophy often appears, especially enlargement of the frontal horns and proximal lateral ventricular bodies. Focal WM necrosis or cavitation is occasionally evident (Pridmore 1993).

## Canavan Disease

Canavan disease (spongiform degeneration of van Bogaert and Bertrand) is a severe, progressive leukoencephalopathy that usually progresses to death within the first 10 years of life. The disease affects all ethnic groups; however, most of the reported patients have been of Ashkenazi Jewish heritage. The disease is caused by a deficiency of the enzyme aspartoacylase. The inheritance is autosomal recessive. Although the disease incidence is not well defined, recently developed genetic screening suggests that the incidence may be 1 in 5000 births in Ashkenazi Jews. This is similar to the incidence of Tay-Sachs disease (Matalon 1995).

The clinical manifestations of Canavan disease are not usually evident at birth, but frequently develop in early infancy. The initial sign of the disease is often developmental delay, which becomes apparent between 3 to 6 months of age. Patients develop macrocephaly, hypoto-

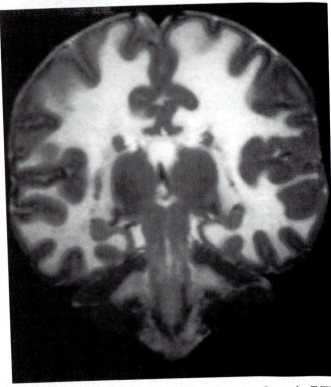

**Figure 14-27 Pelizaeus-Merzbacher disease.** Coronal $T_2$WI shows diffuse increased signal intensity throughout the supratentorial and cerebellar white matter. Head circumference was normal in size.

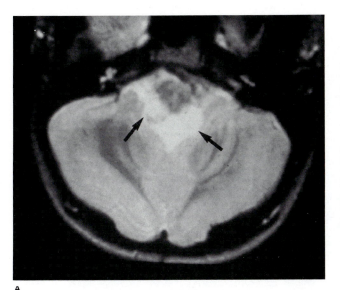
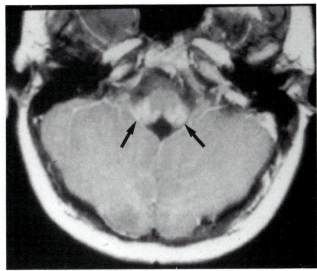

A                                                                B

*Figure 14-28* **Alexander's disease.** Fifteen-year-old male with biopsy proven Alexander's disease and a sister with the same disease. **A.** Axial T$_2$WI shows increased signal intensity in the restiform bodies (inferior cerebellar peduncles) of both sides of the medulla oblongata (arrows). **B.** Axial CEMR shows bilateral enhancement of the restiform bodies (arrows).

nia, and head lag. Developmental milestones are not reached. Hypotonia is eventually replaced by spasticity. Seizures, optic atrophy, and gastroesophageal reflux often occur (Matalon 1995). Three clinical variants have been described. The congenital form is most severe and presents within weeks of birth. Death occurs rapidly. The infantile form is most common and is usually evident by 6 months of age. Death occurs by 4 years of age. In the juvenile form, children may develop normally to 4 or 5 years of age followed by neurological deterioration to death by adolescence (Toft 1993).

The clinical manifestations are caused by marked accumulation of *N*-acetyl-L-aspartate (NAA) in the brain, as a result of the inherited deficiency of the enzyme aspartoacylase. This interferes with the normal myelination process. This is the only known disease with a defect in NAA metabolism (Matalon 1995).

On gross pathological examination, the WM is soft and gelatinous. There is no clear demarcation between gray and white matter. Histologically, prominent vacuolization is present in the WM, especially in the subcortical region. The numerous vacuoles measure up to 100 μm in diameter and appear empty. Normal myelin is absent. On electron microscopy, the vacuoles appear to be caused by swollen astrocytes and splitting of thin myelin lamellae (Lake 1992).

The clinical diagnosis is made by the demonstration of elevated NAA in urine or blood. Absent aspartoacylase can be demonstrated in cultured skin fibroblasts. Brain biopsy is no longer necessary to make the diagnosis (Matalon 1995).

Neuroimaging may suggest the diagnosis in a patient who presents with macrocephaly. CT demonstrates diffuse symmetrical low attenuation in the subcortical and deep WM. MRI demonstrates diffuse WM low signal intensity on T$_1$WI and high signal intensity on T$_2$WI (Fig. 14-29) (Marks 1991; Brismar 1990). Subcortical U fibers are not spared, unlike most other leukodystrophies (Marks 1991; McAdams 1990; Matalon 1995). The internal capsule and corpus callosum may be partially spared. Atrophy may be present, especially late in the illness (Brismar 1990). Late onset (juvenile form) patients may present with high T$_2$ signal intensity in the basal ganglia before abnormal WM is apparent (Toft 1993). MR proton spectroscopy demonstrates elevated cerebral NAA levels that can help establish the diagnosis (Grodd 1991; Marks 1991). In addition to Canavan disease, the differential diagnosis of nonhydrocephalic macrocephaly includes Alexander's disease, Tay-Sachs disease, metachromatic leukodystrophy, glutaric acidemia, autosomal dominant megaloencephaly, and several other neurodegenerative disorders (Matalon 1995).

Other than Canavan disease, there are several enzyme deficiency disorders that affect the developing brain (Table 14-4). In all these enzyme deficiency disorders there is arrested or delayed myelination rather than dysmyelination. These disorders result in varying degrees of severe neonatal atrophy. Early detection may help in correcting the metabolic end result on the brain tissue, with clinical improvement.

In nonketotic hyperglycemia caused by dysfunction of the glycine-clearing enzyme system, there is defective metabolism of glycine. In neonates this results in delayed or arrested myelination. Affected children pre-

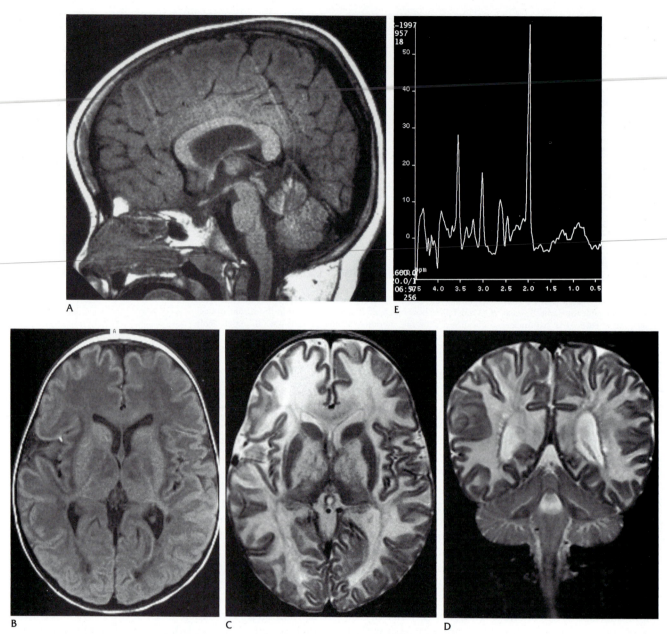

***Figure 14-29*** **Canavan disease.** Sagittal **(A)** and axial **(B)** T$_1$WI at 2 years of age show the white matter to be essentially unmyelinated except for portions of the corpus callosum and the internal capsules. The patient is macrocephalic. **C.** Axial T$_2$WI on the same patient as in **A** and **B** shows diffuse increased signal intensity throughout the cerebral hemispheric white matter, as well as the internal capsules and portions of the thalami and globus pallidi. **D.** Coronal T$_2$WI in another patient of similar age, shows the diffuse supratentorial increased signal intensity of the white matter, but with cerebellar involvement as well. Note that the subcortical U fibers are involved as are the deep white matter fibers. **E.** In a 3-year-old female patient proton spectroscopy performed with an echo time of 20 msec utilizing a STEAM technique with TR of 1600 msec, 2 single voxels. The very tall peak at 2 ppm is elevated *N*-acetyl-L-aspartate level.

sent with seizures and abnormal muscle tone and reflexes. Without treatment, there is developmental delay, and death follows within 5 years of onset. On both CT and MR, atrophy is found in addition to decreased or absent myelination and apparent thinning of the corpus callosum.

Defective myelination is also seen in maple syrup urine disease, galactosemia, and phenylketonuria. The accumulation of polypeptides results in defective myelin formation and spongy degeneration. The CT and MR findings may mimic those of Canavan disease.

## Table 14-4  Enzyme Deficiencies and Neonatal Atrophy

Nonketotic hyperglycemia
Methylmalonic acidemia
Propionic acidemia
Maple syrup urine disease
Tyrosinemia
Phenylketonuria
Hyper-β-alanemia

## Cockayne's Syndrome

Cockayne's syndrome (type 4 sudanophilic leukodystrophy, dwarfism with retinal atrophy, and  deafness) is a rare, recessively inherited condition, in which there appears to be a failure of DNA repair. The children are normal at birth, but later develop mental retardation, a thickened microcephalic skull, abnormal facial appearance, skin photosensitivity, kyphosis, and dwarfism with large hands and feet. Neurological features include sensory neural deafness, optic atrophy, cataracts, cerebellar ataxia, and demyelinating sensory and motor peripheral neuropathy, as well as pigmentary retinal degeneration. Death usually occurs by the third decade, at which time there is marked spasticity,

nystagmus, ataxia, seizures, and choreoathetosis. On MRI and CT there is often patchy CNS demyelination (Fig. 14-30) and on CT there is both basal ganglionic and other sites of calcification. Pathologically the brain is small, the meninges are thickened, there is optic nerve atrophy, basal ganglia calcifications are present, and the ventricles and sulci are atrophically dilated. The demyelination has been called "leopard skin" because of its bands of demyelination.

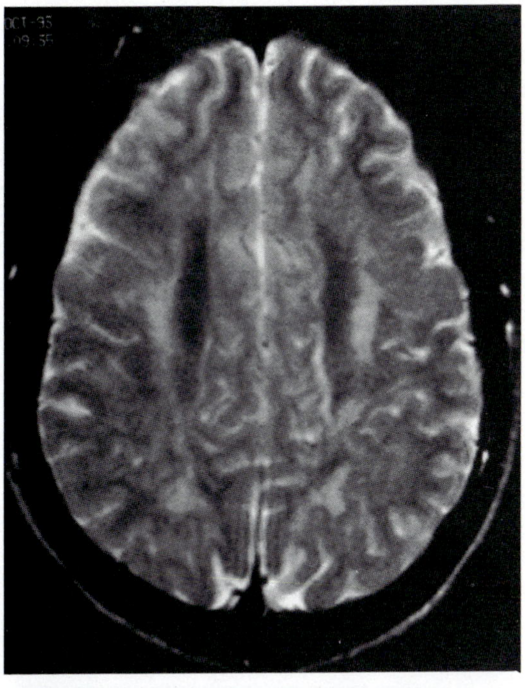

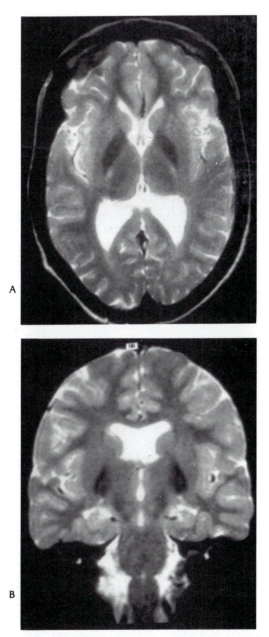

*Figure 14-31*  **18q deletion syndrome.** Eighteen-year-old female. Axial **(A)** and coronal **(B)** T$_2$WI show mild ventriculomegaly involving the atria and the frontal horns of the lateral ventricles. There is decreased white matter volume and a slight diffuse increase in signal intensity within the white matter.

*Figure 14-30*  **Cockayne's syndrome.** Axial T$_2$WI demonstrates the "leopard-skin" demyelination as bands of increased and decreased signal within the white matter. The findings are diffuse.

Soffer and coworkers reported the neuropathological findings in one of two siblings born to consanguineous parents (Soffer 1979). The siblings were of different sexes, and the inheritance appears to be that of an autosomal recessive. The pathology of the white matter showed almost total loss of oligodendroglia, atrophy of the white matter with patchy demyelination of myelinated fibers. There was severe cerebellar cortical degeneration leading to atrophy, and there were also pigmentary changes present in the globus pallidus.

## 18q Deletion Syndrome

18q deletion syndrome is a chromosomal abnormality characterized by partial deletion of the distal long arm of chromosome 18. Features include mental retardation and developmental delay, craniofacial dysmorphism, growth deficiency, limb anomalies, and eye movement disorders, as well as genital hypoplasia. A reduction in cerebral white matter with delayed myelination has been described at autopsy in this syndrome. In the series of Loevner and coworkers, 10 of 16 patients had abnormal white matter (Loevner 1996). Diffuse, bilateral symmetrical deep white matter hyperintensity on $T_2WI$ (Fig. 14-31) in the periventricular region was found in 8 out of 16 cases. Subcortical white matter changes were present in 4 of 16. Abnormal $T_2$ hypointensity in the basal ganglia and thalami were present in 11 of 16. One of the theories behind the manifestations of the 18q deletion syndrome is that white matter abnormalities may be related to one of two genes for myelin basic protein, which have been deleted along with the missing segment of chromosome 18.

For Leigh's disease please see chapter 6.

## MAGNETIC RESONANCE SPECTROSCOPY

The physics of MRS and MRI are fundamentally the same. In general, in vivo MRS obtains resonance signals from molecules in the tissue cells, whereas in vivo MRI obtains resonance signals limited to intracellular and extracellular water and some lipids. MR signals can be displayed as a function of frequency (spectrum) or gray-scale value (image). Spatial localization is achieved through magnetic field gradients in detecting water (imaging) or biochemical compounds in the body (spectroscopy). The difference is in the timing of the applied gradients. MRI uses gradients during the readout or acquisition portion of the pulse sequence, and MRS does not apply a gradient during the acquisition period to preserve frequency information (chemical shift resolution) in a spectrum (Cousins 1995). The nuclei with an odd number of protons and neutrons

such as H-1, P-31, and C-13 have a magnetic moment interacting with magnetic fields. Because of the relatively high biological concentrations and sensitivity to detection compared with other nuclei, H-1 MRS with water suppression technique is most commonly used. Since the energy emitted from the resonating nuclei is linearly proportional to the magnetic field strength and because of inherent limitations due to nucleus sensitivity and biochemical concentrations, MRS preferably needs the highest possible magnetic field strength available. Major brain metabolites that could be identified on MRS are choline, a cell membrane metabolite; phosphocreatin and creatin, energy metabolites; N-acetylaspartate, a metabolite within neurons and perhaps oligodendroglia; lactate, a by-product of metabolism, primarily of anaerobic metabolism; and other proton-containing compounds within the brain tissue (Fig. 14-32). The role of proton MRS has been investigated in brain tumors, metabolic diseases, stroke, and head injuries (Zimmerman 1998). It is believed that MRS can determine the degree of malignancy and differentiate tumorous from non-tumorous disease (Prost 1997; Schimzu 1997).

## FUNCTIONAL MRI (fMRI)

Functional MRI demonstrates cortical activation based on the principles of the blood oxygen level dependent (BOLD) technique. The normal resting cortical blood flow has a high level of deoxyhemoglobin, and activated cortex has a relative increase in oxyhemoglobin due to the increased blood flow associated with an increase in metabolic demand by the functioning neurons (Ogawa 1989). Subtracting the resting state from the activated state and superimposing the signal intensity change on the MRI of the cortex gives graphic evidence of activation. Clinical applications have been in neurosurgical operative procedures where knowledge of the cortical activation is imperative for the safe resection of brain tumors and arteriovenous malformations, and the resection of the temporal lobe for temporal lobe epilepsy (Zimmerman 1998).

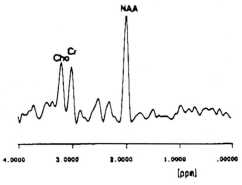

***Figure 14-32*** **Normal MRS.**

# References

ADAMS R, VICTOR M, MANCALL EL: Central pontine myelinolysis: A hitherto undescribed disease occurring in alcoholic and malnourished patients. *Arch Neurol Psychiatry* 81:154–172, 1959.

ADAMS RA, VICTOR M: Multiple sclerosis and allied demyelinative diseases. *Principles of Neurology* 5th ed. New York, McGraw-Hill, 1993.

AICARDI J: The inherited leukodystrophies: A clinical overview. *J Inher Metab Dis* 16:733–743, 1993.

ALLEN I, KIRK J: Demyelinating diseases. *Greenfield's Neuropathology* New York, Oxford University, 1992.

ARNOLD DL, MATTHEWS PM, FRANCIS GS, et al. Proton magnetic resonance spectroscopic imaging for metabolic characterization of demyelinating plaques. *Ann Neurol* 31: 235–241, 1992.

AUBORG P: Adrenoleukodystrophy and other peroxisomal diseases. *Curr Opinion Genet Develop* 4:407–411, 1994.

BALAKRISHNAN J, BECKER PS, KUMAR AJ, et al: Acquired immunodeficiency syndrome: Correlation of radiologic and pathologic findings in the brain. *Radiographics* 10: 201–215, 1990.

BARKER PB, LEE RR, MCARTHUR JC: AIDS dementia complex: Evaluation with proton MR spectroscopic imaging. *Radiology* 195:58–64, 1995.

BARTH PG, HOFFMAN GF, JAEKEN J, et al: L-2-hydroxyglutaric acidemia: A novel inherited neurometabolic disease. *Ann Neurol* 32:66–77, 1992.

BAUM PA, BARKOVICH AJ, KOCH TK, et al: Deep gray matter involvement in children with acute disseminated encephalomyelitis. *AJNR* 15:1275–1283, 1994.

BELMAN AL, COYLE PK, ROQUE C, et al: MRI findings in children infected by *Borrelia burgdorferi*. *Pediatr Neurol* 8:428–431, 1992.

BEREK K, WAGNER M, CHEMELLI AP, et al: Hemispheric disconnection in Marchiafava-Bignami disease: Clinical, neuropsychological and MRI findings. *J Neurosci* 123:2–5, 1994.

BOTS ML, VAN SWIETEN JC, BRETELER MM, et al: Cerebral white matter lesions and atherosclerosis in the Rotterdam study. *Lancet* 341:1232–1237, 1993.

BRAFFMAN BH, ZIMMERMAN RA, TROJANOWSKI JQ, et al: Brain MR: Pathologic correlation with gross and histopathology. 2. Hyperintense white-matter foci in the elderly. *AJR* 151:559–566, 1988.

BRETELER MMB, VAN AMERONGEN NM, VAN SWIETEN JC, et al: Cognitive correlates of ventricular enlargement and cerebral white matter lesions on magnetic resonance imaging: The Rotterdam study. *Stroke* 25:1109–1115, 1994a.

BRETELER MMB, VAN SWIETEN JC, BOTS ML, et al: Cerebral white matter lesions, vascular risk factors and cognitive function in a population based study: The Rotterdam study. *Neurology* 44:1246–1252, 1994b.

BRISMAR J, BRISMAR G, OZAND P: Canavan disease: CT and MR imaging of the brain. *AJNR* 11:805–810, 1990.

BRODERICK DR, WIPPOLD FJ, CLIFFORD DB, et al: White matter lesions and cerebral atrophy on MR images in patients with and without AIDS dementia complex. *AJR* 161:177–181, 1993.

BUDKA H: The definition of HIV-specific neuropathology. *Acta Pathol Japan* 41:182–191, 1991.

CALDEMEYER KS, SMITH RR, HARRIS TM, et al: MRI in acute disseminated encephalomyelitis. *Neuroradiology* 36:216–220, 1994.

CASSEDY KJ, EDWARDS MK: Metabolic and degenerative diseases of childhood. *Topics Mag Reson Imag* 5:73–95, 1993.

CASTELLOTE A, ROIG M, VASQUEZ E, et al: MR in adrenoleukodystrophy: Atypical presentation as bilateral frontal demyelination. *AJNR* 16:814–815, 1995.

CHANG CM, NG HK, CHAN YW, et al: Postinfectious myelitis, encephalitis and encephalomyelitis. *Clin Exp Neurol* 29: 250–262, 1992a.

CHANG KH, CHA SH, HAN MH, et al: Marchiafava-Bignami disease: Serial changes in corpus callosum on MRI. *Neuroradiology* 34:480–482, 1992b.

CHARNESS ME: Brain lesions in alcoholics. *Alcoholism: Clin Exp Res* 17:2–11, 1993.

CHEN TC, HINTON DR, LEICHMAN L, et al: Multifocal inflammatory leukoencephalopathy associated with levamisole and 5-fluorouracil: Case report. *Neurosurgery* 35:1138–1143, 1994.

CHRISTIANSEN P, LARRSON HBW, THOMSEN C et al: Age dependent white matter lesions and brain volume changes in healthy volunteers. *Acta Radiologica* 35:117–122, 1994.

CHRYSIKOPOULOS HS, PRESS GA, GRAFE MR, et al: Encephalitis caused by human immunodeficiency virus: CT and MR imaging manifestations with clinical and pathologic correlation. *Radiology* 175:185–191, 1990.

CORN BW, YOUSEM DM, SCOTT CB, et al: White matter changes are correlated significantly with radiation dose. *Cancer* 74:2828–2835, 1994.

PERCY AK, ODREZIN GT, et al: Globoid cell leukodystrophy: Comparison of neuropathology with magnetic resonance imaging. *Acta Neuropathol* 88:26–32, 1994.

POWER C, KONG PA, CRAWFORD TO, et al: Cerebral white matter changes in acquired immunodeficiency syndrome dementia: alterations of the blood-brain barrier. *Ann Neurol* 34:339–350, 1993.

PRIDMORE CL, BARAISTER M, HARDING B, et al: Alexander's disease: Clues to diagnosis. *J Child Neurol* 8: 134–144, 1993.

PROST BS, HAUGHTON V, LI S-J. Brain tumors: Localized H-1 MR spectroscopy at 0.5T. *Radiology* 204:235–238, 1997.

RAFTO SJ, MILTON WJ, et al: Biopsy confirmed CNS lyme disease: MR appearance at 1.5 T. *AJNR* 11:482–484, 1990.

REIDER-GROSSWASSSER I, BORNSTEIN N: CT and MRI in late onset metachromatic leukodystrophy. *Acta Neurol Scand* 75:64–69, 1987.

RODRIGUEZ M, SCHEITHAUER B: Ultrastructure of multiple sclerosis. *Ultrastructural Pathol* 18:3–13, 1994.

SASAKI M, SAKURAGAWA N, et al. MRI and CT findings in Krabbe disease. *Pediatr Neurol* 7:283–288, 1991.

SCHMIDT R, FAZEKAS F, OFFENBACHER H, et al: Neuropsychologic correlates of MRI hyperintensities: A study of 150 normal volunteers. *Neurology* 43:2490–2494, 1993.

SEITELBERGER F: Neuropathology and genetics of Pelizaeus-Merzbacher disease. *Brain Pathol* 5:267–273, 1995.

SHANLEY DJ: Mineralizing microangiopathy: CT and MRI. *Neuroradiology* 37:331–333, 1995.

SHAPIRO E, LOCKMAN L, KNOPMAN D, et al: Characteristics of the dementia in late-onset metachromatic leukodystrophy. *Neurology* 44:662–665, 1994.

SHIMIZU H, KUMABE T, TOMINAGA T, et al: Noninvasive evaluation of malignancy of brain tumors with proton MR spectroscopy. *AJNR* 17:737–747, 1996.

SHIMOMURA C, MATSUI A, CHOC H, et al: Magnetic resonance imaging in Pelizaeus-Merzbacher disease. *Pediatr Neurol* 4:124–125, 1988.

SILVERSTEIN AM, HIRSH DK, TROBE DK, et al: MR imaging of the brain in five members of a family with Pelizaeus-Merzbacher disease. *AJNR* 11:495–499, 1990.

SOFFER D, GROTSKY HW, RAPIN I, et al: Cockayne syndrome: Unusual neuropathological findings and review of the literature. *Ann Neurol* 6:340–348, 1979.

SPENCE MW, CALLAHAN JW: Sphingomyelin-cholesterol lipidoses: The Niemann-Pick group of diseases, Scriver CR, Beaudet AL, Sly WS, Valle D (eds). *The Inherited Basis of Metabolic Disease*. New York, McGraw-Hill, 1989, chap 6.

STILLMAN AE, KRIVIT W, SHAPIRO E, LOCKERMAN L, et al: Serial MR after bone marrow transplantation in two patients with metachromatic leukodystrophy. *AJNR* 15: 1929–1932, 1994.

TAYBI H, LACHMAN RS: *Radiology of Syndromes, Metabolic Disorders, and Skeletal Dysplasias*. Chicago: Year Book Medical, 1990, p. 592.

THOMAS DJ, PENNOCK JM, HAJNAL JV, et al: Magnetic resonance imaging of spinal cord in multiple sclerosis by fluid-attenuated inversion recovery. *Lancet* 341:593–594, 1993.

THORPE JW, HALPIN SF, et al: A comparison between fast and conventional spin-echo in the detection of multiple sclerosis lesions. *Neuroradiology* 36:388–392, 1994.

TOFT PB, GEIB-HOLTORFF R, ROLLAND MO, et al: Magnetic resonance imaging in juvenile Canavan disease. *Eur J Pediatr* 152:750–753, 1993.

VALK J, VAN DER KNAAP MS: *Magnetic Resonance of Myelin, Meylination, and Myelin Disorders*. New York, Springer-Verlag, 1989.

VALK PE, DILLON WP: Radiation injury of the brain. *AJNR* 12:45–62, 1991.

VANHANEN SL, RAININKO R, SANTAVUORI P: Early differential diagnosis of infantile neuronal ceroid lipofuscinosis, Rett syndrome, and Krabbe disease by CT and MR. *AJNR* 15:1443–1453, 1994.

VAN SWIETEN JC, VAN DEN HOUT JHW, et al: Periventricular lesions in the white matter on magnetic resonance imaging in the elderly. *Brain* 114:761–774, 1991.

WANG PJ, YOUNG C, LIU HM, et al: Neurophysiologic studies and MRI in Pelizaeus-Merzbacher disease: Comparison of classic and connatal forms. *Pediatr Neurol* 12:47–53, 1995.

WEINSHENKER BG: Natural history of multiple sclerosis. *Ann Neurol* 36:S6–S11, 1994.

WENGER DA: Research update on lysosomal disorders with special emphasis on metachromatic leukodystrophy and Krabbe disease. *Apmis Suppl 40* 101:81–87, 1993.

WIESTLER OD, LEIBE SL, SPIEGEL H, et al: Neuropathology and pathogenesis of HIV encephalopathies. *Acta Histochemica* 42:S107–114, 1992.

YETKIN FZ, FISCHER ME, PAPKE RA, et al: Focal hyperintensities in cerebral white matter on MR images of asymptomatic volunteers: Correlation with social and medical histories. *AJR* 161:855–858, 1993.

YLIKOSKI A, ERKINJUNTTI T, RAININKO R, et al: White matter hyperintensities on MRI in the neurologically nondiseased elderly. *Stroke* 26:1171–1177, 1995.

YUH WTC, SIMONSON TM, D'ALESSANDRO MP, et al: Temporal changes of MRI findings in central pontine myelinolysis. *AJNR* 16:975–977, 1995.

ZIMMERMAN RA, BILANINK LT, HUNTER JV: MR diffusion imaging in CNS infections. Presented at ASNR annual meeting. May 17–21, 1998.

ZIMMERMAN RA, HASELGROVE JC, WANG Z, et al: Advances in pediatric neuroimaging. *Brain Dev* 20:275–289, 1998.

# 15 THE BASE OF THE SKULL: SELLA AND TEMPORAL BONE

*Krishna C.V.G. Rao*
*Hector Robles*

## CONTENTS

The skull base is formed of membranous bone and cartilage perforated by nerves, arteries, and veins. The base of the skull consists of the anterior, middle, and posterior compartments. The floor of the anterior cranial fossa is formed laterally by the roof of the orbits and in the midline by the cribriform plate. The bony components of the floor of the middle cranial fossa are

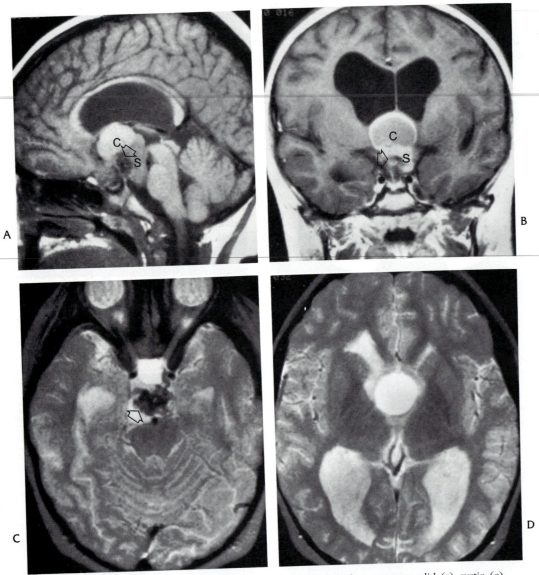

***Figure 15-38*** **Craniopharyngioma.** Sagittal T$_1$-weighted MR (**A**) demonstrates solid (s) cystic (c) and calcification (arrowhead) within the tumor. Adjacent axial T$_2$-weighted MR (**B,C**). Hypointense signal from calcific component (arrow) and hyperintense solid and cystic component with the tumor. Gd-DTPA–enhanced coronal T$_1$-weight MR (**D**) demonstrates enhancement of capsule of the cyst (arrow) and the solid portion of the tumor. Hypointense signal of calcification (long arrow).

gible signal intensity. The appearance of the cysts varies (Fig. 15-38). Some are isointense with CSF in T$_1$WI and T$_2$WI; those with a high protein content are slightly hyperintense with respect to CSF. Hemorrhagic cysts containing subacute blood have high signal intensity in T$_1$WI or T$_2$WI (Chakeres 1989). Papillary squamous craniopharyngiomas are predominantly solid and round, whereas adamantinous craniopharyngiomas have lobulated shape with hyperintense cyst contents and tend to encase vessels (Sartorati-Schefer 1997).

## Meningioma

Meningiomas arise on the dural surface of the anterior clinoid processes, diaphragma sellae, tuberculum, dor-

sum sellae, or cavernous sinuses. Many suprasellar and parasellar meningiomas have characteristic features which permit a specific diagnosis on CT. Globular calcification, which is less common in parasellar meningiomas than it is in meningiomas elsewhere, and hyperostotic bone adjacent to the tumor are more characteristic of meningiomas than they are of other parasellar neoplasms (Fig. 15-39) (Lee 1976).

The matrix of a meningioma enhances homogeneously on CECT (Fig. 15-40) (Daniels 1981). Rarely meningiomas have cystic hypodense areas within them (Russell 1980). They may encroach on the suprasellar cistern, displace the brain, invaginate in the temporal lobe, enlarge the cavernous sinus, or, very commonly,

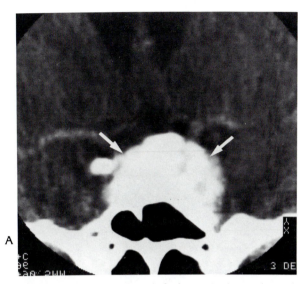
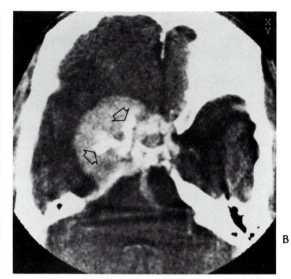

**Figure 15-39**  Densely calcified **meningioma** (arrows) on coronal CECT (**A**). Axial CECT demonstrates a parasellar meningioma that contains dense globular calcifications (open arrows) (**B**). *(From Daniels 1985a.)*

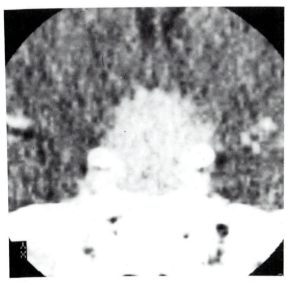

**Figure 15-40**  **Meningioma** on coronal CT. Homogeneously enhancing without calcification, the tumor could be mistaken for a pituitary adenoma. *(From Daniels 1985a.)*

extend through the diaphragma sellae into the pituitary fossa. Their margins are well defined and smoothly marginated. Cerebral edema may be present when the brain is compressed. The attachment of the meningioma to the dural surface is usually broad, sessile, and eccentrically located with respect to the sella. Meningiomas that lack calcification and hyperostosis are more difficult to distinguish from adenomas and other parasellar tumors (Fig. 15-41).

Because most meningiomas are approximately isointense with brain in $T_1WI$ or $T_2WI$, they can be missed unless a contrast-enhanced study is obtained. After in-

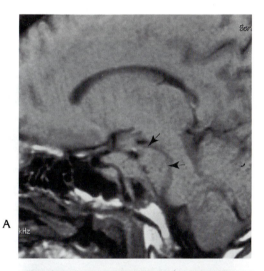
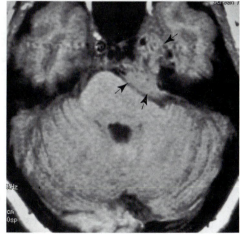

**Figure 15-41**  **Meningioma** involving cavernous sinus. Axial (**A**) and sagittal (**B**) $T_1$-weighted MR. Isointense mass involving the left cavernous sinus, adjacent clivus, and petrous apex (arrows). *(Continued on next page)*

WOLPERT SM, OSBORNE M, ANDERSON M, et al: The bright pituitary gland—A normal MR appearance in infancy. *AJNR* 9:1–3, 1988.

YEAKLEY JW, KULKARNI MV, MCARDLE CT, et al: High-resolution MR imaging of juxtasellar meningiomas with CT and angiographic correlation. *AJNR* 9:279–285, 1988.

YOUNG SC, GROSSMAN RI, GOLDBERG HI, et al: MR of vascular encasement in parasellar masses: Comparison with angiography and CT. *AJNR* 9:35–38, 1988.

YOUSEM DM, ARRINGTON JA, ZINREICH SJ: Pituitary adenomas: Possible role of bromocriptine in intratumoral hemorrhage. *Radiology* 170:239–243, 1989.

YUH WTC, WRIGHT DC, BARLOON TJ, et al: MR imaging of primary tumors of trigeminal nerve and Meckel's cave. *AJNR* 9:655–670, 1988.

ZELLER JR, CERLETTY JM, RABINOVITCH RA, et al: Spontaneous regression of a post-partum pituitary mass demonstrated by computed tomography. *Arch Intern Med* 142: 373–374, 1982

# SECTION B: TEMPORAL BONE

Evaluation for hearing loss or tinnitus almost always includes imaging of the temporal bone. A variety of congenital and acquired disease processes may involve the external, middle, or inner ear structures as well as the cerebellopontine angle cistern, and the auditory pathway of the central nervous system (Weissman 1996; Swartz 1996; Mark 1993) (Table 15-3A).

## HEARING LOSS

Hearing loss could result from sensory-neural component (SNHL), which involves the soft tissues includ-ing the acoustic nerve, from sound conduction of the osteocartilagenous elements defined as conductive hearing loss (CHL), or may be mixed (MHL) resulting from a combination of both of the above elements. Tinnitus is usually associated with a vascular pathology. Tinnitus may occasionally be associated with hearing loss.

Recognition of sound is a complex process. The auricle funnels the sound into the external auditory canal. Vibrations of the tympanic membrane are then transmitted through the ossicular chain, with the foot plate of the stapes transmitting these vibrations to the oval window within the lateral part of the inner ear. The inner ear consists of an outer bony labyrinth and an inner membranous labyrinth filled with fluid, as well as neural elements. The membranous labyrinth consists of the cochlea, the vestibule, and the semicircular canals.

## Table 15-3A   Hearing Loss: Disease Entities Associated with Different Types of Hearing Loss

| | SENSORINEURAL HEARING LOSS | CONDUCTIVE HEARING LOSS | MIXED HEARING LOSS |
|---|---|---|---|
| CONGENITAL | 1. Cochlear and vestibular dysplasia Mondini deformity/Michel anomaly<br>2. Vestibular aqueduct syndrome<br>3. Perilymphatic fistula | 1. Atresia or absent external auditory canal<br>2. Ossicular anomalies<br>3. Congenital cholesteatoma<br>4. Persistent stapedial artery | 1. Otosclerosis<br>2. Osteogenesis imperfecta<br>3. Osteopetrosis |
| TRAUMA | 1. Fractures of the temporal bone<br>2. Cochlear concussion | 1. Ossicular disruption<br>2. Hemotympanum<br>3. Perforated tympanic membrane | |
| INFLAMMATORY | 1. Labyrinthitis<br>2. Sarcoidosis<br>3. Viral meningitis<br>4. Carcinomatous meningitis | 1. Acquired cholesteatoma<br>2. Middle ear infection<br>3. Myringosclerosis | |
| NEOPLASMS | 1. Acoustic neuroma<br>2. Meningioma<br>3. Epidermoid tumor<br>4. Glomus tympanicum<br>5. Lipoma<br>6. Neuroma of cranial nerves 5, 9, 10 | 1. Glomus tympanicum<br>2. Facial nerve neuroma<br>3. Meningioma<br>4. Labyrinthine schwannoma<br>5. Langerhans' cell histiocytosis<br>6. Osteoma | |
| MISCELLANEOUS | 1. Brain stem glioma<br>2. Vascular malformation<br>3. Ischemia/hemorrhage<br>4. Multiple sclerosis | | 1. Paget's disease<br>2. Fibrous dysplasia |

## Table 15-3B    Lesions Associated with Tinnitus:

1. Glomus tympanicum tumor
2. Labyrnthine schwannomas
3. Aberrant internal carotid artery
4. Dehiscent jugular bulb
5. Vascular tympanic membrane
6. Stenosis of the internal carotid artery
7. Hemangioma
8. Arteriovenous malformation
9. Arteriovenous fistula

The cochlea converts the sound waves to neural stimuli of different frequency and pitch by the movement of the fluid within the 2¾ circular component containing small hair cells—the organ of Corti. This is connected to the sensory fibers of the auditory nerve, which determines the pitch of the sound. Neurons in the basal turn recognize high pitch, and apical turn neurons detect low-pitch sounds. The neurons join to form the cochlear division of the eighth cranial nerve. Within the internal auditory canal the cochlear division is situated in the anteroinferior quadrant of the canal. The nerve, along with the vestibular component, traverses the cerebellopontine angle cistern and the brainstem, terminating in the ventral and dorsal cochlear nuclei within the pontomedullary junction. Neural fibers connect these nuclei to the ipsilateral and contralateral superior olivary nuclei, lateral lemniscus, inferior colliculi, and medial geniculate body. These are connected to the auditory center in the superior temporal gyrus, which receives input from both sides. The vestibule and the semicircular canal convey information about movement. Both combine to determine the equilibrium and direction of sound. Based on the type of hearing loss determined by other clinical tests such as audiography and evoked auditory brainstem response, it is possible to determine whether it is due to neural elements (SNHL), an osseous element, or a combined pathology. This determines the decision to evaluate with CT (ideal for demonstrating osseous abnormalities) or with MR (fluid or soft tissue abnormalities).

## TINNITUS

Pulsatile tinnitus, described as a constant noise synchronous with the cardiac cycle, may be subjective or objective. Tinnitus may be associated with hearing loss. The underlying pathology is often a vascular retrotympanic mass (Table 15-3B). CT is useful in identifying the presence of the mass. MR and occasionally angiography may be necessary.

CT with submillimeter spatial resolution, a slice thickness of 2 mm or less, a wide CT number range, "bone detail" reconstruction programs, target reconstruction, and high-quality image reformations is effective in evaluating temporal bone pathology (Shaffer 1980; Turski 1982). CT has replaced pluridirectional tomography because of its superior low-contrast resolution, which permits visualization of middle ear muscles, ligaments, and the tympanic membrane; inflammatory disease; and neoplasms (Mafee 1983a). There is nearly equivalent bony resolution, resulting in precise evaluation of the ossicles, otic capsule, fractures, and otodystrophies.

Magnetic resonance imaging when combined with CEMR is superior to CT in evaluating cerebellopontine angle cisterns and internal auditory canals (Valvassori 1988; Swartz 1989). Because bone produces negligible MR signal, imaging of the internal auditory canal and demonstration of the cranial nerves within the internal auditory and facial nerve canals are accomplished consistently (Daniels 1984, 1985). MR is excellent for imaging acoustic neurinomas (Kingsley 1985; Saeed 1994). CEMR increases the sensitivity of MR for cerebellopontine angle and intracanalicular tumors because most of these tumors enhance intensely (Curati 1986; Daniels 1987c; Swartz 1989; Brogan 1989).

## TECHNICAL ASPECTS

### Temporal Bone CT Scanning

Scanning in two planes, usually axial and coronal, is required for optimal demonstration of temporal bone structures (Table 15-4). The axial scan plane is kept parallel to the infraorbitomeatal line to avoid scanning

## Table 15-4   Imaging Parameters in Evaluating the Temporal Bone

CT

    Both axial and coronal CT obtained at 1-mm contiguous sections through the entire
      petrous portion of the temporal bone

    The field of view is kept at 16 cm.

    Imaged in bone window algorithm with window width of 3000 and window level of 600.

    In most instances IV contrast is not necessary.

MRI

    Spin-echo sagittal $T_1$-weighted and axial spin-density $T_2$-weighted MR to cover entire head.

    Surface coil imaging of the temporal region in the axial and coronal $T_1$-weighted sequence with a small
      field of view at 16-cm width.

    Gd-DTPA–enhanced axial and coronal $T_1$-weighted section with fat suppression, 3-mm thick without inter-
      slice gap.

    Occasionally gradient sequence may be useful, especially when evaluating for vascularity.

---

the eyes, and the coronal plane is kept nearly perpendicular to the axial plane with the patient supine in a hanging head position or prone with the neck extended. Other gantry angulations for axial and coronal scans have been suggested for evaluating specific intratemporal structures (Chakeres 1983). Specialized views, such as semiaxial, sagittal, and Stenvers, have been advocated but usually not necessary given the three-dimensional projections that can be obtained with both CT and MR.

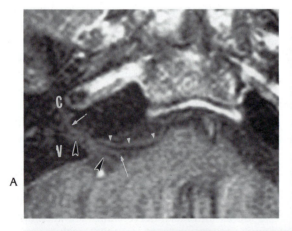

A

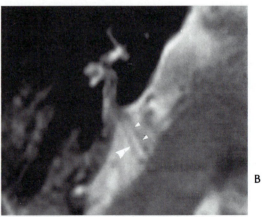

B

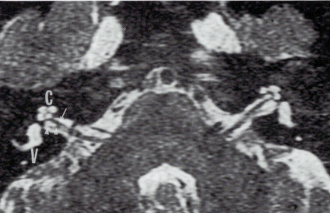

C

**Figure 15-77   Normal internal auditory canal.**
The IAC can be evaluated with different MR pulse sequences. Axial $T_1$-weighted MR (**A**) demonstrates the facial nerve (small arrowheads), cochlear nerve (arrow), and vestibular nerve (large arrowheads) within the right cerebellopontine angle cistern and medial portion of internal auditory canal. $T_2$-weighted axial MR (**B**) shows the facial (small arrowheads) and the cochlear-vestibular nerve (large arrowhead). Axial GRE sequence (**C**) shows the cochlear and vestibular nerves. *(Continued on next page)*

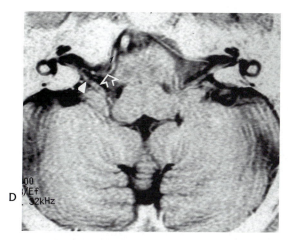

**Figure 15-77 (continued)** Reverse image of long TR (12,000), long TE (200) (**D**) demonstrating the nerve (arrowhead) and vascular loop (open arrow).

## Temporal Bone MR Imaging

In evaluating the internal auditory canals 3-mm-thick contiguous axial and coronal images through the temporal bones are obtained (Table 15-4). An SE pulse sequence with a short repetition time (TR) of 600 to 800 msec and a short echo time (TE) of 20 to 25 msec, a $256 \times 256$ matrix, and two excitations provides excellent contrast and detail, especially if an intravenous contrast agent is used. For contrast enhancement, Gd-DTPA (0.1 mmol/kg) is intravenously injected. Acoustic neurinomas, cerebellopontine angle meningiomas, and other benign tumors intensely enhance in $T_1$WI (e.g., acoustic neuromas enhance as much as 60 percent). $T_1$-weighted gradient-echo images are excellent for defining the neural and vascular structures in the jugular foramen. Such images are obtained with a single-slice acquisition technique, 3-mm-thick sections, a $256 \times 256$ matrix; four excitations, a TR of 100, a TE of 15, a 90° flip angle, and flow compensation (Daniels 1988a). However, this sequence tends to have excessive artifacts and is replaced with $T_2$-weighted fast spin echo imaging.

In short TR and TE MR images ($T_1$WI), the cranial nerves are almost isointense with brain, in contrast to the hypointense signal from the temporal bone or CSF (Fig. 15-77). In long TR and TE MR images ($T_2$WI), the nerves appear hypointense in contrast to the bright signal from CSF. The increased resolution provided by surface coil imaging improves the visualization of the individual cranial nerves (Daniels 1985) (Fig. 15-78). $T_2$-weighted fast spin-echo sequences using phased array coils and maximum intensity projection as well as three-dimensional Fourier transform techniques allows for detailed visualization of the middle and inner ear structures (Brogan 1991; Tien 1992; Stillman 1994; Guirado 1995; Schmalbrock 1995). Although these techniques allow for detailed imaging of soft tissue and

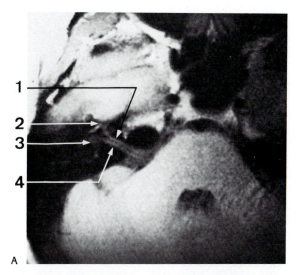

1. facial nerve  2. geniculate ganglion  3. vestibule  4. superior vestibular nerve

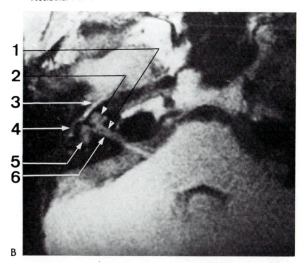

1. cochlear nerve  2. cochlea  3. greater superficial petrosal nerve  4. horizontal segment of facial nerve  5. vestibule  6. inferior vestibular nerve

**Figure 15-78 Cranial nerves in the internal auditory canal** demonstrated on surface coil MRI. Axial short $T_1$WI identify nerves in the upper (**A**) and lower (**B**) parts of the canal.

fluid within the temporal bone, contrast enhancement with Gd-DTPA when combined with fat suppression is useful when evaluating the jugular foramen or the petrous apex. Long Tr/Te sequence has been advocated in demonstrating small tumors without contrast (Allen 1996; Fukui 1996).

## NORMAL ANATOMY

The temporal bone is composed of the styloid process and the tympanic, mastoid, squamous, and petrous portions. The tympanic portion forms the anterior and inferior walls of the bony external auditory canal. The mastoid portion forms the posterior wall of the exter-

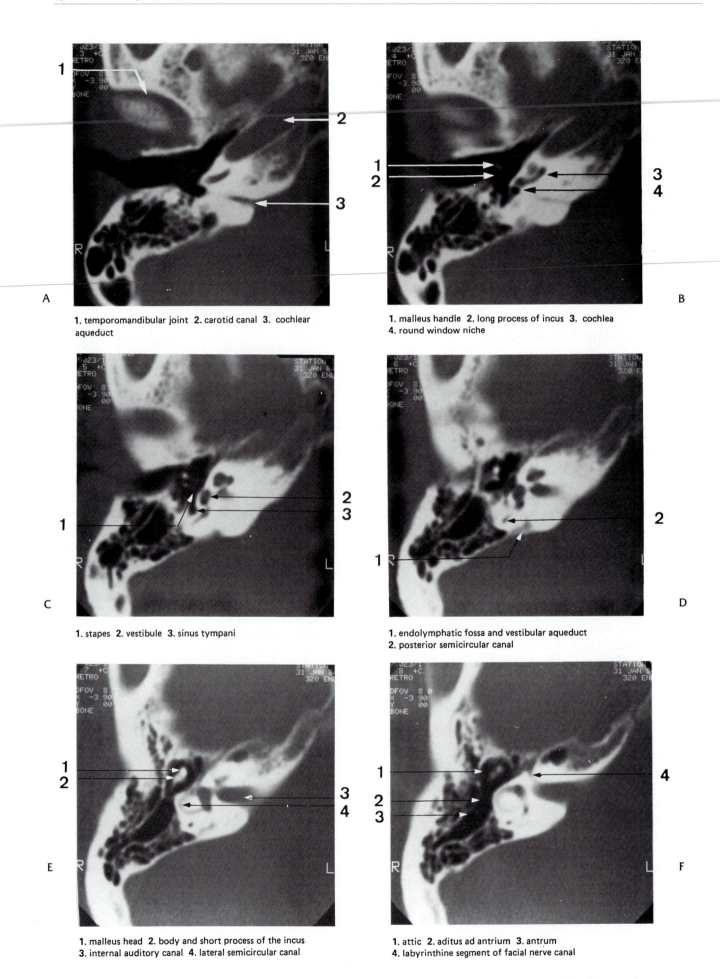

A

**1.** temporomandibular joint  **2.** carotid canal  **3.** cochlear aqueduct

B

**1.** malleus handle  **2.** long process of incus  **3.** cochlea
**4.** round window niche

C

**1.** stapes  **2.** vestibule  **3.** sinus tympani

D

**1.** endolymphatic fossa and vestibular aqueduct
**2.** posterior semicircular canal

E

**1.** malleus head  **2.** body and short process of the incus
**3.** internal auditory canal  **4.** lateral semicircular canal

F

**1.** attic  **2.** aditus ad antrium  **3.** antrum
**4.** labyrinthine segment of facial nerve canal

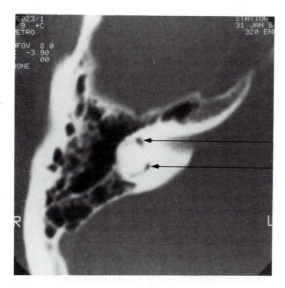

G

**1. superior semicircular canal  2. common crus between superior and posterior semicircular canals**

***Figure 15-79*** Normal axial 1.5-mm-thick contiguous CT scans of the **right ear** from posterior to anterior (**A** to **G**).

nal canal and the middle ear and contains the mastoid air cells and mastoid antrum. The squamous portion superiorly is part of the calvarium, and the petrous portion is a wedge-shaped bone that contains the inner ear. Detailed anatomy of the temporal bone on CT and MR has been described (Chakeras 1983; Swartz 1983a; Brogan 1989); the key landmarks of the temporal bone on CT are emphasized (Figs. 15-79, 15-80).

## External Auditory Canal

The shape of the external auditory canal is variable (Virapongse 1983). Its medial two-thirds is bony, whereas the rest is cartilaginous. The tympanic membrane forms the sloping medial end of the canal.

## Middle Ear

The middle ear is an air-filled chamber that can be subdivided into the epitympanic recess (attic) above the tympanic annulus, the hypotympanum below it, and the mesotympanum medial to it. The eustachian tube provides a communication between the widest (anterior) part of the hypotympanum and the nasopharynx. The epitympanic recess communicates with the mastoid antrum posteriorly through the aditus ad antrum. The mastoid is variably pneumatized depending on hereditary factors and childhood middle ear infections.

The ossicles transmit sound from the tympanic membrane through the middle ear to the oval window. The malleus handle attaches to the tympanic membrane, and the head articulates with the body of the incus, which is immediately behind it in the epitympanum. The incus

has a long process, which articulates with the stapes, and a short process. The malleus and incus appear as an ice cream cone on axial CT scans, with the malleus head representing the ice cream ball and the short process of the incus representing the cone. The stapes is the smallest of the ossicles. Its two crura and a footplate in the oval window resemble a stirrup. CT shows the stapedial crura but seldom the obliquely oriented footplate, which is only 0.05 to 0.1 mm thick centrally.

The complex posterior wall of the middle ear, including the round window niche, sinus tympani, pyramidal eminence, and facial recess, is best visualized in axial CT sections (Swartz 1983a). The tensor tympani muscle, the stapedius muscle, and ligaments in the posterior middle ear also can often be identified on high-resolution CT scans.

## Labyrinth

The bony labyrinth is located in the inner ear. The membranous labyrinth, which contains primarily perilymph and an endolymphatic space surrounded by perilymph in the cochlea, is inside the bony labyrinth. Sound waves transmitted through the ossicular chain are transferred through the oval window to the perilymph and the organ of Corti in the endolymphatic space to produce the sensation of sound. The cochlea resembles a snail with 2½ to 2¾ turns. The basal turn of the cochlea in the medial wall of the tympanic cavity forms the cochlear promontory in the middle ear. The round window is an opening in the basal turn of the cochlea and is covered by a membrane. The cochlear aqueduct, which is parallel to and below the internal auditory canal, connects the cochlea and the posteromedial surface of the petrous pyramid to equilibrate perilymph with the CSF. Posterior and slightly superior to the cochlea, the bony inner ear contains lateral, posterior, and superior semicircular canals, which are connected to the vestibule. The semicircular canals are perpendicular to each other. The posterior semicircular canal is parallel to the posterior surface of the petrous pyramid, which is oriented at approximately 45° to the coronal plane.

## Internal Auditory Canal

The internal auditory canal is usually oriented in a nearly coronal plane. The porus acousticus is the medial end of the internal auditory canal. The posterior lip of the porus is well defined, whereas the anterior wall blends with the petrous apex. The internal auditory canal contains the facial (VII) and cochlear (VIII) nerves anteriorly, separated by the falciform crest and the superior and inferior divisions of the vestibular (VIII) nerve posteriorly.

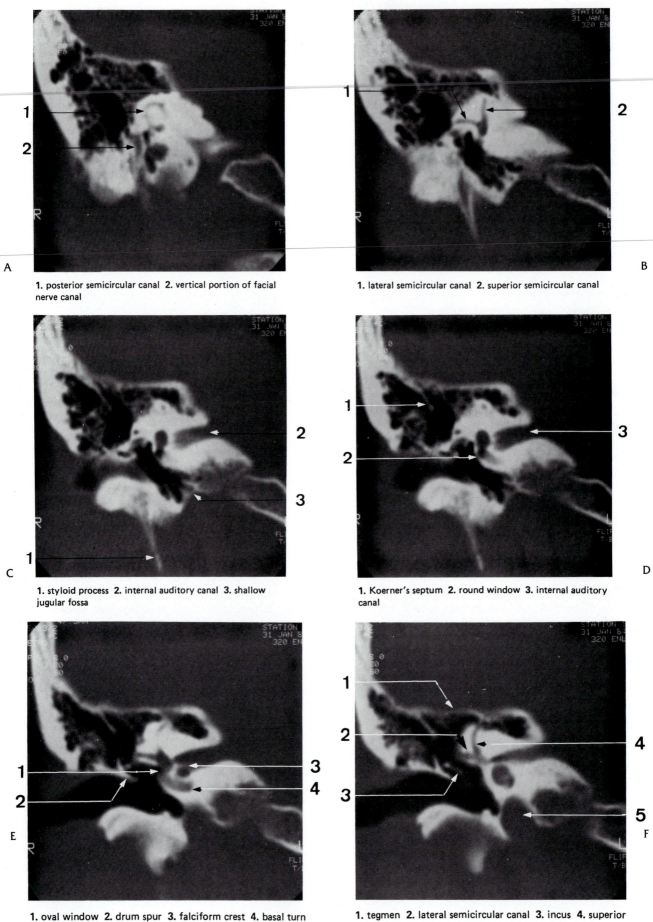

A

1. posterior semicircular canal  2. vertical portion of facial nerve canal

B

1. lateral semicircular canal  2. superior semicircular canal

C

1. styloid process  2. internal auditory canal  3. shallow jugular fossa

D

1. Koerner's septum  2. round window  3. internal auditory canal

E

1. oval window  2. drum spur  3. falciform crest  4. basal turn of cochlea

F

1. tegmen  2. lateral semicircular canal  3. incus  4. superior semicircular canal  5. carotid canal

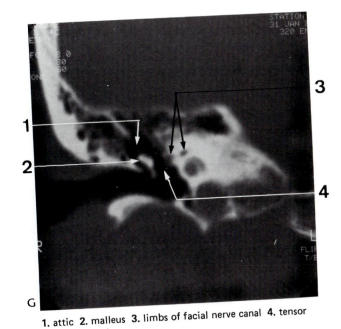

**G**

**1.** attic **2.** malleus **3.** limbs of facial nerve canal **4.** tensor tympani muscle

*Figure 15-80*   Normal coronal 1.5-mm-thick contiguous CT scans of the right ear from posterior to anterior (**A** to **G**).

demonstrating cranial nerves IX through XI in the jugular foramen, the inferior petrosal sinus, and the jugular bulb, with the vascular structures having high signal intensity (Fig. 15-81) (Daniels 1985, 1988*a*).

## CONGENITAL ANOMALIES

Congenital malformations of the ear usually affect the inner ear or the middle and external ear but not usually both, except in a few specific conditions such as maternal ingestion of thalidomide, chromosomal abnormalities, and craniofacial dysplasias (Hanafee 1980). The inner ear forms during the second and third months from the otocyst, which arises from ectodermal thickening on the side of the head. The auricle, ossicles, and external auditory canal develop from the first and second branchial arches and the first branchial groove. The endoderm-lined first pharyngeal pouch forms the tympanic cavity and eustachian tube. Pneumatization of the mastoid begins in the seventh to eighth fetal month and may continue into adulthood. The cartilaginous otic capsule ossifies in the fifth fetal month.

### External and Middle Ear

Except for isolated minor soft tissue malformations of the pinna and external auditory canal, bony anomalies usually coexist in the external canal and middle ear. The bony external auditory canal may be partially filled with soft tissue, hypoplastic, or nonexistent (Fig. 15-82). The degree of hypoplasia correlates with mastoid pneumatization; normal pneumatization generally indicates a less severe anomaly. When the external canal is atretic, the length of the atretic segment correlates with the severity of ossicular malformation. The temporomandibular joint is usually deformed in patients with congenital anomalies of the external ear. The glenoid fossa may be flattened, and the distance from the condyle to the tympanic bone may be markedly increased (Wright 1982). Other middle ear anomalies that occur with external canal atresia include a deformed fused incus and malleus, complete or partial absence of the ossicles, and aplasia of the middle ear (Bergstrom 1980). Many of these anomalies are associated with hearing loss (Weissman 1996; Dahlen 1997).

A common CT finding in these anomalies is a bony plate replacing the tympanic membrane. The middle ear cavity is usually smaller than normal and often is not pneumatized. CT may show a misshapen bony mass instead of normal ossicles, fusion of the malleus handle to the atresia plate, no osseous covering over the facial nerve in the middle ear, partial absence of the ossicles, or variable mastoid development and pneumatization. The tympanic portion of the temporal bone may by hypoplastic. In less severe anomalies,

*Figure 1*

**nerve ca**

row) in a

ternal auc

### Inner l

Several n

with an

lumped :

tional we

The rare

osseous a

The vestibular aqueduct, which is the bony canal for the endolymphatic duct, originates in the vestibule and curves superiorly, posteriorly, and then inferiorly to the posterior surface of the temporal bone.

The facial (VII) nerve has a complex course through the temporal bone. It enters into the anterosuperior portion of the internal auditory canal, exits from the anterolateral end of the canal, and extends anteriorly to the geniculate ganglion, which is above the cochlea and is the site where the greater superficial petrosal nerve originates. The facial nerve then reverses its course, passing along the medial wall of the middle ear under the lateral semicircular canal. Posterior to the middle ear at the level of the sinus tympani, the nerve turns approximately 90° to exit inferiorly at the stylomastoid foramen and then continues into the parotid gland. The locations of the geniculate ganglion and of the horizontal and vertical portions of the facial nerve are easily identified on CT. MR can demonstrate the facial nerve within its canal (Teresi 1987*a,b*).

### Jugular Foramen

The jugular foramen is posterior and lateral to the petrous segment of the temporal bone and its posterior wall is formed by the occipital bone. The jugular foramen is divided into a small anteromedial pars nervosa containing the glossopharyngeal (IX) nerve, the Jacobson nerve, and the inferior petrosal sinus. The larger posterolateral pars vascularis contains the jugular bulb and the vagus (X) and spinal accessory (XI) nerves. The right jugular foramen is often larger than the left, because the right jugular vein and sigmoid sinus are larger. CT is superior to MR in demonstrating the osseous margin of the jugular foramen, whereas CEMR is superior to CT in

*Fig*

low

ear

lar

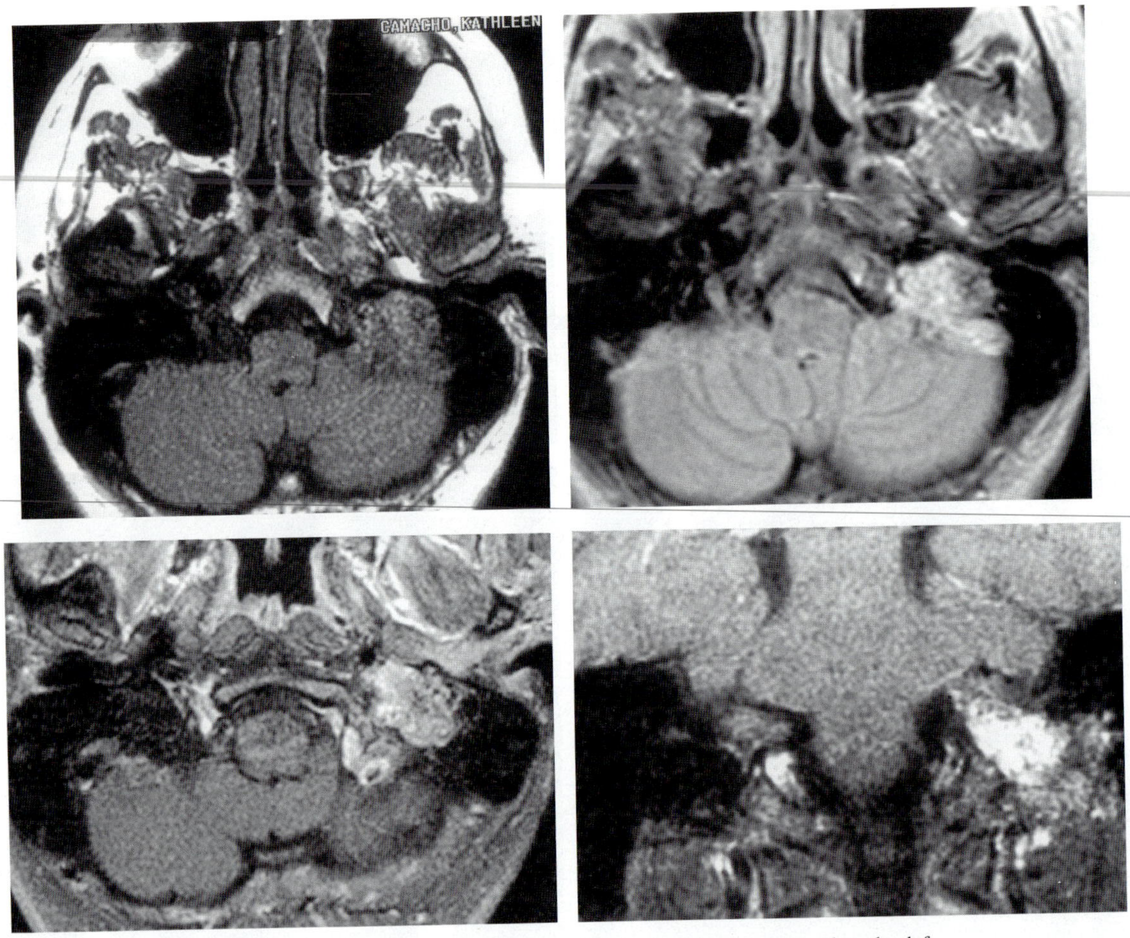

**Figure 15-99**   MR in **glomus tumor.** Axial T₁-weighted MR (**A**) shows a large mass within the left jugular foramen consisting of hyperintense and hypointense punctate signal and appearance similar to "salt and pepper." T₂-weighted MR (**B**) demonstrates a similar appearance. The bright areas represent tumor as well as vascularity of the tumor. Axial (**C**) and coronal (**D**) Gd-DTPA–enhanced T₁-weighted MR. The extent of the enhancing tumor is well demarcated between these two planes.

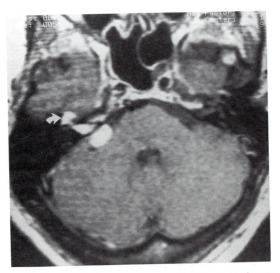

**Figure 15-100**   **Facial nerve tumor** on axial T₁-weighted MRI with intravenous Gd-DTPA. Note the tumor's intensely enhancing extracanalicular and intracanalicular components and a tumor involving the geniculate ganglion (curved arrow). *(From Daniels 1988b.)*

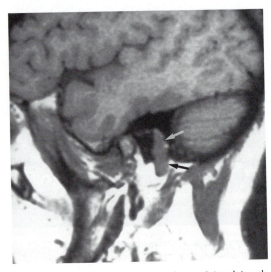

**Figure 15-101**   **A facial nerve tumor** (arrows) involving the vertical portion of the facial nerve is shown on sagittal T₁-weighted MRI.

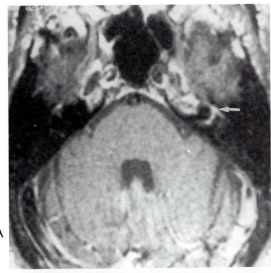

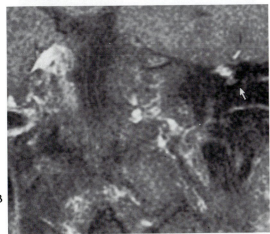

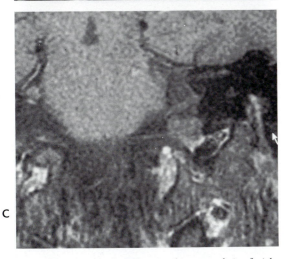

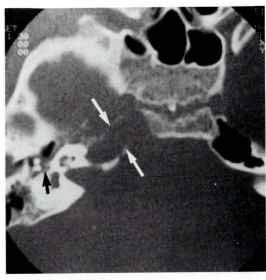

***Figure 15-103*** **Rhabdomyosarcoma** in a 12-year-old boy with right-sided hearing loss. Axial CT demonstrates petrous apex destruction (white arrows) and a tumor in the middle ear (black arrow). *(From Shaffer 1985.)*

***Figure 15-102*** Abnormally enhancing but normal-size facial nerve (arrow) in a patient with **ipsilateral Bell's palsy** is demonstrated on axial T$_1$-weighted MRI with intravenous Gd-DTPA. Coronal Gd-DTPA–enhanced MR, (**B**) posterior and (**C**) anterior sections, demonstrates the enhancing facial nerve (arrow) in a patient with Bell's palsy. The nerve is not enlarged.

mass or bone erosion is related to the course of the facial nerve. On MR, facial nerve tumors appear as soft tissue masses which follow the course of the facial nerve and show intense enhancement with intravenous gadolinium (Figs. 15-100, 15-101) (Daniels 1987*b*). This enhancement is nonspecific because facial nerve inflammation in, for example, Bell's palsy is associated with facial nerve enhancement (Daniels 1989). However, in Bell's palsy the abnormal facial nerve is a normal size (Fig. 15-102). In differentiating enhancing facial nerve tumors from high-signal-intensity fatty marrow and fat below the skull base, it is helpful to compare T$_1$-weighted SE images with and without Gd-DTPA.

## MALIGNANT TUMORS

When squamous cell carcinoma occurs in the middle ear, it usually results from spread from the external auditory canal (Chen 1978). Adenocarcinomas and their variants are also rare in the middle ear (Adam 1982). The diagnosis of malignant tumor is often delayed, since the tumor may masquerade as chronic inflammatory disease.

Rhabdomyosarcoma, usually of the embryonal type, is the most common soft tissue sarcoma in children, and the ear is the most common site after the orbit and nasopharynx (Fig. 15-103) (Schwartz 1980).

A soft tissue mass in the middle ear that destroys bone characterizes most primary middle ear malignancies and aggressive benign processes such as infection. The primary role of CT in malignant tumors of the temporal bone is in staging rather than in the differential diagnosis.

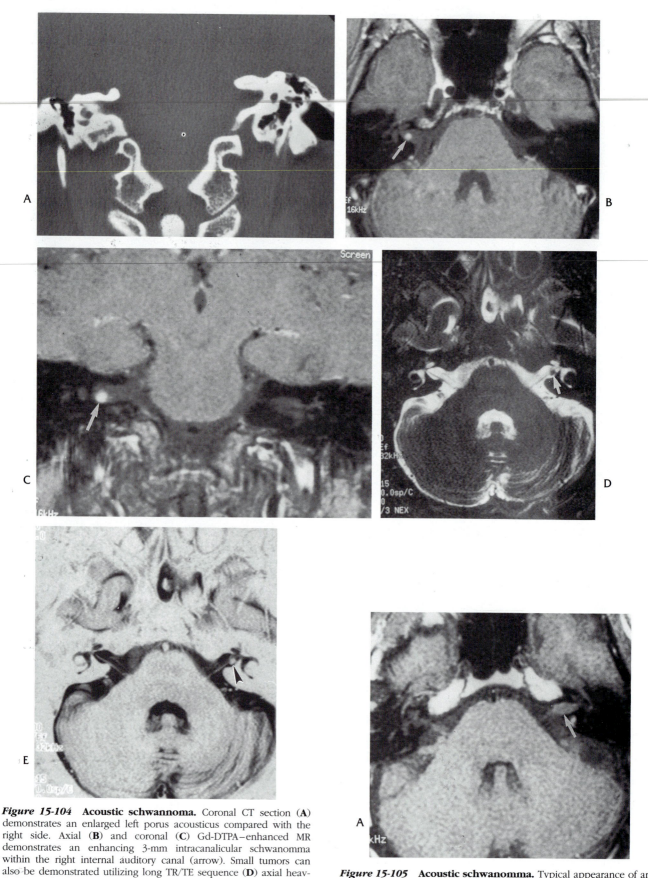

**Figure 15-104  Acoustic schwannoma.** Coronal CT section (**A**) demonstrates an enlarged left porus acousticus compared with the right side. Axial (**B**) and coronal (**C**) Gd-DTPA–enhanced MR demonstrates an enhancing 3-mm intracanalicular schwanomma within the right internal auditory canal (arrow). Small tumors can also be demonstrated utilizing long TR/TE sequence (**D**) axial heavily T₂-weighted MR. Reversed image (**E**) demonstrates a 2-mm tumor within the left IAC.

**Figure 15-105  Acoustic schwanomma.** Typical appearance of an intracanalicular tumor seen in (**A**) T₁-weighted MR as a soft tissue mass with homogenous enhancement *(Continued on next page)*

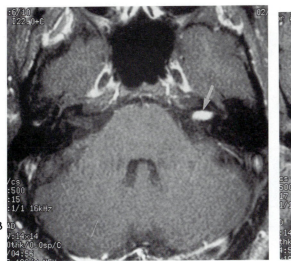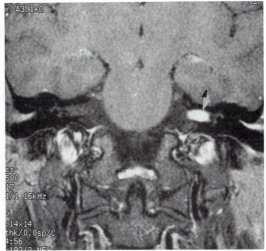

*Figure 15-105 (continued)*    in both (**B**) axial and (**C**) coronal planes (arrow).

# Inner Ear

## VESTIBULAR SCHWANNOMA

These benign tumors arise from Schwann cells, especially those near Scarpa's ganglion of the superior vestibular nerve. The tumors frequently arise in the internal auditory canal and grow medially into the cistern. Expansion of the bony canal, particularly its medial end, is a common feature of most vestibular schwannomas (acoustic neurinomas). They are slow in growth, and most have a cerebellopontine angle mass by the time of diagnosis. Bilateral schwannomas are common with neurofibromatosis. Patients with vestibular schwannomas present with a variety of symptoms due to compression of the cochlear division and vascular compromise. The symptoms include gradually progressive sensorineural hearing loss with poor discrimination, dizziness or true vertigo, tinnitus, facial nerve paralysis, pain, decreased corneal sensation, and brainstem signs.

MR has replaced CT and CT gas cisternography previously utilized in evaluating small intracanalicular schwannomas. With MR when combined with contrast studies, even small intracanalicular acoustic neurinomas can be demonstrated effectively. In evaluating patients with sensorineural hearing loss CEMR (Figs. 15-104, 15-105) (Gentry 1987; Mafee 1987; Armington 1988; Press 1988; Valvassori 1988; Swartz 1989) or MR with long TR/TE is equally effective in demonstrating even small lesions (Allen 1996, Fukui 1996). With intravenous Gd-DTPA, relatively fast T1-weighted imaging sequences can be used to identify vestibular schwannoma, which typically enhance intensely (Figs. 15-106, 15-107) (Breger 1987; Haughton 1988). A small percentage of acoustic schwannomas, primarily in the cerebellopontine angle cistern and porous acoustics,

may have a cystic component within the tumor or surrounding the tumor (Fig. 15-108). The shape of an acoustic neuroma is based on its location. Intracanalicular neuromas are usually identified as small rounded masses or may follow the entire volume of the canal. These are best identified with gadolinium-enhanced coronal and axial sections. Small intracanalicular neuromas have hypointense lesions in T2-weighted images. When the tumor extends medially beyond the porous acousticus, into the cerebello-pontine angle cistern, it has the shape of an ice cream cone lying on its side, with flaring of the porous. Larger tumors within the cerebellopontine angle (CPA) cistern may deform the brain-stem and the cisternal space. Cystic changes within the tumor are seen in nearly 15 percent of the extracanalicular schwannomas. Nearly 5 percent of acoustic schwannomas are associated with an arachnoid cyst within the CPA cistern. Rarely, an acoustic neuroma may involve the labyrinth either by direct extension of an intracanalicular schwannoma or as a primary lesion within the labyrinth (Mafee 1990). The intralabyrinthine schwannomas usually involve the cochlear division and less often the vestibular division. On CT and MR, the tumor is seen as a soft tissue mass. On CT of the temporal bone, erosion of the promontory obstruction of the round window and widening of the basal turn of cochlea are the key findings (Mafee 1990). On gadolinium-enhanced MR, the mass enhances homogeneously (Doyle 1994). Differentiation from glomus tympanicum and other neurogenic and vascular lesions is difficult. The MR examination is therefore effective, fast, and safe. CT should be reserved for cases in which visualization of osseous structures is crucial, such as congenital anomalies, trauma, otodystrophies, inflammatory disease, and some tumors that primarily affect the temporal bone.

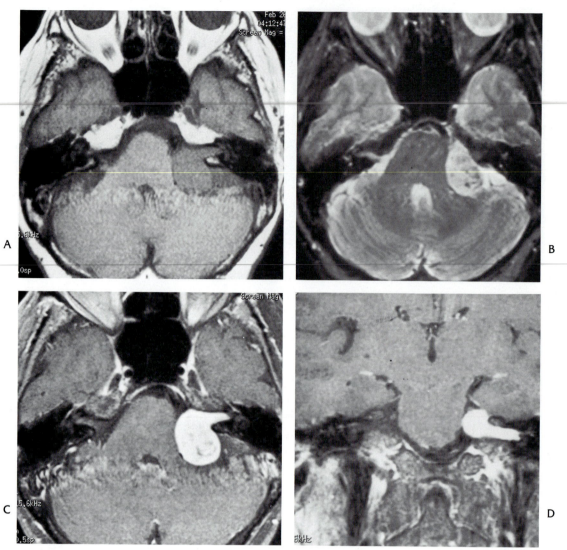

**Figure 15-106  Large intracanalicular and cerebellopontine angle schwanomma.** Axial (**A**) T₁-weighted MR demonstrates a mild hypointense mass within the IAC spilling into the cerebellopontine angle cistern. (**B**) T₂-weighted MR demonstrates mild hypointense signal with punctate areas of decreased signal (**C**) axial (**D**) coronal gadolinium enhanced MR demonstrates homogeneous enhancement of the tumor. Note the widening of the cisternal space. The enhancing tumor has appearance of an ice cream cone on its side.

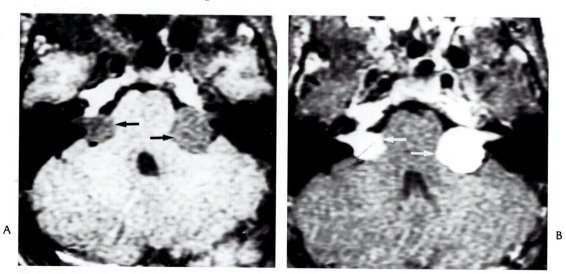

**Figure 15-107  Bilateral large acoustic neurinomas** (arrows) without (**A**) and with (**B**) intravenous gadolinium in a patient with neurofibromatosis. Axial T₁WI demonstrates that the tumors are slightly less intense than the normal brainstem (**A**) and are markedly enhancing (**B**).

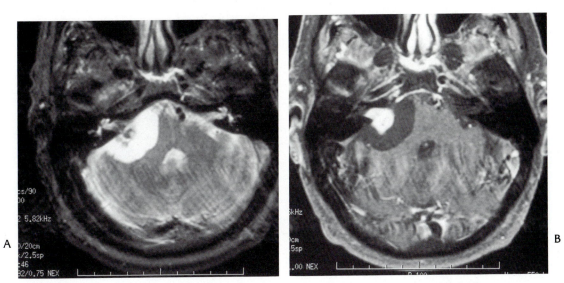

**Figure 15-108** **Cystic schwanomma.** Axial (**A**) $T_2$-weighted MR demonstrates a focal ill-defined mass with calcification extending into the right internal auditory canal, surrounded by cyst with CSF signal intensity. Gd-DTPA–enhanced $T_1$-weighted MR (**B**) demonstrates a vestibular schwanomma surrounded by an arachnoid cyst.

## MENINGIOMA

Meningiomas, which arise along the posterior surface of the petrous portion of the temporal bone, must be differentiated from the more common acoustic neurinomas (Valavanis 1981). It is less common for meningiomas to arise from ectopic arachnoid granulations in the temporal bone (Guzowski 1976).

On CT, a meningioma appears as a uniformly enhancing mass in the cerebellopontine angle cistern. Meningiomas resemble acoustic neurinomas only superficially. A meningioma has a sessile broad-based attachment to the petrous bone, which is atypical of acoustic neurinoma, and rarely enlarges the internal auditory canal. Frequently, meningiomas cause hyperostosis or have dense focal calcifications that can be better shown with CT than with MR (Fig. 15-109). On MR, meningiomas have a signal intensity similar to that of brain in $T_1$WI and variable in $T_2$WI (Fig. 15-110) (Gentry 1987). Meningiomas enhance intensely with intravenous Gd-DTPA (Breger 1987; Haughton 1988). The identification of a small amount of enhancing tissue that extends from the meningioma along a dural surface, "the dural tail," is due to either dural reaction or tumor extension. This finding if present differentiates a meningioma from an acoustic neurinoma, since the latter is not associated with the tail sign (Fig. 15-111) (Goldsher 1990). In cases that are not easily differentiated by CT or MR, angiography is indicated to distinguish the characteristic blush and dural blood supply of a meningioma from the more subtle changes of a vestibular schwannoma.

## EPIDERMOID AND DERMOID TUMORS

Epidermoid tumors, also called congenital or primary cholesteatoma, arise from ectodermal cell rests at multiple intracranial sites, including the cerebellopontine angle cistern, the petrous apex, and the middle ear, or elsewhere in the temporal bone. Epidermoid tumor is the third most common cerebellopontine angle mass. It may produce a variety of symptoms, depending on the exact location of the mass and its extension to the surrounding structures. CT is a reliable way to detect epidermoid tumors since their keratin content gives them lower density than brain has on NCCT and

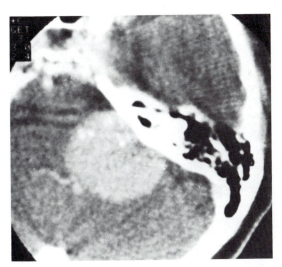

**Figure 15-109** A **meningioma** presents as a homogeneously enhancing round mass with punctate calcifications in the cerebellopontine angle cistern on CECT.

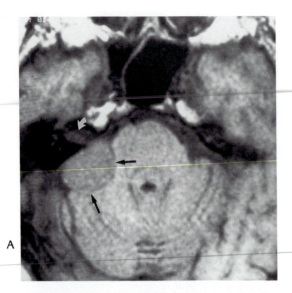

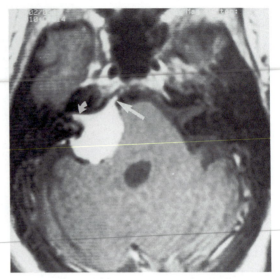

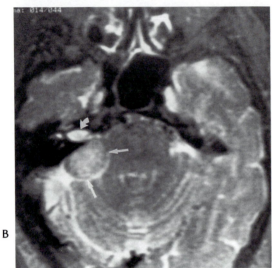

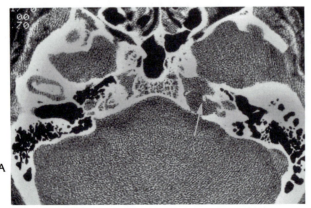

*Figure 15-111* Enhancing **cerebellopontine angle meningioma** on axial T₁-weighted MRI with intravenous Gd-DTPA. The tumor extending into the internal auditory canal (curved arrow) and along the dura (straight arrow) is evident.

*Figure 15-110* **Cerebellopontine angle meningioma** (straight arrows) that is less intense than the brainstem and CSF on axial T₁-weighted (**A**) and T₂-weighted (**B**) MRI is shown. The tumor is centered posterior to the internal auditory canal (curved arrow) containing cranial nerves VII and VIII and CSF.

CECT. Smooth or scalloped borders are typical (Latack 1985) (Fig. 15-112). In MR, epidermoids have negligible or low-intensity signals in T₁WI and high-intensity signals in T₂WI (Fig. 15-113) (Gentry 1987; Griffin 1987). Typically, epidermoids do not enhance with Gd-DTPA. A cerebellopontine angle epidermoid can be differentiated from an arachnoid cyst utilizing FLAIR or diffusion weighted MR (Fig. 15-114).

The differential diagnosis of a petrous apex epidermoid includes schwannoma, meningioma, glomus tumor, metastasis, petrositis, histiocytosis, cholesterol granuloma, and mucocele (Gacek 1980) (Table 15-5). With CT, the smooth bone erosion and lack of enhancement differentiate epidermoid tumors from most other masses except mucocele and cholesterol granu-

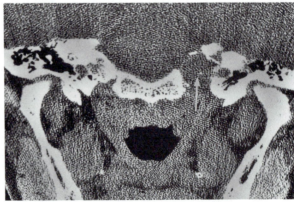

*Figure 15-112* **Epidermoid tumor.** Axial (**A**) and coronal (**B**) CT demonstrates mildly hypodense mass in the left petrous apex with thin bony margin (arrow). *(Continued on next page)*

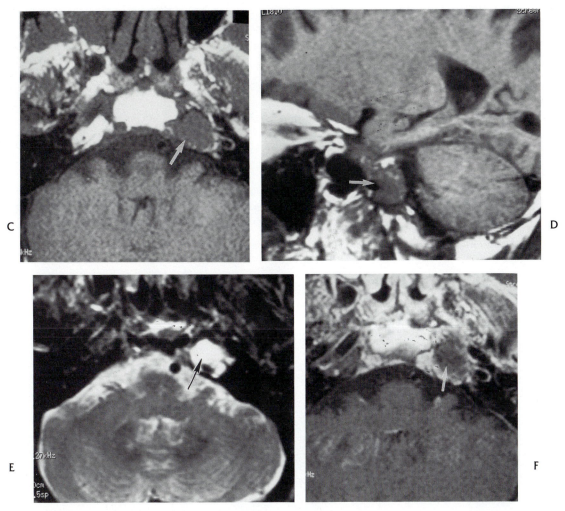

**Figure 15-112 (continued)**   Axial (**C**) and sagittal (**D**) T$_1$-weighted MR shows an isointense signal mass (arrow). Hyperintense signal (**E**) in T$_2$-weighted MR (arrow). The mass does not enhance (**F**) in Gd-DTPA–enhanced T$_1$-weighted MR.

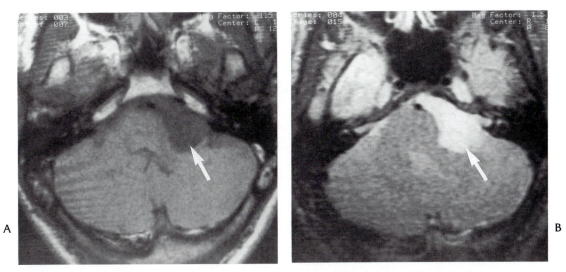

**Figure 15-113**   **Cerebellopontine angle epidermoid** (arrow) isointense with CSF and displacing the brainstem is demonstrated on axial T$_1$-weighted (**A**) and t$_2$-weighted (**B**) MRI. *(From Daniels 1988b.)*

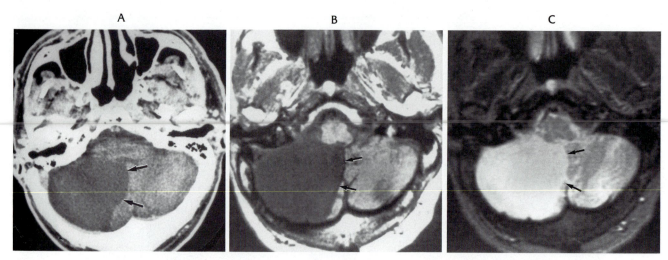

**Figure 15-114** **Large posterior fossa arachnoid cyst** (arrows) with mass effect appearing isodense and isointense with CSF is identified on axial CT (**A**) and $T_1$- and $T_2$-weighted MRI (**B** and **C**).

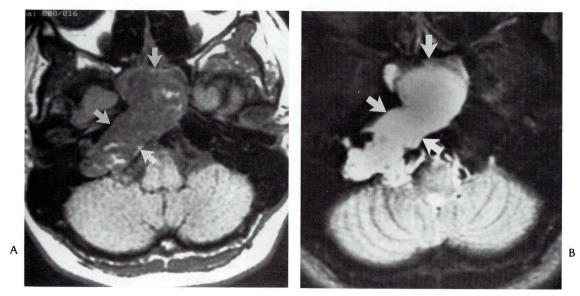

**Figure 15-115** **Petrous apex and sphenoid epidermoid** (arrows) are characterized by predominantly low-intensity and high-intensity signals on $T_1$-weighted (**A**) and $T_2$-weighted (**B**) MRI.

loma. In MR, epidermoids at the petrous apex (Fig. 15-115) can be differentiated from cholesterol granulomas, which typically have high signal intensity in $T_1$WI and $T_2$WI as a result of old hemorrhage (Gomori 1985; Gentry 1987; Griffin 1987; Greenberg 1988).

## OTHER TUMORS

*Schwannomas* or *neurinomas* of the fifth, seventh, ninth, tenth, eleventh, or twelfth cranial nerves may erode bone in the inner ear. Schwannoma of the fifth cranial nerve characteristically can amputate the petrous apex. Neurinomas of the seventh cranial nerve arising in the intracanalicular segment of the nerve expand the internal canal exactly the same way as an acoustic schwannoma. Neurinomas of the ninth, tenth, and eleventh cranial nerves enlarge the jugular fossa in the manner of a glomus tumor, but without irregular margins (Fig. 15-116). Similarly, neurinomas of the twelfth cranial nerve have a similar appearance, mildly hypointense on $T_1$WI, bright on $T_2$WI, and enhancement following CEMR (Fig. 15-117). On CT and MR, neurinomas enhance homogeneously but less than glomus tumors, which are extremely vascular (Breger 1987; Daniels 1987*b*). A neurinoma may be small or bulky, hypointense on $T_1$WI, hyperintense on $T_2$WI with homogenous enhancement of the tumor. Cyst or necrosis is seen as a hypointense signal on the Gd-DTPA enhanced MR (Fig. 15-117).

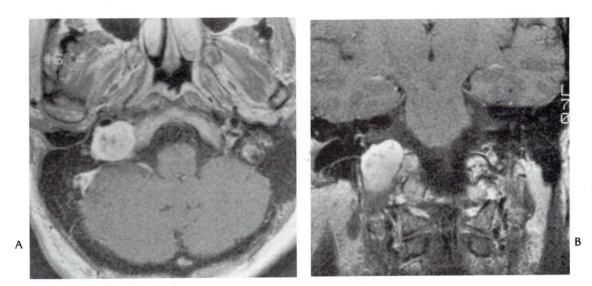

***Figure 15-116*** **CN X schwanomma.** Axial (**A**) and coronal (**B**) Gd-DTPA–enhanced T$_1$-weighted MR demonstrates a homogenously enhancing mass within the jugular foramen characteristic of a schwanomma.

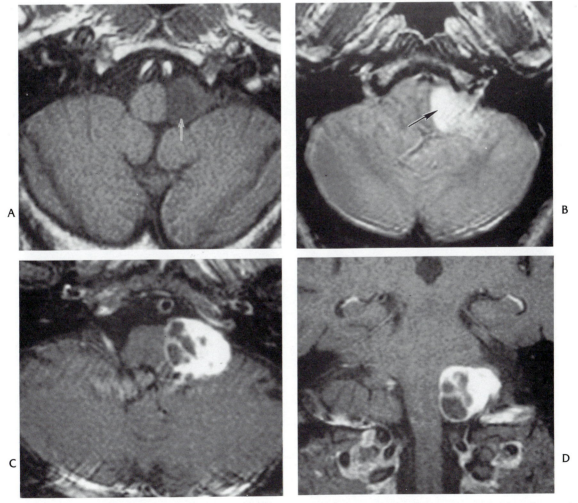

***Figure 15-117*** **CN XII schwanomma.** T$_1$-weighted axial MR (**A**) demonstrates a hypointense signal mass adjacent to the medulla with widening of the left hypoglossal canal (arrow). The mass (**B**) is bright in T$_2$-weighted MR (arrow). Axial (**C**) and coronal (**D**) Gd-DTPA–enhanced MR demonstrates a large schwanomma with a cystic component.

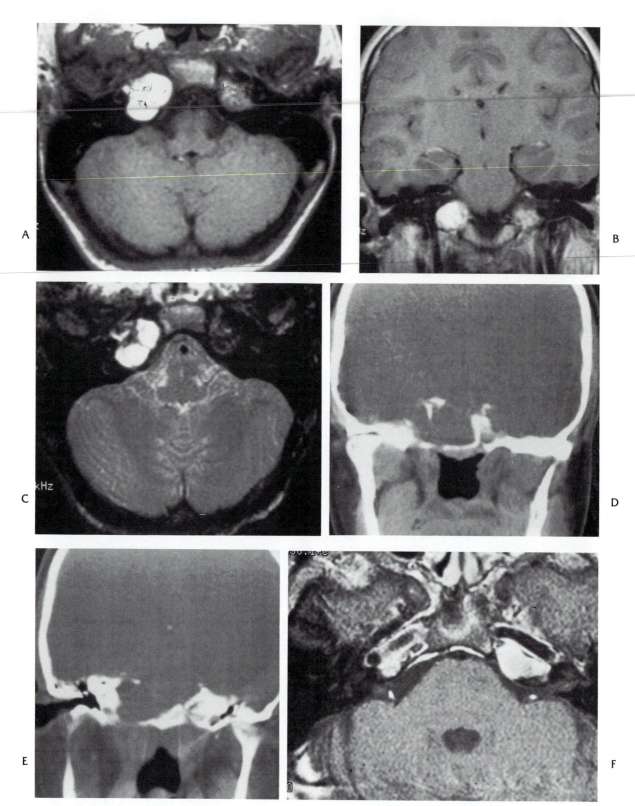

***Figure 15-118***   **Cholesterol granuloma.** Axial (**A**) and coronal (**B**) T$_1$-weighted MR. T$_2$-weighted axial MR (**C**) demonstrates a mass which has hyperintense signal in all pulse sequences. The T$_2$-weighted MR also demonstrates focal hypointense signal from an old hemorrhage. Coronal CT (**D,E**) demonstrates the soft tissue mass with erosion of the petrous apex (arrow). This is typical of a cholesterol granuloma or chocolate cyst. T$_1$-weighted MR (**F**). Compare with normal variation in the amount of fat in the petrous apex.

A *cholesterol granuloma* (giant cholesterol cyst) may be mistaken for an epidermoid tumor in the petrous apex, middle ear, or mastoid. It usually results from obstructed ventilation, poor drainage, or hemorrhage. Cholesterol granulomas, unlike epidermoid tumors, contain cholesterol crystals, giant cells, and dark or yellow material lined by fibrous connective tissue, whereas epidermoids contain pale and flaky material. CT shows a mass that smoothly erodes bone and has a density nearly isodense to the brain and therefore higher than that of an epidermoid (Lo 1984). MR often shows a cholesterol granuloma with high-intensity signals in $T_1WI$ and $T_2WI$ from old hemorrhage and methemoglobin formation (Fig. 15-118) (Gomori 1985; Gentry 1987; Griffin 1987; Greenberg 1988).

*Mucocele* is another process which, like a cholesterol granuloma or epidermoid, erodes the bone and occasionally destroys bone in the petrous apex. Since a mucocele arises in an apex air cell, CT usually shows a pneumatized air cell on the opposite side. Ipsilaterally, the mastoid air cells may be fluid-filled (Osborn 1979). Mucocele in the petrous apex, similar to that in the sphenoid sinus, is bright on both $T_1$- and $T_2$-weighted images, although occasionally may be isointense on $T_1$-weighted MR.

*Hemangiomas* are rare tumors which occur in the internal auditory canal or any portion of the temporal bone. Characteristic features, including spokelike trabeculations or phleboliths, can be demonstrated with CT in some cases (Lo 1984; Curtin 1987).

*Fibroosseous tumors*, including chondroma and osteoma, affect the inner ear as well as other portions of the temporal bone. Metastatic involvement of the inner ear occurs through direct extension or hematogenous spread of tumor. A tumor can extend directly to the inner ear from a nasopharyngeal carcinoma, a meningeal carcinomatosis, or an adjacent intracranial malignancy. *Hematogenous metastasis* to the temporal bone usually occurs late in the course of disease, as does lymphoma. This may spread along the dural surface and may mimic a meningioma (Fig. 15-119). In most cases the destructive metastatic lesions are from tumors such as carcinomas of the breast, prostate, lung, and kidney. The petrous apex contains marrow spaces which may trap circulating tumor cells, but the otic capsule and well-pneumatized bone are not often involved (Schuknecht 1968).

## INFLAMMATORY DISEASE

### External Ear

Except for the so-called malignant form, otitis externa is seldom evaluated with imaging studies. The malignant appellation refers to the aggressive course of *Pseudomonas aeruginosa* infection in elderly diabetics and immune suppressed patients. Malignant external otitis is divided into an early stage characterized by soft tissue changes without bone destruction and an advanced stage with spread of infection and bone destruction (Mendez 1979).

Pain, drainage from the ear, impaired hearing, and granulation tissue in the external auditory canal occur in both stages. Facial nerve paralysis, other cranial nerve palsies, and temporomandibular joint involvement occur late. Long-term systemic antibiotic therapy

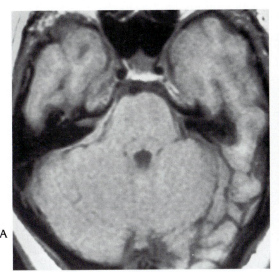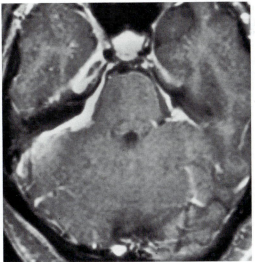

*Figure 15-119*   **Skull base lymphoma.** Axial $T_1$-weighted MR (**A**) demonstrates dural thickening. Gd-DTPA–enhanced $T_1$-weighted MR (**B**) demonstrates homogenous enhancement of the dura, as well as the pituitary gland from lymphoma. Similar appearance may be seen with leukemia.

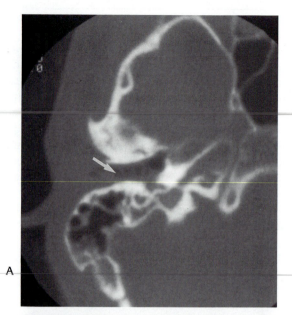

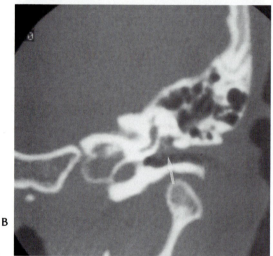

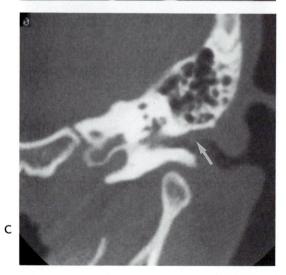

*Figure 15-120* **Malignant otitis externa.** Axial (**A**) and adjacent coronal (**B,C**) MR demonstrates soft tissue mass extending from the pinna into the external and middle ear, destroying the bone and ossicles (arrow).

and local surgical debridement are used to treat this condition. CT findings in malignant external otitis include abnormal soft tissue in the external auditory canal, middle ear, and mastoid; destruction of bone in the external canal and skull base; and a mass in the nasopharynx and subtemporal space (Fig. 15-120). CT findings of malignant external otitis are not specific. The nasopharyngeal inflammatory mass may be mistaken radiographically for malignant tumor since the infection crosses fascial planes. The CT abnormalities are easily interpreted only with the typical clinical findings. In these patients, CT is effective in evaluating bone destruction as well as soft tissue spread in the ear and subtemporal space. Nuclear scanning more effectively defines the extent of active infection in patients who are being treated for malignant external otitis. Technetium 99m bone scanning is more sensitive than CT in detecting bony involvement. Gallium 67 citrate scans can determine the activity of an infection under treatment (Strashun 1984).

## Middle Ear

**CHOLESTEATOMA**   Temporal bone cholesteatoma, a stratified squamous epithelium-lined cyst filled with keratin debris, is usually a complication of inflammatory disease but rarely is a congenital neoplasm arising from epithelial rests. The incidence of congenital cholesteatoma is less than 2 percent. Congenital cholesteatoma in the middle ear appears as a pearly mass behind an intact tympanic membrane in a patient with no history of middle ear inflammatory disease.

Acquired cholesteatomas usually occur in patients with a history of otitis media. Retraction of the par flaccida portion of the tympanic membrane, tympanic membrane perforation, and migration of epithelial cells into the middle ear cause most acquired cholesteatomas (Nager 1977; Swartz 1984a). Dysfunction of the eustachian tube, poor pneumatization of the mastoid, and hereditary factors are contributory. The epithelial cells produce a cyst, which accumulates keratin debris. Bone destruction results in most cases because of collagenase activity of the cholesteatoma or associated inflammatory disease. CT is the most accurate means of determining the extent of disease before surgical treatment is planned. CT demonstrates the soft tissue mass in the middle ear, air-fluid levels, erosion of the tegmen and lateral semicircular canal, and the posterior wall of the middle replacing imaging with pluridirectional tomography (Shaffer 1984). Characteristically, CT shows a soft tissue mass in Prussak's space with bone erosion, particularly involving the drum spur (scutum) and the long process of the incus (Fig. 15-121). In an extensive cholesteatoma there may be

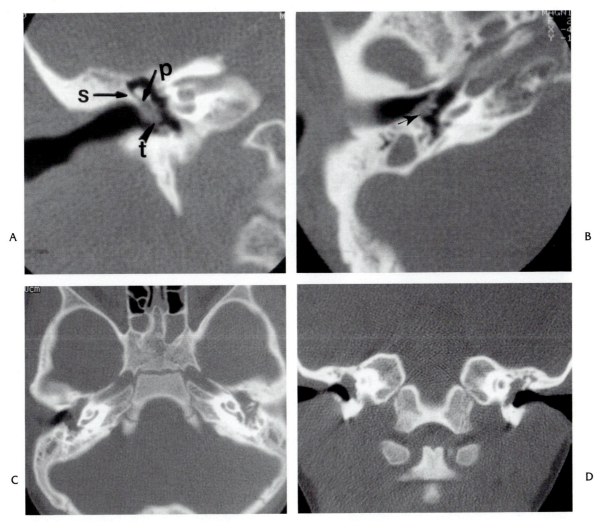

***Figure 15-121*** **Cholesteatoma.** Coronal (**A**) and axial (**B**) CT demonstrates a soft tissue mass between the scutum (S) and the malleus in Prussak's space (P), sparing the sinus tympani. Axial (**C**) and coronal (**D**) CT in a 3-year-old child with bilateral congenital cholesteatoma.

erosion of the lateral semicircular canal, the lateral attic wall, and occasionally the tegmen tympani. In a partially opacified middle ear and mastoid, movement of fluid between axial and coronal scans and air-fluid levels help distinguish fluid from mass.

Granulation tissue from chronic infection, which often coexists with cholesteatoma, cannot be differentiated reliably from cholesteatoma by means of CT numbers. CT may show calcification (tympanosclerosis) or retraction of the tympanic membrane (Swartz 1983*b*, 1984*a*). In a patient previously operated on for cholesteatoma, it is difficult to determine the recurrence or residual cholesteatoma from surgical scarring. In a modified radical mastoidectomy, a mastoidectomy cavity is created with or without an intact canal wall. CT in a postoperative patient is useful in identifying recurrent cholesteatoma or granulation tissue and evaluating ossicular reconstruction. Baseline axial CT scans

3 to 6 months after surgery may be helpful in patients who have residual cholesteatoma or those having mastoidectomy with an intact canal who have a higher risk of developing a recurrent cholesteatoma (Johnson 1984).

**MASTOIDITIS**    Acute otomastoiditis is seldom reviewed by imaging studies, but when there is evidence of complication, such as coalescent mastoiditis or intracranial spread of infection, CT or MR is indicated (Mafee 1985*c*; Holliday 1989). CT is also useful in studying patients who have chronic middle ear infections without clinical evidence of cholesteatoma (Mafee 1986).

### Inner Ear

Labyrinthitis ossificans, or bone filling the inner ear, is most commonly due to suppurative labyrinthitis but may result from trauma, severe otosclerosis, surgery,

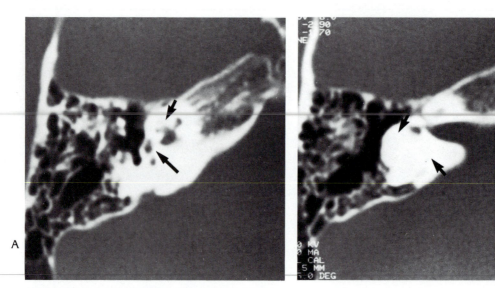

**Figure 15-122** **Postinfectious labyrinthitis ossificans** in a deaf 8-year-old boy. Axial CT (**A,B**) demonstrates bone that obliterates most of the cochlear turns (short arrow, **A**), vestibule (long arrow, **A**), and semicircular canals (arrows, **B**). *(From Shaffer 1985.)*

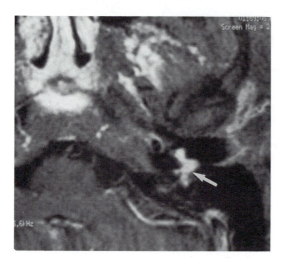

**Figure 15-123** Axial Gd-DTPA–enhanced T$_1$-weighted MR demonstrates intense enhancement of a **schwanomma** within the left labyrinth.

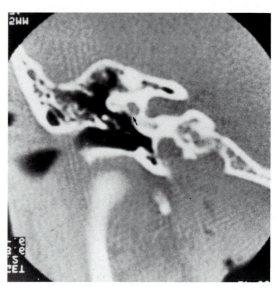

**Figure 15-124** **Otosclerotic reclosure of the oval window** (arrow) on coronal CT. The patient had a history of stapedectomy and a wire loop prosthesis. *(Courtesy of Kedar N. Chintapalli, M.D., San Antonio.)*

or tumors (Hoffman 1979). Labyrinthitis ossificans has a characteristic appearance with a decreased luminal size and sclerosis of the affected ear structures (Fig. 15-122). The affected ear usually has no auditory or vestibular function ("dead ear"). Acute labyrinthitis is a clinical diagnosis without radiographic findings, usually as a complication of otomastoiditis resulting from involvement of the oval window. It presents with acute onset of hearing loss and vertigo. On CT a fluid-filled density may be seen within the labyrinth. On T$_1$-weighted CEMR, mild enhancement may be present. If there is intense enhancement of the membranous labyrinth, it is more likely from labyrinthine schwanomma (Fig. 15-123).

Petrositis is an infection of petrous apex air cells secondary to middle ear and mastoid infection. The majority of individuals, without air cells in the petrous apices, do not develop petrositis. The classic clinical presentation of petrositis is pain along the fifth cranial nerve distribution and sixth cranial nerve palsy (Gradenigo's syndrome). Air cell opacification, middle

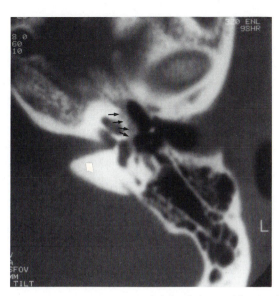

**Figure 15-125** Young woman with left-sided mixed hearing loss and a history of **otosclerosis.** Demineralized areas of the cochlear capsule are seen with cochlear otosclerosis (arrows).

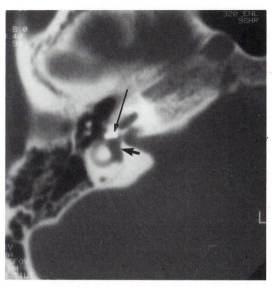

**Figure 15-126** Patient dizzy after placement of a **stapes prosthesis.** The metal prosthesis (long arrow) is positioned too far into the anterior vestibule (short arrow).

ear disease, and bone destruction are important CT findings in patients with petrositis. Infection in any portion of the temporal bone can cause meningitis, lateral sinus thrombosis, and epidural, subdural, or brain abscess.

## OTODYSTROPHIES: OTOSCLEROSIS

Otosclerosis, a disease of unknown etiology, is responsible for hearing loss and tinnitus, particularly in young white women. The dense endochondral layer of the bony labyrinth is replaced by foci of thick vascular bone. Otosclerosis may be hereditary and is frequently bilateral. Stapedial otosclerosis (fenestral otoslcerosis), the more common form, fixes the stapes footplate in the oval window, causing conductive hearing loss. CT shows lytic (spongiotic) changes early and sclerotic reparative changes later. CT may show bone obliterating the oval window niche (Fig. 15-124) (Swartz 1984b; Mafee 1985a).

Small otosclerotic foci can produce hearing loss without radiographic abnormalities. When otosclerosis involves the otic capsule and cochlea in addition to the stapes, sensorineural as well as conductive hearing loss (mixed hearing loss) may be present.

The CT diagnosis of otosclerosis is not precise. The semiaxial projection perpendicular to the plane of the oval window provides the best view of the stapes footplate. However, with this projection, each ear must be scanned separately. CT demonstrates replacement of the oval or round windows with bone in moderately advanced cases. The improved contrast resolution of CT compared with pluridirectional tomography allows more accurate identification of the lytic foci in the otic capsule. Advanced cochlear otosclerosis has been demonstrated on CT as a lucent halo of small demineralized foci around the cochlea (Fig. 15-125). The CT appearance of cochlear otosclerosis is quite specific, except for differentiation from osteogenesis imperfecta (Mafee 1985b). Other processes, such as tumor, infection, and Paget's disease, produce lucent areas in the petrous portion of the temporal bone but do not affect the otic capsule primarily.

CT is also useful in studying the poststapedectomy ear when there has been sudden or progressive hearing loss. Ankylosis of the prosthesis in the oval window or posttraumatic dislocation can be identified. Dislocation is demonstrated as a displacement of the prosthesis away from the oval window or protrusion into the vestibule, producing vertigo (Fig. 15-126).

# References

ADAM W, JOHNSON JD, PAUL DJ, et al: Primary adenocarcinoma of the middle ear. *AJNR* 3:67–76, 1982.

ALLEN RW, HARNSBERGER HR, SHELTON C, et al.: Low-cost high resolution FSE MR of acoustic schwannoma: an alternative to enhanced conventional spin-echo MR. *Am J Neuroradiol* 17:1205–1210, 1996.

ANDERSON P, DIEHL J, MARAVILLA K, et al: Computerized axial tomography with air contrast of the cerebellopontine angle and internal auditory canal. *Laryngoscope* 91:1083–1097, 1981.

ANDERSON R, OLSON J, DORWART P, et al: CT air-contrast scanning of the internal auditory canal. *Ann Otol Rhino Laryngol* 91:501–504, 1982.

ARMINGTON WG, HARNSBERGER HP, SMOKER WRK, et al: Normal and diseased acoustic pathway: Evaluation with MR imaging. *Radiology* I67:509–515, 1988.

BATSAKIS JG: *Tumors of the Head and Neck,* 2d ed, Baltimore, Williams & Wilkins, 1979.

BERGSTROM L: Pathology of congenital deafness-present status and future priorities. *Ann Otol Rhinol Laryngol* 89 (Suppl 74):31–42, 1980.

BERLINGER NT, KOUTROUPAS S, ADAM S, et al: Patterns of involvement of the temporal bone in metastatic and systemic malignancy. *Laryngoscope* 90:619–627, 1980.

BIRD CP, HASSO AN, STEWART EC, et al: Malignant primary neoplasms of the ear and temporal bone studied by high-resolution computed tomography. *Radiology* 149:170–174, 1983.

BREGER RK, PAPKE RA, POJUNAS KW, et al: Benign extraaxial tumors: Contrast enhancement with Gd-DTPA. *Radiology* 163:427–429, 1987.

BROGAN M, CHAKERAS DW: Computed tomography and magnetic resonance imaging of the normal anatomy of the temporal bone. *Semin Ultrasound CT MR* 10:179–194, 1989.

BROGAN M, CHAKERES DW, SCHMALBROCK P: High resolution 3DFT MR imaging of the endolymphatic duct and soft tissues of the otic capsule. *AJNR* 12:1–11, 1991.

CHAKERES DW, SPIEGEL PK: A systematic technique for comprehensive evaluation of the temporal bone by computed tomography. *Radiology* 146:97–106, 1983.

CHEN WFK, DEHNER LP: Primary tumors of the external and middle ear: I. Introduction and clinicopathologic study of squamous cell carcinoma. *Arch Otolaryngol* 104:247–252, 1978.

CURATI WL, GRAIF M, KINGSLEY DPE, et al: Acoustic neuromas: Gd-DTPA enhancement in MR imaging. *Radiology* 158:447–451, 1986.

CURTIN HIP, WOLFE P, SNYDERMAN N: The facial nerve between the stylomastoid foramen and the parotid: Computed tomographic imaging. *Radiology* 149:165–169, 1983.

CURTIN HD, JENSEN JE, BARNES L JR, et al: "Ossifying" hemangiomas of the temporal bone: Evaluation with CT. *Radiology* 164:831–835, 1987.

DAHLEN T, HARNSBERGER HR, GRAY SD, et al: Overlapping thin section fast spin-echo MR of the large vestibular aqueduct syndrome. *AJNR Am J Neuroradiol* 18:67–75, 1997.

DAMSMA H, MALI WPTM, ZONNEVEID FW: CT diagnosis of an aberrant internal carotid artery in the middle ear. *J Comput Assist Tomogr* 8:317–319, 1984.

DANIELS DL, HERFKINS R, KOEHLER PR, et al: Magnetic resonance imaging of the internal auditory canal. *Radiology* 151:105–108, 1984.

DANIELS DL, SCHENCK JF, FOSTER T, et al: Surface-coil magnetic resonance imaging of the internal auditory canal. *AJNR* 6:487–490, 1985.

DANIELS DL, BREGER RK, STRANDT JA, et al: "Truncation" artifact in MR images of the internal auditory canal. *AJNR* 8:793–794, 1987*a*.

DANIELS DL, CZERVIONKE IF, et al: Facial nerve enhancement in MR imaging. *AJNR* 8:605–607, 1987*b*.

DANIELS DL, MILLEN SJ, MEYER GA, et al: MR detection of tumor in the internal auditory canal. *AJNR* 8:249–252, 1987*c*.

DANIELS DL, HAUGHTON VM, NAIDICH T: *Cranial and Spinal Magnetic Resonance Imaging. Atlas and Guide,* New York, Raven, 1987*d*.

DANIELS DL, CZERVIONKE LF, PECH P, et al: Gradient recalled echo MR imaging of the jugular foramen. *AJNR* 9:675–678, 1988*a*.

DANIELS DL, HAUGHTON VM, CZERVIONKE LF: MR of the skull base, in Bradley WG, Stark D (eds), *Magnetic Resonance Imaging,* St Louis, Mosby 1988*b*.

DANIELS DL, CZERVIONKE LF, MILLEN SJ, et al: MR imaging of facial nerve enhancement in Bell palsy or after temporal bone surgery. *Radiology* 171:807–809, 1989.

DOLANIK D: Temporal bone fractures. *Semin Ultrasound CT MR* 10:262–279, 1989.

DOYLE KJ, BRACKMANN DE: Intralabyrinthine schwannoma. *Otolaryngol Head Neck Surg* 110:517–523, 1994.

EELKEMA E, CURTIN HIP: Congenital anomalies of the temporal bone. *Semin Ultrasound CT MR* 10:195–212, 1989.

ENZMANN DP, O'DONOHUE J: Optimizing MR imaging for detecting small tumors in the cerebellopontine angle and internal auditory canal. *AJNR* 8:99–106, 1987.

FUKUI MB, WEISMAN JL, CURTIN HD, et al. $T_2$-weighted MR characteristics of internal auditory canal masses. *Am J Neuroradiol* 17:1211–1218, 1996.

GACEK RR: Evaluation and management of primary petrous apex cholesteatoma. *Otolaryngol Head Neck Surg* 88:519–523, 1980.

GENTRY LP, JACOBY CG, TURSKI PA, et al: Cerebellopontine angle—Petromastoid mass lesions: Comparative Study of diagnosis with MR imaging and CT. *Radiology* 162:513–520, 1987.

GOLDSHER D, LITT AW, PINTO RS, et al: Dural "tail" associated with meningiomas on Gd-DTPA-enhanced MR images. *Radiology* 176:447–450, 1990.

GOMORI JM, GROSSMAN RI, GOLDBERG HI, et al: Intracranial hematomas imaging by high-field MR. *Radiology* 157:87–93, 1985.

GREENBERG JI, OOT RF, WISMER G, et al: Cholesterol granuloma of the petrous apex: MR and CT evaluation. *AJNR* 9:1205–1214, 1988.

GRIFFIN C, DELAPAZ R, ENZMANN E: MR and CT correlation of cholesterol cysts of the petrous bone. *AJNR* 8:825–829, 1987.

GUINTO FC JR, GARRABRANT EC, RADCLIFFE WB: Radiology of the persistent stapedial artery. *Radiology* 105:365–369, 1972.

GUIRADO CR, MARTINEZ R, ROIG F, et al: Three dimensional MR of the inner ear with steady state free precession. *AJNR* 16:1909–1913, 1995.

GUZOWSKI J, PAPARELLA MM, RAO KN, et al: Meningiomas of the temporal bone. *Laryngoscope* 84:1141–1146, 1976.

HANAFEE WN, BERGSTROM L: Radiology of congenital deformities of the ear. *Head Neck Surg* 2:213–221, 1980.

HAUGHTON VM, RIMM AA, CZERVIONKE LF, et al: Sensitivity of MR imaging of benign extra-axial tumors. *Radiology* 166:829–833, 1988.

HOFFMAN RA, BROOKLER KH, BERGERON RT: Radiologic diagnosis of labyrinthitis ossificans. *Ann Otol Rhinol Laryngol* 88:253–257, 1979.

HOLLAND B, BRANT-ZAWADZKI M: High-resolution CT of temporal bone trauma. *AJNR* 5:291–295, 1984.

HOLLIDAY RA, REEDE DL: MRI of mastoid and middle ear disease. *Radiol Clin North Am* 27:283–299, 1989.

JACKLER RK, LUXFORD M, HOUSE WF. Congenital malformation of the inner ear: A classification based on embryogenesis. *Laryngoscope* 97:2–14, 1987.

JOHNSON DW: Air cisternography of the cerebellopontine angle using high-resolution computed tomography. *Radiology* 151:401–403, 1984a.

JOHNSON DW, HASSO AW, STEWART CE, et al: Temporal bone trauma: High-resolution computed tomographic evaluation. *Radiology* 151:411–415, 1984b.

JOHNSON DW: CT of the postsurgical ear. *Radiol Clin North Am* 22:67–76, 1984c.

KASEFF LG: Tomographic evaluation of trauma to the temporal bone. *Radiology* 93:321–327, 1969.

KINGSEY DPE, BROOKS GB, LEUNG AWL, et al: Acoustic neuromas: Evaluation by magnetic resonance imaging. *AJNR* 6:1–5, 1985.

LARSON TC, REESE DF, BAKER HL, et al: Glomus tympanicum chemodectomas: Radiographic and clinical characteristics. *Radiology* 163:801–806, 1987.

LATACK JI, KARTUSH JM, KEMINK L, et al: Epidermoidomas of the cerebellopontine angle and temporal bone: CT and MR aspects. *Radiology* 157:361–366, 1985.

LEE SH, LEWIS E, MONTOYA JH, et al: Bilateral cerebellopontine angle air-CT cisternography. *AJNR* 2:105–106, 1981.

LEVENSON MJ, PARISIER SC, JACOBS M, et al: The large vestibular aqueduct syndrome in children. *Arch Otolaryngol Head Neck Surg* 115:54–58, 1989.

LO WW, SOLTI-BOHMAN LG, BRACKMANN DE, et al: Cholesterol granuloma of the petrous apex: CT diagnosis. *Radiology* 153:705–711, 1984.

LO WW, SOLTI-BOHMAN L, MCELVEEN JT JR: Aberrant carotid artery radiologic diagnosis with emphasis on high-resolution computed tomography. *Radiographics* 5:98–993, 1985.

MCCAFFREY TV, MCDONALD TJ: Histiocytosis X of the ear and temporal bone. Review of 22 cases. *Laryngoscope* 89:173–1742, 1979.

MAFEE ME, KIMAR A, YANNIAS DA, et al: Computed tomography of the middle ear in the evaluation of cholesteatomas and other soft tissue masses: Comparison with pluridirectional tomography. *Radiology* 148:465–472, 1983a.

MAFEE ME, VALVASSORI GE, SHUGAR MA, et al: High resolution and dynamic sequential computed tomography: Use in the evaluation of glomus complex tumors. *Arch Otolaryngol* 109:691–696, 1983b.

MAFEE MF, HENDRICKSON GC, et al: Use of CT in stapedial otosclerosis. *Radiology* 156:709–714, 1985a.

MAFEE MF, VALVASSORI GE, DEITCH RL, et al: Use of CT in the evaluation of cochlear otosclerosis. *Radiology* 156:703–708, 1985b.

MAFEE MF, SINGLETON EL, VALVASSORI GE, et al: Acute otomastoiditis and its complications: Role of CT. *Radiology* 155:391–397, 1985c.

MAFEE MF, AIMI K, KAHEN H, et al: Chronic otomastoiditis: A conceptual understanding of CT findings. *Radiology* 160:193–200, 1986.

MAFEE MF. Acoustic neuroma and other acoustic nerve disorders: Role of MRI and CT, analysis of 238 cases. *Semin Ultrasound, CT and MR* 8:256–263, 1987.

MAFEE MF, LACHENAUER CS, KUMAR A, et al. CT and MR imaging of intralabyrinthine schwannoma: Report of two cases and review of the literature. *Radiology* 174:395–400, 1990.

MAFEE MF, CHARLETTA D, KUMAR A, et al: Large vestibular aqueduct and congenital sensorineural hearing loss. *AJNR* 13:805–809, 1992.

MARK AS, SELTZER S, HARNSBERGER HR: Sensorineural hearing loss: More than meets the eye? *AJNR* 14:37–45, 1993.

MAYER TE, BRUECKMANN H, SIEGERT R, et al: High resolution CT of the temporal bone in dysplasia of the auricle and external auditory canal. *AJNR Am J Neuroradiol* 18:53–65, 1997.

MENDEZ G JR, QUENCER RM, POST MJD, et al: Malignant external otitis: A radiographic-clinical correlation. *AJR* 132:957–961, 1979.

NAGER GT, Cholesteatoma of the middle ear: pathogenesis and surgical indication, in McCabe BF, Sade J, Abramson M (eds). *Cholesteatoma: First International Conference*, Birmingham Ala. *Aesculapis* 1977, pp 193–203.

OLSON WL, DILLON WP, KELLY WM, et al: MR imaging of paragangliomas. *AJNR* 7:103–1042, 1986.

OSBORN AG, PARKIN JL: Mucocele of the petrous temporal bone. *AJR* 132:680–681, 1979.

PETASNICK JP: Tomography of the temporal bone in Paget's disease. *AJR* 105:838–843, 1969.

PHELPS PD, LLOYD GAS: Course of the facial nerve in congenital ear deformities. *Acta Radiologica Diagn* 22(fasc 4):475–583, 1981a.

PHELPS PD, LLOYD GAS: The radiology of carcinoma of the ear. *Br J Radiol* 54:103–109, 1981b.

PHELPS PD, SHANKER L, HAWKE M: Imaging case of the month: Radiological features of glomus tympanicum and glomus jugulare. *J Otolaryngol* 120:225–227, 1991.

PRESS GA, HESSLINK JR. MR imaging of cerebellopontine angle and internal auditory canal lesions at 1.5T. *AJNR* 9:241–251, 1988.

SCHMALBROCK P, PRUSKI J, SUN L, et al: Phased array RF coils for high resolution MRI of the ear and brainstem. *J Comput Assist Tomogr* 19:8–14, 1995.

SCHWARTZ RH, MOROSSAGHI N, MARION ED. Rhabdomyosarcoma of the middle ear. A wolf in sheep's clothing. *Pediatrics* 65:1131–1132, 1980.

SHAFFER KA, VOIZ DJ, HAUGHTON VM: Manipulation of CT data for temporal bone imaging. *Radiology* 137:825–829, 1980.

SOM PM, REEDE DL, BERGERON RT, et al: Computed tomography of glomus tympanicum tumors. *J Comput Assist Tomogr* 7:1447, 1983.

STILLMAN AE, REMLEY K, et al: Steady state free precession imaging of the internal ear. *AJNR* 15:348–350, 1994.

STRASHUN AM, NEGATHEIM M, GOLDSMITH SJ: Malignant external otitis: Early scintigraphic detection. *Radiology* 150:541–545, 1984.

SWARTZ JD: High resolution computed tomography of the middle ear and mastoid: I. Normal radioanatomy including normal variations. *Radiology* 148:44–54, 1983a.

SWARTZ JD, GOODMAN RS, RUSSELL KB, et al: High resolution computed tomography of the middle ear and mastoid: II. Tubotympanic disease. *Radiology* 148:455–459, 1983b.

SWARTZ JD: Cholesteatomas of the middle ear: Diagnosis, etiology and complications. *Radiol Clin North Am* 22:15–36, 1984a.

SWARTZ JD, FAERBER EN, WOLFSON RJ, et al: Fenestral otosclerosis: Significance of preoperative CT evaluation. *Radiology* 151:703–707, 1984b.

SWARTZ JD: *Imaging of the Temporal Bone,* New York, Thieme, 1986a.

SWARTZ JD, LANSMAN AK, BERGER AS, et al: Stapes prosthesis: Evaluation with CT. *Radiology* 158:17–182, 1986b.

SWARTZ JD: Current imaging approach to the temporal bone. *Radiology* 171:309–317, 1989.

SWARTZ JD: Sensorineural hearing deficit: A systematic approach based on imaging findings. *Radiographics* 16:561–574, 1996.

TIEN RD, FELSBERG GJ, FERRIS NJ, et al: Fast spin-echo high resolution MR imaging of the inner ear. *Am J Roentgenol* 159:395–398, 1992.

TERESI L, LUFKIN R, WORTHAM D, et al: MR imaging of the intratemporal facial nerve using surface coils. *AJNR* 8:49–54, 1987a.

TERESI L, LUFKIN R, NITTA K, et al: MRI of the facial nerve: Normal anatomy and pathology. *Semin Ultrasound CT MR* 8:240–255, 1987b.

TURSKI E, NORMAN D, DEGROOT J, et al: High-resolution CT of the petrous bone: Direct vs. reformatted images. *AJNR* 3:391–394, 1982.

VALAVANIS A, SCHUBIGER O, HAYEK J, et al: CT of meningiomas on the posterior surface of the petrous bone. *Neuroradiology* 22:111–121, 1981.

VALVASSORI GE, MAFEE MF, DOBBEN GD: Computerized tomography of the temporal bone. *Laryngoscope* 92:562–565, 1982.

VALVASSORI GE, MORALES FG, PALACIOS E, et al: MR of the

normal and abnormal internal auditory canal. *AJNR* 9:115–119, 1988.

VIRAPONGSE C, SARWAR M, SASAKI C, et al: High-resolution computed tomography of the osseous external canal: Normal anatomy. *J Comput Assist Tomogr* 7:486–492, 1983.

VOGL T, BRUNING R, SCHEIDEL H, et al: Paragangliomas of the jugular bulb and carotid body: MR imaging with short sequences and Gd-DTPA enhancement. *AJR* 153:583–587, 1989.

WEISSMAN JL: Hearing loss. *Radiology* 199:593–611, 1996.

WEISSMAN JL, HIRSCH BE: Beyond the promontory: The multifocal origin of glomus tympanicum tumors. *AJNR* 19:119–122, 1998.

WRIGHT JW JR: Trauma of the ear. *Radiol Clin North Am* 12:527–532, 1974.

WRIGHT JW JR, WRIGHT JW III, HICKS G: Polytomography and congenital anomalies of the ear. *Ann Otol Rhinol Laryngol* 91:480–484, 1982.

ZIMMERMAN RA, BILANIUK LT, HACKNEY DB, et al: Magnetic resonance imaging in temporal bone fracture. *Neuroradiology* 29:246–251, 1987

# SECTION C: BASE OF THE SKULL

Apart from the specific pathological processes involving the sellar and parasellar regions and the temporal bone, a variety of other lesions may also involve the anterior, middle, and posterior cranial regions of the skull base (Table 15-5). These include congenital, neoplastic, infectious, or traumatic etiologies. The lesions may originate from (1) structures below the skull base which then invade the cranial fossa and intracranial contents, (2) neoplasms primarily involving the bones forming the skull base, and (3) intracranial lesions with extracranial extension through the neurovascular foramen or by direct extension. Although it is occasionally difficult to identify the initial site of origination, both CT and MR imaging are important in defining the extent of the lesion and the involvement of vital neurovascular structures and in surgical planning.

## LESIONS OUTSIDE THE SKULL BASE

The most common entities invading the skull base are malignant tumors of the head and neck. These include squamous cell carcinoma, adenoid cystic carcinoma, and lymphoma. Involvement of the skull base is often by local extension or by hematogenous and lymphatic pathways (Fig. 15-127). Tumors may also invade the skull base or the intracranial compartment along perineural or endoneural spaces through the various foramina within the base of the skull (Laine 1990). Systemic neoplasm may involve the skull base, the rest of the calvaria, and spread within the brain parenchyma. Metastases from renal and thyroid neoplasms tend to be vascular. Hemorrhage is not unusual. Metastases enhance significantly both in CT and

**Table 15-5  Neoplasms Involving the Skull Base**

Tumors that may involve any portion of skull base
  Metastases from squamous cell carcinoma
  Lymphoma
  Malignant melanoma
  Fibrous histiocytoma
  Giant cell tumor
  Osteoblastoma
  Osteogenic sarcoma
  Chondromyxoid fibroma
  Meningioma
  Hemangioma
  Lymphangioma
  Lipoma
  Extramedullary plasmacytoma

Tumors specifically involving anterior skull base
  Esthesioneuroblastoma
  Schwannoma from CN I
  Spread of tumor from sinonasal region

Parasellar and middle cranial skull base tumors
  Neurinomas (CN III to CN VI)
  Schwannomas (CN III to CN VI)
  Rhabdomyosarcoma
  Chordoma
  Cholestrol granuloma
  Epidermoid tumors

Posterior cranial skull base tumors
  Chordomas
  Epidermoid tumors
  Glomus jugulare tumor
  Neurinoma (CN IX to CN XII)
  Vestibular schwannoma

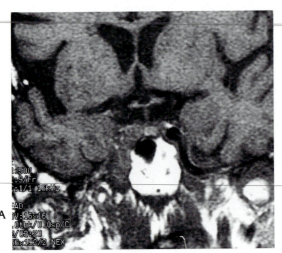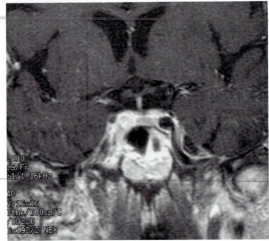

**Figure 15-127** **Metastasis from adenocystic carcinoma** involving the left cavernous sinus. Coronal $T_1$-weighted MR (**A**) demonstrates a soft tissue mass invading the right cavernous sinus. Enhancement of the mass (**B**) is seen with the enhancement involving the trigeminal nerve within the Meckel's cave.

MR. Metastases from prostate tend to involve the extradural compartment (Fig. 15-128), whereas other types of metastasis may not only destroy the normal bony matrix but also invade the dura (Fig. 15-129). CT is useful in demonstrating the osseous involvement. Gadolinium-enhanced MR is necessary in demonstrating the perineural spread of tumor or the local extension into the cranial cavity if the bony vault has been involved. In most instances the tumor within the cranial vault is confined by the dura. The tumor as well as the adjacent dura may demonstrate enhancement with gadolinium-enhanced MR. Edema of the adjacent brain parenchyma and rarely gyral enhancement may be present, probably due to venous congestion.

## Perineural Spread of Tumor

Perineural spread of tumor is best evaluated with MR following intravenous Gd-DTPA. Subtle bone involvement may be difficult to visualize in MR studies and requires CT in both the axial and coronal planes. Perineural invasion of head and neck tumors most often involves the mandibular division (V3) of the trigeminal nerve (CN V), the facial nerve (CN VII), the hypoglossal nerve (CN XII), and less often the other cranial nerves. MR studies should include $T_1$WI followed by fat-suppressed, Gd-DTPA–enhanced MR (Fig. 15-130). Primary tumors that involve the anterior cranial fossa include meningioma, lymphoma, osteoid osteoma, osteogenic fibroma, and esthesioneuroblastoma.

## Esthesioneuroblastoma

This is a rare neuroectodermal tumor also known as *olfactory neuroblastoma*. It arises from nasal epithelium within the cribriform plate, the adjacent upper part of the nasal septum, and extends intracranially as an extradural mass. Invasion of the brain parenchyma is uncommon. It usually is seen in adolescent age group (below the age of 20 years) although a second peak is seen at 50 years and beyond (Olsen 1983). The tumor may be entirely within the nasal cavity, but more often it extends intracranially through the cribriform plate. On CT the tumor usually has a solid appearance, and enhances homogenously following IV contrast. In MR the tumor has a hypointense signal in $T_1$-weighted images and a hyperintense signal in both spin-density and $T_2$-weighted images with homogenous enhancement in gadolinium-enhanced MR (Derdeyn 1994). Cystic degeneration and calcification within the tumor may occasionally be present. In fact the presence of a cystic component in the intracranial portion of the tumor is presumed to be a pathognomic MR finding (Som 1994). Similar cysts may also be seen in meningioma and in malignant schwannoma. Angiography demonstrates tumor blush in the majority of cases.

Rarely, when the tumor is purely extracranial within the nasal cavity, on the basis of imaging studies, differentiation from other neoplasms such as squamous cell carcinoma or cystic adenocarcinoma and from juvenile angiofibroma may be difficult.

Malignant schwannoma of the "zero cranial nerves" is a rare neoplasm with similar location and imaging characteristic, presumed to arise from the primary olfactory nerve fibers within the nasal mucosa (Fig. 15-131) (Hillstrom 1990, Donnelly 1992). Presumably necrotic degeneration and calcification are more common. The appearance is very similar to esthesioneuroblastoma. They are usually seen in females between the ages of 10 and 30 years.

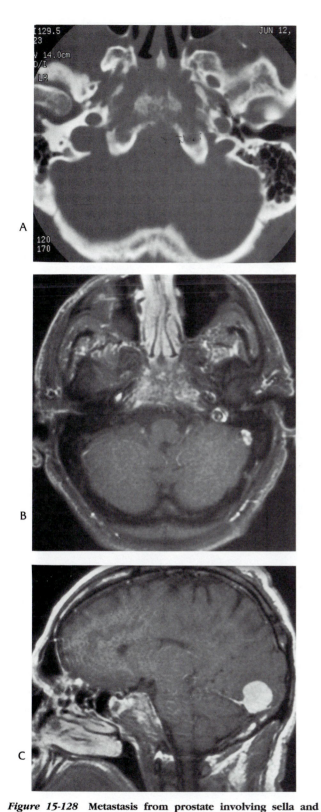

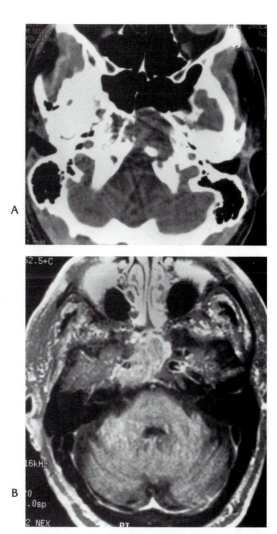

**Figure 15-129  Plasmacytoma involving the sella.** Axial CT section (**A**) demonstrates destruction of the floor of sella by plasmacytoma. Gd-DTPA–enhanced MR (**B**) demonstrates moderate enhancement of the mass.

**Figure 15-128  Metastasis from prostate involving sella and clivus.** Axial CT (**A**) demonstrates bony erosion of the clivus (arrow). Axial (**B**) and sagittal (**C**) Gd-DTPA–enhanced MR demonstrates ill-defined enhancement of the clivus and floor of sella. Incidental enhancing meningioma of the tentorium with dural tail (arrow).

**Figure 15-130  Perineural spread of tumor.** Axial T₁-weighted MR (**A**). Gd-DTPA–enhanced T₁-weighted MR (**B**) demonstrates enhancement of the V2 division of trigeminal nerve from intracranial extension of squamous cell carcinoma. ▶

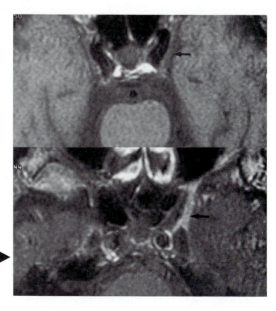

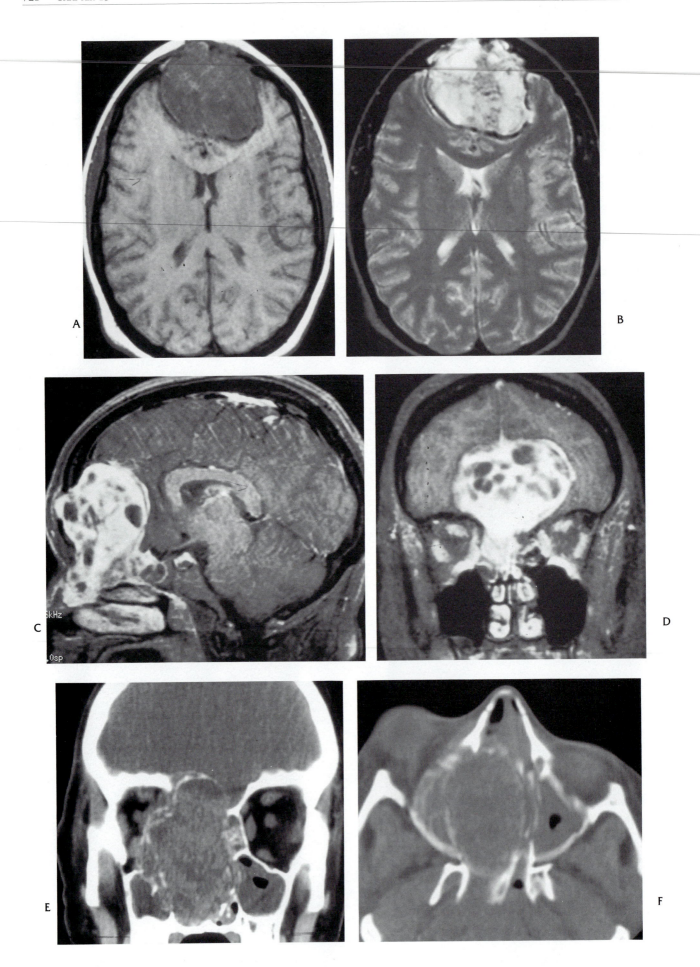

◀*Figure 15-131* **Malignant schwannoma.** Large hypointense signal mass in the frontal region with bony erosion (**A**). The mass has predominantly bright signal (**B**) in $T_2$-weighted MR. Calcification is present around the periphery of the tumor as well as within the mass. Sagittal (**C**) and coronal (**D**) Gd-DTPA−enhanced images demonstrate intense enhancement with multiple foci of hypointensity from cystic necrosis. Enhancement of the dural margin indicates an extradural tumor. Axial (**E**) and coronal (**F**) CT in another patient with nonossifying fibroma. A large soft tissue mass with destruction of midline floor of anterior cranial fossa and intracranial extension is present. The appearance is similar to CT findings in esthesioneuroblastoma and the malignant schwannoma.

## LESIONS WITHIN THE SKULL BASE

Both benign and malignant conditions may affect the skull base. In the older age group, metastasis from systemic primary cancer is the most common cause of a destructive bone lesion (Fig. 15-129). Malignant lesions include entities pathologically classified as sarcomas consisting of chondroid, fibrous, osteogenic, or mixed elements (Brown 1994; Sato 1996) and giant cell tumors (Silver 1996). Except for minor differences, all these neoplasms present as an expansile lesion, with destruction of the outer or inner table of the skull and an associated soft tissue component. *Chondrosarcoma* is commonly seen along the lateral aspects of the skull base, adjacent or overriding the suture. The more common lateral site is the petrooccipital suture (Fig. 15-132). On CT the tumor appears as an expansile bony mass with erosion or destruction of the cortical bone. Tumors show varying degrees of enhancement. In MR they are isointense or mildly hyperintense in $T_1$-weighted MR and hyperintense with varying extent of hypointense signal from calcification, and they demonstrate nonhomogeneous enhancement. *Chondromyxoid fibroma* may appear as a soft tissue mass involving the skull base. Similar to chondromas and chondrosarcoma they are usually seen close to the suture line (Fig. 15-133). In MR they appear as a hypointense soft tissue mass with disruption of the cortical margins and in $T_2$-weighted MR, they appear bright. *Osteogenic sarcoma* may often be seen following radiation therapy or as a primary lesion. It is usually found during middle age. On CT osteogenic sarcoma presents as a soft tissue mass with destructive bony margins. Occasionally there may be amorphous or irregular calcification, which may be central or discrete throughout the tumor. In MR osteogenic sarcoma appears as a hypointense or intermediate signal intensity. The nonossified areas appear as hyperintense signal in $T_2$-weighted MR (Fig. 15-134). Giant cell tumor is usually a benign tumor (osteoclastoma) and occasionally can be aggressive. They are usually associated with Paget's disease.

In CT giant cell tumor presents as a mass with destructive bone changes or remodeling of the bone. These tumors enhance moderately in CECT. Similarly in MR they appear as a hypointense or isointense mass with enhancement in Gd-DTPA−enhanced MR (Fig. 15-135). There are no characteristic features helpful in differentiating an osteogenic sarcoma from a chondromyxoid fibroma or a chondroblastoma. A solitary

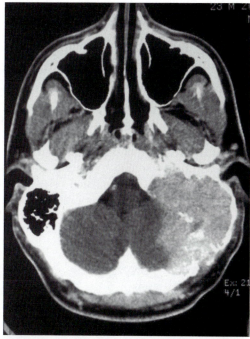

A

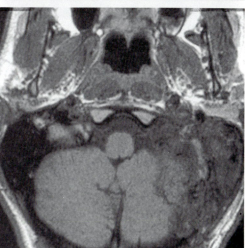

B

*Figure 15-132* **Chondrosarcoma.** CECT (**A**) demonstrates a large ▶ mildly hyperdense mass involving the right basiocciput and adjacent petrous segment of temporal bone. $T_1$-weighted axial (**B**) and spin-density weighted *(Continued on next page)*

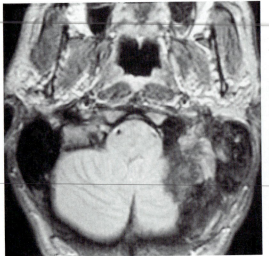

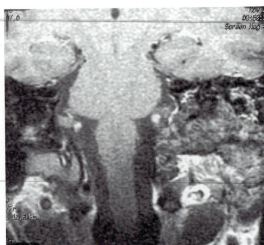

C

D

*Figure 15-132 (continued)* (**C**) MR. The mass has a nonhomogenous appearance with admixture of dark and bright signal. Coronal (**D**) and axial (**E**) T₁-weighted MR demonstrates nonhomogeneous enhancement of the tumor.

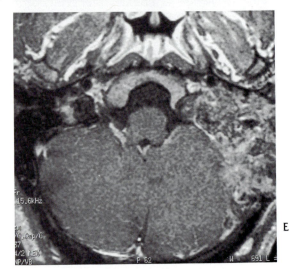

E

metastasis may have a similar appearance. CT is useful in demonstrating the expansile soft tissue mass arising within the bone, with a disrupted thin rim of cortical bone. CT-guided biopsy is useful in determining the histological characteristics of the neoplasm. Solid or heterogeneous enhancement is common. Giant cell tumors may not show intrinsic spiculated osseous or cartilaginous elements. From the above description it is evident that tumors with different cellular characteris-

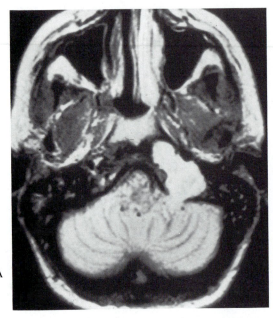

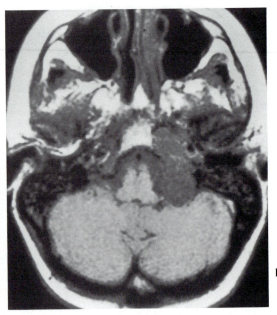

A

B

*Figure 15-133* **Chondromyxoid fibroma.** Axial T₁-weighted MR (**A**). Axial spin-density–weighted MR (**B**). A mass involving the petrous apex and adjacent clivus demonstrates a hypointense signal in T₁-weighted MR and bright signal in spin-density image.

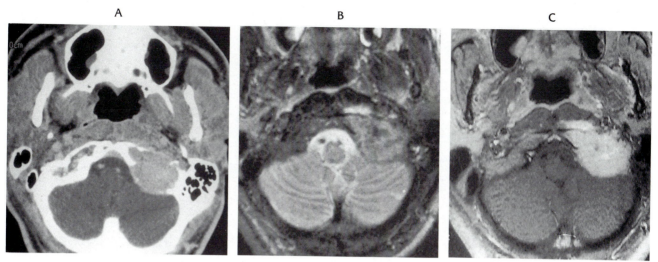

**Figure 15-134   Osteogenic sarcoma.** CECT (**A**) shows a mildly enhancing destructive bone lesion involving the basiocciput and occipital condyle (arrow). $T_2$-weighted MR (**B**) demonstrates an isointense mass. Intense enhancement in Gd-DTPA–enhanced MR (**C**).

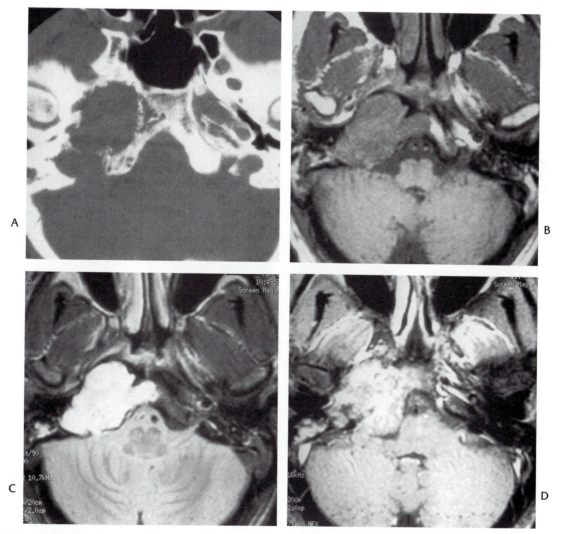

**Figure 15-135   Giant cell tumor.** Axial CT (**A**) demonstrates a large lytic area with moth-eaten appearance in the right temporal region. The mass is hypointense in $T_1$-weighted MR (**B**), hyperintense in spin-density–weighted MR (**C**) and enhanced in Gd-DTPA–enhanced MR (**D**). Apart from the enhancement characteristic, similar appearance may be seen in epidermoid tumor.

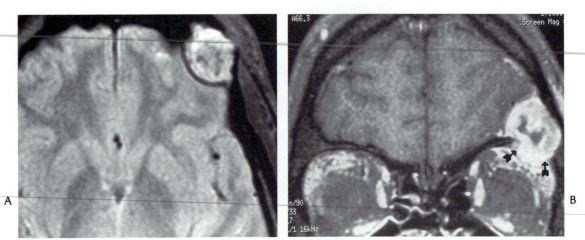

***Figure 15-136*** **Intradiploic dermoid.** Spin-density–weighted axial MR (**A**) demonstrates an extradural hyperintense signal lesion involving the lateral aspect of roof of orbit. Coronal Gd-DTPA–enhanced MR (**B**) demonstrates intense marginal enhancement of the neoplasm with destruction of the roof of the orbit (arrows). This is the most common site of intradiploic dermoid.

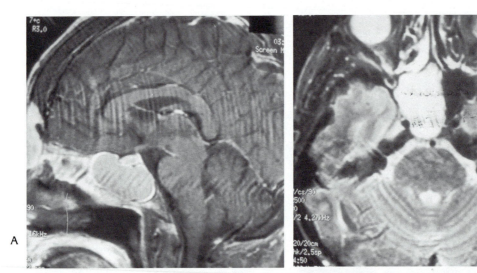

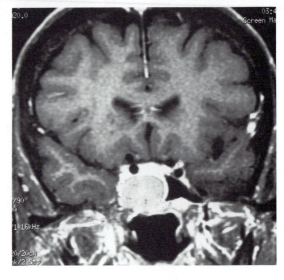

***Figure 15-137*** **Mucocele of the sphenoid sinus.** Sagittal $T_1$-weighted MR (**A**). Axial spin-density–weighted MR (**B**) demonstrates a hyperintense signal mucocele of the sphenoid sinus with bright signal in both sequences. Coronal Gd-DTPA–enhanced MR (**C**) in another patient with sphenoid sinus mucocele demonstrates enhancement of the capsule of the mucocele which extends into the sella.

tics may appear similar, with minor differences both on CT and MR (Table 15-6). The purpose of imaging studies is to define the extent of the bony lesion and identify vascular structures that may be compromised by the tumor. MR does not usually add additional information, except if the tumor is adjacent to a major dural venous sinus. MRA or MRV should be obtained if there is suspicion of invasion or encasement of the vascular channels by the tumor. In almost all cases biopsy of the tumor is necessary to arrive at the histological diagnosis.

Benign lesions that involve the skull base include fibrous dysplasia, fibroosseous masses, Paget's disease, bone dysplasias, and intradiploic tumors such as dermoid (Fig. 15-136), epidermoid, and hemangiomas. The benign character of the lesion is based primarily on an expansile intradiploic mass, but often without erosion or destruction of the inner and outer plate. Signal intensities depend on the amount of fat, fibrous tissue, and vascularity within the mass.

Inflammatory lesions other than those described in the section on temporal bone may be secondary to infection extending from the adjacent head and neck region. Mucocele occurs following obstruction of the orifice of the sinus. Mucocele may involve the petrous apex region as well as the sphenoid sinus. Mucocele or petrous apicitis may have an appearance similar to a cholesterol cyst, bight in both $T_1$- and $T_2$-weighted MR. Mucocele in the sphenoid sinus is usually hyperintense in both $T_1$- and $T_2$-weighted MR (Fig. 15-137) or appears as an enlarging mass expanding the sinus, and not enhancing following Gd-DTPA. Lymphoma may involve the sphenoid or other paranasal sinuses. It has a hypointense signal in $T_1$-weighted MR, is mildly hyperintense in $T_2$-weighted MR, and demonstrates intense enhancement in Gd-DTPA–enhanced $T_1$-weighted MR (Fig. 15-138).

## Neurofibromatosis

Patients with NF 1 type neurofibromatosis may show parenchymal hamartomas, gliomas of the optic nerve, or neuroma of the cranial nerves. Osseous changes are in the form of enlarged foramen in the spinal axis resulting from dural ectasia. A similar phenomena involving the skull bone is thinning or absence of the greater wing of the sphenoid bone resulting in mild ophthalmoplegia. In most cases the dura is intact. Usually the temporal lobe of the brain herniates into the orbit. It may present as an isolated finding (Fig. 15-139).

## Paget's Disease

Paget's disease produces chronic progressive changes in the skeletons of middle-age and elderly adults. A lytic phase characterized by loss of bone is followed by a sclerotic phase characterized by coarse thickened trabeculae. The skull and, less frequently, the temporal bones may be affected. Temporal bone involvement usually causes conductive hearing loss if the stapes becomes fixed in the oval window or sensorineural hearing loss if the cochlea is involved. Paget's disease of the temporal bone usually is accompanied by severe skull involvement.

In Paget's disease, temporal bone changes are usually lytic. Demineralization begins medially in the petrous pyramid and progresses laterally. The dense otic capsule bone is the last to be affected (Fig. 15-140). The diagnosis of Paget's disease is made by identifying calvarial changes in association with the lytic changes in the temporal bone. The lytic areas in the temporal bone cannot be distinguished from otosclerosis, metastases, or luetic osteitis.

## Fibrous Dysplasia

Fibrous dysplasia is a congenital osseous disorder of unknown etiology in which cancellous bone is replaced by fibrous tissue that erodes and expands normal cortical bone from within. There are monostotic and polyostotic subtypes. There is a variable amount

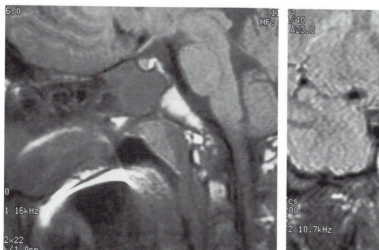
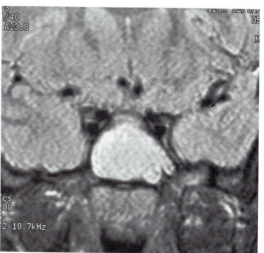

*Figure 15-138* **Lymphoma involving the sphenoid sinus.** $T_1$-weighted MR (**A**) shows a hypointense mass expanding the sella. Gd-DTPA–enhanced MR (**B**) demonstrates homogeneous enhancement of the tumor.

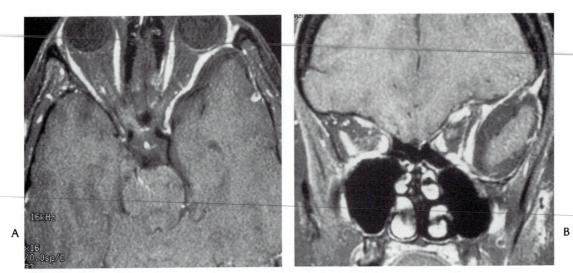

***Figure 15-139*** **Empty orbit in patient with neurofibroma.** Axial (**A**) and coronal (**B**) Gd-DTPA–enhanced MR demonstrates absence of greater wing of the sphenoid, enhancing dura. Proptosis is due to herniation of temporal lobe herniation and transmitted CSF pulsation.

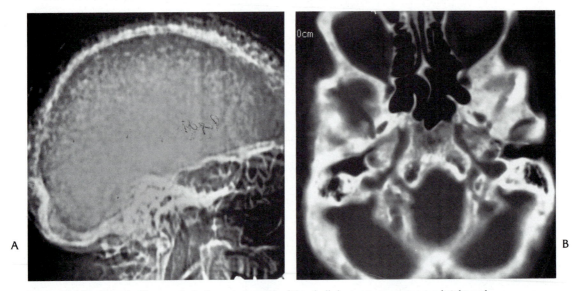

***Figure 15-140*** **Paget's disease.** Sagittal scout view (**A**) of the skull demonstrates extensive bright and dark areas within a thickened calvaria from Paget's disease. Axial CT (**B**) demonstrating the bony changes involving the petrous region.

of metaplastic bone formation, and so fibrous dysplasia can have a cystic, isodense, or a "ground glass" appearance, depending on the proportion of bony and soft tissue elements. Any skull bone may be involved, although the sphenoid bone, frontal bone, and temporal bone are more often involved (Fig. 15-141). When fibrous dysplasia occurs in the sinuses or temporal bones, the lesion usually is osteomatoid, appearing as a uniformly dense region of expanded bone. Patients often present with mastoid prominence and hearing loss caused by narrowing of the external auditory

canal or middle ear (Nager 1982). On CT, fibrous dysplasia of the temporal bone is usually characterized by homogeneous dense thickened bone, which may narrow the external auditory canal and middle ear. The uncommon lucent foci caused by fibrosis may have an expanded cortex (Fig. 15-142). In MR the lesion is hypointense in $T_1$-weighted images. Depending on the pattern of bony trabeculae, cellularity, and presence or absence of cystic or hemorrhagic component, the lesion may be isointense, hyperintense, or heterogeneous in appearance (Jee 1996). Gadolinium-

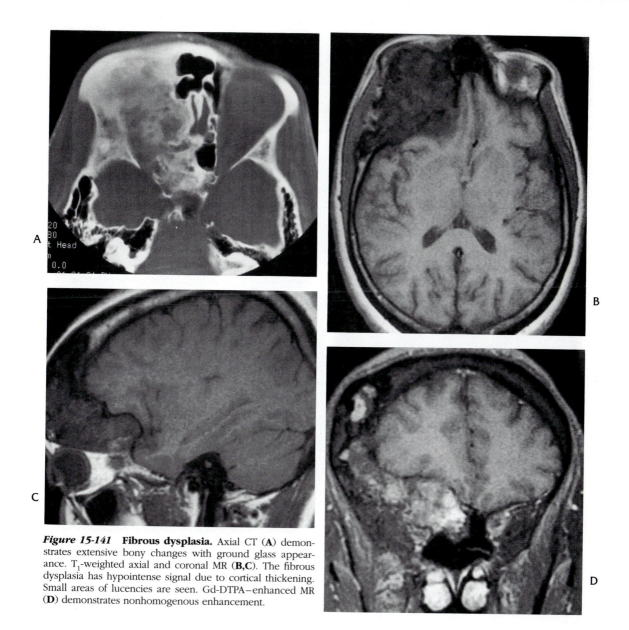

**Figure 15-141 Fibrous dysplasia.** Axial CT (**A**) demonstrates extensive bony changes with ground glass appearance. T$_1$-weighted axial and coronal MR (**B,C**). The fibrous dysplasia has hypointense signal due to cortical thickening. Small areas of lucencies are seen. Gd-DTPA–enhanced MR (**D**) demonstrates nonhomogenous enhancement.

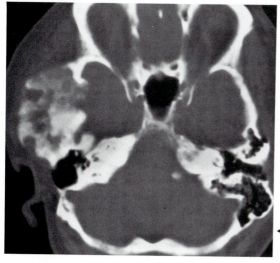

enhanced–T$_1$-weighted MR may show areas of enhancement. The differential diagnosis includes metastasis, meningioma, Paget's disease, osteosarcoma, ossifying fibroma, and osteopetrosis. Malignant degeneration, although rare, should be suspected if a large expansile lesion with characteristic findings of expanded thickened bone and areas of intense enhancement is present (Fig. 15-143).

Hemangiomas of the calvaria may also expand the diploic space and in plain x-rays have appearance of

◀ **Figure 15-142 Fibrous dysplasia.** Axial CT demonstrates focal expansion of the temporal bone with combination of solid and cystic component. This should not be mistaken for a malignant tumor.

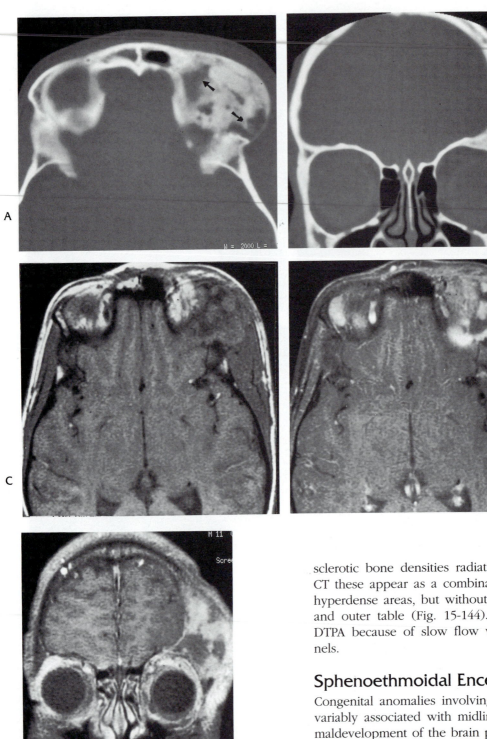

***Figure 15-143*  Fibrous dysplasia with malignant degenera-tion.** Axial (**A**) and coronal (**B**) CT demonstrates a cystic component (arrow) within an expansile sclerotic bone lesion involving the roof and lateral wall of the orbit. Axial $T_1$-weighted MR (**C**) demonstrates a heterogeneous isointense and hypointense signal within the fi-brous dysplasia. Axial (**D**) and coronal (**E**) Gd-DTPA–enhanced MR demonstrates nonhomogeneous enhancement of the expansile bone lesion.

sclerotic bone densities radiating from the center. In CT these appear as a combination of hypodense and hyperdense areas, but without disruption of the inner and outer table (Fig. 15-144). They enhance in Gd-DTPA because of slow flow with the vascular chan-nels.

## Sphenoethmoidal Encephalocele

Congenital anomalies involving the skull base are in-variably associated with midline clefts and associated maldevelopment of the brain parenchyma. Encephalo-cele results from absence of the osseous component of the skull base with herniation of the intracranial brain parenchyma. It is most common in the anterior skull base associated with absence of the cribriform plate. Sphenoethemoid encephalocele is a common example. The encephalocele may present as a mass within the nasal cavity. MR is excellent in demonstrating the brain herniation and associated bony defect (Fig. 15-145). CT in the axial and coronal planes is useful to demon-strate the bony defect and for surgical planning.

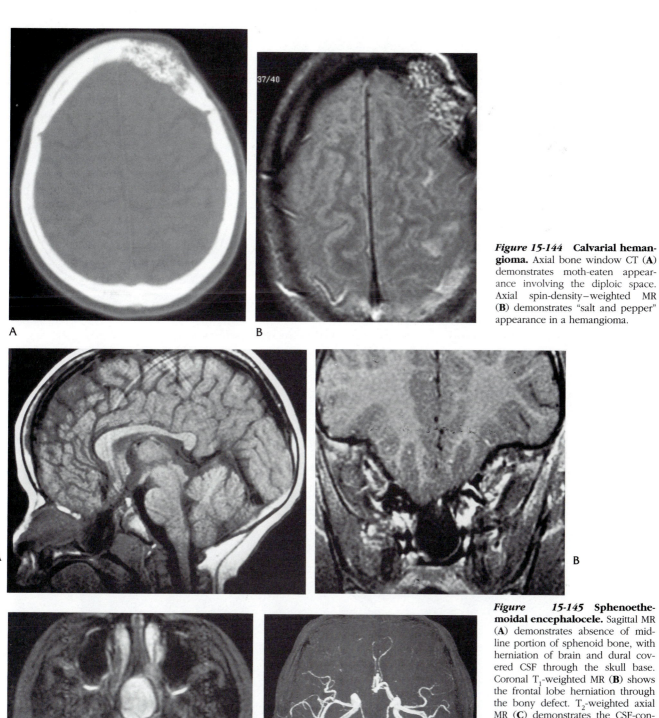

*Figure 15-144* **Calvarial hemangioma.** Axial bone window CT (**A**) demonstrates moth-eaten appearance involving the diploic space. Axial spin-density–weighted MR (**B**) demonstrates "salt and pepper" appearance in a hemangioma.

*Figure 15-145* **Sphenoethemoidal encephalocele.** Sagittal MR (**A**) demonstrates absence of midline portion of sphenoid bone, with herniation of brain and dural covered CSF through the skull base. Coronal $T_1$-weighted MR (**B**) shows the frontal lobe herniation through the bony defect. $T_2$-weighted axial MR (**C**) demonstrates the CSF-containing cyst within the nasopharynx. Three-dimensional TOF MRA (**D**) demonstrates the associated absence of the right proximal segment of anterior cerebral artery. CT in another case of sphenoethemoidal encephalocele. *(Continued on next page)*

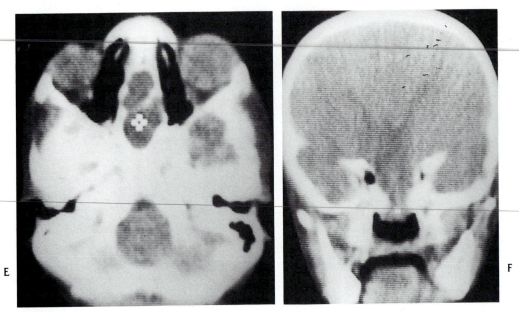

**Figure 15-145 (continued)**    Axial (**E**) and coronal (**F**) CT demonstrates soft tissue mass (*) extending through a bone defect.

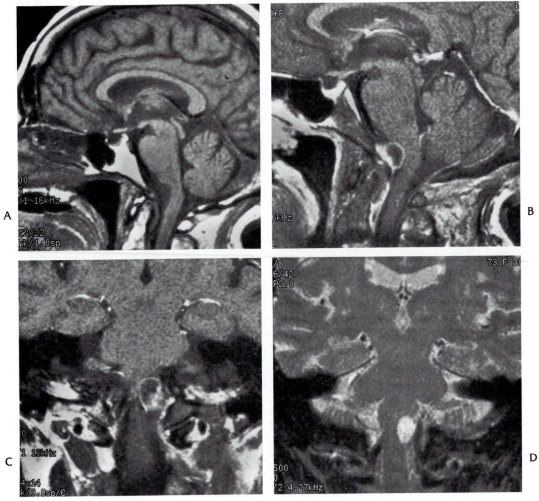

**Figure 15-146    Synovial cyst.** Sagittal MR demonstrates a soft tissue mass deforming the cervicomedullary junction (arrow) (**A**). Sagittal (**B**), and coronal (**C**) Gd-DTPA–enhanced MR demonstrates an isoin- tense mass with capsular enhancement. $T_2$-weighted coronal MR (**D**). The mass is hyperintense.

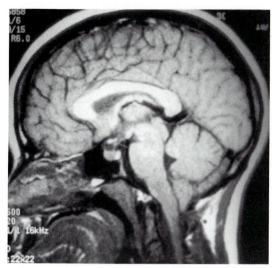

*Figure 15-147*  **Ectopic position of cerebellar tonsil.** Chiari type 1 anomaly associated with low position of the tonsil.

## Synovial Cyst: Craniocervical Junction

Synovial cysts are benign cystic masses usually due to degenerative changes in joints with synovial lining. As such they are common in the spinal region arising adjacent to facet joints (Reginster 1994; Quaghebaur 1992; Patel 1988). Synovial cyst may be seen at the occipitocervical region involving the condylar process of the occiput and the Atlas vertebrae (Fig. 15-146). Depending on their size they may cause compression of the cervicomedullary junction. They appear as an extra dural cystic mass, which has an isointense or hypointense signal on $T_1$WI and hyperintense signal on $T_2$WI. Enhancement of the cyst capsule is not uncommon and is probably related to chronic inflammation. These cysts may mimic an extraaxial abscess, a small arachnoid cyst, or a schwannoma. Characteristic MR finding is helpful in diagnosis.

Pigmented villonodular synovitis (PVNS) may also involve the craniocervical junction. Similar to PVNS in other synovial joints, punctate areas of hypointense signal in $T_2$WI represent areas of microcalcification or hemosiderine from hemorrhage.

## Tonsillar Ectopia

Ectopic position of the cerebellar tonsils is often associated with Chiari type 1 anomaly (Fig. 15-147). However, tonsillar ectopia may be seen in patients who have had prior diversion of the CSF pathways, either with a cyst-subarachnoid shunt or drainage of an intracranial cyst with a cyst-peritoneal shunt.

## Table 15-6    Imaging Characteristics of Selected Skull Base Lesions

| TUMOR TYPE | CT | $T_1$-WEIGHTED MR | $T_2$-WEIGHTED MR | Gd-DTPA–ENHANCED MR |
|---|---|---|---|---|
| Cholesterol granuloma | Hypodense, nonenhancing | Bright | Bright; dark areas if Hg within cyst | No enhancement |
| Epidermoid | Hypo- or isodense | Hypo- or isointense | Bright | No enhancement |
| Chordoma | Soft tissue mass Ca$^{2+}$ often present | Heterogeneous; hypo- or isointense | Heterogeneous; hypo- or hyperintense | Heterogeneous enhancement |
| Meningioma | Hyperdense or isodense; intense enhancement | Isointense | Hypointense | Homogeneous enhancement |
| Acoustic | Isodense | Isointense | Hyperintense | Homogeneous |
| Glomus tumor | Soft tissue density; intense enhancement | Hypointense | Heterogeneous "salt/pepper" appearance | Heterogeneous enhancement |
| Giant cell tumor | Bone destruction; spiculated bone | Hypointense | Heterogeneous bright areas | Heterogeneous enhancement |
| Osteogenic sarcoma | Enlarged diploic space; extensive bone erosion | Hypointense | Hyperintense heterogeneous | Heterogeneous Enhancement |
| Chondro-sarcoma | Hypodense or mixed; usually within suture lines | Hypointense | Heterogeneous | Heterogeneous Enhancement |

# References

BROWN E, HUG EB, WEBER AL: Chondrosarcoma of the skull base. *Neuroimag Clin North Am* 4:929–316, 1994.

DERDEYN CP, MORAN CJ, WIPPOLD FJ, et al: MRI of esthesioneuroblastoma. *J Comput Assist Tomogr* 18:16–21, 1994.

DONNELLY MJ, SALER MH, BLAYNEY AW: Benign nasal schwannoma. *J Laryngol Otol* 105:186–190, 1992.

HILLSTROM RP, ZARBO RJ, JACOBS JR: Nerve cell tumor of the paranasal sinuses: Electron microscopy and histopathologic diagnosis. *Otol Head Neck Surg* 102:257–263, 1990.

JEE WH, CHOI KH, PARK JM, SHINN KS: Fibrous dysplasia: MR imaging characteristics with radiopathologic correlation. *AJR* 167:153–1527, 1996.

LAINE FJ, BRAUN IF, JENSEN ME, et al: Perineural tumor extension through the foramen ovale: Evaluation with MR imaging. *Radiology* 174:65–71, 1990.

NAGER GT, KENNEDY DW, KIPSTEIN E: Fibrous dysplasia: A review of the disease and its manifestations in the temporal bone. *Ann Oto Rhinol Laryngol* (suppl) 92:5–52, 1982.

OLSEN KD, DESANTO WL: Olfactory neuroblastoma. Biologic and clinical behavior. *Arch Otolaryngol* 109:797–802, 1983.

PATEL SC, SANDERS WP: Synovial cyst of the cervical spine: Case report and review of the literature. *AJNR* 9:602–603, 1988.

QUAGHEBAUR G, JEFFREE M: Synovial cyst of the high cervical spine causing myelopathy. *AJNR* 13:981–983, 1991.

REGINSTER P, COLLIGNON J, DONDELINGER RF: Synovial cysts of the lumbar spine: CT and MRI correlation. *Eur Radiol* 4:332–335, 1994.

SILVERS AR, SOM PM, BRANDWEIN M, et al: Role of imaging in the diagnosis of giant cell tumor of the skull base. *AJNR* 17:1392–1395, 1996.

SOM PM, LIDOV M, BRANDWEIN M, et al: Sinonasal esthesioneuroblastoma with intracranial extension: Marginal tumor cysts as a diagnostic MR finding. *AJNR* 15:1259–1262, 1994.

## ACKNOWLEDGMENT

The present authors would like to acknowledge the original material written by David L. Daniels, Katherine A. Shaffer, and Victor M. Haughton, which forms the basis of the present chapter.

# 16 THE ORBIT

*Larissa T. Bilaniuk*

*Robert A. Zimmerman*

## CONTENTS

Major advances have been achieved in the diagnosis of orbital and visual pathway lesions, first with the application of computed tomography to the evaluation of the orbit (Forbes 1980, 1982; Trokel 1979; Jacobs 1980) and then with the application of magnetic resonance (Sullivan 1986; Bilaniuk 1987; Atlas 1987*a;* Bilaniuk 1994) to the evaluation of the orbit. Both CT and MR provide excellent anatomic detail (Figs. 16-1 through 16-4) and information regarding the presence, location, and extent of intraorbital lesions as well as the involvement of the orbit by lesions arising in the adjacent bone and paranasal sinuses (Mancuso 1978; Weber 1978; Som 1985). Until recently, CT was the first procedure to be performed, with MR playing a complementary role. At present, CT or MR is performed first, depending on the clinical picture. CT remains the procedure of choice in cases of acute trauma, acute

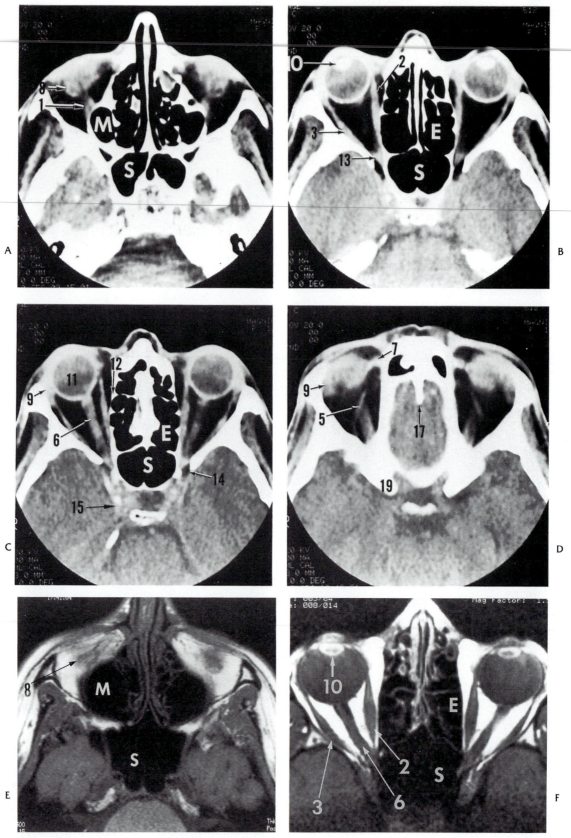

*Figure 16-1*    A-J caption on facing page.

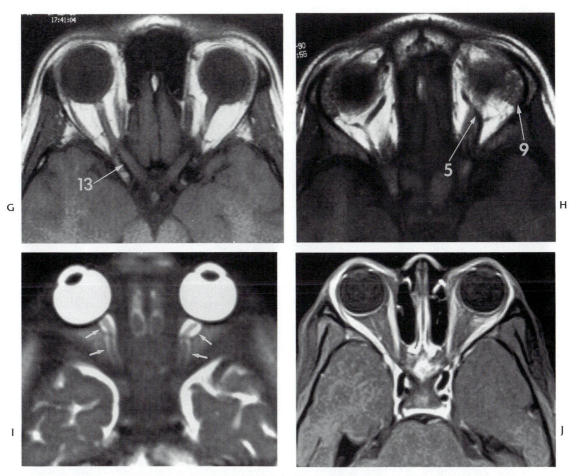

***Figure 16-1*** (CT: **A–D**; MR: **E–H**) **Normal orbit, axial plane,** inferior to superior. 1 = inferior rectus, 2 = medial rectus, 3 = lateral rectus, 4 = superior rectus, 5 = superior ophthalmic vein, 6 = optic nerve, 7 = superior oblique, 8 = inferior oblique, 9 = lacrimal gland, 10 = lens, 11 = vitreous, 12 = lamina papyracea, 13 = optic canal, 14 = superior orbital fissure, 15 = cavernous sinus, 16 = floor of orbit, 17 = crista galli, 18 = cribriform plate, 19 = anterior clinoid, 20 = planum sphenoidale, 21 = inferior orbital fissure, 22 = levator palpebrae superioris, 23 = ophthalmic artery, 24 = III, $V^1$, VI cranial nerves, 25 = $V^2$ and foramen rotundum, M = maxillary sinus; E = ethmoid sinus; S = sphenoid sinus; C = chiasm; CA = carotid artery; P = pituitary gland. **I.** Normal axial HASTE image through the midorbits shows the optic nerve sheath complexes distinguishing the subarachnoid space and the actual optic nerves. Also there is excellent demonstration of the globes with clear outline of the anterior chambers, lenses, and posterior chambers. **J.** Axial MR through the midorbit after contrast enhancement and fat saturation. There is normal contrast enhancement of the rectus muscles. Note that the fat is slightly hypointense compared with the muscle.

infection, or a bony lesion or abnormality. CT of the orbit is a well-established technique. It is more widely available than MR, easier to perform and interpret, and less susceptible to motion artifacts, and it provides better bony detail. However, a tremendous upsurge in the number of MR scanners and new software and surface coil developments (Breslau 1995) as well as the utilization of paramagnetic contrast agents with fat suppression (Tien 1991; Hendrix 1990) have made MR a serious competitor of CT. Thin sections in multiple planes with high resolution can now be obtained with MR without the penalty of longer scanning times. In some categories of orbital disease MR shows clear advantages over CT. MR provides better characterization of

ocular, vascular, hemorrhagic, and bone marrow lesions (Rebsamen 1993) and more precisely delineates visual pathway lesions and other lesions with extraorbital extension. Familiarity with the advantages and disadvantages of each technique is important in deciding on the proper sequencing of diagnostic studies and leads to a customized approach in the evaluation of orbital abnormalities.

## TECHNIQUE

The examination of the orbit by CT or MR should be tailored to the clinical problem at hand but also should be anatomically complete. Thin sections are obtained

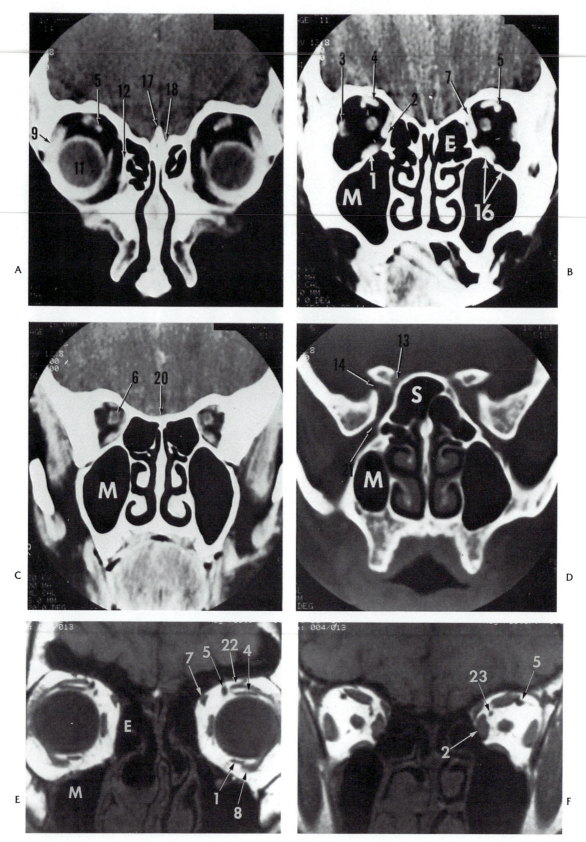

***Figure 16-2***   **A–H caption on facing page.**

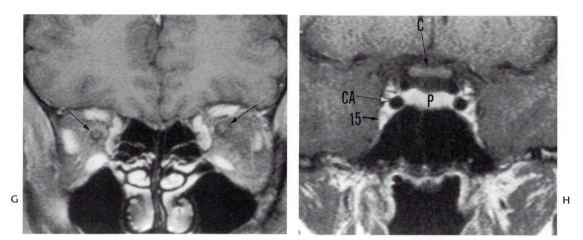

**Figure 16-2** (CT: **A–D**; MR: **E–H**) **Normal orbit, coronal plane,** anterior to posterior. See legend for Fig. 16-1. **G.** Coronal orbital image following contrast enhancement and fat saturation. There is normal enhancement of the extraocular muscles. The presence of hypointense CSF (arrows) around the optic nerves permits identification of the optic nerve sheath complexes. Note that the intraconic fat is hypointense to the muscles.

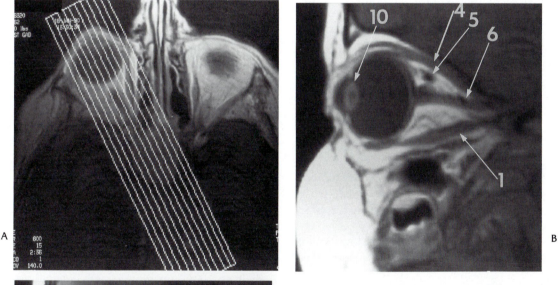

**Figure 16-3  Normal orbit:** MRI, sagittal plane. **A.** The position of the sagittal slices is indicated by white lines on an axial image of the orbits. **B.** Sagittal section, $T_1WI$ (600/15; 3 mm) obtained along the long axis of the orbit demonstrates the entire optic nerve, intraorbital, intracanalicular, and intracranial. See legend for 16-1. **C.** Sagittal section, $T_1WI$ (600/15; 4 mm thick) shows a tortuous optic nerve which would have been difficult to demonstrate in its entirety on other planes. The superior and inferior rectus muscles are also shown on this plane.

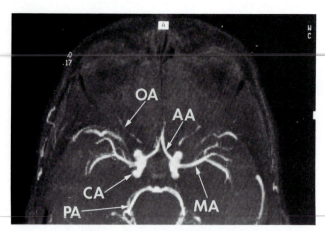

*Figure 16-4* **Magnetic resonance angiography,** compressed image (3D acquisition; TR 35 msec, TE 7 msec, matrix 256 × 256). OA = ophthalmic artery; CA = carotid artery; MA = middle cerebral artery; AA = anterior cerebral artery; PA = posterior cerebral artery.

routinely in at least two planes. The entire orbit is encompassed, along with the adjacent portions of the brain, the cavernous sinus, and portions of the paranasal sinuses and facial and nasopharyngeal soft tissues. Familiarity with the history and clinical results leads to proper planning and thus a more efficient and successful imaging study. It is also important to anticipate sedation when children, retarded patients, or claustrophobic patients are being evaluated.

The adequacy of an imaging examination of the orbit can be assured only if the study is carefully monitored and if images that are marred by motion or artifacts are repeated. After completion of the examination, the study must be carefully reviewed. Such a review is best done on a diagnostic display console so that the sections can be examined for the osseous and soft tissue structures at a variety of window widths with different window levels. To obtain a permanent film record of a CT study, two settings are recommended: one for soft tissue and the other for bony detail. Unless a technique for fat suppression or surface coil correction is used, a window level and width manipulation may be also necessary for viewing and filming of MR images to optimally visualize both the superficial and deep structures of the orbit.

## Computed Tomography

Contiguous thin sections, generally 3 mm thick in the transverse plane and 5 mm thick in the coronal plane, are obtained routinely (Baleriaux-Waha 1977; Hoyt 1979; Osborn 1980; Tadmor 1978; Unsold 1980a; Wing 1979) (Figs. 16-1A–D, 16-2A–D). The search for a small lesion, or optimal visualization of the optic-nerve-sheath complex, may require 1- to 15-mm-thick

sections. Provided that the patient has not moved during the examination, such thin sections also permit reformation in other planes, such as the sagittal, as well as three-dimensional reconstruction, which is useful in the evaluation of congenital or posttraumatic facial-orbital deformities (Vannier 1987). The authors' experience indicates that examination is necessary in the transverse plane, usually at an angulation of −10° to the orbitomeatal baseline (Fig. 16-1A–D) and that the initial examination should be made both before and after the injection of an adequate amount of iodinated contrast material. Oblique reformation, which allows one to follow the plane of the optic nerve (Unsold 1980a) or that of the superior ophthalmic vein, may be of value in specific cases.

A recently developed CT technology, spiral CT, permits rapid volumetric data acquisition and reconstruction of images in any plane (Zimmerman 1991; Coleman 1994). This technique is faster than conventional CT, and so there is less likelihood of motion artifacts. The need for patient sedation is decreased, and it entails a lower radiation dose.

Because of its sinuous course in two places, the appearance and course of the optic nerve depend on the thickness and plane of the CT section as well as the direction of gaze (Unsold 1980b). Unsold recommends a negative angulation of −20° to the orbitomeatal baseline with the eye in the upgaze position to stretch the nerves and have their course parallel to the plane of section.

## Magnetic Resonance Imaging

Patients considered for MR scanning must be screened for ferromagnetic orbital foreign bodies (Kelly 1986; Williamson 1994), vascular clips, and prosthetic material as well as electronic devices (New 1983; Otto 1992; Shellock 1994). Imaging centers generally have lists of devices and materials that are contraindicated for MR imaging. One such list has been published (Shellock 1988) (see Chap. 3).

Certain forms of eye makeup contain iron oxides and can produce artifacts on images (Fig. 16-5); the oxides can also be attracted toward the magnet and accumulate on it (Wright 1985). Patients should be instructed not to wear any eye makeup on the day of the study or to remove it before the MR examination.

Careful explanation of what the orbital MR study entails can ensure a successful examination. To avoid artifacts caused by globe motion in scans requiring shorter scanning times, the patient should be asked to relax but gaze in one direction. To avoid eye strain in longer scanning sequences, the patient should be asked to keep the eyes closed but consciously try not

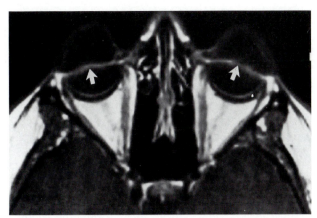

***Figure 16-5*** Artifact on MR created by **eye makeup.** An axial T₁WI (600/22) shows a prominent high-intensity line (arrows) crossing each globe and prominent distortion of the anterior aspect of the globes. This was caused by an eyeliner.

duced by the relaxing magnetization (generally a surface coil). To obtain thin sections with high spatial resolution in short scanning times, the surface coil should be of a size that allows it to primarily capture signal from the orbits (Shenck 1985). This is particularly important for short TR/TE spin-echo sequences, which provide the best morphological detail. The orbit has such good inherent soft tissue contrast that a short TR/TE sequence (T₁WI) with 3-mm-thick sections can be obtained in about 2 minutes of scanning time with the number of excitations being just one (NEX = 1). Long TR/short TE (PDWI) and long TR/long TE spin-echo sequences (T₂WI) that provide information that helps characterize lesions take longer and may be obtained either with an orbital surface coil or a head receiving coil, preferably a quadrature head coil. Numerous pulse sequences other than the routine spin echo are available and may be utilized in special circumstances (Atlas 1987*b*, 1988; Dixon 1984; Simon 1988; Keller 1987) (Table 16-1). Recently introduced half-Fourier single-shot turbo-spin-echo (HASTE) technique requires only 1.2 seconds per slice and provides good images of the globes and the optic nerves (Fig. 16-1I). Three-dimensional or time-of-flight acquisitions are utilized for the imaging of vessels. Magnetic resonance angiography permits excellent delineation of major vessels; even the ophthalmic artery can be demonstrated (Fig. 16-4).

to wander with the globes. Children and retarded, uncooperative, or severely claustrophobic patients generally require sedation. Sedated patients should be carefully monitored while in the magnet. This is done with equipment specially designed for the magnetic environment.

MR scanning of the orbits involves the use of two coils: one for transmitting the imaging pulse sequence (whole body coil) and one for receiving the signals in-

## Table 16-1    Orbital MR Techniques

| INDICATION | COIL | SEQUENCE | PLANE |
|---|---|---|---|
| Routine morphology (cong./trauma) | Surface coil | SE short TR, short TE TR 600 ± 100; TE 15 msec | Axial, coronal 3-mm-thick sections |
| Morphology of orbital roof, floor, and optic canal | Surface coil | SE short TR, short TE TR 600 ± 100; TE 15 msec | Sagittal along long axis of orbit; coronal |
| Tissue characterization | Head or surface coil | SE long TR/short TE long TR/long TE 2500–3000/ 20–90 | Axial, coronal (3- to 5-mm-thick sections) |
| Contrast enhancement ocular, orbital, periorbital lesions | Surface coil | Fat suppression (if not available, careful wide window photography) | Axial, coronal and/or sagittal |
| Contract enhancement if orbital lesion with intracranial extent | Head coil | Short TR/short TE; fat suppression for orbital component | Axial, coronal, and/or sagittal |
| Intravascular flow; thrombosis | Head coil | Gradient echo | Axial, coronal |
| Vascular malformation or vascular lesions | Head coil | MRA | Axial, coronal |
| Thin sections of optic nerve sheath complex | Head coil | 3-dimensional acquisition | Reconstruct in any plane (1-mm-thick sections) |
| Avoid high intensity from orbital fat | | STIR | Axial, coronal, and/or sagittal |

The rationale for the use of contrast material is the same as that for contrast-enhanced CT (CE CT): to characterize and delineate ocular and orbital mass lesions and lesions that extend beyond or into the orbit. Because it may be difficult to delineate contrast-enhanced high-intensity lesions within high-intensity orbital fat, some form of fat-suppression technique is required (Keller 1987) (Fig. 16-1J).

Proper interpretation of MR images requires familiarity with numerous artifacts that can occur during scanning. These artifacts are listed and discussed in several publications (Pusey 1986; Hahn 1988; Clark 1988). The chemical shift artifact is of particular importance in orbital scanning because it can be misinterpreted as an anatomic structure or a pathological process, particularly in the case of optic nerve sheath complex or superior ophthalmic veins. The artifact, which consists of a black band on one side and a bright band on the other side of a structure (Fig. 16-6), results from the fact that fat and water protons are found in different electron environments and therefore resonate at slightly different frequencies (Babcock 1985).

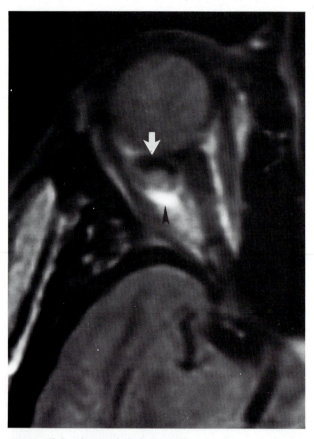

***Figure 16-6*** **Chemical shift MR artifact** demonstrated adjacent to a probable small hemangioma on an axial PDWI. It consists of a black stripe (white arrow) anterior to the small mass and a bright stripe (arrowhead) posterior to the mass.

# NORMAL ANATOMY OF THE ORBIT

## Orbital Walls

The orbit is a pyramidal bony compartment that houses the eyeball and its functional components (extraocular muscles, blood vessels, nerves, lacrimal gland, and fat) (Tadmor 1978; Last 1968). The orbital walls separate the intraorbital components from the surrounding brain and facial structures (Hesselink 1978).

The roof of the orbit (Fig. 16-2) is formed for the most part by the orbital plate of the frontal bone and separates the orbit from the anterior cranial fossa. The lacrimal gland (Figs. 16-1, 16-2) forms the lacrimal fossa in the superolateral aspect of the orbit. Overall, the bone that forms the roof of the orbit is relatively thin. To a variable extent, the frontal sinus and sometimes the ethmoid sinuses extend into the roof of the orbit (Fig. 16-2E). The posterior component of the roof of the orbit that is formed by the lesser wing of the sphenoid may also contain air cells derived from either the posterior ethmoidal cells or the sphenoid sinus.

The floor of the orbit (Figs. 16-2, 16-3) is composed primarily of the orbital plate of the maxilla. It has a triangular shape, with contributions from portions of the zygoma and the palatine bone. The infraorbital nerve and the infraorbital vessels course in the infraorbital groove and the infraorbital canal in the floor of the orbit. The orbital floor is thin, except at its most anterior margin, where the orbital rim is formed; the rim is a thicker osseous structure that is in continuity below with the anterior wall of the maxillary sinus. The floor of the orbit separates the intraorbital structures from the maxillary sinus (Fig. 16-2), which lies beneath.

The lateral wall of the orbit is formed by the zygoma (Figs. 16-1, 16-2) anteriorly and the greater wing of the sphenoid posteriorly (Figs. 16-1, 16-2). The lateral orbital wall is the thickest and strongest of the orbital walls. Lateral to this structure lies the temporal fossa, which contains the temporalis muscle.

The medial wall (Figs. 16-1, 16-2) is the thinnest component of the orbital walls. It serves to separate the orbital contents from the ethmoid and sphenoid air cells. Contributions to the structure of the medial wall are made by the maxilla, the lacrimal bone, the ethmoid bone, and the body of the sphenoid. The largest component is the one contributed by the ethmoidal orbital plate (lamina papyracea).

## Orbital Fissures and Canals

At the apex of the pyramidal structure of the orbit lie three openings that communicate with adjacent extraorbital areas (Daniels 1995).

The optic canal (Figs. 16-1, 16-2) is formed by the sphenoid bone and serves to conduct the optic nerve and the ophthalmic artery between the orbit and the middle cranial fossa. The optic nerve is surrounded by a small subarachnoid space that contains cerebrospinal fluid and is surrounded by the arachnoid. In the optic canal the ophthalmic artery lies beneath the optic nerve. The roof of the optic canal measures 10 to 12 mm in length and is formed by the lesser wing of the sphenoid. The medial wall of the optic canal is formed by the body of the sphenoid bone, whereas inferior and lateral walls are formed by the roots of the lesser wing of the sphenoid (optic strut), which also separates the optic canal from the superior orbital fissure.

The superior orbital fissure (Fig. 16-2) is a space between the greater and lesser wings of the sphenoid. It is separated medially from the optic canal by the optic strut. Transmitted through the superior orbital fissure between the middle cranial fossa and the orbit are the ophthalmic veins; the third, fourth, and sixth cranial nerves; and the first division of the fifth cranial nerve.

The inferior orbital fissure (Fig. 16-2) permits communication between the orbit and the pterygopalatine and infratemporal fossae. Through it runs the zygomatic nerve and the communication between the inferior ophthalmic vein and the pterygoid venous plexus. The maxilla, the palatine bone, and the greater wing of the sphenoid bone contribute to its margins.

## Periosteum

Periosteum, also referred to as *periorbita*, lines the bones of the orbit and is in communication with the periosteum (dura mater) covering the intracranial compartment through the various fissures. An intricate system of connective tissue septa exists throughout the orbital fat and provides support for the orbital structures (Koornneef 1979). The septum orbitale (Fig. 16-1) is a periosteal reflection from the anterior orbital margin that is continuous with the tarsal plates. It serves to separate the orbit into preseptal and postseptal components. The intraorbital fat is limited anteriorly by the orbital septum. The eyelids lie anterior to the orbital septum.

## Orbital Soft Tissue

The wall of the globe consists of three layers. The innermost—the retina—contains the nerve elements that allow visual perception. The middle layer consists of the choroid, ciliary body, and iris. These three components are also referred to as the *uvea* and have vascular, nutritive, and temperature-regulating functions. The outermost layer is a fibrous protective coat that constitutes the sclera and, anteriorly, the transparent cornea. The lens (Figs. 16-1, 16-3) is a transparent crystalline body approximately 1 cm in diameter that transmits and focuses light; it lies between the iris and the vitreous humor (Figs. 16-1, 16-3). Between the cornea and the lens is a space containing the aqueous humor that is divided by the iris into an anterior chamber and a posterior chamber.

The optic nerve (Figs. 16-1 through 16-3), which is the second cranial nerve, extends from the papilla on the posterior surface of the globe to the optic chiasm. Its length is 35 to 50 mm, with the intraorbital component 20 to 30 mm, the intracanalicular portion 4 to 9 mm, and the intracranial portion 3 to 6 mm. The diameter of the optic nerve is approximately 3 to 4 mm. Running beneath the optic nerve as it enters the optic canal from the intracranial compartment is the ophthalmic artery, which remains beneath the optic nerve in its intracanalicular segment and initial intraorbital segment and then crosses medially, usually over (approximately 80 percent) the nerve. Surrounding the optic nerve sheath complex throughout its intraorbital course is the central orbital fat.

Six extraocular muscles (Figs. 16-1 through 16-3) insert on the sclera: the medial and lateral recti, the superior and inferior recti, and the superior and inferior oblique muscles. The superior rectus is the longest, 40 mm, with the medial, lateral, and inferior recti being of progressively shorter length. The medial rectus has the largest diameter of the ocular muscles. The superior oblique muscle is the thinnest muscle and lies in the superomedial aspect of the orbit. The levator palpebrae superioris muscle lies just under the roof of the orbit as a thin flat structure above the superior rectus. It attaches to the skin of the upper eyelid. Below the superior rectus muscle lies the superior ophthalmic vein, below which lies the optic nerve. The lateral rectus lies adjacent to the periosteum of the lateral orbital wall, and only anteriorly does a slight amount of fat intervene between the periosteum and the muscle. The medial rectus is separated from the lamina papyracea by some orbital fat. The posterior portion of the inferior rectus muscle lies in contact with the floor of the orbit, but its anterior portion is separated from the roof of the maxillary sinus by orbital fat.

Orbital fat (Figs. 16-1 through 16-3) fills the space that is not occupied by the globe, nerves, muscles, or vessels. It extends from the orbital septum anteriorly and from the optic nerve to the orbital walls. It is divided by an incomplete intermuscular membrane into a central portion and a more peripheral (extramuscular) portion. The periphery fat lies between the periosteum of the orbital walls and the rectus muscles. The orbital fat is crossed by an extensive network of connective tissue septa (Koornneef 1977).

The superior ophthalmic vein (Figs. 16-1 through 16-3) forms at the root of the nose, at the juncture of the frontal and angular veins, and enters the orbit, passing around the trochlea for the superior oblique muscle. After coursing posterosuperiorly for a very short segment, it passes posterolaterally into the muscle cone and comes to lie adjacent to the inferior surface of the superior rectus muscle. It then turns posteromedially to course between the superior rectus and lateral rectus muscles. At the orbital apex, it is joined by the inferior ophthalmic vein and enters the superior orbital fissure (Bilaniuk 1977). After it passes through the superior orbital fissure, it joins the cavernous sinus. The diameter of the superior ophthalmic vein varies

from 2 to 3.5 mm and can change with head position. Asymmetry may be present in a normal patient.

A small space filled with cerebrospinal fluid surrounds the optic nerve. The space lies within a meningeal sheath and extends from the optic canal forward to the papilla. The size of the space varies, and its degree of communication with the chiasmatic cistern also may vary (Haughton 1980). Entrance of both Pantopaque (Tabaddor 1973) and air (Tenner 1968) has been reported at the time of myelography and pneumocephalography. Radiographic visualization of the space has not been a regular phenomenon and has

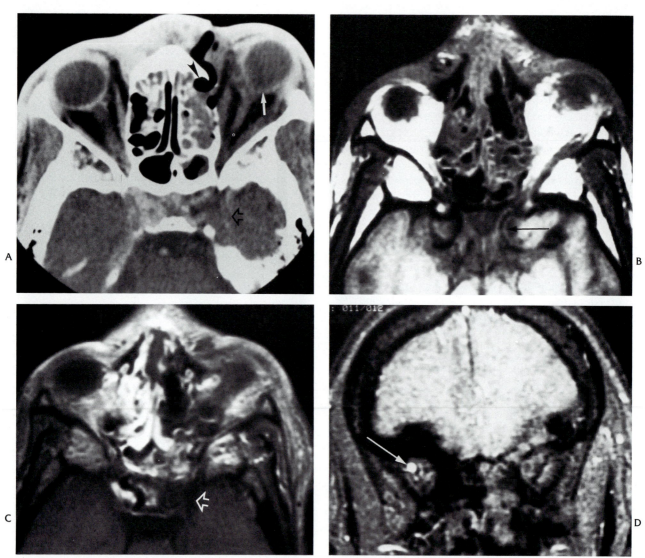

***Figure 16-7*** Paranasal sinus **mucormycosis** with extension into the orbit and cavernous sinus in a diabetic 19-year-old man. **A.** Axial CE CT. Ethmoid sinuses are opacified, and there is air (arrowhead) escaping from the left ethmoid sinus because of destruction of the lamina papyracea. There is proptosis and tenting of the left globe (white arrow). Inflammatory process surrounds the globe and has produced irregularity of the rectus muscles. The left cavernous sinus (open arrow) has not opacified with contrast material. **B.** Axial MRI

obtained 1 day later. The left intracavernous internal carotid artery (arrow) is of decreased caliber and has a thickened wall, indicating inflammation. **C.** CE MR shows lack of normal enhancement in the left cavernous sinus (arrow). There is swelling of the left facial tissues. **D.** Coronal gradient echo MRI (TR 150/TE 15, flip angle 50°) shows no evidence of flow in the left superior ophthalmic vein (compare with the normal right superior ophthalmic vein, arrow).

carried the risk of optic nerve injury (Tabaddor 1973). Water-soluble intrathecal contrast medium opacifies the intracranial subarachnoid space, putting into relief the structures which lie within, such as the optic chiasm. Opacification of the perioptic subarachnoid space has been recognized on CT after the intrathecal injection of metrizamide (Fox 1979; Manelfe 1978; Jinkins 1986). However, the subarachnoid space surrounding the optic nerve can be seen frequently on coronal T$_2$-weighted MR images without the injection of contrast material. The multiplanar capability of MR, particularly in sagittal scans along the long axis of the orbit, permits visualization of the optic nerve even when it is tortuous (Fig. 16-3) (Bilaniuk 1990a). High-resolution CT and MR, without and with intravenously injected contrast material, have obviated the need for intrathecal contrast instillation for the evaluation of possible optic nerve pathology.

## ORBITAL INFLAMMATION

## Bacterial Infection

Bacterial infection of the orbit is most often due to sinus infection, a foreign body, skin infection, or bacteremia (Krohel 1982). Fungal infection, such as aspergillosis or mucormycosis, can produce extensive osteomyelitis and tends to occur in diabetic (Fig. 16-7) or immunocompromised patients (McGill 1980; Zinreich 1988). The orbital septum, the reflected periosteum from the anterior bony margin of the orbit, functions as a barrier that prevents preseptal cellulitis from extending back into the orbital

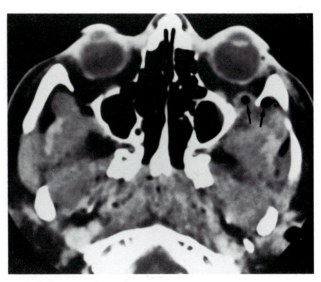

**Figure 16-9** **Orbital abscess** secondary to maxillary sinus infection which resulted from tooth extraction. Axial NCCT demonstrates air entering the orbit posterolaterally. The air collection in the orbit is contained by soft tissue reaction. There is loss of tissue planes in the infratemporal fossa.

soft tissues (Fig. 16-8) (Kaplan 1976). However, eventually the postseptal portion of the orbit may become involved by bacterial infection transmitted through the orbital septum. Also, the infection may extend into the orbit proper along venous pathways, along fissures (Fig. 16-9), or through the orbital wall and then through the periosteum (Fig. 16-7).

The chief clinical manifestation of orbital infection is swelling and redness of the eyelids—either edematous swelling or actual cellulitis. In either situation, adequate physical examination of the eye is often difficult or impossible, and the extent of the infection cannot be delineated or its source determined clinically.

The absence of valves in the facial veins (including the orbit and the paranasal sinuses) leads to the free transmission of elevated pressure between the sinus and the orbit. In children and adolescents, orbital infection is most often a concomitant of sinusitis. Increased pressure in the sinus cavity is transmitted to the orbit and causes preseptal edema. Septic thrombophlebitis leads to cellulitis and may lead to orbital cellulitis. Direct extension of infection through congenital osseous dehiscences or involvement of the thin bony walls of the orbit by osteomyelitis can lead to the formation of a subperiosteal abscess (Fig. 16-10, 16-11). The orbital periosteum is loosely attached except at the suture line, so that subperiosteal collections are easily formed. In a young child with ethmoid sinusitis, the subperiosteal collection forms along the medial orbital wall and produces lateral proptosis of the globe (Fig. 16-11). In an adolescent or adult with frontal sinusitis, the subperiosteal collection is in the

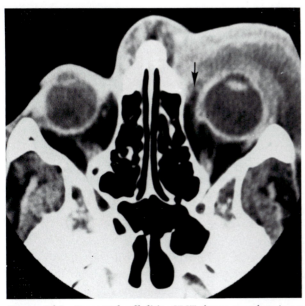

**Figure 16-8** **Preseptal cellulitis.** CECT shows an enhancing mass anterior to orbital septum (arrow) with normal retrobulbar fat.

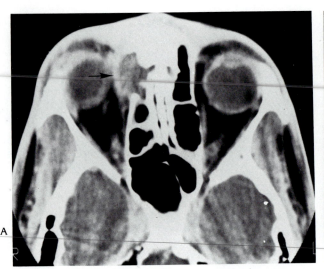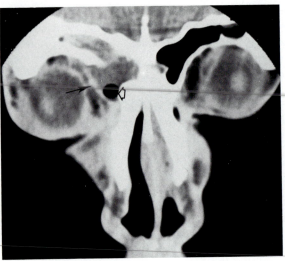

**Figure 16-10   A,B. Subperiosteal abscess** on CECT. Soft tissue density extending from the right fronttoethmoid sinus into the orbit. Note focal defect in the nonexpanded sinus wall, enhancing the periosteal lining (arrow) and air within abscess (open arrow).

superior aspect of the orbit and produces anterior and downward displacement of the globe.

Both CT and MR show the extent of involvement of soft tissues by infection; however, CT is more precise in demonstrating the bony changes (osteitis or erosion). Zimmerman (1980*a*) reported a series of 18 patients with orbital infection with or without cerebral

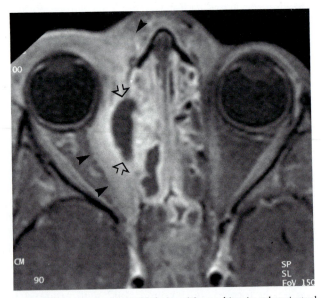

**Figure 16-11**   Right **ethmoidal sinusitis** resulting in subperiosteal abscess and orbital cellulitis. Axial CEMR with fat suppression results in definition of a subperiosteal abscess (open arrows) which is of low intensity. This results in marked lateral displacement and enlargement of the right medial rectus muscle (arrowheads). There is bilateral ethmoidal sinusitis which is more severe on the right.

complications who were studied with CT. All cases of acute orbital cellulitis showed preseptal swelling, and the majority showed proptosis, scleral thickening, subperiosteal abscesses, and occasionally infection of the peripheral surgical space. Intracranial complications such as frontal lobe cerebritis and epidural inflammation are well shown by CT and MR. Soft tissue scarring of the retrobulbar space can be seen years after bacterial orbital cellulitis. In patients with trauma or a foreign body, CT not only localizes the radiodense foreign body but also demonstrates intraorbital, subperiosteal, and intracranial abscesses (Zimmerman 1980*a*; Bilaniuk 1984).

Infection within the orbit proper can be classified as (1) intraconic, within the muscle cone (central surgical space), (2) extraconic, extrinsic to the intermuscular fibrous septum (within the peripheral surgical space), or (3) subperiosteal, between the orbital wall and its periosteal covering. Most cases of postseptal cellulitis are limited to the extraconal space (Towbin 1986). Infection of the central surgical space obliterates the soft tissue planes that exist normally between the optic-nerve-sheath complex, the orbital fat, and the rectus muscles. The intraconic fat shows abnormal density on CT and abnormal intensity on MR. Infection in the peripheral surgical space obliterates the plane between the rectus muscles, the peripheral fat, and the wall of the orbit. Infection in the subperiosteal space is demonstrated by displacement of the contrast-enhanced periosteal membrane away from the orbital wall (Fig. 16-10). The infection may be limited to one structure of the orbit, such as the lacrimal sac, which can become markedly distended by pus (Fig. 16-12).

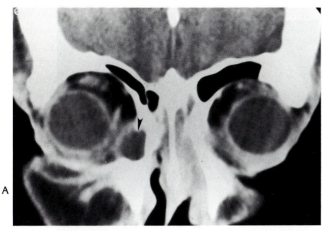 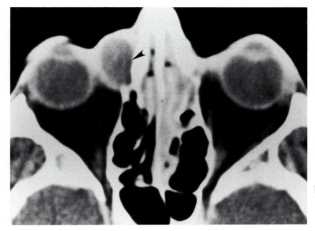

*Figure 16-12* **Dacryocystitis** with pyocele formation. Coronal **(A)** and axial **(B)** CECT show marked dilatation of the right lacrimal sac (arrowhead).

The lacrimal sac can also become enlarged as a result of obstruction, which can be secondary to a tumor (Fig. 16-13).

Both CT (Handler 1991) and MR are very helpful in the evaluation of patients with orbital infection. Treatment of orbital infection, whether medical or surgical, must be timely, specific, and sufficient. It is imperative that the disease process be recognized quickly and

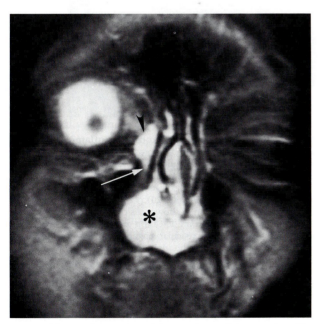

*Figure 16-13* **Obstruction** of the nasolacrimal duct produced by a **chondroid nasal tumor.** A coronal MRI (3000/90; 5 mm) shows a dilated lacrimal sac (arrowhead), a dilated nasolacrimal duct (arrow) extending inferiorly from the sac, and an expansile nasal tumor (asterisk). On this $T_2$WI both the tumor and the sac show increased intensity. On CE MR (not shown) the tumor enhanced, but not the lacrimal sac or the nasolacrimal duct.

treated aggressively and that operative drainage be carried out whenever indicated. A diffuse inflammatory process or small subperiosteal collections can be treated medically and followed with imaging studies. Larger subperiosteal abscesses must be drained, often along with the offending infected sinuses. The dangers of epidural or subdural empyemas, meningitis, or cavernous sinus thrombosis are real and carry with them, even in the antibiotic era, significant morbidity and mortality (Kaplan 1976; Clayman 1991). Once infection has extended into the cavernous sinus or beyond, MR is the procedure of choice. MR demonstrates and characterizes the cavernous sinus better and is more sensitive in showing a thrombosis (Fig. 16-7) and intracranial sites of inflammation. The consequences of inadequate treatment remain potentially catastrophic because blindness and death may result from meningitis, vasculitis, and extensive brain infection. The consequences of cerebritis and cerebral abscess formation, even when the condition is adequately treated, may include seizures, motor weakness, and psychological aberrations.

## Idiopathic Orbital Inflammation (Pseudotumor)

Between the ages of 10 and 40, the most common cause of an intraorbital mass is idiopathic orbital inflammation (orbital pseudotumor) (Bernardino 1977). The classic clinical triad includes proptosis, pain, and impaired ocular motility. To a variable degree there may also be diplopia, decreased vision, papillitis, and retinal striae. The symptomatology and clinical signs simulate those of an intraorbital tumor. Orbital pseudotumor is one of the most common causes of unilateral exophthalmos (Bernardino 1977), but bilaterality is common (Rothfus 1984; Dresner 1984).

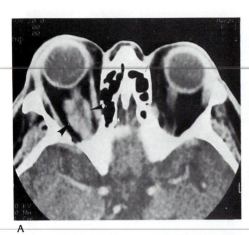

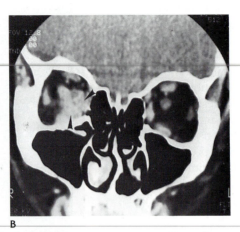

*Figure 16-17 A,B. Pseudotumor* on CECT. Enhancing irregular intraconal mass (arrowheads) surrounding the right optic nerve.

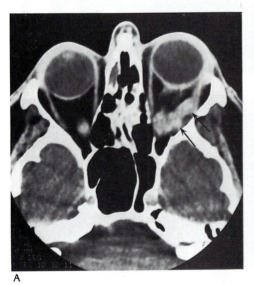

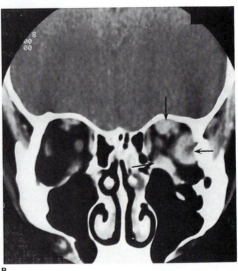

*Figure 16-18 Pseudotumor* on CECT. Involvement of left superior, lateral, and inferior rectus muscles (arrows) demonstrated on a coronal image. Note sparing of the left medial rectus, in contrast to thyroid myositis.

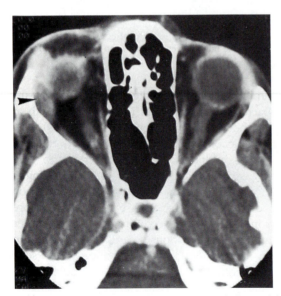

*Figure 16-19 Pseudotumor* on CECT. Mass in right lacrimal fossa (arrowhead) as the sole manifestation of pseudotumor.

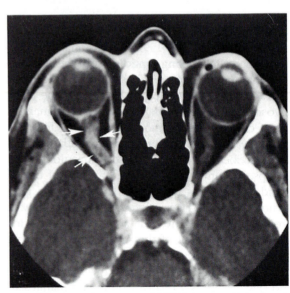

*Figure 16-20 Pseudotumor* on CECT. Enhancing thickening along the periphery of the right optic nerve/sheath complex ("tram-track" sign), mimicking optic nerve meningioma (arrows).

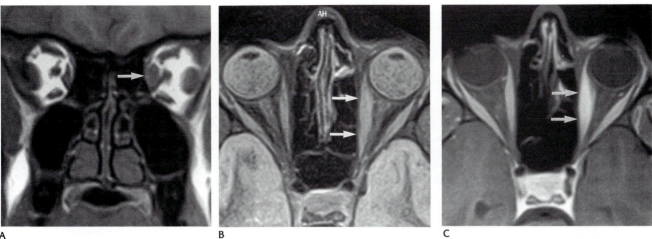

A   B   C

***Figure 16-21*** **Myositis** of the left medial rectus muscle. **A.** Coronal $T_1$-weighted MR shows enlarged left medial rectus muscle (arrows). **B.** Axial inversion recovery MR image again demonstrates well de-lineated but enlarged left medial rectus muscle (arrows). **C.** Axial MR following contrast enhancement and fat suppression shows increased enhancement of the enlarged left medial rectus muscle (arrows). The muscle is well defined and the adjacent fatty tissue appears normal in intensity.

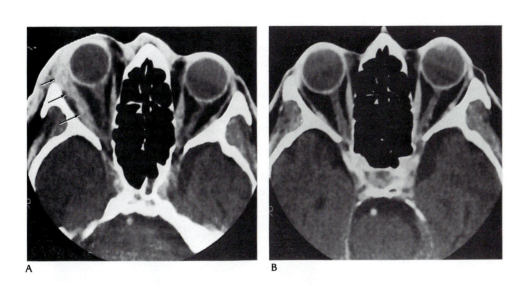

A   B

***Figure 16-22*** **Pseudotumor** on CECT. **A.** Enlarged right lateral rectus with involvement of inser-tion and lacrimal gland (arrows), on presentation. **B.** After steroid therapy, there was total resolu-tion.

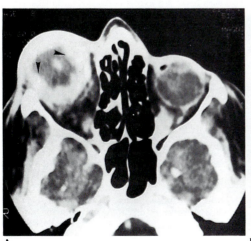

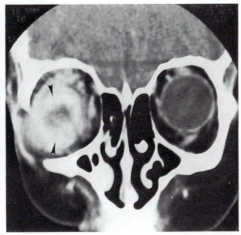

A   B

***Figure 16-23*** **A,B.** **Endoph-thalmitis-periophthalmitis.** CECT shows markedly thickened, enhancing ill-defined sclera with streaky densities in retrobulbar fat. Lobulated thickened soft tissue within the peripheral vitreous (arrowheads) indicates endoph-thalmitis.

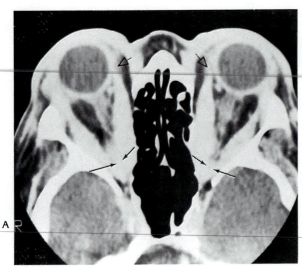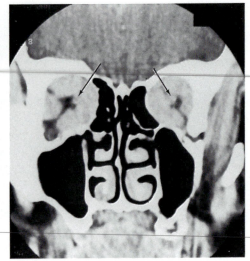

*Figure 16-24*   **A,B. Thyroid ophthalmopathy.** Bilateral marked enlargement of all extraocular muscles with typical tapering at insertions (open arrowheads). Streaky increased densities in fat can be seen in severe thyroid ophthalmopathy as well as pseudotumor. Note compression of optic nerves at the orbital apex on axial **(A)** and coronal **(B)** NCCT (arrows).

including lymphoma and metastatic carcinoma (breast), as well as retrobulbar hemorrhage. MR aids in the differential diagnosis by specifically identifying blood products. Also, metastatic breast carcinoma usually becomes hyperintense on $T_2$-weighted spin-echo images, whereas a pseudotumor is typically hypointense (Atlas 1987*a*).

## Thyroid Exophthalmos

The exophthalmos of Graves' disease is of unknown etiology. Inflammatory infiltration and proliferation of connective tissue occur in the soft tissues of the orbit, especially the extraocular muscles (Alper 1977).

The histopathological picture of the muscles in Graves' disease is similar to that found in idiopathic orbital inflammation (Jones 1979). It is possible that autoimmune responses cause both the thyroid exophthalmos of Graves' disease and the changes associated with idiopathic orbital inflammation. Most easily recognized is the massive swelling of the extraocular muscles (Fig. 16-24), which may be enlarged volumetrically up to eight times their normal size. Infiltration of the muscles by lymphocytes, plasma cells, and mast cells and deposition of hydrophilic mucopolysaccharides account for their enlargement. When the condition occurs in association with thyrotoxicosis, the orbital fat content may be increased (Peyster 1986) (Fig. 16-25). However, increased orbital fat may also be seen in Cushing's disease or syndrome and in obesity (Cohen 1981; Carlson 1982). The increase in volume of the orbital tissues produces proptosis. Ulceration of the

cornea, occlusion of the central retinal vein or artery, and compressive optic neuropathy may be seen as a result. Muscle dysfunction occurs, and ocular motility is impaired. Pain is usually not a feature of thyroid ophthalmopathy, unlike with idiopathic orbital inflammation, where pain is a significant symptom.

The exact incidence of thyroid exophthalmos is not known. It occurs in both hyperthyroid and euthyroid patients. It may precede clinical hyperthyroidism. Its presentation is usually bilateral; it is unilateral in 5 to 10 percent of cases (Rothfus 1984; Peyster 1986). The

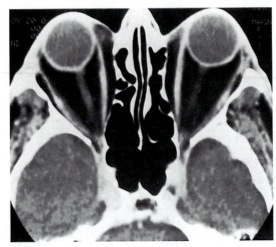

*Figure 16-25*   **Thyroid ophthalmopathy.** NCCT shows bilateral proptosis with a marked increase in orbital fat, bowing the orbital septum and separating the medial rectus from the medially bowed lamina papyracea.

classic, mild form is characterized clinically by a prominent stare, mild proptosis, eyelid retraction, and lid lag (Alper 1977). This is most frequently found associated with thyrotoxicosis in young females, and it is bilateral. Most often the patient is asymptomatic (Alper 1977). Typically, the more severe clinical form occurs in middle-aged patients and is associated with the gradual onset of severe proptosis and varying degrees of ophthalmoplegia. Thyrotoxicosis is usually present. Overall, women predominate in the incidence of both thyroid disease (4:1) and Graves' exophthalmos (Alper 1977). However, the female predominance decreases with age (Rootman 1988).

Soon after the introduction of CT, its efficacy in the study of Graves' disease was recognized (Brismar 1976; Enzmann 1976). This was followed by reports of studies correlating CT results with the pathological and clinical features of Graves' ophthalmopathy (Enzmann 1979; Trokel 1981). Eventually quantitative CT methods were developed for the evaluation of extraocular muscles and orbital fat (Feldon 1982; Forbes 1986). More recently Nugent (1990) reported the clinical and quantifiable nonvolumetric high-resolution CT data from 142 orbits of patients with Graves' orbitopathy and from 40 orbits of subjects without Graves' disease.

Graves' disease accounts for more cases of unilateral and bilateral exophthalmos in the adult than does any other single disease entity (Enzmann 1976; Jacobs 1980). Although an imaging study, either CT or MRI, is not always necessary for the diagnosis of Graves' disease, it is useful in indicating the degree of muscle involvement and in identifying bilaterality when there is ophthalmopathy without clinical or laboratory evidence or a history of thyroid disease (Enzmann 1979; Nugent 1990). CT is preferred to MR in presurgical evaluation, since it provides the greatest detail about the bony walls. CT or MR is useful for evaluating the results of orbital decompressive surgery. In the transverse section, the inferior and superior recti are cut tangentially (Fig. 16-1). These muscles are better evaluated either in the coronal projection (Fig. 16-2) or on reformed sagittal CT sections. In a direct sagittal CT section, the inferior and superior recti are visualized in their entire length, and so minimal changes of Graves' disease can be recognized (Wing 1979). The muscles can be demonstrated easily in multiple planes and characterized according to $T_2$ relaxation time (Oshnishi 1994) with MRI without having the patient assume an uncomfortable position, not the case with CT. The plane of sectioning can be optimized for each muscle or for the optic nerve sheath complex. Also, MR provides better resolution and the ability to identify the optic nerve sheath complex when there is crowding of structures at the orbital apex as a result of the enlarged muscles.

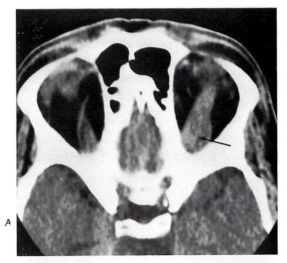

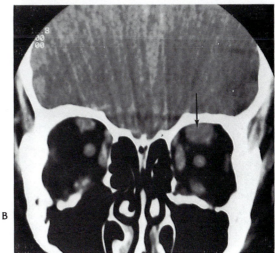

***Figure 16-26*** **Thyroid ophthalmopathy.** Isolated enlargement of the left superior rectus muscle (arrow) on axial **(A)** and coronal **(B)** NCCT.

Enzmann (1979) reported the CT findings in 107 hyperthyroid and 9 euthyroid patients with thyroid ophthalmopathy. CT revealed bilateral involvement (Fig. 16-24) in 85 percent, unilateral involvement (Fig. 16-26) in 5 percent, and no abnormality in 10 percent. Seventy percent of Enzmann's patients with bilateral involvement had symmetrical muscle disease, whereas 30 percent had asymmetrical muscle involvement. Most commonly, all four of the recti mentioned above were involved (Fig. 16-24). The inferior and medial recti were involved in approximately three-fourths of the cases and had the most severe degree of enlargement, whereas the superior and lateral recti were involved in approximately half the cases and had a lesser degree of enlargement. Indeed, any or all extraocular muscles may be involved in nearly any combination. However, if isolated lateral rectus enlargement exists, another etiology is suggested. Enzmann (1979) found a rough linear parallel between the clinical assessment of the degree of ophthalmopathy and the severity of muscle enlargement. However, no correlation was found between the degree of muscle enlargement and the degree of abnormal thyroid function. Enzmann pointed out that in 6 of 12 patients who had given a clinical impression of unilateral disease, CT revealed the presence of bilateral disease.

Forbes (1986) found a higher frequency of abnormal changes on CT in hyperthyroid patients with Graves' disease without clinical ophthalmopathy than had previously been reported. He obtained pixel-calibrated measurements of muscle and fat in the orbits of 72 patients with Graves' disease and found abnormal measurements in 87 percent of those with clinically detectable ophthalmopathy and in 70 percent of hyperthyroid patients without clinical eye signs. Overall, the medial and inferior muscles were the most fre-

quently involved. Among patients with ophthalmopathy, 46 percent had both muscle enlargement and fat increase and 8 percent had only an increase in fat. Among the seven patients with unilateral clinical ophthalmopathy, six were found on CT to have abnormalities in the contralateral orbit.

In his study, Nugent (1990) obtained measurements directly from CT scans. He and his coworkers found muscle enlargement in all their patients with ophthalmopathy, but especially in those with optic neuropathy. In this study the superior muscle group was most frequently involved (63.4 percent), followed by medial (61.3 percent) and inferior (57 percent) recti. The most common pattern was involvement of all five muscles that were measured. Solitary involvement was most frequent in the superior muscle group (6.3 percent). Enlargement of the optic nerve sheath and the superior ophthalmic vein was noted in cases of optic neuropathy.

## Optic Neuritis

Optic neuritis, an inflammatory infectious or demyelinating process involving any part of the optic nerve, is clinically diagnosed on the basis of loss of visual acuity and visual field changes. It may be associated with inflammation in other portions of the visual pathway or more extensive intracranial inflammation. Most frequently, optic neuritis is a manifestation of multiple sclerosis (Sandberg-Wollheim 1990; Brodsky 1994), but it may represent other disease entities, among them vasculitis (Sklar 1996). High-resolution contrast-enhanced CT and particularly contrast-enhanced MR can demonstrate changes that are due to optic neuritis: swelling and contrast enhancement (Merandi 1991) (Figs. 16-27, 16-28, 16-29). The process also can be

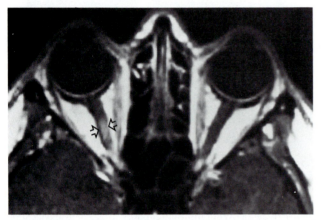

***Figure 16-27*** Right **optic neuritis** in a 26-year-old woman. Axial CE MR (600/22; Gd-DTPA) shows enhancement of the intraorbital optic nerve (arrows) on the right side.

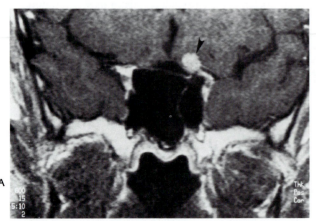
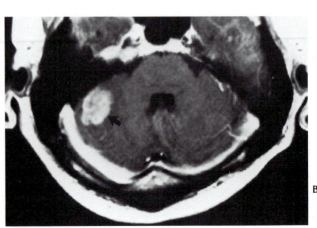

***Figure 16-28*** Left **optic neuritis** in a 38-year-old man with multiple sclerosis. **A.** CE MR (600/15; Gd-DTPA) shows enlarged prominently enhancing intracranial portion of the left optic nerve (arrowhead). **B.** CE MR of the posterior fossa reveals a large region (arrow) of abnormal contrast enhancement in the periphery of the right cerebellar hemisphere; it was thought to represent a demyelinating plaque.

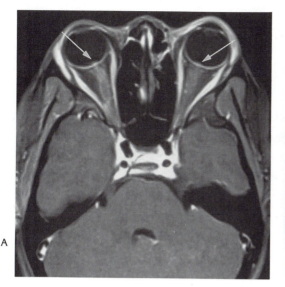 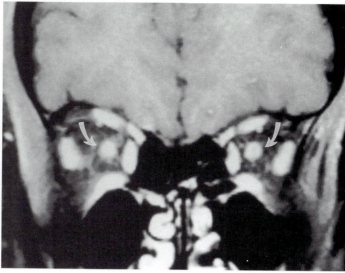

*Figure 16-29*  **Bilateral optic neuritis with papillitis. A.** Prominent enlargement of the optic nerve sheath complexes as well as optic nerve heads (arrows). **B.** Coronal CEMR with fat saturation reveals enlargement and prominent enhancement of both optic nerve sheath complexes (arrows).

shown to involve the chiasm (Bilaniuk 1993). In such instances, the enlarged chiasm needs to be differentiated from chiasmal sarcoidosis (Walker 1990; Carmody 1994) and chiasmal neoplasms.

## ORBITAL TRAUMA

A blow to the face or head may result in injury to the osseous orbit and the orbital soft tissues. An overlying soft tissue hematoma may preclude adequate physical examination of the orbit. In such circumstances, CT is a useful adjunct in demonstrating the presence or absence of underlying osseous and soft tissue injury (Figs. 16-30, 16-31). CT is the procedure of choice because of its ability to show bone detail and acute hemorrhage and demonstrate foreign bodies. MR is contraindicated whenever the mode of injury is uncertain and there is a possibility of a ferromagnetic foreign body. Also, on MR, acute orbital hemorrhage may be difficult to detect, and differentiation between air bubbles and bone fragments may be difficult. However, MR can be a useful adjunct in the evaluation of orbital trauma by providing information on anatomic disruption (Fig. 16-32) in multiple planes as well as demonstrating associated intracranial traumatic lesions if they have occurred and which initially may not be clinically apparent. Also, MR can demonstrate a chronic or subacute intramuscular hemorrhage (Fig. 16-33), which on CT may appear as a mass. Fractures of the orbit are classifiable as external (e.g., a tripod fracture of the zygoma and anterior orbital rim) (Fig. 16-34) or internal

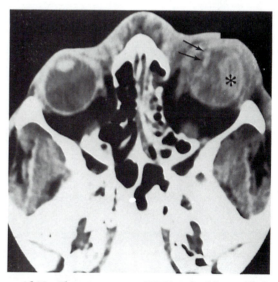

*Figure 16-30*  **Blunt trauma** on NCCT. Left globe is filled with hemorrhage (asterisk). Lens is disrupted (arrows). Note that a medial wall blowout fracture has opacified the left ethmoid sinus.

(a blowout fracture into the ethmoid or maxillary sinuses) (Figs. 16-31 and 16-35 through 16-38). In fractures of the orbital floor it is more often the tethering of the muscles caused by prolapsed orbital fat and the connective tissue (Fig. 16-36), rather than the actual entrapment of the muscles, that results in abnormalities of ocular motility (Koornneef 1977, 1979). Both CT and MR are able to demonstrate herniation of the soft tissue contents into the maxillary sinus (Grove 1978;

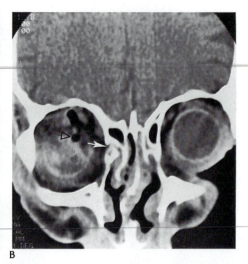

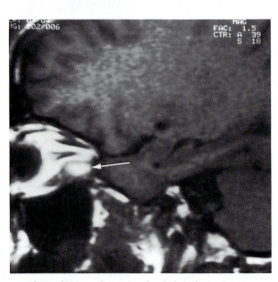

**Figure 16-31 Blowout fracture. A,B.** Medial wall fracture with ruptured globe. Axial **(A)** and coronal **(B)** NCCT demonstrates right medial wall blowout fracture (arrow) and orbital emphysema. Signs of ruptured globe include distortion of normal shape with intravitreal hemorrhage and intraocular air (open arrow). The lens cannot be identified. Note extensive preseptal hemorrhage (asterisk).

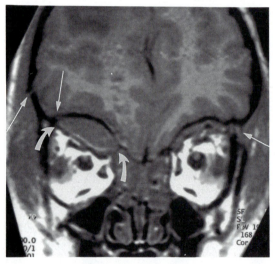

**Figure 16-32 Craniofacial trauma.** Coronal MR (T₁WI) reveals calvarial and orbital fractures (arrows). In addition there are bilateral superior subperiosteal hematomas, much larger on the right side (curved arrows).

**Figure 16-33 Hemorrhage in the left inferior rectus muscle.** Sagittal MR (T₁WI) demonstrates the hemorrhage (arrow) within the inferior rectus muscle.

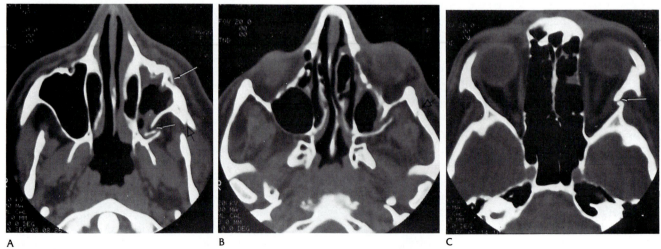

**Figure 16-34 A–C. Tripod fracture.** Axial NCCT demonstrates fractures involving anterior and lateral walls of the right maxillary sinus (arrows) and widening of the frontozygomatic suture (open arrow). Note intact pterygoids.

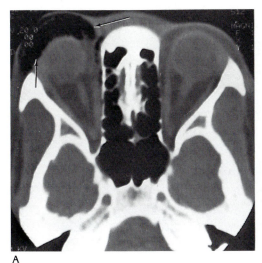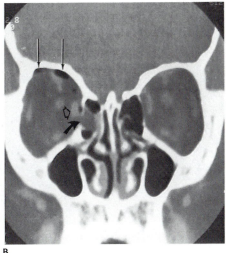

*Figure 16-35* **A,B. Medial wall fracture.** Medial orbital wall fracture (curved arrow) is best demonstrated in coronal CT **(B)**, with soft tissue and fat herniating into the right ethmoid. Medial rectus is in its normal position (open arrow). Extensive orbital emphysema is also present (straight arrows).

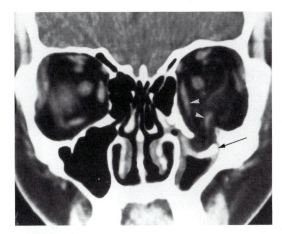

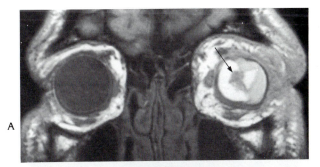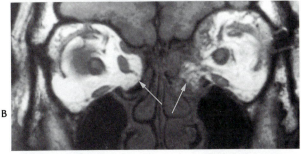

*Figure 16-36* **Blowout fracture** of the left orbital floor. Coronal CT obtained just posterior to the globes reveals a blowout fracture on the left with inferior displacement of the fracture fragment (arrow). The orbital fat has prolapsed through the defect in the floor. There is rotation and tethering of the inferior rectus muscle (arrowhead) and the medial rectus muscle (arrowhead). Note the prominent elongation of the medial rectus muscle compared with the normal side.

*Figure 16-37* **Rupture of the left globe with avulsion of the optic nerve head. A.** Coronal MRI, $T_1WI$ (600/20) shows a smaller squared-off left globe filled with blood. The central irregular hypodensity (arrow) within the globe represents the avulsed optic nerve head. There is hemorrhage and swelling of the tissues lateral to the globe. **B.** Coronal MRI, $T_1WI$ (600/20) posterior to that shown in **A** reveals bilateral medial blowout fractures (arrows), the old one on the right and the acute one on the left. Hemorrhage and edema obscure the left superior oblique and medial rectus muscles and produce an irregular reticular pattern in the orbital fat. As a result of the herniation of the fat through the fracture in the medial wall of the left orbit, the orbital structures are pulled toward the midline. Two fractures (arrows) are present in the lateral wall of the left orbit.

Hammerschlag 1982; McArdle 1986). CT also may detect an unsuspected fracture of the orbital apex (Unger 1984).

In addition to damage to the bony orbit, trauma of sufficient force and direction can lead to damage to the globe and optic nerve. Rupture of the globe is most often associated with blows to the lateral aspect of the orbit that strike the globe just anterior to the lateral wall. CT and MR demonstrate the deformity of the eyeball and the presence of intraocular hemorrhage (Figs. 16-30, 16-31, 16-37, 16-39). Direct damage to the optic nerve and perioptic bleeding (Fig. 16-38) within the subarachnoid, subdural, and/or intradural spaces can lead to loss of vision as a result of either the primary optic nerve injury or secondary optic nerve injury by vascular compression or vascular injury. Fractures in the vicinity of the optic foramen, especially those associated with local subperiosteal hemorrhage, may compress the optic nerve focally. This is an indication for emergency decompression. Intradural hemorrhage in

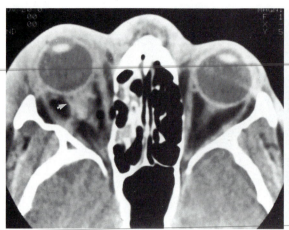

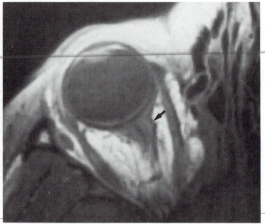

*Figure 16-38*    Orbital trauma with **perioptic hemorrhage** on the right. **A.** Axial CT shows an irregular retrobulbar hemorrhage (arrow) which obscures the optic nerve sheath complex. There is also proptosis of the right globe and swelling of the lids. There is soft tissue thickening at the insertions of the medial and lateral rectus muscles. A small amount of air has escaped into the medial extraconic space through a fracture in the medial wall of the right orbit. **B.** Axial MRI, $T_1WI$ (600/20) reveals retrobulbar irregular hypodensity (arrow) which is consistent with recent hemorrhage. The optic nerve sheath complex is obscured by the hemorrhage.

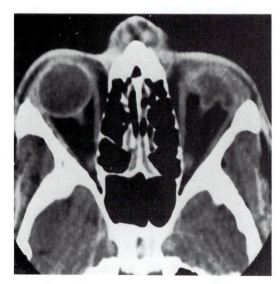

*Figure 16-39* **Perforated globe.** Left globe on axial CT is markedly decreased in size and has an abnormal configuration after a perforating injury, indicating rupture.

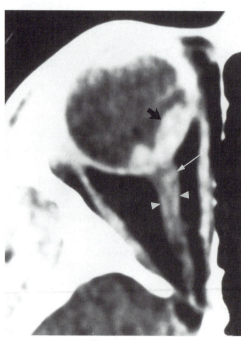

*Figure 16-40* **Posttraumatic hemorrhages.** Axial CT shows retinal detachment (black arrow) and intraneural (white arrow) and perioptic (subarachnoid) hemorrhage (arrowheads).

the optic nerve sheath occurs most frequently at the apex of the orbit, where there is a close relationship between the tendinous ring of Zinn (the site of the origin of recti) and the dura mater which divides at this site into the sheath of the optic nerve, the periorbita, and the orbital connective tissue system. The medial part of the tendinous ring is inserted into the cleft formed by the splitting of the dura into the periorbita and the perioptic sheath (Whitnall 1921). Intraneural optic nerve hemorrhage also occurs at the apex of the orbit. Subarachnoid and subdural hemorrhages occur more frequently just posterior to the papilla, where

they are associated with subhyaloid retinal hemorrhages (Lindberg 1973) (Fig. 16-40).

## Foreign Bodies

Localization of an intraorbital foreign body by routine radiographic means may be difficult. To facilitate surgical planning for removal, it is necessary to localize the

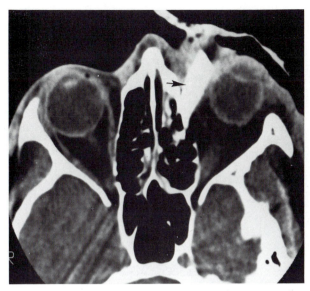

**Figure 16-41 Glass foreign body.** Axial CT demonstrates large high-attenuation glass foreign body (arrows) just medial to the left globe, leaving he globe intact.

foreign body accurately. This is easier with radiodense foreign bodies, as they are well shown on routine x-rays and CT (Figs. 16-41 through 16-43). However, CT is clearly superior to conventional radiography in demonstrating the precise anatomic location of foreign bodies within the globe and their sequelae (ruptured globe, retinal detachment, lens disruption, or vitreal hemorrhage) in patients who may be difficult to examine clinically (Sevel 1983). In addition, unsuspected fragments, retrobulbar or intracranial in location, often are detected by CT. Three-dimensional CT reconstructions are particularly helpful in the precise localization of fragments and foreign bodies (Fig. 16-42). Prognostic information may also be obtained by CT in penetrating injuries of the globe (Sternberg 1984; Brown 1985; Weisman 1983). Double penetration of the globe and optic nerve injury by foreign bodies are relevant to surgical planning and prognosis.

With a nonopaque foreign body (Fig. 16-44), such as a sponge or a wood splinter, CT or MR may show only

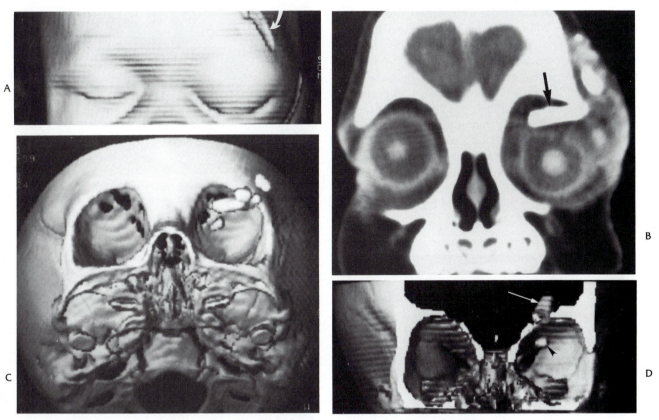

**Figure 16-42 Fracture and foreign body in the orbit and frontal lobe** resulting from the fall of an 8-month-old child onto a shot glass. **A.** A 3D reconstruction of the soft tissues reveals prominent swelling of the left eyelid and a wound (arrow) in the supraorbital region. **B.** Coronal CT reveals a large linear foreign body (arrow) which was a large fragment of the shot glass. There is rupture of the globe (it has lost its normal round configuration), as can be seen on the right. Prominent soft tissue swelling, hemorrhage, and other foreign bodies are identified in the lateral aspect of the orbit. **C.** A 3D bony reconstruction demonstrates well the multiple foreign bodies in the left orbit. They were found to represent fragments of glass. **D.** A 3D reconstruction shows well the site of the orbital roof penetration and two foreign bodies, one representing a bony fragment and a larger one representing glass (arrow). In addition, a deeper foreign body (arrowhead) can be identified intraorbitally.

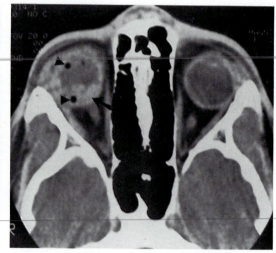

**Figure 16-43  A,B. Intraocular foreign body.** Metallic foreign body on coronal image **(A)** in vitreous, with secondary intraocular hemorrhage and air. Note subretinal hemorrhage (arrow) and air (arrowheads) on the axial CT **(B).**

what appears to be focal air (Roberts 1992; Herman 1993; Ho 1996; McGuckin 1996), or in the case of subacute or chronic trauma with foreign body, a granulomatous reaction with mass and enhancement (Macrae 1979) (Fig. 16-45). The density of a wooden foreign body depends on the hydration of the wood and ranges from very hypodense (Fig. 16-46) to the density of soft tissues. In a patient who presents with proptosis or with evidence of a granulomatous reaction in the vicinity of the orbit, consideration should be given to a forgotten trauma produced by an intraorbital foreign body. In such a case, CT is capable of revealing metallic fragments and radiodense foreign bodies such as pencil lead and glass. MR is contraindicated in patients suspected of having a ferromagnetic ocular or orbital foreign body (Kelly 1986).

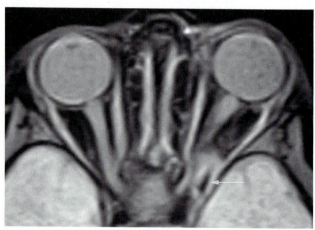

**Figure 16-45  Penetrating injury** to the left orbit with retained foreign body. Axial FLAIR image reveals a hypointense foreign body (arrow) crossing from the orbital apex through the superior orbital fissure into the anterior aspect of the left cavernous sinus. The child fell running in a field and the foreign body is believed to be organic material. The image shows it surrounded by soft tissue reaction.

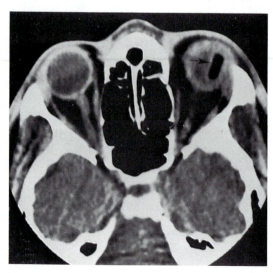

**Figure 16-44  Intraocular sponge** on CT. Intraocular air density (arrow) indicates a retained surgical sponge in the left globe.

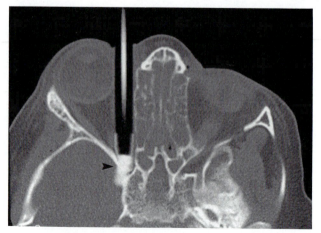

**Figure 16-46  Penetrating trauma** to the right orbit secondary to a pencil. Axial CT shows a pencil lying along the medial aspect of the right orbit, and the eraser of the pencil (arrow) crosses from the orbital apex into the region of the cavernous sinus.

## VASCULAR LESIONS

### Capillary Hemangioma

Capillary hemangiomas are the most common vascular tumors of childhood, usually appearing within the first 2 weeks of life, with a female predominance. They are nonencapsulated infiltrative tumors that consist of abnormal blood vessels and endothelial cells (Plesner-Rasmussen 1983). They usually show a growth spurt during the first 6 months, reach a plateau within 1 to 2 years, and then involute by the sixth or seventh year (Flanagan 1979). The lesions can be very large and thus can produce prominent enlargement of the bony orbit. Because these lesions involute spontaneously and often do not require treatment, it is important to differentiate them from other lesions. MR is helpful in this regard, since it demonstrates the internal architecture of these lesions (Bilaniuk 1990*c*). On CT, the lesions have irregular margins and enhance prominently and at times may be difficult to differentiate from rhabdomyosarcomas. MR reveals hemangiomas to be heterogeneous and vascular. The lesions have slightly higher intensity than does muscle and contain signal voids as a result of vessels on $T_1WI$ (Figs. 16-47, 16-48). They are hyperintense to fat on $T_2WI$ and show contrast enhancement. By demonstrating vessels within the hemangioma, MR provides more specific information than does CT.

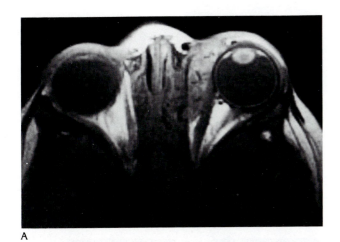

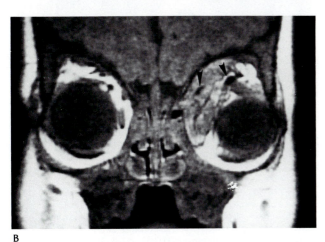

**Figure 16-47  Capillary hemangioma** in the left orbit of an 11-week-old boy. **A.** Axial MRI, $T_1WI$ (600/20) demonstrates a heterogeneous extraconic mass in the medial aspect of the left orbit. It contains linear signal voids within it, indicating vessels. **B.** Coronal MR, $T_1WI$ (600/20) shows a finely lobulated mass which has produced enlargement of the left bony orbit. Again demonstrated are signal voids (arrowheads) within the mass, indicating vessels.

### Cavernous Hemangioma

Cavernous hemangiomas show a female predominance and occur most frequently during the third and fourth decades of life (Harris 1978). They are characterized by a slowly progressive course. The symptoms consist of proptosis and difficulty with extraocular motility. Cavernous hemangioma is one of the most common benign intraorbital lesions (Forbes 1982) and is most often located within the muscle cone (Figs. 16-49 through 16-51), although some can be extraconal (Fig. 16-52).

Cavernous hemangiomas consist of large, dilated endothelium-lined vascular channels. They are considered by some not to be hemangiomas but actually to represent venous malformations (Mulliken 1988). They are encompassed by a fibrous pseudocapsule. The arterial blood supply is not prominent, and blood flow is relatively stagnant. Thus, thrombosis is not uncommon. Spontaneous hemorrhage is not a feature of this lesion. Phlebolith formation with calcification is rare (Fig. 16-49).

Imaging studies demonstrate a cavernous hemangioma as a homogeneous mass, usually within the muscle cone, with smooth margins and generally uniform contrast enhancement (Figs. 16-49, 16-52) (Davis 1980). However, a scan obtained during or immediately after the injection of contrast material may show heterogeneity caused by opacification of the large vascular channels within the lesion (Bilaniuk 1990*b*) (Fig. 16-51). On nonenhanced studies, the hemangioma appears as a dense mass on CT; on MR, it is isointense to muscle on $T_1WI$ and hyperintense to muscle on $T_2WI$. These lesions often do not deform the globe when abutting it, distinguishing hemangioma

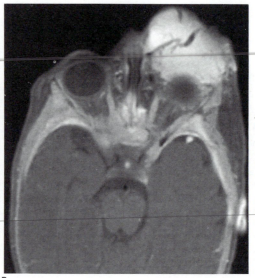

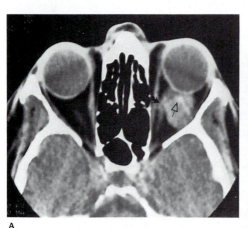

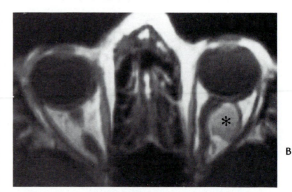

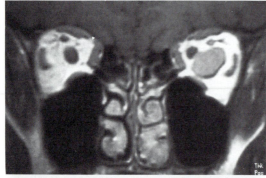

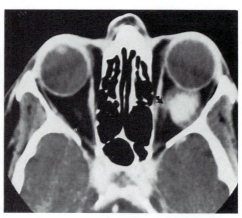

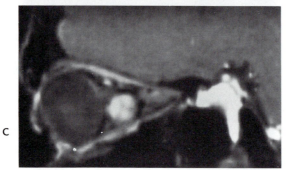

*Figure 16-48* Large **capillary hemangioma** of the left orbit. **A.** MR ($T_2$WI) shows a very large lobulated mass in the anterior aspect of the left orbit. The mass displaces the globe posteriorly. Within the mass there are hypointense curvilinear structures which represent vessels. **B.** CEMR with fat suppression shows the large capillary hemangioma which has enhanced and contained large vessels in its midportion.

*Figure 16-49* **A,B. Intraconal hemangioma.** NCCT **(A)** demonstrates a well-circumscribed intraconal mass deviating the right optic nerve (curved arrow) medially. Note artifacts emanating from a calcified phlebolith (open arrow) within the mass. Note absence of deformity of the posterior globe. Mass enhances homogeneously on CE CT **(B).**

*Figure 16-50* Presumed **cavernous hemangioma. A.** Axial CEMR (600/15 with Gd-DTPA). A well-marginated mass (asterisk) displaces the left optic nerve medially. It shows slight hypointensity in relationship to the fat. **B.** Coronal CEMR (600/15 with Gd-DTPA) shows the well-defined mass displacing the optic nerve superomedially. **C.** Contrast-enhanced fat-suppressed gradient-echo 3D acquisition reconstructed in the sagittal plane shows a slightly heterogeneous high-intensity mass inferior to the optic nerve.

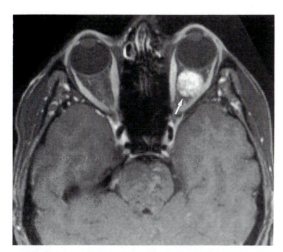

**Figure 16-51** **Cavernous hemangioma** of the left orbit. Axial CEMR with fat suppression reveals a mildly lobulated round contrast enhancing mass (arrow) in the left orbit. The mass does contain fine internal septations.

from many retrobulbar metastases (Fig. 16-53). Lymphoma is similarly a soft mass which often does not deform the globe. Expansion of the adjacent orbital wall is common, but bone destruction does not occur and, if present, suggests a more aggressive lesion. The detection on CT of a calcified phlebolith is an infrequent but highly suggestive characteristic of this lesion. In Davis' series (1980), 83 percent of the cavernous hemangiomas were intraconic, with 67 percent being lateral to the optic nerve; 22 percent of his cases extended to the orbital apex. Even small hemangiomas, if located at the apex, may produce visual symptoms. On CT, but more so on MR, it is possible to demarcate a cavernous hemangioma from the adjacent optic nerve and muscles. This is important in planning for operative removal. Because a cavernous hemangioma is encapsulated, it is easily peeled off from the extraocular

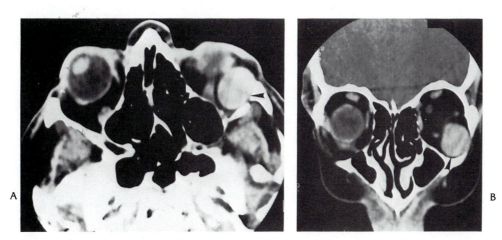

**Figure 16-52** **A,B. Extraconal hemangioma.** Well-circumscribed, homogeneously enhancing mass (arrowhead) in the inferolateral aspect of the left orbit is outside the muscle cone on axial **(A)** and coronal **(B)** CECT.

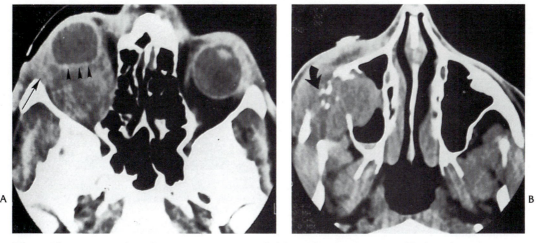

**Figure 16-53** **Metastatic melanoma** on NCCT. **A.** A slightly nonhomogeneous mass fills the right orbit, infiltrates the lacrimal gland (arrow), and deforms the posterior aspect of the globe (arrowheads). **B.** Mass destroys the right malar eminence (curved arrow) and erodes into the maxillary sinus.

muscles and the optic nerve. These tumors show no tendency to recur or undergo malignant transformation (Jones 1979). It is important to differentiate hemangioma from lymphangioma of the orbit, a lesion that is not easily removed surgically, frequently recurs, and is more often extraconic, ill defined, and less homogeneous in its enhancement.

## Lymphangioma

Lymphangiomas occur in the orbit despite there being no lymphatic tissue in the postseptal portions of the normal orbit. They most likely represent hamartomas (Jones 1979). Their histopathological spectrum includes dilated lymphatic vessels, clusters of dysplastic blood vessels, new and old blood products, lymphocytic aggregates, bundles of smooth muscle fibers, and loose connective tissue septa (Rootman 1986; Graeb 1990). The lesions are unencapsulated and often cross anatomic compartments. However, in Davis' series (1980) most of the lesions were extraconic. Lymphangiomas usually present during early childhood. In Graeb's (1990) series of 13 lymphangiomas, 11 occurred in children and 10 presented before age 6 years. Although lymphangiomas are relatively hemodynamically isolated, they show a great tendency for hemorrhage. The usual presentation of deep lesions is that of sudden proptosis caused by hemorrhage that can compress the optic nerve. In such situations emergency decompression is required. Imaging studies, particularly MR, are helpful in showing the relationship of the lesion to the optic nerve (Figs. 16-54, 16-55). On CT and MR, the lymphangiomas appear as irregularly marginated, multilobulated, poorly defined

lesions (Figs. 16-54 through 16-56) that may be heterogeneous (Fig. 16-57) and that enhance partially. The regions of enhancement correlate with the sites of the venous channels from which the hemorrhages originate (Graeb 1990). Localization of these sites is impor-

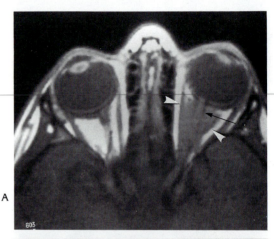

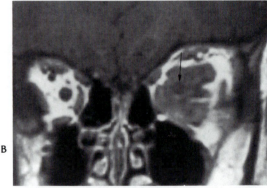

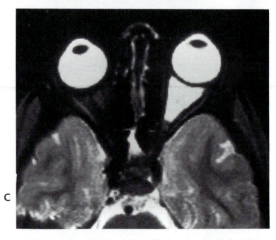

**Figure 16-55** Extensive **lymphangioma** in the left orbit in a 4-year-old girl. **A.** An axial $T_1WI$ (600/15) shows a conically shaped mass (arrowheads) encasing the left optic nerve (arrow). **B.** CE MR (600/15 with Gd-DTPA) reveals partial enhancement of the mass and shows well the lobulated nature of the lymphangioma. The nerve (arrow) can be identified. **C.** An axial $T_2WI$ (3000/80) reveals the lesion to be of high intensity.

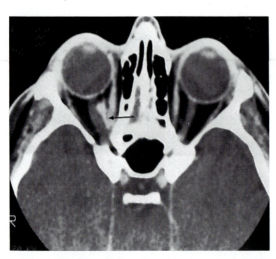

**Figure 16-54** **Lymphangioma.** NCCT: High-attenuation region of acute hemorrhage (arrow) in an ill-defined intraconal mass along the right optic nerve.

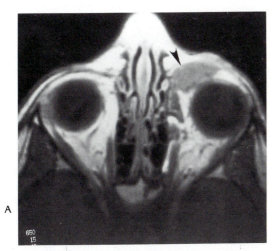
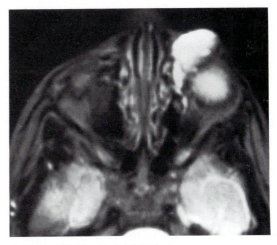

*Figure 16-56* **Lymphangioma** in a 3-year-old boy. **A.** Axial CE MR (600/15 with Gd-DTPA) shows a somewhat irregular low-intensity mass (arrowhead) in the anteromedial aspect of the left orbit. **B.** Axial T$_2$WI (3000/90) shows increased intensity in the mass.

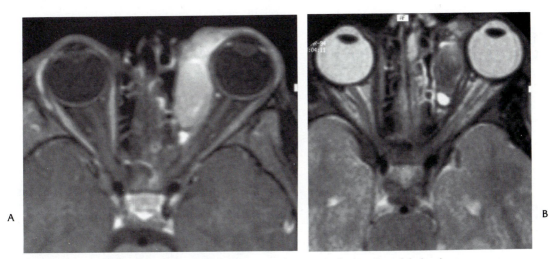

*Figure 16-57* **Lymphangioma** of the left orbit. **A.** Axial MR T$_1$WI shows a large lobulated mass extending and widening the medial extraconic space of the left orbit. It is hyperintense on T$_1$ consistent with hemorrhage. **B.** Axial T$_2$WI at a similar plane to that shown in **A** shows that a large portion of the left medial extraconic mass has become hypointense, indicating hemorrhage with methemoglobin being present within the red blood cells.

tant for surgical planning. MR is more specific than CT in identifying old blood products and showing the various components of a lymphangioma. At times the lesion may consist of a single giant cyst. Some lymphangiomas may be extensive, filling and expanding the bony orbit.

## Varix

Vascular malformations of the venous system are infrequently occurring orbital lesions which include orbital varices and varicoceles. They are characterized by the production of intermittent exophthalmos, most often associated with activities that produce an increase in venous pressure (coughing, straining, the Valsalva maneuver). This type of response does not occur with lymphangiomas and helps to differentiate them clinically from varices. The lack of valves within the jugular vein allows back pressure to be transmitted to the orbital veins and the venous malformation. The distention of vascular spaces within the venous malformation produces the exophthalmos. Recurrent episodes of extreme proptosis have been reported to lead to blindness in up to 15 percent of patients with orbital varix.

Some varices may hemorrhage (Fig. 16-58). Other causes of intermittent exophthalmos are bleeding into lymphangiomas, sinus infection with edema of the orbital soft tissue, and allergic edema. Venous varicocele formations associated with arteriovenous fistulas, carotid-cavernous in nature, are usually pulsatile and do not regress in size.

Routine skull radiographs are usually normal, although phleboliths may be present within the varix. Orbital venography was the most useful diagnostic modality (Bilaniuk 1977) before the advent of high-resolution CT. CT and MR clearly demonstrate the location of the soft tissue mass of a varix (Figs. 16-58, 16-59) and characterize it by showing enlargement of the varix with the Valsalva maneuver (Rubin 1995) and diminution in its size with the Muller maneuver. Alternatively, varix can be documented by its appearance and disappearance on CT with changes in head position. (Varix becomes evident when the neck is hyper-

extended to position the head for coronal scans.) By showing a signal void within the dilated veins, MR confirms the vascular nature of the lesion and helps differentiate it from morphologically similar lesions such as plexiform neurofibroma and orbital fibrosis. However, if the flow is very slow, or there is stagnation of blood within the varix, then the signal may be increased.

## Carotid-Cavernous Fistula

A communication between the internal carotid artery (or branches of the external carotid artery) and the cavernous sinus leads to the development of a fistula in which the veins are under arterial pressure. Valveless venous intercommunication between the cavernous sinus and the superior ophthalmic vein leads to a transmission of arterial pressure into the veins of the orbit. Proptosis, motility disturbances, pulsating exophthalmos (with a bruit), and suffusion of the globe, sclera, and conjunctiva are the hallmarks of a carotid-cavernous fistula. The etiology is most often trauma (Fig. 16-60), but fistulas may occur spontaneously, either secondary to atherosclerotic disease or from communications between the dural branches of the external carotid artery and the basilar venous plexus (dural arteriovenous malformations) (Figs. 16-62, 16-63). The

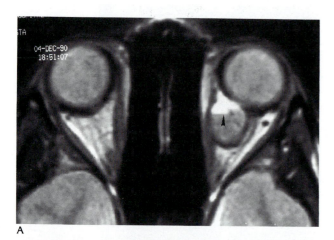

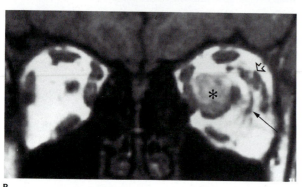

**Figure 16-58** A 14-year-old girl with **varix. A.** Axial MRI (3000/30) shows a mass with a fluid level (arrowhead) between blood products. The mass displaces the left optic nerve laterally. **B.** A coronal T₁WI (600/15) reveals a somewhat lobulated heterogeneous mass (asterisk) which displaces the optic nerve laterally. The higher intensity within the mass is due to methemoglobin. An irregular portion of the varix (open arrow) is located in the lateral portion of the orbit and extends to the lateral rectus. There is also an enlarged lateral connecting vein (arrow).

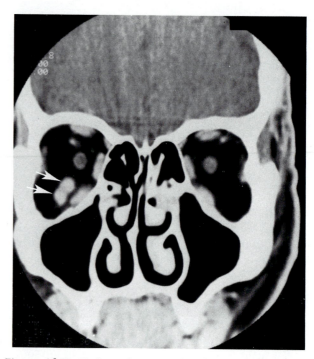

**Figure 16-59** **Varix,** inferior ophthalmic vein. Coronal CECT demonstrates a "double-barrel" enlarged inferior ophthalmic vein (arrows), consistent with a tortuous venous varix.

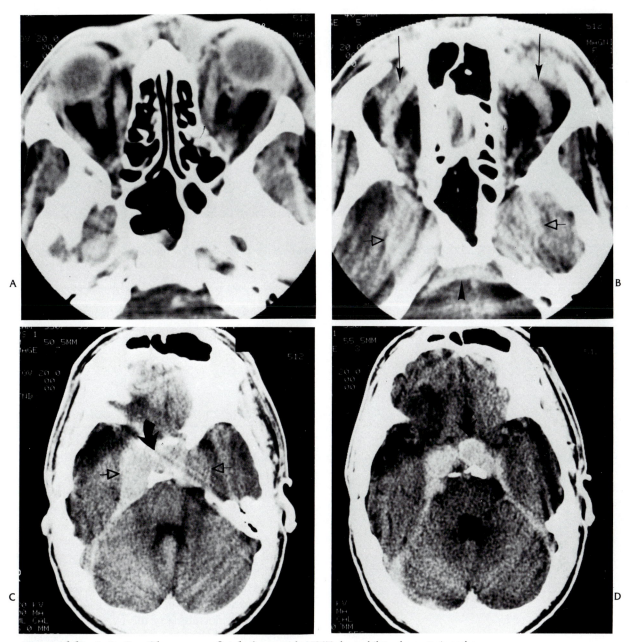

***Figure 16-60*** **A–D. Carotid-cavernous fistula** (traumatic). NCCT shows bilateral proptosis and engorgement of all muscles with markedly enlarged superior ophthalmic veins bilaterally (arrows). The cavernous sinuses are bulging (open arrows), and there appears to be an intrasellar and suprasellar mass (curved arrows). The basilar venous plexus is also engorged (arrowhead).

exophthalmos and ocular symptoms that accompany the fistula are usually ipsilateral to the site of the fistula but are contralateral in 10 percent and may be bilateral, since intercavernous sinus connections exist.

Although carotid arteriography remains the definitive method for demonstrating the site of a fistula and its pattern of venous drainage (Zimmerman 1977), CT and MR are contributory in the initial diagnosis of cases that are not clinically obvious or typical. Enlargement of the

superior ophthalmic vein, engorgement of the rectus muscles, proptosis, and distention of the involved cavernous sinus can be demonstrated on CT (Figs. 16-60, 16-62) and MR (Figs. 16-61 and 16-63), especially with MR angiography (MRA) (Fig. 16-61B). While traumatic fistulas require surgical or neurointerventional treatment, dural fistulas may thrombose spontaneously. The differential diagnosis of an enlarged superior ophthalmic vein is shown in Table 16-2.

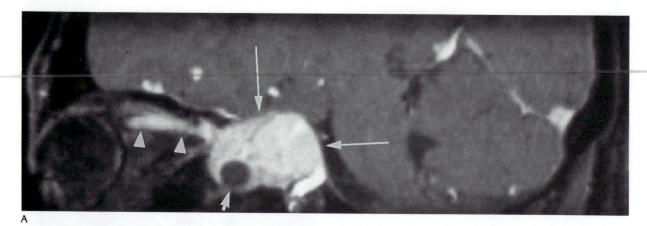

A

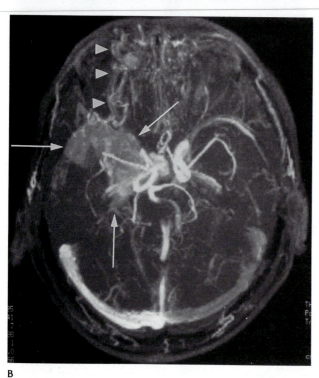

B

***Figure 16-61*** Right **carotid cavernous fistula. A.** A sagittal reconstruction from a 3D TOF MRA shows a venous aneurysm (arrows) in the region of the cavernous sinus and also an enlarged superior ophthalmic vein (arrowhead). The inferior portion of the venous aneurysm contains a a collapsed balloon (empty arrow). **B.** Axial MRA shows a markedly dilated vein occupying the anterior portion of the right middle cranial fossa as well as enlarged and tortuous veins (arrows) within the right orbit.

## Table 16-2   Etiologies of Enlarged Superior Ophthalmic Vein

Carotid-cavernous fistula
  Traumatic
  Dural fistula (AVM)
Varix
Superior ophthalmic vein or cavernous sinus thrombosis
Orbital apex mass (compressing vein)
Thyroid opthalmopathy
Idiopathic orbital inflammation
Capillary hemangioma
Normal variant

# OCULAR TUMORS

## Ocular Melanoma

Both benign and malignant melanomas arise intraocularly from the uveal tract. Extraocular extension through the vortex veins occurs in approximately 13 percent of ocular melanomas (Starr 1962). Local recurrence of the melanoma after exenteration is extremely high if extraocular extension has already occurred. The diagnosis of melanoma as a primary tumor in the orbit requires the exclusion of a primary intraocular focus and an extracranial primary site (Jones 1979).

Malignant melanoma of the uveal tract (iris, choroid, ciliary body) is the most common intraocular malignancy in adults (Shields 1977), predominantly occurring in whites and rare in African Americans (Shields 1977; Yanoff 1975). Primary malignant melanoma of the choroid is nearly always unilateral. Melanomas usually occur in older patients and are uncommon in the pediatric population. The clinical presentation varies from visual field defects or decreased visual acuity to pain or inflammation.

On CT, melanoma usually presents as a focal mass of slight hyperdensity which projects into the vitreous (Fig. 16-64). These tumors may show slight enhancement (Mafee 1985; Peyster 1985). The shape of the mass varies from polypoid (Fig. 16-64) to flat or crescentic (Fig. 16-65); associated retinal detachment is common and often requires intravenous contrast for CT differentiation (Fig. 16-66) or $T_2WI$ for MR (Fig. 16-

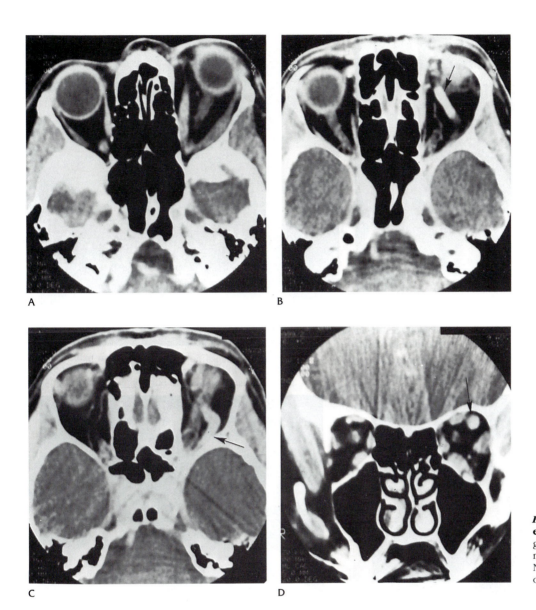

***Figure 16-62***  **A–D. Dural cavernous fistula** on CECT. The left globe is proptotic, and extraocular muscles on the left are engorged. Note the enlarged left superior ophthalmic vein (arrow).

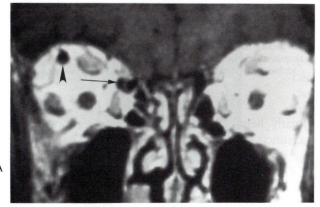

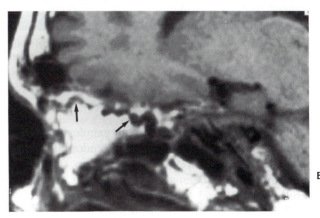

***Figure 16-63***  **Dural cavernous fistula** with right orbital varix and enlargement of the right superior ophthalmic vein. **A.** Coronal CEMR (600/15 with Gd-DTPA). A prominent varix (arrow) is present in the medial extraconic space of the right orbit. The right superior oph-

thalmic vein (arrowhead) is prominently enlarged. Compare with the normal one on the left side. The rectus muscles show normal enhancement. **B.** A sagittal CEMR demonstrates the large varicose vein (arrows).

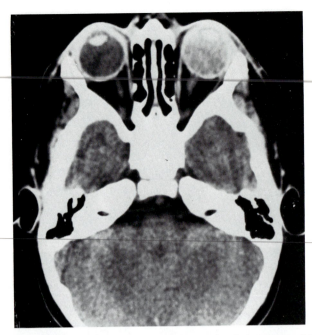

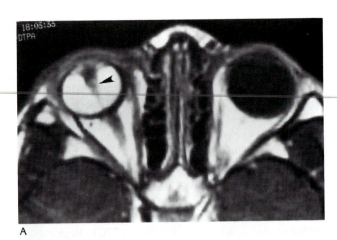

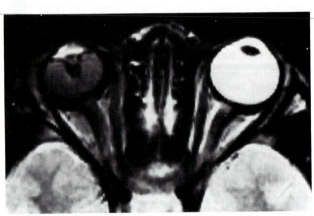

*Figure 16-78*  **Coats' disease** on NCCT. Uniformly hyperdense left globe presenting as leukokoria. Absence of calcifications helps distinguish this condition from retinoblastoma.

fluid accumulation causing retinal detachment. Males (80 percent) of ages 6 to 8 years are typically affected (Reese 1976). CT demonstrates relatively homogeneous hyperdensity involving the entire vitreous cavity (Fig. 16-78) secondary to lipoproteinaceous exudate underlying a (usually) total retinal detachment (Sherman 1983). Calcification is nearly always absent, although tiny foci of calcified cholesterol plaques may rarely be seen on funduscopy. Features distinguishing this entity from retinoblastoma include an older age at presentation, an exclusively unilateral occurrence, lack of calcification or enhancement, and absence of extraocular spread (Haik 1985). CT or MR can therefore obviate the need for globe exenteration in these patients and instead lead to appropriate laser therapy. Coats' disease is the primary entity to distinguish from retinoblastoma in the differential diagnosis. MR is superior to CT in differentiating the two entities and in the case of Coats' disease demonstrates the lipoproteinaceous subretinal exudate which characteristically is hyperintense to the vitreous on both $T_1WI$ and $T_2WI$ (Mafee 1987, 1990).

## Persistent Hyperplastic Primary Vitreous

Persistent hyperplastic primary vitreous (PHPV) results from failure of involution of the embryonic intraocular vascular system. Imaging studies demonstrate a linear or triangular density, the residual hyaloid vascular system with connective tissue, extending from the poste-

*Figure 16-79*  **Persistent hyperplastic primary vitreous** with microphthalmic globe. **A.** Axial MRI, $T_1WI$ (600/20) reveals a smaller globe on the right with a shallow anterior chamber and an abnormal lens from which triangularly shaped tissue (arrowhead) extends posteriorly. This tissue represents persistence of the hyaloid vascular system. There is complete retinal detachment. The left globe appears normal. **B.** Axial $T_2WI$ (3000/90) shows an abnormally deformed and small lens. The tissue extending posteriorly from the lens is of markedly decreased intensity. The probable subretinal fluid has decreased in intensity.

rior aspect of the lens to the back of the globe (Fig. 16-79). There also may be associated retinal detachment as a result of recurrent hemorrhage. A hyaloid remnant may be difficult to differentiate from retinal detachment when it is complete. PHPV is unilateral and noncalcified. There usually is microphthalmos (Haik 1985), deformity of the globe and lens, increased density or intensity of the vitreous body, and enhancement of the band of tissue that extends between the lens and the posterior globe (Magill 1990). Without contrast enhancement the band of tissue may be difficult to detect on CT, but it is seen as a band of low intensity on MR images (Fig. 16-79). When PHPV is bilateral, it is usually part of optic dysplasia such as Norrie's disease (congenital progressive oculoacoustic cerebral degeneration).

## Norrie's Disease

Norrie's disease is a rare X-linked inherited disease that is transmitted by females but affects only males (Liberfarb 1985). The disease involves mental deterioration and progressive loss of vision and hearing. The eye abnormalities include retinal detachment with hemorrhage, retrolental mass, and lens abnormalities.

## Retinopathy of Prematurity

Retinopathy of prematurity, or retrolental fibroplasia, is usually seen in premature infants who receive high oxygen concentrations. Recent literature suggests that the high oxygen concentration in inspired air is not a requisite for the development of this entity (Patz 1985). Bilateral retinal detachments with variable enhancement and occasional calcification may be seen. Microphthalmia has also been described (Haik 1985).

## Ocular Toxocariasis

*Toxocara canis* infestation can present with leukokoria and retinal detachment secondary to endophthalmitis. "Pseudomicrophthalmia" (Haik 1985) from focally thickened sclera with enhancement is common. CT may also demonstrate a nonenhancing hyperdense mass occupying most of the vitreous cavity (Edwards 1985). MR may demonstrate the larval granuloma as a hyperintense mass on both $T_1WI$ and $T_2WI$ (Mafee 1990).

# GLOBE SHAPE ABNORMALITIES

## Coloboma

Colobomas are congenital defects in the retina, choroid, iris, optic nerve, and/or lens which result from deficient closure of the fetal optic fissure along the inferonasal aspect of the globe and optic nerve (Simmons 1983). The posterior globe and optic nerve are most commonly affected. The defect is transmitted as an autosomal dominant trait with variable penetrance, occurring bilaterally in 60 percent of cases. Visual field defects and decreased visual acuity are present. MR and CT (Fig. 16-80) demonstrate defects in the posterior globe extending into the optic nerve (Bilaniuk 1992). Microphthalmia and retinal cysts may accompany optic nerve colobomas. CT and MR are useful in identifying retinal cysts posterior to the globe and in revealing any central nervous system (CNS) abnormality which can be associated with these lesions, such as encephalocele or callosal agenesis (Corbett 1980).

## Staphyloma

Staphylomas are acquired defects in the wall of the globe that result in protrusion of either the cornea or the sclera. These defects are lined with iris or choroid tissue. In severe myopia, accompanying staphylomas typically are seen as focal bulges in the posterior surface of the globe on the temporal side of the optic disk (Anderson 1983). Anterior staphylomas can be seen in inflammatory entities such as rheumatoid arthritis.

## Axial Myopia

Axial myopia is characterized by an enlarged anteroposterior diameter of the globe (Fig. 16-81). Anterior protrusion may be noted and may result in proptosis

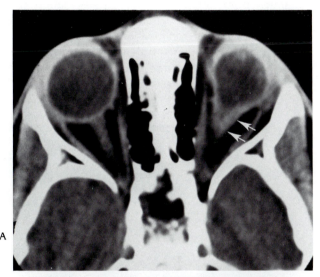

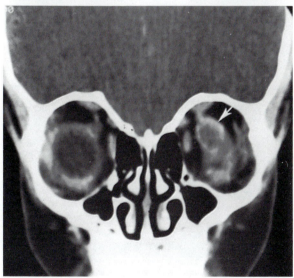

*Figure 16-80* **A,B.** Microphthalmos with **coloboma.** Conical defect in posterior globe extending into optic nerve (arrows) seen on axial **(A)** and coronal **(B)** CT in a microphthalmic globe.

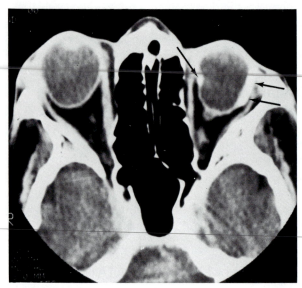

*Figure 16-81* **Myopia,** status postscleral banding on CT. Both globes have a myopic configuration. High-density structures at the periphery of the left globe (arrows) with waistlike deformity represent scleral bands placed for prior retinal detachment.

percent of cases and is caused by maldevelopment of aqueous humor outflow channels in the anterior chamber angle. Glaucoma in a child results in an enlarged globe (Fig. 16-82). Macrophthalmos may be unrelated to intraocular pressure, however, and can be seen as an isolated entity secondary to massive intraocular tumor or in association with neurofibromatosis.

## Microphthalmos

Anophthalmia results when there is failure of the optic pit to deepen to form a vesicle or when an optic vesicle forms and then degenerates. Complete failure of eye development is extremely rare, and only a histological examination can differentiate between anophthalmia and severe microphthalmia. Microphthalmia (Fig. 16-83) may occur as an isolated finding, but much more often it is seen in association with other ocular (Fig. 16-80), craniofacial, and systemic abnormalities (Smith 1983; Albernaz 1997). It is seen in 75 percent of patients with trisomy-13 syndrome and is commonly associated with mental retardation.

(Brodey 1983). Axial myopia is distinguished from staphyloma by the absence of a focal bulge in an elongated globe. Retinal detachment and staphyloma may accompany the myopic globe.

## Buphthalmos

Buphthalmos, or congenital glaucoma, is usually detected because of clouding or enlargement of the cornea or because the child is insensitive to light (Gittinger 1984). It is unilateral in approximately 25

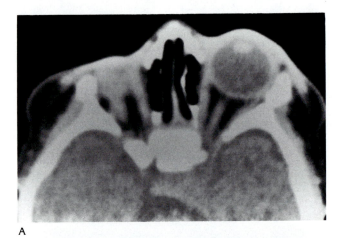

A

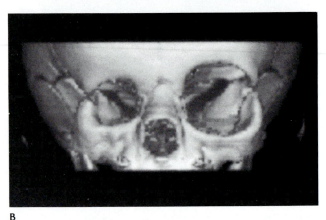

B

*Figure 16-83* Right **microphthalmos** in a 7-week-old girl. **A.** Axial CT fails to reveal a normal globe on the right. The right bony orbit is small. **B.** Three-dimensional CT reconstruction of the facial skeleton reveals marked hypoplasia of the right bony orbit.

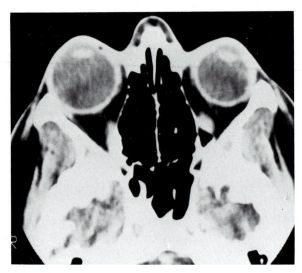

*Figure 16-82* **Buphthalmos.** CT shows macrophthalmic right globe in a patient with glaucoma.

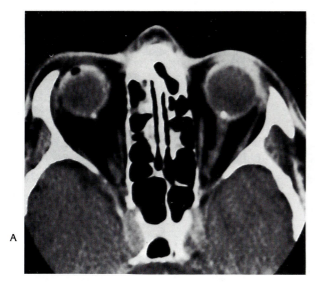
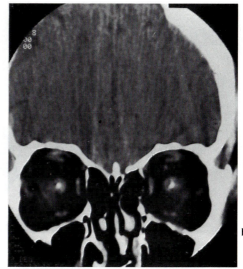

**Figure 16-84** **A,B.** Bilateral **optic nerve drusen.** Axial **(A)** and coronal **(B)** CT demonstrates round, focal calcification at the optic disks, diagnostic of optic nerve drusen.

Microphthalmia with cyst results when there is malformation of the globe with incomplete closure of the fetal fissure. The disorganized cystic neuroectodermal tissue prolapses into the orbit and may be larger than the globe itself (Bilaniuk 1992).

## GLOBE CALCIFICATIONS

The etiology of calcification in the globe is varied (Hedges 1982; Turner 1983), and the differential diagnosis is highly dependent on the age of the patient (Table 16-3). In an infant or young child (up to 3 years of age), any focal calcification in the globe must be considered a retinoblastoma until proved otherwise. The contralateral eye must be examined thoroughly for calcification, since up to one-third of retinoblastomas are bilateral (Fig. 16-73). Calcification is seen in up to 95 percent of cases (Bullock 1977). Other etiologies of globe calcification in a child include astrocytic hamartoma, a nodular mass frequently associated with tuberous sclerosis (Fig. 16-74). Choroidal osteoma is a rare tumor that usually is seen in young women as a focal area of calcification near the optic disk (Hedges 1982).

In adults, the most common cause of focal calcification in the globe is optic nerve drusen. These lesions are commonly bilateral (Fig. 16-84) and represent benign accumulations of hyalinelike material beneath the surface of the optic disk (Hedges 1982; Ramirez 1983). Funduscopically, drusen can masquerade as papilledema. Although frequently asymptomatic, optic nerve drusen can be associated with visual field defects in up to 80 percent of cases (Savage 1985). It is interesting that visual field defects typically occur in areas not corresponding

to the funduscopic location of the drusen (Savage 1985). The etiology of optic nerve drusen is not clearly established, but drusen is considered to represent a developmental anomaly or degenerative process (Ramirez 1983). There is a familial tendency for the development of these lesions.

Phthisis bulbi is an end-stage calcified, shrunken globe which is blind. Extensive calcification is seen on CT, or ringlike hypointensity on MR, in a small, irregularly shaped globe (Fig. 16-85). Etiologies include trauma, recurrent retinal hemorrhage, prior surgery, chronic ocular inflammation (Fig. 16-86), and radiation.

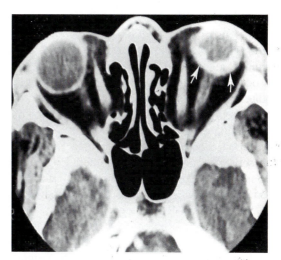

**Figure 16-85** **Phthisis bulbi** on CT. Small left globe with extensive choroidal calcification (arrows) in a patient many years after trauma to the globe.

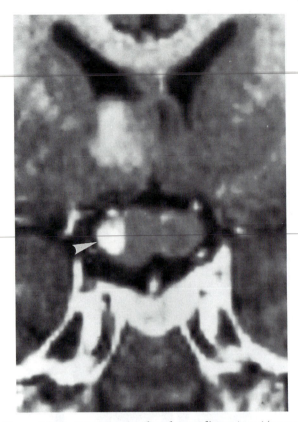

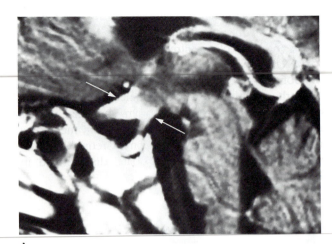

A

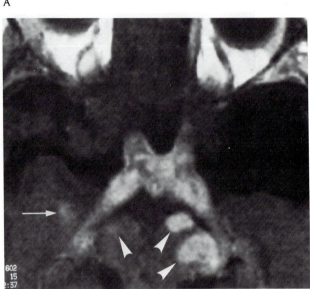

B

**Figure 16-90** Extensive **visual pathway glioma** in a 14-year-old girl with neurofibromatosis. Coronal CE MR (600/15; Gd-DTPA) shows markedly enlarged chiasm that enhances (arrowhead) on the right. There is also a partially enhancing hypothalamic mass.

percent by age 20. There is an association with neurofibromatosis, and as the techniques for detection of the visual pathway gliomas have improved, so has the percentage of association, in some series reaching more than 50 percent (Stern 1980). Aoki (1989) detected optic nerve glioma in 19 of 53 patients with neurofibromatosis type 1. The symptoms of an intraorbital optic glioma include progressive nonpulsatile exophthalmos, limitation of eye movement, optic atrophy, and papilledema. The proptosis precedes a decrease in vision and the onset of strabismus. Histologically, these lesions are low-grade astrocytomas.

CT represented a major breakthrough in the diagnostic evaluation of visual pathway gliomas (Byrd 1978; Peyster 1983; Rothfus 1984) because for the first time the tumors were directly visualized not only in the orbit but also intracranially. A significant number of optic gliomas are part of a more extensive disease process that involves the more posterior visual pathways, including not only the optic nerve but the optic chiasm, optic tract, lateral geniculate body, and optic radiations (Figs. 16-89 through 16-91). It has been the authors' experience that unsuspected involvement of

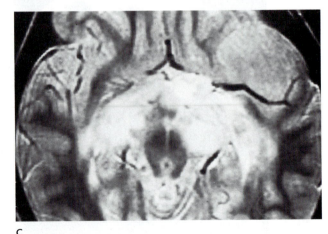

C

**Figure 16-91** Extensive **visual pathway glioma** in a 5-year-old girl with neurofibromatosis. **A.** Sagittal CE MR shows a hyperintense enlarged chiasm (arrows). **B.** Axial CE MR (600/15; 3 mm; Gd-DTPA) shows a glioma in both intracranial optic nerves, the chiasm, and the optic tracts, as well as sites of contrast enhancement in the medial right temporal lobe (arrow) and the midbrain (arrowheads). **C.** Axial $T_2WI$ (3000/45) shows extensive abnormal hyperintensity in the region of the chiasm, optic tracts, and lateral geniculate bodies in brain adjacent to these structures.

the visual pathways can be present in a significant number of these patients (Bilaniuk 1989). In addition to better showing the extent of visual pathway gliomas, MR demonstrates the spectrum of brain abnormalities that can occur secondary to neurofibromatosis (Braffman 1988). Also, imaging modalities are helpful in the differential diagnosis of orbital lesions occurring in patients with neurofibromatosis. Plexiform neurofibroma, the most frequent orbital manifestation of neurofibromatosis (Zimmerman 1983), is shown on CT (Fig. 16-92) (Reed 1986), but is much better delineated and characterized by MR (Burk 1987) (Figs. 16-93, 16-94).

Optic gliomas appear most often as nodular or fusiform enlargements of the optic nerve or as uniform enlargements (Fig. 16-95), most of which show at least some contrast enhancement (Figs. 16-89, 16-90, 16-91, 16-96, 16-97). Optic nerve gliomas show a variable pattern on imaging, reflecting their different growth patterns. They may grow within the optic nerve, expanding it (Figs. 17-89, 17-95, 17-96), or they may grow within the nerve as well as extraneurally, encircling the nerve (Fig. 17-97). In addition, these gliomas may be associated with arachnoidal hyperplasia, which may be confused with meningioma on biopsy (Cooling 1979). MR with the use of $T_1$- and $T_2$-weighted sequences (Fig. 16-98) and contrast enhancement with fat suppression is the best modality for the characterization of optic gliomas (Imes 1991). Bilateral involvement (Figs. 16-89, 16-90, 16-91, 16-95), which in some cases is clinically unsuspected, may be diagnostic of neurofibromatosis. Intracranially, visual pathway gliomas are better delineated with MR, showing increased intensity

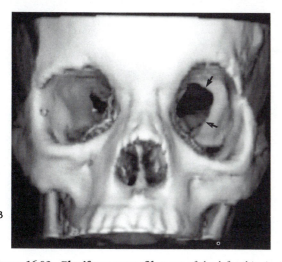

**Figure 16-92** **Plexiform neurofibroma** of the left orbit. **A.** Axial CT shows abnormally wide left superior orbital fissure (black arrows) due to dysplasia of the greater wing of the sphenoid. In addition there is extensive thickening of tissues of the lid (white arrow) and the left temporalis fossa due to the infiltration by a plexiform neurofibroma. **B.** A 3D reconstruction of the bony structures of the face shows the markedly expanded superior orbital fissure (arrows).

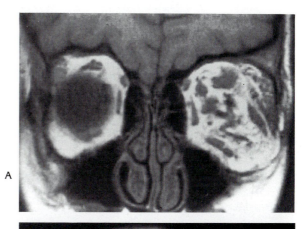

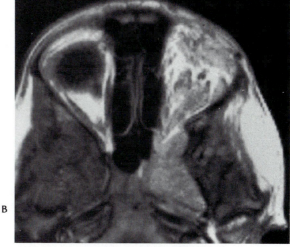

**Figure 16-93** Extensive **plexiform neurofibroma** in an 11-year-old girl who had enucleation. **A.** Coronal MRI, $T_1$WI (600/15) reveals multiple small irregular masses throughout the fat of the left orbit. These are portions of a plexiform neurofibroma. **B.** Axial CE MR (600/15; Gd-DTPA) demonstrates the intraorbital as well as the cavernous sinus component of the plexiform neurofibroma.

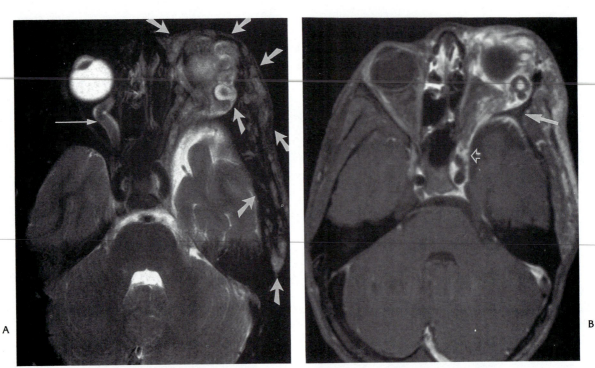

***Figure 16-94*** **Plexiform neurofibroma,** MR. Extensive plexiform neurofibroma in a patient with neurofibromatosis. **A.** Axial T$_2$WI shows lobulated and serpiginous infiltrative mass (arrows) involving the left temporalis muscle and infiltrating most of the left orbit. There is dysplasia of the left orbit with hypoplastic greater wing of the sphenoid. Because of the dysplasia of the left sphenoid wing, there is more anterior extent of the left middle cranial fossa. There is hyperintense CSF anterior to the left temporal lobe. Also noted is enlargement of the right optic nerve (arrow) indicating optic glioma. **B.** CEMR: Axial image at the same level as that shown in **A** with fat suppression shows enhancement of the neurofibroma and better demonstrates the infiltration of the soft tissues by the neurofibroma. Arrow points to the hypoplastic left wing of the sphenoid. There is extension of the neurofibroma into the left cavernous sinus (arrowhead).

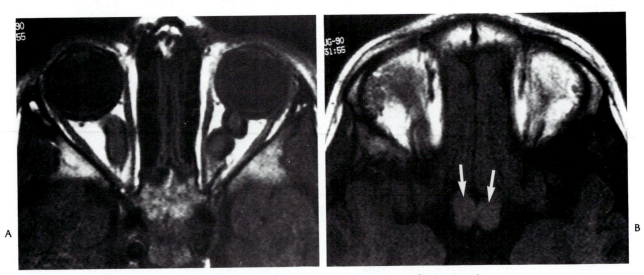

***Figure 16-95*** **Bilateral optic nerve gliomas** in a 4-year-old boy. **A.** Axial MRI, T$_1$WI (600/15; 3 mm) shows enlargement of both optic nerves. **B.** Axial MRI, T$_1$WI (600/15; 3 mm) obtained superior to that shown in **A** shows the two large optic nerves (arrows) joining to form the chiasm.

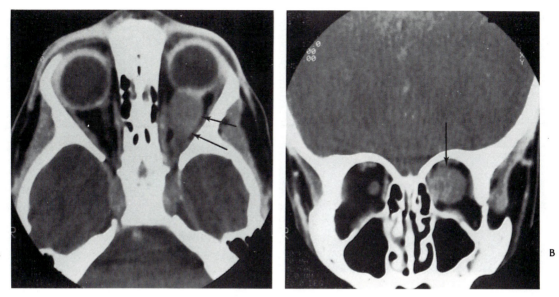

***Figure 16-96***  **A,B.** Contrast-enhancing **optic glioma.** Massive lobulated enlargement of the left optic nerve (arrow) in axial **(A)** and coronal **(B)** CECT. Note slight flattening of globe.

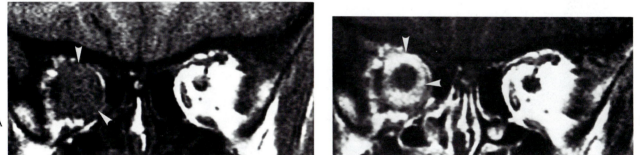

***Figure 16-97***  Right **optic nerve glioma** in a 6-year-old boy. **A.** Coronal MRI, T$_1$WI (600/15; 3 mm) shows a large mass (arrowheads) which occupies most of the right intraconic space. **B.** Coronal CE MR (600/15; 3 mm; Gd-DTPA) obtained at the same level shown in **A** shows that a thick rim of tumor (arrowheads) has enhanced but surrounds a central portion which does not show enhancement. The central portion is about three times as large as the normal optic nerve sheath complex on the left.

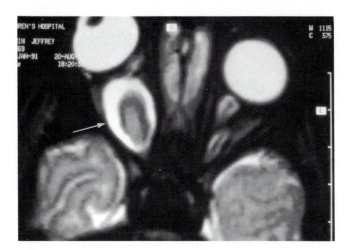

***Figure 16-98***  Right **optic glioma.** Axial MR, T$_2$WI shows a large right optic nerve sheath complex (arrow) due to an optic nerve glioma. The glioma shows heterogeneous intensity pattern.

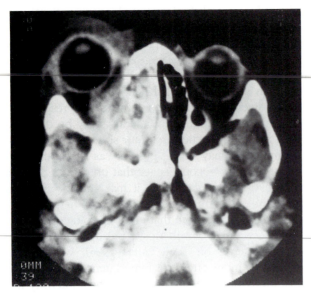

**Figure 16-115** **Neuroblastoma metastases.** Destructive mass involving the right medial orbit and the ethmoid sinus causes proptosis on CE CT.

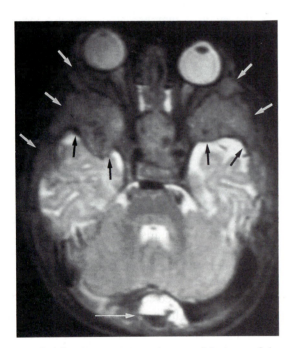

**Figure 16-116** MRI: T$_2$WI: Extensive **neuroblastoma** of the cranial base shows marked bony expansion (short arrows) of the anterior cranial base. There is extensive involvement of the entire sphenoid bone. There is also a metastatic focus to the torcular Herophili, and as typically can be seen, there is evidence of hemorrhage resulting in a fluid-fluid level which is indicated by a long horizontal white arrow.

and 16-118 through 16-121). A minority of metastatic lesions are discrete and well circumscribed. Metastatic retrobulbar carcinoma from breast carcinoma has been relatively common in the authors' experience. This

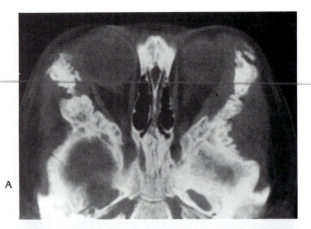

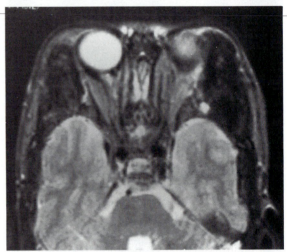

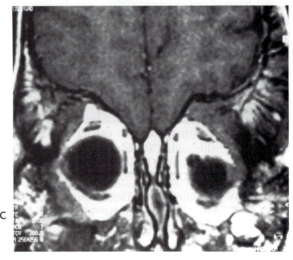

**Figure 16-117** Extensive residual bony and soft tissue changes in a patient 5 years after treatment for **metastatic neuroblastoma.** The patient is 10 years old. **A.** An axial CT performed through the midportion of the orbits shows highly abnormal lateral orbital walls. It can also be faintly seen that there is increased soft tissue adjacent to the left lateral bony orbital wall. **B.** An axial MR, T$_2$WI (2500/90) shows that there is primarily hypointensity in the regions of the abnormal bones. **C.** A coronal MR, T$_1$WI (700/22) reveals markedly expanded bony orbital walls with multiple striations. In addition, there is prominent soft tissue in the superolateral extraconic portions of the orbits. The bony orbits themselves are deformed and show an increased vertical diameter. There also is hypotelorism.

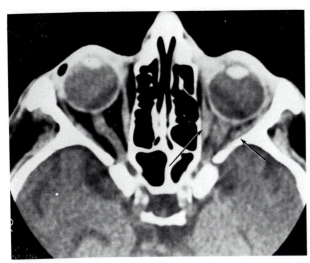

**Figure 16-118   Metastatic breast carcinoma.** CE CT shows extraconal masses in the left orbit (arrows) with secondary enophthalmos, typical of scirrhous breast carcinoma metastasis.

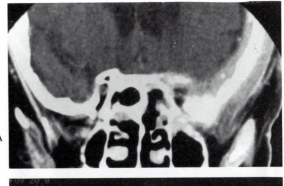
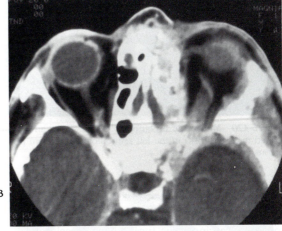
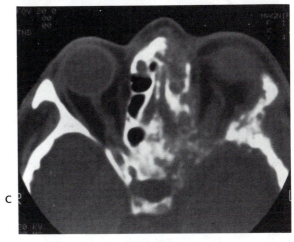

**Figure 16-119   Metastatic breast carcinoma. A.** Coronal CE CT. Irregular bony destruction and contrast-enhanced tumor are present in the apex of the left orbit and in the lateral wall of the left middle cranial fossa. **B.** Axial CE CT shows extensive tumor in the medial and lateral wall of the left orbit and in the anterior wall of the left middle cranial fossa. **C.** Axial CT with wide window setting shows the moth-eaten pattern of bony destruction in the left ethmoid sinus and left orbit.

most often appears on CT or MR as a diffusely infiltrative contrast-enhancing mass lesion without clear-cut margins. At times metastases may have an appearance similar to that seen with extensive orbital pseudotumor. MR is of some help in differentiating these entities (Atlas 1986). Metastatic breast carcinoma shows increased intensity on $T_2WI$, whereas most pseudotumors are of decreased intensity (Atlas 1986). However, there are tumors that are hypointense on $T_2WI$; one of these is the carcinoid tumor (Braffman 1987). When the metastasis is from a scirrhous carcinoma, the fibrous response produces enophthalmos (Fig. 16-118).

In children, orbital metastases most often involve the walls of the orbit. The tumors extend subperiosteally into the orbital space. Neuroblastoma frequently presents with simultaneous metastases to both orbits (Rootman 1988) (Fig. 16-117) but often also presents as unilateral metastatic disease (Fig. 16-115). The bone is infiltrated, and the orbital periosteum is displaced (Zimmerman 1980b; Bilaniuk 1990a). Imaging studies show mixed lytic and hyperostotic bone changes, spiculated periosteal bone reaction, and obliteration of adjacent paranasal sinuses. These bone changes are different from those produced by localized histiocytosis (previously referred to as eosinophilic granuloma) where there is sharply defined bone destruction. However, histiocytosis may also be diffuse and infiltrative (Fig. 16-125), and then it may be similar to that of neuroblastoma. In addition to revealing the bone changes, CT and MR demonstrate the subperiosteal portion of the neuroblastoma, which shows contrast enhancement (Zimmerman 1980b). The orbital tumor in neuroblastoma may be hyperdense on NCCT because of

hemorrhage within the tumor. MR is more specific in identifying the blood products within the tumor. There may be extensive residual bony changes even many years after treatment of a neuroblastoma (Fig. 16-117).

Distant metastases to the orbital bones and paranasal sinuses also occur in adults and may resemble pedi-

BILANIUK LT, ZIMMERMAN RA: Facial trauma, in Dalinka MK, Kaye JJ (eds): *Radiology in Emergency Medicine,* New York, Churchill Livingstone, 1984, pp 135–155.

BILANIUK LT, ATLAS SW, ZIMMERMAN RA: MRI of the orbit. *Radiol Clin North Am* 25:509–528, 1987.

BILANIUK LT, ZIMMERMAN RA, GUSNARD DA, PACKER RJ, SUTTON LN, ATLAS SW, HACKNEY DB, GOLDBERG HI, GROSSMAN RI, SCHUT L, RORKE LB: MR imaging of the visual pathway gliomas. *Radiology* (RSNA '89 Abstracts) 173P:85, 1989.

BILANIUK LT: Magnetic resonance imaging: Orbital anatomy, in Newton TM, Bilaniuk LT (eds): *Radiology of the Eye and Orbit,* New York, Raven Press, 1990a, pp 4.1–4.12.

BILANIUK LT, ZIMMERMAN RA, NEWTON TH: Magnetic resonance imaging: Orbital pathology, in Newton TM, Bilaniuk LT (eds): *Radiology of the Eye and Orbit,* New York, Raven Press, 1990b, pp 5.1–5.84.

BILANIUK LT, ZIMMERMAN RA, GUSNARD DA: MR of head and neck hemangiomas. *Radiology* (RSNA '90 Abstracts) 177P:256, 1990c.

BILANIUK LT, FARBER M: Imaging of developmental anomalies of the eye and orbit. *AJNR* 13:793–803, 1992.

BILANIUK LT, ZIMMERMAN RA, SAVINO PJ: Visual pathways, in Kelly WM (ed): *Cranial Neuropathy, Neuroimaging Clinics of North America* 3:71–83, 1993.

BILANIUK LT, RAPOPORT RJ: Magnetic resonance imaging of the orbit. *Top Magn Reson Imaging* 6(3):167–181, 1994.

BRAFFMAN BH, BILANIUK LT, EAGLE RC, et al: MR imaging of a carcinoid tumor metastatic to the orbit. *J Comput Assist Tomogr* 11:891–894, 1987.

BRAFFMAN BH, BILANIUK LT, ZIMMERMAN RA: The central nervous system manifestations of the phakomatosis on MR. *Radiol Clin North Am* 26:773–800, 1988.

BRANT-ZAWADZKI M, ENZMANN DR: Orbital computed tomography: Calcific densities of the posterior globe. *J Comput Assist Tomogr* 3:503–505, 1979.

BREASLAU J, DALLEY RW, TSURUDA JS, et al: Phased-array surface coil MR of the orbits and optic nerves. *AJNR* 16:1247–1251, 1995.

BRISMAR J, DAVIS KR, DALLOW RL, BRISMAR G: Unilateral endocrine exophthalmos. Diagnostic problems in associated with computed tomography. *Neuroradiology* 12:24, 1976.

BRODEY PA, RANDEL S, LANE B, FISCH AE: Computed tomography of axial myopia. *J Comput Assist Tomogr* 7:484–485, 1983.

BRODSKY MC, BECK RW: The changing role of MR imaging in the evaluation of acute optic neuritis. *Radiology* 192:22–23, 1994.

BROWN GC, TASMAN WS, BENSON WE: BB-gun injuries to the eye. *Ophthal Surg* 16:505–508, 1985.

BROWN GC, WEINSTOCK F: Arterial macroaneurysm on the optic disk presenting as a mass lesion. *Ann Ophthalmol* 17:519–520, 1985.

BULLOCK JD, CAMPBELL RJ, WALKER RR: Calcification in retinoblastoma. *Invest Ophthalmol Vis Sci* 16:252–255, 1977.

BULLOCK JD, YANES B: Metastatic tumors of the orbit. *Ann Ophthalmol* 12:1392–1394, 1980.

BURK DL, BRUNBERG JA, KANAL E, et al: Spinal and paraspinal neurofibromatosis: Surface coil MR imaging at 1.5T[1]. *Radiology* 162:797–801, 1987.

BYRD SE, HARDWOOD-NASH DC, FITZ CR, BARRY JF, ROGOVITZ DM: Computed tomography of intraorbital optic nerve gliomas in children. *Radiology* 129:73–78, 1978.

CABANIS EA et al: Computed tomography of the optic nerve: II. Size and shape modifications in papilledema. *J Comput Assist Tomogr* 2:150–155, 1978.

CARLSON RE, SCHERIBEL KW, HERING PI, WOLIN L: Exophthalmos, global luxation, rapid weight gain: Differential diagnosis. *Ann Ophthalmol* 14:724–729, 1982.

CARMODY RF, MAFEE MF, GOODWIN JA, et al: Orbital and optic pathway sarcoidosis: MR findings. *AJNR* 15:775–783, 1994.

CLARK JA, KELLY WM: Common artifacts encountered in magnetic resonance imaging. *Radiol Clin North Am* 26:893–920, 1988.

CLAYMAN GL, ADAMS GL, PAUGH DR, et al: Intracranial complications of paranasal sinusitis: A combined institutional review. *Laryngoscope* 101:234–239, 1991.

COHEN BA, SOM PM, HAFFNER PH, FRIEDMAN AH: Steroid exophthalmos. *J Comput Assist Tomogr* 5:907–908, 1981.

COLEMAN LT, ZIMMERMAN RA: Pediatric craniospinal spiral CT: Current applications and future potential. *Sem Ultrasound CT MRI* 15:148–155, 1994.

COOLING RJ, WRIGHT JE: Arachnoid hyperplasia in optic nerve glioma: Confusion with orbital meningioma. *Br J Ophthalmol* 63:596–599, 1979.

CORBETT J, SAVINO PJ, SCHATZ NJ, ORR LS: Cavitary developmental defects of the optic disc. *Arch Neurol* 37:210–213, 1980.

DAMADIAN R, ZANER JK, HOR D: Human tumors by NMR. *Physiol Chem Phys* 5:381–402, 1973.

DANIELS DL, MARK LP, MAFEE MF, et al: Osseous anatomy of the orbital apex. *AJNR* 16:1929–1935, 1995.

DAVIS KR, HESSELINK JR, DALLOW RL, GROVE AS Jr: CT and ultrasound in the diagnosis of cavernous hemangioma and lymphangioma of the orbit. *CT: J Comput Assist Tomogr* 4:98–104, 1980.

DIXON WT: Simple proton spectroscopic imaging. *Radiology* 153:189–194, 1984.

DRESNER SC, ROTHFUS WE, SLAMOVITZ TL, KENNERDELL JS, CURTIN HD: Computed tomography of orbital myositis. *AJR* 143:671–674, 1984.

EDWARDS MG, PORDELL GR: Ocular toxocariasis studied by CT scanning. *Radiology* 157:685–686, 1985.

ENZMANN D, DONALDSON SS, MARSHALL WH, KRISS JP: Computed tomography in orbital pseudotumor (idiopathic orbital inflammation). *Radiology* 120:597–601, 1976.

ENZMANN DR, DONALDSON SS, KRISS JP: Appearance of Graves' disease on orbital computed tomography. *J Comput Assist Tomogr* 3:815–819, 1979.

ERLY WK, CARMODY RF, DRYDEN RM: Orbital histiocytosis X. *AJNR* 16:1258–1261, 1995.

FELDON SE, WEINER JM: Clinical significance of extraocular muscle volumes in Graves' ophthalmopathy: A quantitative computed tomographic study. *Arch Ophthalmol* 100:1266–1269, 1982.

FLANAGAN JC: Vascular problems of the orbit. *Ophthalmology* 86:896–913, 1979.

FLANDERS AE, ESPINOSA GA, MARKIEWICZ DA, HOWELL DD: Orbital lymphoma: Role of CT and MR. *Radiol Clin North Am* 25:601–613, 1987.

FONT RF, GAMEL JW: Adenoid cystic carcinoma of the lacrimal gland: A clinicopathologic study of 79 cases, in Nicholson DH (ed): *Ocular Pathology Update.* New York, Masson Publishing, 1980, pp 277–283.

FORBES GS, SHEEDY PF, WALLER RR: Orbital tumors evaluated by computed tomography. *Radiology* 136:101–111, 1980.

FORBES G: Computed tomography of the orbit. *Radiol Clin North Am* 20:37–49, 1982.

FORBES G, GORMAN CA, BRENNAN MD, GEHRING MD, ILSTRUP DM, EARNEST F IV: Ophthalmopathy of Graves disease: Computerized volume measurements of the orbital fat and muscle. *AJNR* 7:641–656, 1986.

FOX AJ, DEBRUN G, VINUELA F, ASSIS L, COATES R: Intrathecal metrizamide enhancement of the optic nerve sheath. *J Comput Assist Tomogr* 3:653–656, 1979.

GITTINGER JW: *Ophthalmology: A Clinical Introduction.* Boston, Little, Brown, 1984.

GOLDBERG RA, ROOTMAN J, CLINE RA: Tumors metastatic to the orbit: A changing picture. *Surv Ophthalmol* 35(1):1–24, 1990.

GOMORI JM, GROSSMAN RI, SHIELDS JA, AUGSBURGER JJ, JOSEPH PJH, DE SIMONE D: Choroidal melanomas: Correlation of NMR spectroscopy and MR imaging. *Radiology* 158:443–445, 1986.

GONVERS M: Temporary silicone oil tamponade in the management of retinal detachment with proliferative vitreoretinopathy. *Am J Ophthalmol* 100:239–245, 1985.

GRAEB DA, ROOTMAN J, ROBERTSON WD, LAPOINTE JS, NUGENT RA, HAY EJ: Orbital lymphangiomas: Clinical, radiologic, and pathologic characteristics. *Radiology* 175:417–421, 1990.

GROVE AS Jr, TADMOR R, NEW PFJ, MOMOSE KJ: Orbital fracture evaluation by coronal computed tomography. *Am J Ophthalmol* 85:679–685, 1978.

HAHN EJ, CHU WK, COLEMAN PE, ANDERSON JC, DOBRY CA, IMRAY TJ, HAHN PY, LEE SH: Artifacts and diagnostic pitfalls on magnetic resonance imaging: A clinical review. *Radiol Clin North Am* 26:717–735, 1988.

HAIK BG, SAINT LOUIS L, SMITH ME, ABRAMSON DH, ELLSWORTH RM: Computed tomography of the nonrhegmatogenous retinal detachment in the pediatric patient. *Ophthalmology* 92:1133–1142, 1985.

HAMMERSCHLAG SB, HUGHES S, O'REILLY GV, NAHEEDY MH, RUMBAUGH CL: Blow-out fractures of the orbit: A comparison of computed tomography and conventional radiography with anatomical correlation. *Radiology* 143:487–492, 1982.

HANDLER LC, DAVEY IC, HILL JC, et al: The acute orbit: Differentiation of orbital cellulitis from subperiosteal abscess by computerized tomography. *Neuroradiology* 33:15–18, 1991.

HARRIS GJ, JAKOBIEC FA: Cavernous hemangioma of the orbit: A clinicopathologic analysis of ninty-six cases, in Jakobiec FA (ed): *Ocular and Adnexal Tumors,* Birmingham, Ala., Aesculapius, 1978, pp 741–781.

HAUGHTON VM, DAVIS KP, HARRIS GJ, HO JC: Metrizamide optic nerve sheath opacification. *Invest Radiol* 15:343–345, 1980.

HEDGES TR, POZZI-MUCELLI R, CHAR DH, NEWTON TH: Computed tomographic demonstration of ocular calcification: Correlations with clinical and pathologic findings. *Neuroradiology* 23:15–21, 1982.

HENDRIX LE, et al: MR imaging of optic nerve lesions: Value of gadopentetate dimeglumine and fat-suppression technique. *AJR* 11:749, 1990.

HERMAN M, VALKOVA Z: Intraorbital wood foreign bodies. *Radiology* 188:878, 1993.

HESSELINK JR et al: Computed tomography of the paranasal sinus and face. I. Normal anatomy. *J Comput Assist Tomogr* 2:559–567, 1978.

HESSELINK JR, WEBER AL, NEW PFJ, DAVIS KR, ROBERSON GH, TAVERAS JM: Evaluation of mucoceles of the paranasal sinuses with CT. *Radiology* 133:397–400, 1979*a.*

SANDBERG-WOLLHEIM M, BYNK EH, CRONQUIST S, HOLTAS S, PLATZ P, RYDER LP: A long-term prospective study of optic neuritis: Evaluation of risk factors. *Ann Neurol* 27:386–393, 1990.

SAVAGE GL, CENTARO A, ENOCH JM, NEWMAN NM: Drusen of the optic nerve head: An important model. *Ophthalmology* 92:793–799, 1985.

SERGOTT RC, GLASER JS, CHARYULU K: Radiotherapy for idiopathic inflammatory pseudotumor: Indications and results. *Arch Ophthalmol* 99:853–856, 1981.

SEVEL D, KRAUSZ H, PONDER T, CENTENO R: Value of computed tomography for the diagnosis of a ruptured eye. *J Comput Assist Tomogr* 7:870–875, 1983.

SHELLOCK FG: MR imaging of metallic implants and materials: A compilation of the literature. *AJR* 151:811–814, 1988.

SHELLOCK FG, KANAL E. Re: Metallic foreign bodies in the orbits of patients undergoing MR imaging: Prevalence and value of radiography and CT before MR. *AJR* 162:985–986, 1994.

SHENCK JF, HART HR Jr, FOSTER TH, EDELSTEIN WA, BOTTOMLEY PA, REDINGTON RW, HARDY CJ, ZIMMERMAN RA, BILANIUK LT: Improved MR imaging of the orbit at 1.5 T with surface coils. *AJNR* 6:193–196, 1985.

SHERMAN JL, MCLEAN IW, BRAILLIER DR: Coat's disease: CT—pathologic correlation in two cases. *Radiology* 146:77–78, 1983.

SHIELDS JA; Current approaches to the diagnosis and management of choroidal melanomas. *Surv Ophthalmol* 21:443–463, 1977.

SIMMONS JD, LAMASTERS D, CHAR D: Computed tomography of ocular colobomas. *AJR* 141:1223–1226, 1983.

SIMON J, SZUMOSKI J, TOTTERMAN S, KIDO D, EKHOLM S, WICKS A, PLEWES D: Fat-suppression MR imaging of the orbit. *AJNR* 9:961–968, 1988.

SKLAR EML, SCHATZ NJ, GLASER JS, et al: MR of vasculitis-induced optic neuropathy. *AJNR* 17:121–128, 1996.

SMITH CG, GALLIE BI, MORIN JD: Normal and abnormal development of the eye, in Crawford JS, Morin JD (eds): *The Eye in Childhood*. New York, Grune & Stratton, 1983.

SOLOWAY HB: Radiation-induced neoplasms following curative therapy for retinoblastoma. *Cancer* 12:1984–1988, 1966.

SOM PM, SHUGAR JMA: The CT classification of ethmoid mucoceles. *J Comput Assist Tomogr* 4:199–203, 1980.

SOM PM: CT of the paranasal sinuses. *Neuroradiology* 27:189–201, 1985.

SOM PM, DILLON WP, FULLERTON GD, ZIMMERMAN RA, RAJAGOPALAN B, MARON Z: Chronically obstructed sinonasal secretions: Observations on T1 and T2 shortening. *Radiology* 172:515–520, 1989.

STARR H, ZIMMERMAN L: Extrascleral extension and orbital recurrence of malignant melanomas of the choroid and ciliary body. *Int Ophthalmol Clin* 2:369, 1962.

STERN J, JACOBIEC FA, HOUSEPIAN EM: The architecture of optic nerve gliomas with and without neurofibromatosis. *Arch Ophthalmol* 98:505–511, 1980.

STERNBERG P, DE JUAN E, MICHELS RG, AUER C: Multivariate analysis of prognostic factors in penetrating ocular injuries. *Am J Ophthalmol* 98:467–472, 1984.

SULLIVAN JA, HARMS SE: Surface coil MR imaging of orbital neoplasms. *AJNR* 7:29–34, 1986.

TABADDOR K: Unusual complications of iophendylate injection myelography. *Arch Neurol* 29:435–436, 1973.

TADMOR R, NEW PFJ: Computed tomography of the orbit with special emphasis of coronal sections: 1. Normal anatomy. *J Comput Assist Tomogr* 2:24–34, 1978.

TENNER NS, TROKEL SL: Demonstration of the intraorbital portion of the optic nerves by pneumoencephalography. *Arch Ophthalmol* 79:572–573, 1968.

TIEN RD, CHU PK, HESSELINK JR, et al: Intra- and paraorbital lesions: Value of fat-suppression MR imaging with paramagnetic contrast enhancement. *AJNR* 12:245–253, 1991.

TOWBIN R, HAN BK, KAUFMAN RA, BURKE M: Post-septal cellulitis: CT in diagnosis and management. *Radiology* 158:735–737, 1986.

TROKEL SL, HILAL SK: CT scanning in orbital diagnosis, in Thompson HS (ed): *Topics in Neuro-ophthalmology*. Baltimore, Williams & Wilkins, 1979, pp 336–346.

TROKEL SL, JAKOBIEC FA: Correlation of CT scanning and pathologic features of ophthalmic Graves' disease. *Ophthalmology* 88:553–564, 1981.

TURNER RM, GUTMAN I, HILAL SK, BEHRENS M, ODEL J: CT of drusen bodies and other calcific lesions of the optic nerve: Case report and differential diagnosis. *AJNR* 4:175–178, 1983.

UNGER J: Orbital apex fractures: The contribution of computed tomography. *Radiology* 150:713–717, 1984.

UNSOLD R, NEWTON TH, HOYT WF: Technical note—CT examination of the optic nerve. *J Comput Assist Tomogr* 4:560–563, 1980a.

UNSOLD R, DEGROOT J, NEWTON TH: Images of the optic nerve: Anatomic CT correlation. *AJR* 135:767–773, 1980b.

VANNIER MW, MARSH JL, KNAPP RH: Three-dimensional reconstruction from CT scans: Disorders of the head. *Appl Radiol* 16:117–127, 1987.

VERMESS M, HAYNES BF, FANCI AS, WOLFF SM: Computed assisted tomography of the orbital lesions in Wegener's granulomatosis. *J Comput Assist Tomogr* 2:45–48, 1978.

WALKER FO, et al: Chiasmal sarcoidosis. *AJNR* 11:1205, 1990.

WEBER AL, TADMOR R, DAVIS R, ROBERSON G: Malignant tumors of the sinuses. *Neuroradiology* 16:443–448, 1978.

WEISMAN RA, SAVINO PJ, SCHUT L, SCHATZ NJ: Computed tomography in penetrating wounds of the orbit with retained foreign bodies. *Arch Otolaryngol* 109:265–268, 1983.

WHITNALL SE: *The Anatomy of The Human Orbit*. London, Frowder, Hodder and Stoughton, 1921.

WILLIAMSON MR, ESPINOSA MC, BOUTIN RD, et al: Metallic foreign bodies in the orbits of patients undergoing MR imaging: Prevalence and value of radiography and CT before MR. *AJR* 162:981–983, 1994.

WILNER HI, COHN EM, KLING G, JAMPEL RS: Computer assisted tomography in experimentally induced orbital pseudotumor. *J Comput Assist Tomogr* 2:431–455, 1978.

WING SD, HUNSAKER JN, ANDERSON RE, VANDYCK HJL, OSBORN AG: Direct sagittal computed tomography in Graves' ophthalmopathy. *J Comput Assist Tomogr* 3:820–824, 1979.

WRIGHT JE, et al: Optic nerve glioma and the management of optic nerve tumours in the young. *Br J Ophthalmol* 73:967, 1989.

WRIGHT JE, STEWART WB, KROHEL GB: Clinical presentation and management of lacrimal gland tumors. *Br J Ophthalmol* 63:600–606, 1979.

WRIGHT RM, SWIETEK PA, SIMMONS ML: Eye artifacts from mascara in MRI. *AJNR* 6:652, 1985.

YANOFF M, FINE BS: *Ocular Pathology: A Text and Atlas*. Hagerstown, MD, Harper & Row, 1975.

YOUSEM DM, LEXA FJ, BILANIUK LT, ZIMMERMAN RA: Rhabdomyosarcomas in the head and neck: MR imaging evaluation. *Radiology* 177:683–686, 1990.

ZIMMERMAN RA, VIGNAUD J: Ophthalmic arteriography, in Arger PH (ed): *Orbit Roentgenology*. New York, Wiley, 1977, pp 135–169.

ZIMMERMAN RA, BILANIUK LT, LITTMAN P: Computed tomography of pediatric craniofacial sarcoma. *CT: J Comput Tomogr* 2:113–121, 1978.

ZIMMERMAN RA, BILANIUK LT: Computed tomography in the evaluation of patients with bilateral retinoblastomas. *CT: J Comput Tomogr* 3:251–257, 1979.

ZIMMERMAN RA, BILANIUK LT: CT of orbital infection and its cerebral complications. *Am J Roentgenol Radium Ther Nucl Med* 134:45–50, 1980a.

ZIMMERMAN RA, BILANIUK LT: Computed tomography of primary and secondary craniocerebral neuroblastoma. *AJNR* 1:431–434, 1980b.

ZIMMERMAN RA, BILANIUK LT, METZGER RA, et al: Computed tomography of orbital-facial neurofibromatosis. *Radiology* 146:113–116, 1983.

ZIMMERMAN RA, GUSNARD DA, BILANIUK LT: Pediatric craniocervical spiral CT. *Neuroradiology* 34:112–116, 1992.

ZINREICH SJ, KENNEDY DW, MALAT J, et al: Fungal sinusitis: Diagnosis with CT and MR imaging. *Radiology* 169:439–444, 1988.

# 17 THE PARANASAL SINUSES AND NASAL CAVITY

*D. W. Fellows*

*S. J. Zinreich*

## CONTENTS

The paranasal sinuses are air-containing spaces within the facial bones which in part form the floor of the anterior cranial fossa and skull base. These air-containing spaces are located in the frontal bones (the frontal sinuses), the maxillary bones (the maxillary sinuses), the sphenoid bone (the sphenoid sinus), and the ethmoid bones (the ethmoid sinuses). These air sinuses communicate with each other and with the nasal passages through openings under the superior and middle turbinates. They are lined with a thin mucous membrane which is continuous within the nasal cavity.

## TECHNIQUES OF EVALUATION

### Standard Radiographs

Despite the frequency of utilization, standard radiographs offer only limited information because of the problem of structural superimposition. The anteroposterior (AP) and Waters views best demonstrate the frontal and maxillary sinuses. The lateral view best displays the sphenoid sinus. However, the fine bony detail of the ethmoid sinuses is poorly displayed on all views because of overlapping structures. Although of limited value in the evaluation of patients with chronic inflammatory disease, standard radiographs may be of value in the assessment of patients with acute inflammatory disease or aggressive pathology (Zinreich 1990, 1992; White 1991). Here, a single Caldwell or Waters view may be very informative.

823

# Computed Tomography

CT is currently the modality of choice in the evaluation of the paranasal sinuses and the nasal cavity (Zinreich 1990, 1993). Its ability to optimally display bone, soft tissue, and air facilitates accurate definition of regional anatomy and extent of disease. Variation in the regional anatomy of the nasal passages and their communication with the paranasal sinuses pattern are easy to identify prior to surgical intervention (Bolger 1991; Earwaker 1993). In patients with inflammatory disease, imaging in the coronal plane is preferred as the initial screening technique. The coronal plane optimally displays the osteomeatal unit (OMU) and the relationship of the brain and ethmoid roof, and it depicts the relationship of the orbits to the paranasal sinuses. Coronal images correlate with the endoscopic surgical approach and, therefore, should be obtained in patients with inflammatory sinus disease who are surgical candidates (Zinreich 1987). Axial imaging is important in the evaluation of trauma and neoplasms in this region.

The following parameters are useful when evaluating a patient with inflammatory disease of the paranasal sinuses:

- *Patient position:* prone with chin hyperextended
- *Gantry angulation:* perpendicular to the bony palate (Fig. 17-1)
- *Extent of examination:* from the anterior portion of the frontal sinus through the sphenoid sinus (Fig. 17-2)
- *Slice thickness:* 3 mm, contiguous
- *Field of view:* 14 cm

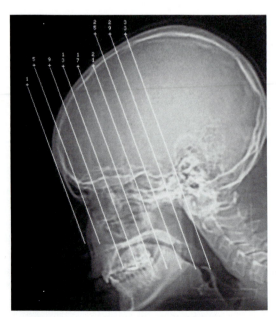

***Figure 17-1*** **Orientation of coronal CT imaging:** gantry angulation. The patient lies prone with chin extended. The gantry is angulated as perpendicular as possible to the hard palate.

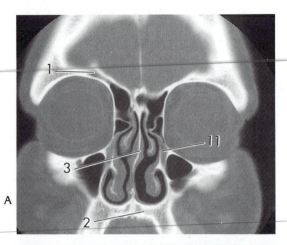

A

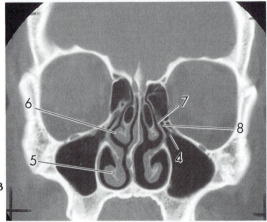

B

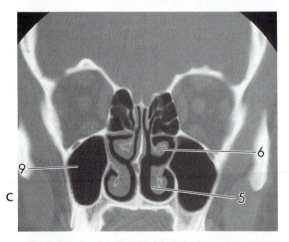

C

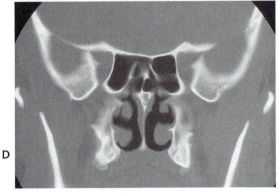

D

*(Continued top of next page)*

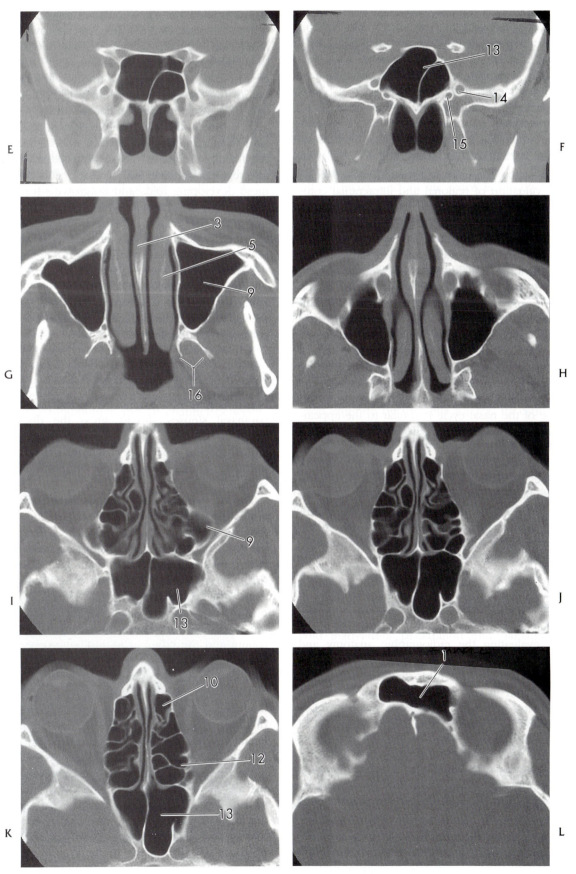

***Figure 17-2*  Coronal CT from anterior to posterior extent
(A–D).** Axial CT (**E–H**). 1, Frontal sinus; 2, hard palate; 3, nasal septum; 4, maxillary sinus ostium; 5, inferior turbinate; 6, middle
turbinate; 7, uncinate process; 8, infundibulum; 9, maxillary sinus;
10, anterior ethmoid air cell; 11, nasolacrimal duct; 12, posterior ethmoid air cell; 13, sphenoid sinus; 14, foramen rotundum; 15, vidian
canal; 16, pterygoid plates.

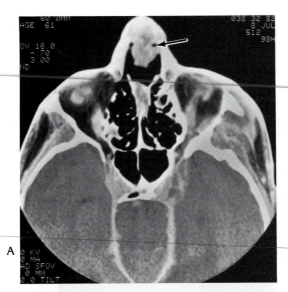

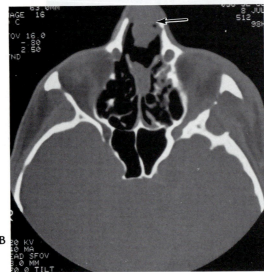

**Figure 17-14    Cocaine granuloma.** Axial CT in (**A**) soft tissue and (**B**) bone window setting, demonstrates a typical soft tissue mass with destruction of the nasal septum associated with cocaine addiction. Similar appearance may be seen in a variety of other chronic granulomatous diseases.

gressive infection are atypical for bacterial pathogens (Som 1993*b*).

### ALLERGIC SINUSITIS

Allergic sinusitis occurs in 10 percent of the population (Harnsberger 1990). It typically produces a pansinusitis with symmetrical involvement (Babbel 1992). CT often shows a nodular mucosal thickening with thickened turbinates (Harnsberger 1990). Air-fluid levels are rare unless bacterial superinfection occurs.

### GRANULOMATOUS SINUSITIS

Whereas many granulomatous diseases (sarcoidosis, tuberculosis, leprosy, foreign body, etc.) can involve the

sinonasal cavity, the most commonly encountered are Wegener's granulomatosis, cocaine granuloma, and idiopathic midline granuloma.

Wegener's granulomatosis is a necrotizing granulomatous vasculitis of unknown etiology. It may present as a localized or systemic form. The sinonasal region is involved in 90 to 95 percent of patients (Allen 1996). CT findings in sinonasal involvement are often nonspecific, but typically there is a nodular soft tissue opacification or mucosal thickening with sclerosis of the thicker bones of the involved sinus and destruction of the thinner septa. Nasal septal perforation may be one of the first distinguishing features in an otherwise nonspecific chronic inflammatory process (Harrison 1987). The maxillary sinus is the most common sinus involved (Youssem 1993). Sphenoid sinus disease, in particular, can spread to the cavernous sinus, orbital apex, and optic canal.

Idiopathic midline granulomas are a group of diseases that are chronic necrotizing inflammatory disorders which are now recognized as being part of the lymphoma spectrum (Harrison 1987). Clinical and radiological manifestations in the paranasal region are often similar to Wegener's granulomatosis. The radiographic hallmark is a destructive mass in the nasal septum, an appearance very similar to that seen in cocaine granuloma (Fig. 17-14).

## Complications of Inflammatory Sinus Disease

### MUCOUS RETENTION CYST

This is a small cyst that most commonly occurs in the maxillary sinus floor in patients with a history of previous inflammatory disease. It occurs in 10 percent of the population and is the result of inflammatory obstruction of a seromucinous gland within the sinus mucosal lining (Laine 1992; Harnsberger 1990). On CT, this appears as a homogenous, well circumscribed hypo- to isodense mass (Fig. 17-15). On MR imaging, it is usually hypointense on $T_1$WI and hyperintense on $T_2$WI.

### MUCOCELE

This is a dilated mucus-filled sinus that is lined by mucous membrane. It is the result of a chronically obstructed sinus ostium with resulting enlargement of bony walls due to mucous secretions filling the sinus cavity (Som 1993*a*; Scuderi 1991). It is most commonly caused by inflammatory obstruction of the ostium, but can also be secondary to trauma, tumors, or surgical manipulation (Scuderi 1991). Sixty-six percent of mucoceles occur in the frontal sinuses with 25 and 10 percent occurring in the ethmoid and maxillary sinuses, respectively. Involvement of the sphenoid sinus is the least common; however, it is not unusual (Dawson 1989; Barat 1990). On CT, this appears as a hypodense, nonenhancing mass that fills and expands the sinus cavity with thinning or erosion of the bony wall (Fig. 17-16). On MR imaging, the appearance is variable due to alterations in protein concentration of the obstructed mucoid secretions. Gadolinium-enhanced MR demonstrates enhancement of the mucosal wall, although the contents usually do not enhance. The relationship of the mucocele to adjacent structures is important. For example, the location of a sphenoid sinus mucocele in relation to the optic nerves is critical in surgical planning. An infected mucocele, a mucopyocele, may demonstrate rim enhancement (Babbel 1992).

## INFLAMMATORY POLYPS

Polyps in the paranasal sinuses result from a local upheaval of the sinus mucosa with mucous membrane hyperplasia secondary to chronic inflammation (Babbel 1992; Som 1993*b*). Allergic sinusitis often plays a role in the formation of polyps. If large or numerous, polyps can cause local problems due to obstruction of the important ostiomeatal channels including the sinus ostia. On CT polyps involving the sinonasal region

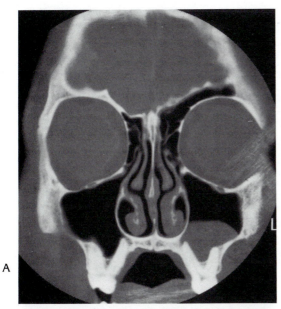

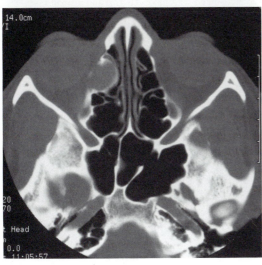

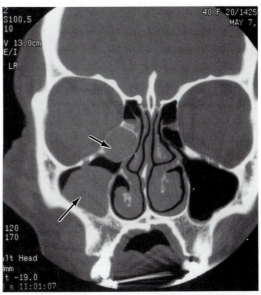

***Figure 17-15*** **Mucous retention cyst. A.** Coronal CT demonstrates a well marginated soft tissue. **B.** On MR retention cysts are usually hypointense in $T_1$-weighted MR and hyperintense in $T_2$-weighted images. Bony changes are usually absent. Axial (**C**) CT in another patient with retention cyst within the right maxillary sinus (arrow) and in an enlarged ethmoid bulla (arrowhead).

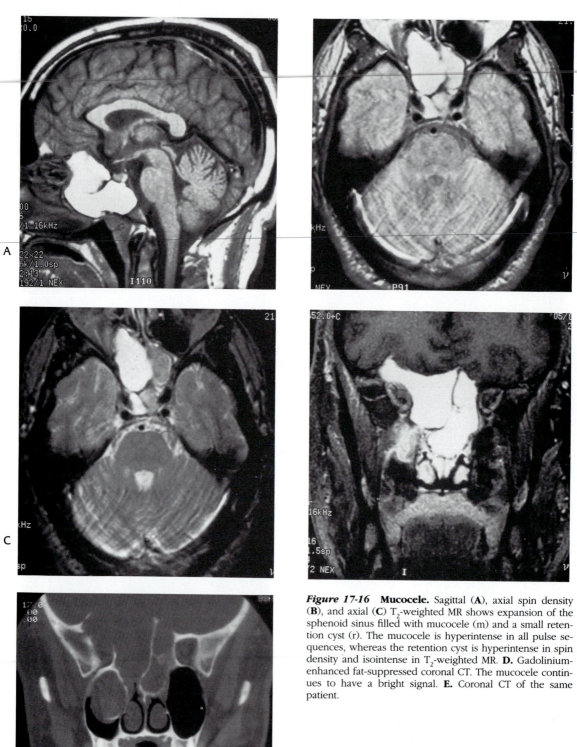

***Figure 17-16*** **Mucocele.** Sagittal (**A**), axial spin density (**B**), and axial (**C**) T$_2$-weighted MR shows expansion of the sphenoid sinus filled with mucocele (m) and a small retention cyst (r). The mucocele is hyperintense in all pulse sequences, whereas the retention cyst is hyperintense in spin density and isointense in T$_2$-weighted MR. **D.** Gadolinium-enhanced fat-suppressed coronal CT. The mucocele continues to have a bright signal. **E.** Coronal CT of the same patient.

appear as bulky soft tissue masses associated with chronic mucosal thickening within the sinus. On MR imaging, polyps are often indistinguishable from mucous retention cysts (Babbel 1991) (Fig. 17-17).

## ORBITAL COMPLICATIONS

About 3 percent of patients with sinusitis, more commonly children, have some form of orbital involvement and orbital manifestations may be the first sign of sinus infection (Buus 1990). Sixty to 84 percent of the cases of orbital infection are caused by complicated sinusitis. (Stammberger 1988; Buus 1990; Hudgins 1993). The ethmoid sinuses are the most common origin, with frontal, sphenoid, and maxillary sinuses in decreasing order of frequency. The ethmoid and maxillary sinuses are present at birth and therefore are the source in younger children. The frontal sinuses are usually detectable radiographically after 6 years, but are not usually significant sources of infection until after 10 years. The sphenoid sinuses likewise develop late and are rarely implicated in the pediatric age group.

CT is the imaging modality of choice when there is clinical evidence of postseptal infection (i.e., when proptosis and limitation of eye movement are present) or when there is failure to improve with antibiotics (Babbel 1992; Messerklinger 1967) (Fig. 17-18). Since the disease can be much more aggressive in the pediatric population, a CT should be considered when there is clinical evidence of preseptal inflammation.

CT reveals diffuse soft tissue density and thickening of the preseptal soft tissues. At this stage there is swelling and redness of the eyelids but no proptosis or limitation of eye movement. As infection spreads from the ethmoid sinus to the orbit, there is inflammation of the orbital periosteum. This becomes thickened and elevated, with accumulation of an inflammatory phlegmon. On CT this appears as an ill-defined, slightly enhancing mass on the sinus and orbital sides of the lamina papyracea. It is limited laterally by the periosteum; however, in more advanced cases it merges with a thickened and enhancing medial rectus muscle, which is displaced laterally. Subsequently, liquefaction may occur in the subperiosteal compartment to form an abscess. This is evident on CT as regions of low density, sometimes with an enhancing rim. The CT finding of low attenuation material surrounded by an enhancing rim suggests the diagnosis of abscess rather than a phlegmon, though the distinction between them can be difficult, given the continuum existing between these two states.

Rare orbital complications of paranasal sinus infection include superior ophthalmic vein (SOV) thrombosis and cavernous sinus thrombosis. SOV thrombosis is suspected on CT scans when there is asymmetrical enlargement of this vessel (best seen on coronal scans) with relative lack of normal enhancement, though thrombus within the lumen can be hyperdense. MR may demonstrate these changes more accurately. Magnetic resonance angiography (MRA), especially phase-contrast techniques, can establish the presence of SOV thrombosis.

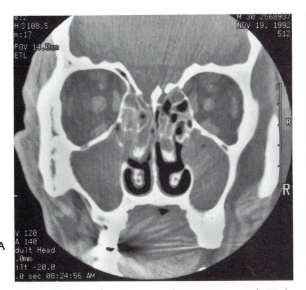
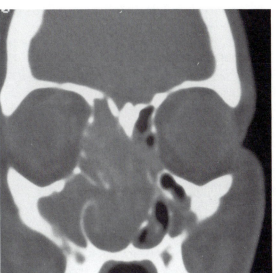

***Figure 17-17*** **Inflammatory polyps. A,B.** Coronal CT demonstrates soft tissue masses within the maxillary and ethmoid sinuses, as well as within the nasal cavity.

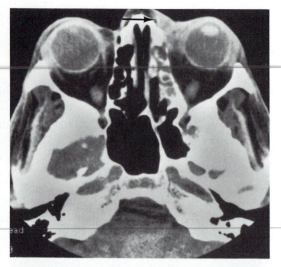

**Figure 17-18  Preseptal orbital cellulitis. A,B.** Contrast-enhanced axial CT demonstrates preseptal enhancing soft tissue (arrow) from adjacent ethmoid sinusitis. **C.** Pre- and postseptal spread of infection in another patient shows preseptal soft tissue swelling (arrowhead) and enhancement of the medial rectus muscle with a small amount of fluid density in the extracoanal space (arrow).

## CAVERNOUS SINUS THROMBOSIS

This condition is evident as fullness of the affected side with convexity of the lateral margin of the cavernous sinus, instead of the normal, slightly concave margin. Gadolinium-enhanced, axial and coronal MR scans would be expected to be more sensitive to the presence of cavernous sinus thrombosis than CT.

## BENIGN NEOPLASMS

There are several soft tissue neoplasms that affect the sinuses (Table 17-1); the more common ones are discussed below. However, it is important to be cognizant of mimics of intrasinus masses such as an encephalocele, or neoplasm which may directly arise within the sinuses or extend into the sinus.

### Inverted Papilloma

These tumors are part of a group called schneiderian papillomas, arising from the sinonasal mucosa. These tumors are uncommon, representing less than 5 percent of all sinonasal tumors (Myers 1990; Hill 1986; Youssem 1990), and occurring most commonly in males from 40 to 70 years. Inverting papillomas arise from the lateral nasal wall in the region of the middle meatus/infundibulum. Small lesions appear as a nonspecific polypoid nasal lesion. When larger, they are expansile masses, causing bone remodeling. They often have a characteristic appearance on coronal CT, with a soft tissue mass extending from the middle meatus into the maxillary antrum (Myers 1990). On CT these tumors are usually well defined with moderate enhancement, and a small amount of calcification may

be present (Fig. 17-19). The MR appearance of inverted papillomas is iso- to slightly hyperintense to muscle on $T_1WI$ images, and they have intermediate signal intensity on $T_2WI$ images (Youssem 1993).

The reported rate of associated malignancy, usually squamous cell carcinoma, is around 10 percent (Wilbur 1987; Hill 1986). Unfortunately, there are no distinctive signal characteristics on MR imaging that differentiate inverted papilloma from various malignant tumors (Youssem 1993). However, the presence of obvious bone destruction should raise this possibility. Inverting papilloma has a strong tendency to recur and requires aggressive resection for a cure. CT is important in diagnosis, showing the full extent of the tumor prior to resection, and also in follow-up, for detection of recurrence.

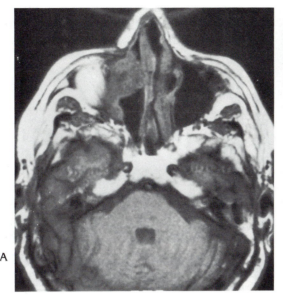

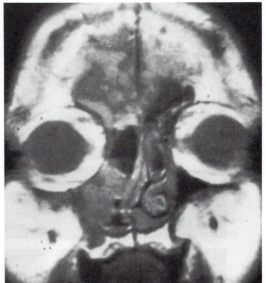

## Juvenile Angiofibroma

The juvenile angiofibroma is a rare, histologically benign, but locally aggressive tumor. It occurs almost exclusively in males usually 10 to 18 years of age. It arises in the margin of the sphenopalatine fossa, and most commonly spreads to the pterygopalatine fossa and then to the nasopharynx. There may be extension into the orbit via the inferior orbital fissure; however, direct extension into the sphenoid, maxillary, and ethmoid sinuses is more common.

Widening of the pterygopalatine fossa is a common and relatively specific radiological finding on both plain film and CT. The bones are often remodeled, with bowing but not frank destruction. Because of its highly vascular nature, intense enhancement of the mass is seen on postcontrast CT (Fig. 17-20). On MRI the mass is of intermediate signal intensity of $T_1$- and $T_2$-weighted sequences, with multiple flow voids usually visible. Both CT and MRI easily demonstrate the extent of tumor, in particular orbital extension. Angiography usually demonstrates significant vascularity within the mass.

## Neurogenic Tumors

These include schwannomas and neurofibroma, both of which may rarely show malignant degeneration. They usually involve the sensory nerves, primarily the maxillary or mandibular division of the trigeminal nerve. Since the olfactory bulb and tract do not have schwann cells, schwannomas of the olfactory nerve have not been described. However, rarely schwannomas may arise from the nerve within the nasal mucosal

*Figure 17-19* **Inverted papilloma.** Axial (**A**) and coronal (**B**) $T_1$-weighted MR demonstrates a soft tissue mass within the right nasal cavity and maxillary sinus. **C.** $T_1$-weighted gadolinium-enhanced MR demonstrates nonhomogeneous enhancement of the inverted papilloma.

surface, which may extend superiorly through the cribriform plate, histologically classified as *zero cranial nerve schwannomas* (Fig. 17-21). Remodeling of the adjacent bone and expansion are common, whereas bone destruction or erosion is rare. If these features are present, it is indicative of malignant degeneration. Cystic degeneration within the mass is not uncommon. On CT it usually appears as a homogenous mass with enhancement on the postcontrast images, except in areas of cystic component. On MR the mass is isointense on $T_1$WI and mild to moderate hyperintense on spin

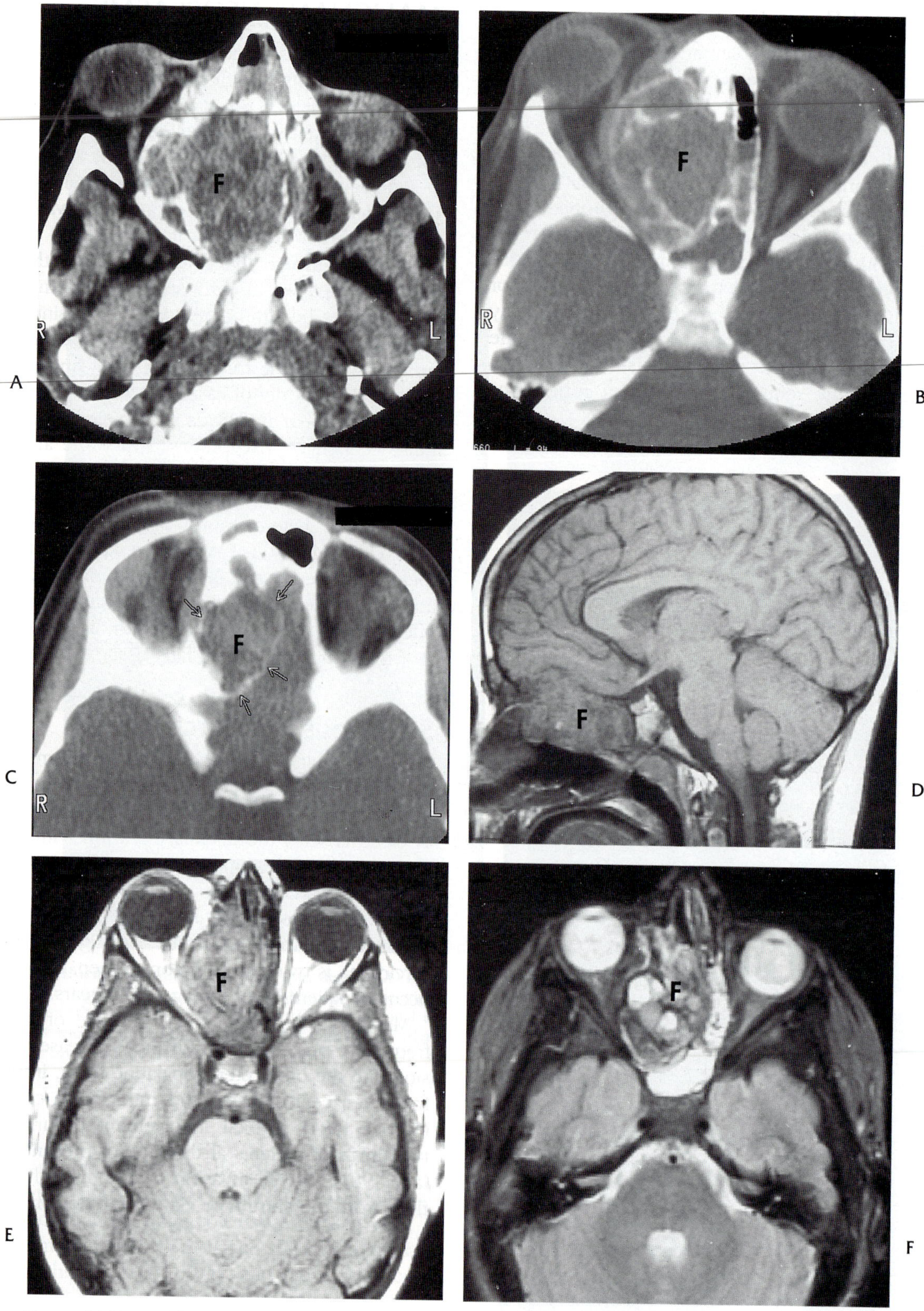

***Figure 17-24*** **Ossifying fibroma. A—C.** An axial CT section demonstrates a large soft tissue mass within the nasal cavity, extending through the cribriform plate. (**F**) A shell of calcium and bone surrounds the mass. Lucent areas in the mass with fluid levels represent multiple abscess formation within the fibroma (arrows). Sagittal (**D**) and axial (**E**) $T_1$-weighted MRs show an isointense mass with ill-defined hypointense signal. *(Continued on next page.)*

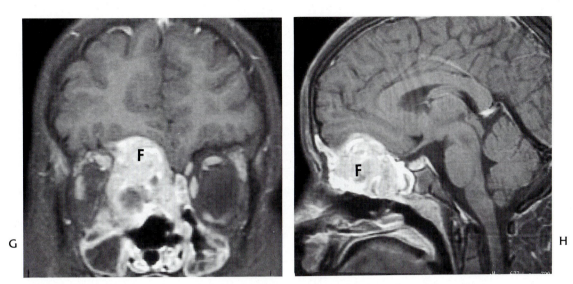

**Figure 17-24 (continued)**    Axial (**F**), coronal (**G**), and sagittal (**H**) gadolinium-enhanced T₁-weighted MRs show intense enhancement of the fibroma. Bright signal areas were multiple abscesses.

Lymph node metastasis at the time of initial presentation is uncommon (Weber 1984).

CT scanning has proved to be helpful in mapping the extent of tumor for surgical planning (Fig. 17-26). On CT, the tumor is usually of homogenous soft tissue density and shows little enhancement with contrast. Areas of necrosis may be present. Aggressive bone destruction, the hallmark of squamous cell carcinoma, is often present. However, early in the course of the disease before bone destruction occurs, the tumor may be indistinguishable from common entities such as chronic sinusitis and inflammatory polyps. Because of the mild enhancement that occurs, contrast administration with CT is of dubious value in assessing carcinomas in the sinonasal cavity. However, contrast material is often useful in evaluating for intracranial spread (Som 1988). One limitation of CT in defining tumor extension is the distinction between tumor and inflammatory reaction within the sinus and adjacent soft tissues, both of which will be soft tissue density. MR imaging has proved to be helpful in this regard. The majority (95 percent) of sinonasal tumors are highly cellular and have low to intermediate signal intensity on T₂WI (Som 1988). By comparison, the coexistent inflammatory changes often have a high water content and are hyperintense on T₂WI. However, more chronic secretions may have varying degrees of T₂ shortening (as described above), which can make this distinction between tumor and inflammatory secretions difficult.

The MR appearance of squamous cell carcinoma is often nonspecific, appearing as a homogeneous mass of low to intermediate signal intensity on both T₁WI and T₂WI (Fig. 17-25). The presence of bone destruction is not reliably detected on MR imaging and often requires CT imaging. The advantage of MR imaging over CT is in the detection of intracranial and intraorbital spread, where gadolinium-DTPA is often helpful. In most instances imaging diagnosis is based on both CT and MR finding.

## Glandular Tumors

This group of tumors arise from either minor salivary glands present in the sinus mucosa or differentiation of stem cells. Approximately 19 percent of malignant tumors of the sinuses fall into this category (Som 1988). The most common entities in this group are adenocarcinomas, which tend to occur in the ethmoid sinuses, and adenoid cystic and mucoepidermoid carcinomas, which are more frequent in the maxillary antrum. Many of these tumors are indistinguishable from the more common squamous cell carcinoma on CT and MR. This group of tumors typically remodels bone, in contradistinction to the marked tendency of squamous cell carcinoma to destroy bone. The glandular tumors, as a group, are more likely to exhibit inhomogeneous areas on both CT and MR because of cystic degeneration, mucous secretion, and necrosis (some may be mostly hyperintense on T₂WI). Orbital involvement can occur by remodeled bone encroaching on orbital contents or via perineural spread. Adenoid cystic carcinoma, in particular, has a propensity for perineural spread, with the infraorbital nerve acting as a possible conduit to the orbit and orbital apex (Fig. 17-26).

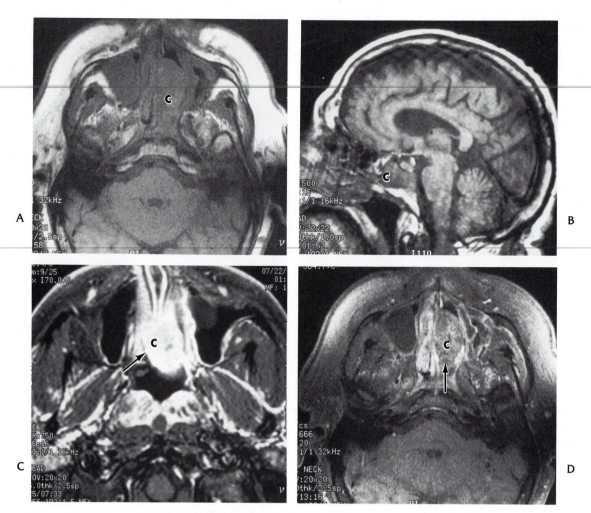

***Figure 17-25*** **Squamous cell carcinoma.** Axial (**A**) and sagittal (**B**) T₁-weighted MRs demonstrate squamous cell carcinoma invading the nasal cavity (T), with chronic mucosal thickening of the maxillary sinus. **C.** Adjacent gadolinium-enhanced MRs demonstrate the enhancing tumor (arrow). **D.** Fat-suppressed T₁-weighted MR is useful in distinguishing the tumor (arrow) from normal enhancing mucosa.

## Lymphoma

When lymphoma involves the paranasal sinuses, it is usually of the non-Hodgkins type and often is associated with systemic involvement. Lymphoma may account for as much as 8 percent of paranasal sinus malignancy (Weber 1984; Som 1988). Usually lymphoma is found in the maxillary antrum or nasal cavity. These tumors tend to be bulky soft tissue masses that may remodel bone. On CT scanning, they are of homogenous, soft tissue density and enhance moderately. On MR, they are of intermediate signal intensity on all sequences (Fig. 17-27).

## Esthesioneuroblastoma

Esthesioneuroblastoma (olfactory neuroblastoma) is an uncommon tumor arising within the olfactory mucosa

in the upper nasal cavity or septum and the cribriform plate region. About 70 percent involve the sinuses (Hill 1986; Som 1988), in particular the ethmoid sinuses. These tumors often present with nasal obstruction or epistaxis (Weber 1984). On CT, these tumors are of homogenous soft tissue density, sometimes with calcification and strong enhancement. Bone destruction may also be a feature. On MR, the tumor is hypointense on T₁WI and hyperintense on T₂WI. The tumor is locally aggressive and has a tendency to spread in the submucosa (Weber 1984). Metastatic involvement of the cervical lymph node chains, as well as more distant sites, often occurs.

## Other Malignant Tumors

*Extramedullary plasmacytoma* represents 2 to 4 percent of sinonasal tumors (Weber 1984; Som 1988), and

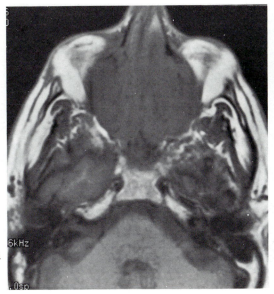

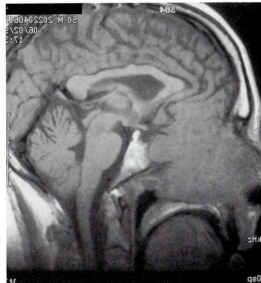

**Figure 17-26   Adenoid cystic carcinoma.** Axial (**A**) and sagittal (**B**) T₁-weighted MR demonstrates a large soft tissue mass (T), replacing the contents of the nasal passage and extending through the cribriform plate (arrow). **C.** In axial T₂-weighted MR the mass has both a solid and cystic component. **D.** Gadolinium-enhanced coronal MR demonstrates intense enhancement of the tumor mass. Superiorly the tumor is contained by the enhancing dural margin.

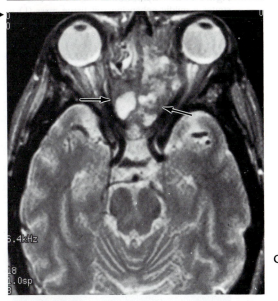

15 percent of them present with proptosis (Wilbur 1987). CT reveals a homogenous, enhancing mass with bone destruction (Fig. 17-28). On MR, these are of intermediate signal intensity on all sequences and may show vascular flow voids.

*Melanoma* occasionally arises in the sinuses, usually classified as neuroendocrine secreting neoplasm. These tumors may destroy or remodel bone and enhance strongly on CT, and some may exhibit high signal intensity components on T₂WI resulting from melanin, which is paramagnetic.

*Rhabdomyosarcoma* is common in the pediatric age group, usually between 2 and 5 years. They usually involve the sinonasal cavity by extension from the primary site within the pharyngeal space. They often extend intracranially associated with bone destruction or displacement. Rhabdomyosarcoma may show homogenous or heterogenous enhancement on CT and MR. (See Chap. 15.)

Other less common tumors that may involve the nasal passage and sinuses by extension from the skull base include chondroma, chondrosarcoma, chordoma, and osteogenic sarcoma. Rarely, other neoplasms, such as neuroendocrine carcinoma, may have imaging characteristics similar to lymphoma or small glandular cell tumors (Fig. 17-29).

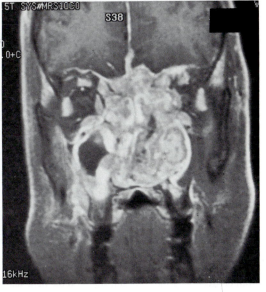

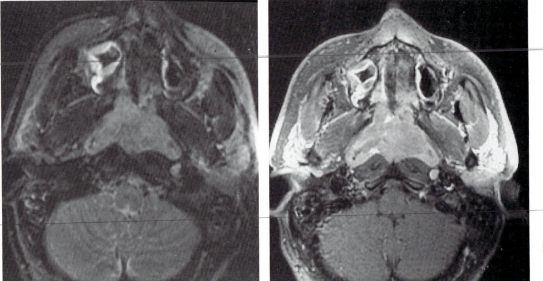

**Figure 17-29 (continued)**   **E.** T$_2$-weighted axial section shows the mass is minimally bright, and (**F**) is bright on gadolinium-enhanced, fat-suppressed T$_1$-weighted MR.

2. *OMU:* Note should be made of the extent of the uncintectomy and removal of the ethmoid bulla. The outline of the middle turbinate should be examined to determine whether a middle turbinetomy has been performed. If so, then careful attention should be paid to both the vertical attachment of the middle turbinate to the cribriform plate as well as the attachment of the basal lamella to the lamina papyracea. Traction applied during the course of middle turbinectomy can inflict damage at these sites.

3. *Lamina papyracea:* Inspection of the entire course of the lamina papyracea should be carried out to evaluate the integrity of this structure. Postoperative dehiscences are not uncommonly found just posterior to the nasolacrimal duct, at the level of the ethmoid bulla and basal lamella attachment.

4. *Sphenoid sinus area:* The margins of the sphenoid sinus should be evaluated for bony dehiscence and/or cephalocele.

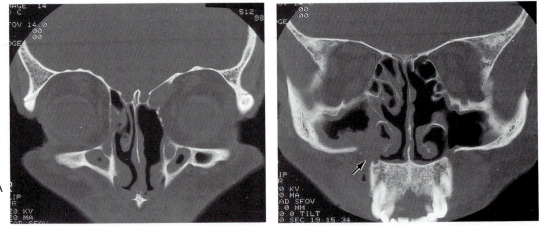

**Figure 17-30   Post-FESS CT appearance. A,B.** Coronal CT section demonstrates postsurgical changes following FESS. The left superior and middle turbinates have been removed. Turbinates on the left side have been removed and passage created to drain the left maxillary sinus and ethmoid sinus. Prior Caldwell-Luc procedure on the right (arrowhead) with persistent obstruction on the right side.

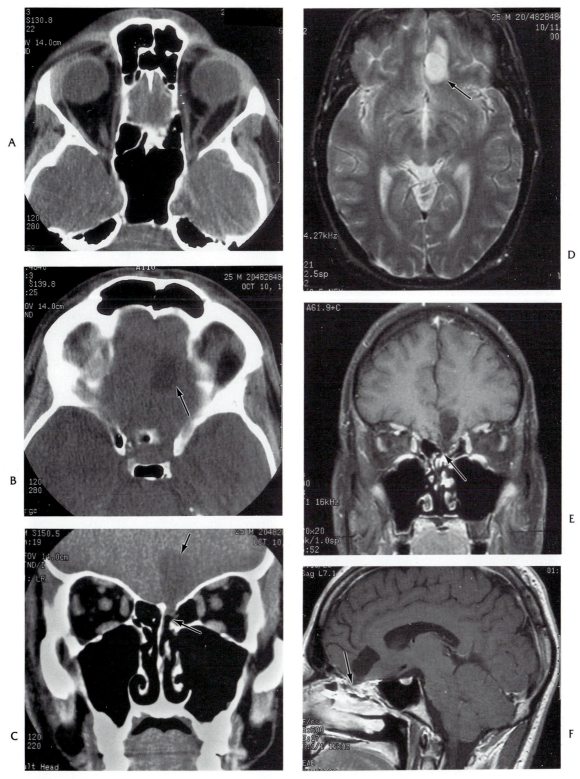

***Figure 17-31***   **CSF rhinorrhea. A,B.** Adjacent axial CT section. **C.** Coronal CT section. A defect within the cribriform plate is present (arrow). An associated hypodensity is seen within the frontal lobe (arrowhead), continuous with the bony defect. **D.** Spin-density-weighted MR demonstrates a focal hyperintense signal with CSF collection in the inferior frontal lobe (arrow). **E.** $T_1$-weighted coronal MR demonstrates the bony defect and the CSF fluid collection (arrow). **F.** Gadolinium-enhanced sagittal $T_1$-weighted MR demonstrates the site of the CSF leak.

# OPERATIVE COMPLICATIONS FOLLOWING ENDOSCOPIC SINUS SURGERY

In general, complications can be divided into minor and major (Hudgins 1993, 1992; Maniglia 1991; Stankiewicz 1989). Minor complications include periorbital emphysema, epistaxis, postoperative nasal synechiae, and tooth pain. Although these all can commonly occur, they are usually self-limited and do not require postoperative radiological evaluation. Major complications are rarer, but can be severely devastating or fatal (Maniglia 1991). Loss of integrity of the lamina papyracea can permit intraorbital fat to herniate into the ethmoid sinuses. Preexisting dehiscence of the lamina papyracea may be due to prior trauma or erosion from chronic sinus disease. *Intraoperative disruption of the lamina papyracea* can occur during resection of the middle turbinate if the ground lamella is resected back to its attachment to the lamina papyracea.

*Direct damage to the extra ocular muscles* such as the medial rectus muscle, superior oblique muscle, or other orbital contents can occur if there is preexisting or intraoperative disruption of the lamina papyracea. Injuries to the orbital contents may result in postoperative diplopia. The etiology of the diplopia can be from muscle entrapment among bone fragments or direct muscle laceration, or it can be secondary to nerve injury. Thin-section axial and coronal CT can be of benefit in evaluation of such cases. Clinically, subconjunctival hemorrhage is often associated with extraocular muscle damage (Neuhaus 1990). If intraorbital and intraocular pressure builds up as a result of an expanding hematoma or air being forced into the orbit from the nasal cavity (via a dehiscent lamina papyracea), then visual impairment or blindness secondary to ischemia can result (Neuhaus 1990).

*Blindness,* temporary or permanent, as a result of injury of the optic nerve can occur during posterior ethmoidectomy if the bony limit of the sinus is violated (Hudgins 1993; Maniglia 1991; Neuhaus 1990). Trauma to the vascular supply of the optic nerve can also result in visual loss.

*Massive hemorrhage* from direct injury to major vessels can occur. Laceration of the internal carotid artery has been reported and is often a fatal complication (Maniglia 1991). Emergent angiography with balloon occlusion of the lacerated artery has been performed. Patients who report severe postoperative headache or photophobia or who have signs to suggest subarachnoid hemorrhage should have a noncontrast head CT. If subarachnoid blood is found, cerebral angiography is recommended to detect vascular injury (Hudgins 1992, 1993).

*Injury to the nasolacrimal duct* can result during anterior enlargement of the maxillary ostium in the middle meatus. Injury to the membranous portion of the duct may be self-limited and remit by spontaneous fistulization into the middle meatus. Stenosis or total occlusion of the nasolacrimal duct can result from more severe injury (Neuhaus 1990).

*Postoperative cerebrospinal fluid leak* is another major complication of FESS (Maniglia 1991; Stankiewicz 1989). These leaks occur following inadvertent penetration of the dura. Extension of the injury to involve the cribriform plate, fovea ethmoidalis, and anterior cranial fossa, as well as the skull base, has been reported (Fig. 17-31). Secondary nasal encephalocele or deep penetration of the cerebrum can be seen following violation of the cranial vault. A CSF leak may not become clinically apparent for up to 2 years after surgery (Hudgins 1993). CSF leaks often close spontaneously with conservative measures (i.e., lumbar drain) (Hudgins 1993). However, if they persist, radionuclide CSF study is indicated. If the radionuclide test is positive (directly or indirectly), then a contrast CT cisternogram is done to define the anatomy and to pinpoint the site of leakage.

# References

Allen N: Wegener's Granulomatosis, in Bennett J, Plum F (eds): *Cecil Textbook of Medicine.* Philadelphia, W. B. Saunders, 1996 pp 1495–1496.

BABBEL R, HARNSBERGER HR, NELSON B, et al: Optimization of techniques of the paranasal sinuses. *AJNR 12:* 849–854, 1991*a.*

BABBEL R, HARNSBERGER HR, NELSON B, et al: Optimization of techniques in screening CT of the sinuses. *AJR* 157:1093–1098, 1991*b.*

BABBEL R, HARNSBERGER H, SONKENS J, et al: Recurring patterns of inflammatory sinonasal disease demonstrated on screening sinus CT. *AJNR* 13(3):903–912, 1992.

BARAT JL, MARCHAL JC, BRACARD S, et al: Mucocele of the sphenoid sinus. *J Neuroradiol* 17:135–141, 1990.

BARKOVICH AJ, VANDERMARCK P, EDWARDS MSB, et al: Congenital nasal masses: CT and MR imaging features in 16 cases. *AJNR* 12:105–116, 1991.

BECKER GD, HILL S: Midline granulomas due to illicit cocaine use. *Arch Otolaryngol Head Neck Surg* 114:90–91, 1988.

BOLGER WE, BUTZIN CA, PARSONS DS: Paranasal sinus bony anatomic variations and mucosal abnormalities: CT analysis for endoscopic surgery. *Laryngoscope* 101:56–64, 1991.

BUUS D, TSE D, FARRIS B: Ophthalmic complications of sinus surgery. *Ophthalmology* 97:612–619, 1990.

CHOW JM, MAFEE MF: Radiologic assessment preoperative to endoscopic sinus surgery. *Otolaryngol Clin N Am* 22:691–701, 1989.

DAWSON RC, HORTON JA: MR imaging of mucocele of the sphenoid sinus. *AJNR* 10:613–614, 1989.

DILLON WP, SOM PM, FULLERTON GD: Hypointense signal in chronically inspissated sinonasal secretions. *Radiology* 174:73–78, 1990.

DOLAN K: Radiology of nasal cavity and paranasal sinuses, in Cummings C, Krouse CJ (eds): *Otolaryngology*—Head and Neck Surgery. Chicago, Mosby Yearbook, 1989, pp 853–862.

DRETTNER B: The obstructed maxillary ostium. *Rhinology* 51:100–104, 1967.

EARWAKER J: Anatomic variants in sinonasal CT. *Radiographics* 13:381–415, 1993.

ECCLES R, ECCLES KSJ: Asymmetry in the autonomic nervous system with reference to the nasal cycle, migraine, anisocoria and Meniers syndrome. *Rhinology* 19:121–125, 1981.

EVANS F, SYDNOR J, MOOR W, MOORE G: Sinusitis of the maxillary antrum. *N Engl J Med* 293(15):735–739, 1975.

FELLOWS D, KING D, CONTURO T, et al: In vitro evaluation of hypointensity in aspergillus colonies. *AJNR* 15:1139–1144, 1994.

GULLANE P, CONLEY J: Carcinoma of the maxillary sinus. A correlation of the clinical course with orbital involvement. *J Otolaryngol* 12:141–145, 1983.

HARNSBERGER H: Imaging for the sinus and nose, in, Som P, Bergeron R (eds): *Head and Neck Imaging Handbook*, Chicago, Mosby Yearbook, 1990, pp 387–419.

HARRISON D: Midline destructive granuloma: Fact or fiction. *Laryngoscopy* 97:1049–1053, 1987.

HILDING AC: The physiology of drainage of nasal mucosa. *Ann Otolaryngol* 53:35–41, 1944.

HILL J, SOBOROFF B, APPLEBAUM E: Nonsquamous tumors of the nose and paranasal sinuses. *Otolaryngol Clin North Am* 19(4):723–739, 1986.

HUDGINS P, BROWNING D, GALLUPS J: Endoscopic paranasal sinus surgery: Radiographic evaluation of severe complications. *AJNR* 13:1161–1167, 1992.

HUDGINS P: Complications of endoscopic sinus surgery—The role of the radiologist in prevention. *Radiol Clin North Am* 31(1):21–32, 1993.

KENNEDY DW, ZINREICH SJ, ROSENBAUM AE, et al: Functional endoscopic surgery: Theory and diagnosis. *Arch Otolaryngol II* 1:576–582, 1985.

LAINE F, SMOKER W: The osteomeatal unit and endoscopic surgery: Anatomy, variations, and imaging findings in inflammatory diseases. *AJR* 159(4):849–857, 1992.

LAINE FJ, KUTA AJ: Imaging the sphenoid bone and basiocciput pathologic considerations. *Semin Ultra CT MRI* 14(3):160–177, 1993.

LANG J: *Clinical Anatomy of the Nose, Nasal Cavity and Paranasal Sinuses.* New York, Theime, 1989.

MANIGLIA A: Fatal and major complications secondary to nasal and sinus surgery. *Laryngoscope* 101:349–354, 1991.

MESSERKLINGER W: On drainage of the normal frontal sinus of man. *Acta Otolaryngol* 673:176–181, 1967.

MOLONEY J, BADHAM N, McRAE A: The acute orbit, preseptal, periorbital cellulitis, subperiosteal abscess and orbital cellulitis due to sinusitis. *J Laryngol Otol* 12:1–8, 1987.

MOSS A, PARSONS V: Current estimates from the National Health Interview Survey, United States-1985. Hyattsville, Maryland, National Center for Health Statistics, 1986.

MYERS EN, FERNAU JL, JOHNSON JT, et al: Management of inverted papilloma: Evaluation with MR imaging. *Laryngoscope* 100:481–490, 1990.

NADAS S, DUVOISIN B, LANDRY M, et al: Concha bullosa: Frequency and appearance on CT and correlation with sinus disease in 308 patients with chronic sinusitis. *Neuroradiology* 37:234–237, 1995.

NEUHAUS R: Orbital complications secondary to endoscopic sinus surgery. *Ophthalmology* 97:1512–1518, 1990.

SCHAEFFER JP: The genesis, development and adult anatomy of the nasofrontal region in man. *Am J Anat* 20:125–43, 1916.

SCUDERI A, BABBEL R, HARNSBERGER H, SONKENS J: The sporadic pattern of inflammatory sinonasal disease including post-surgical changes. *Semin Ultrasound CT MRI* 12(6):575–591, 1991.

SOM P: Sinonasal tumors and inflammatory tissues: Differentiation with MR. *Radiology* 167:803–809, 1988.

SOM P, BERGERON R, in, Som P, Bergeron R (eds): *Head and Neck Imaging Handbook*, 1991, pp 114–224.

ISBN 0-07-037689-1